Companion Animal Zoonoses

Companion Animal Zoonoses

Edited by

J. Scott Weese
DVM, DVSc, DipACVIM

Department of Pathobiology and Centre for Public Health and Zoonoses, Ontario Veterinary College, University of Guelph, Guelph, Ontario, Canada

Martha B. Fulford
BSc, BEd, MA, MD, FRCPC

Division of Infectious Diseases, McMaster University Medical Centre, Hamilton, Ontario, Canada

⊛WILEY-BLACKWELL

A John Wiley & Sons, Inc., Publication

Edition first published 2011
© 2011 Blackwell Publishing Ltd.

Blackwell Publishing was acquired by John Wiley & Sons in February 2007. Blackwell's publishing program has been merged with Wiley's global Scientific, Technical, and Medical business to form Wiley-Blackwell.

Editorial Office
2121 State Avenue, Ames, Iowa 50014-8300, USA

For details of our global editorial offices, for customer services, and for information about how to apply for permission to reuse the copyright material in this book, please see our Website at www.wiley.com/wiley-blackwell.

Library of Congress Cataloging-in-Publication Data

Companion animal zoonoses / [edited by] J. Scott Weese, Martha B. Fulford.
     p. ; cm.
  Includes bibliographical references and index.
    ISBN 978-0-8138-1964-8 (hardcover : alk. paper)
1. Zoonoses. 2. Pet medicine. I. Weese, J. Scott. II. Fulford, Martha B.
  [DNLM: 1. Zoonoses–transmission. 2. Animals, Domestic. 3. Communicable Diseases–veterinary.
4. Disease Reservoirs–veterinary. 5. Disease Transmission, Infectious–prevention & control. WC 950]
  RA639.C66 2011
  614.5'6–dc22

                              2010042170

A catalog record for this book is available from the U.S. Library of Congress.

Set in 9.5 on 11.5 pt Palatino by Toppan Best-set Premedia Limited
Printed and bound in Singapore by Fabulous Printers Pte Ltd

1 2011

Contents

Preface

The concept of zoonotic diseases, those that can be transmitted from animals to humans, has been understood for centuries. Some of the oldest recognized and most devastating infectious diseases have been zoonoses, such as the bubonic plague, and zoonoses have played an important role in human history and development. Traditionally, the main focus has involved food animals, food, water, and wildlife as sources of zoonotic infection. While certainly of importance, those areas do not encompass all zoonotic disease risks, particularly as people in developed countries distance themselves from food animals and nature, and increase their contact with pets.

Companion animals play an important role in the lives of many individuals and are often considered to be members of the family. The majority of households in many countries contain pets, and a large percentage of the population has periodic, if not regular, close contact with a variety of companion animal species. As with any contact between individuals, every animal–human contact carries an inherent risk of pathogen transmission. While the risk is low in most situations, companion–animal-associated zoonoses certainly occur and can range from mild to fatal. Despite the role of companion animals in peoples' lives and the risk of disease transmission, the field of companion animal zoonoses is one that has only received limited attention in veterinary medicine, human medicine, and public health, with attention being focused on a limited range of pathogens such as rabies virus.

There is no standard definition of a *companion animal*, and one could successfully argue that some farm animal species, particularly horses, are also true companion animals. This book, however, is restricted to discussion of issues surrounding household pets, because of the vastly different issues involving species like horses. We had a more difficult time deciding on what household pets to include, as the proliferation of exotic animal species has resulted in diverse types of animals in households. We chose to restrict the focus of this book to common household pets, particularly dogs, cats, rabbits, "pocket pets" (mice, rats, hamsters, gerbils, and guinea pigs), and common reptiles (turtles, nonvenomous snakes, lizards). Other animal species are included periodically in reference to specific issues or past outbreaks, such as the monkeypox outbreak in the United States that was associated with prairie dogs. Purists may argue that "humans are animals too," but for the purposes of this book, "animals" refers to animal species other than humans.

Some nonzoonotic diseases and some with minimal zoonotic disease risks have been included. Concerns are often raised regarding diseases with minimal zoonotic potential, and resources clarifying the lack of risk can be useful. Understanding which diseases are not zoonoses, and the reasons for the lack of risk, can be as important as understanding which diseases do have a zoonotic potential. A major emphasis of this book is on infection control measures to reduce the transmission of zoonotic pathogens in households and veterinary hospitals. An unfortunate reality of the state of science in this field is that evidence-based recommendations are difficult to make because of the paucity of research regarding infection control in companion animals and in households. Whenever possible, recommendations that have been made are based on available evidence. However, many recommendations are expert opinion based on knowledge of pathophysiology, epidemiology, and principles of infection control.

While raising the profile of companion animal zoonoses is important, it can be accompanied by unintended consequences, namely a backlash against pets or inappropriate fear of pet contact. This can lead to unnecessary decisions to remove pets from households or have them euthanized, even in the absence of evidence of the role of pets in a particular disease situation. As an example, increased awareness among physicians, veterinarians, and pet owners of the potential role of pets in the transmission of methicillin-resistant *Staphylococcus aureus* (MRSA) sometimes led to a rapid progression from "pets can't be involved in this disease" to "pets are the root of all evil and should be eliminated." The authors have dealt with many unfortunate situations where removal or euthanasia of a pet was recommended based on little to no evidence suggesting the pet was a source of infection. This book will hopefully fill some of the information void that is currently a major contributor to such problems.

Achieving a balance between pointing out possible risks and benefits of pet ownership is difficult, particularly in the absence of detailed epidemiological data for many diseases. This book raises many issues with respect to the potential for transmission of zoonotic pathogens in households, but hopefully does so in a balanced manner. It is certainly not our intent to raise fears regarding pets and diseases. Rather, we wholeheartedly support the presence of pets in households and fully understand the positive aspects that pets may bring to peoples' lives. Instead of highlighting infectious disease risks as an indication that pet ownership is inherently dangerous, we hope that this information will promote safe and appropriate pet ownership, with a reduction in human and animal illness and an improvement of the undeniable human–animal bond.

J. Scott Weese
Martha B. Fulford

Contributors

Maureen E.C. Anderson, DVM, DVSc, DipACVIM. Department of Pathobiology, Ontario Veterinary College, University of Guelph, Guelph, Ontario, N1G2W1, Canada.

Martha B. Fulford, BSc, BEd, MA, MD, FRCPC. Division of Infectious Diseases, McMaster University Medical Centre, Hamilton, Ontario, L8N3Z5, Canada.

Andrew S. Peregrine, BVMS, DVM, PhD, DipEVPC, MRCVS. Department of Pathobiology, Ontario Veterinary College, University of Guelph, Guelph, Ontario, N1G2W1, Canada.

Jason Stull, VMD, MVPM, DACVPM. Department of Pathobiology, Ontario Veterinary College, University of Guelph, Guelph, Ontario, N1G2W1, Canada.

J. Scott Weese, DVM, DVSc, DipACVIM. Department of Pathobiology and Centre for Public Health and Zoonoses, Ontario Veterinary College, University of Guelph, Guelph, Ontario, N1G2W1, Canada.

Companion Animal Zoonoses

1 Parasitic Diseases

J. Scott Weese, Andrew S. Peregrine, Maureen E.C. Anderson, and Martha B. Fulford

Introduction

Companion animals can harbor a wide range of parasites, some of which are transmissible to humans. The overall burden of human diseases attributable to companion animal-associated parasites is unknown and varies greatly between regions. The risks associated with some are often overstated while others are largely ignored, and the range of illness can extend from mild and self-limited to fatal.

Ascaris lumbricoides

Introduction

A. lumbricoides is a roundworm that has typically been considered host specific to humans; however, there is evidence of infection of dogs and the potential for dogs to be an uncommon source of human infection.

Etiology

As with other intestinal nematodes, *A. lumbricoides* is a nonsegmented, elongated, cylindrical parasite

Companion Animal Zoonoses. Edited by J. Scott Weese and Martha B. Fulford. © 2011 Blackwell Publishing Ltd.

that undergoes sexual reproduction. Like other ascarids, as well as hookworms and *Trichuris*, *A. lumbricoides* undergoes a maturation stage in soil and is therefore sometimes referred to as a geohelminth.[1] Female worms are larger than males and can reach 40 cm in length and 6 mm in diameter.[2]

Life cycle

Adult worms live within the small intestinal lumen of humans and excrete massive numbers of eggs per day. As with other ascarids, eggs are not immediately infective and must mature to infective third-stage larvae in the environment over a period of days. After embryonated eggs are ingested by a human, larvae hatch, penetrate the intestinal mucosa, and reach the liver via portal circulation. After migrating through the liver, the larvae eventually reach the lungs, penetrate the airways, ascend the tracheobronchial tree, and are coughed up and swallowed. They mature into adults in the small intestinal lumen and complete the life cycle. The time from ingestion of infective eggs to development of adults is approximately 8 weeks.[2]

Geographic distribution/epidemiology

A. lumbricoides is one of the most prevalent nematodes in humans and is most common in tropical and subtropical regions, infecting approximately 25% of the world's population.[3-5] Up to 80% of people can be infected in some areas.[1,4,6-9] The regional prevalence varies depending on factors such as climate, sanitation, socioeconomic status, and human behavior. Areas with warm, humid climates facilitate maturation and survival of infective eggs. Poor sanitation leads to an increased risk of contamination of the environment with human feces. Outdoor defecation similarly results in increased likelihood of contamination, and outdoor activities in contaminated areas that are accompanied by suboptimal hand hygiene increase the risk of fecal–oral infection. *A. lumbricoides* eggs can be found in the soil in public places such as parks[10,11] and can survive outdoors for years in favorable environmental conditions.[1] Infections are more common in children.

Some older studies reported the presence of ascarid eggs that could have been *A. lumbricoides* in canine feces.[12,13] More recently, convincing evidence of the presence of *A. lumbricoides* in dogs has been reported. A study of dogs in tea-growing communities in northern India identified *A. lumbricoides* eggs in 18–37% of dogs.[7] In that study, dogs were at increased risk of shedding *A. lumbricoides* if one or more household members regularly defecated outdoors. Simply finding eggs in feces, particularly in an environment where dogs may ingest human feces, does not necessarily indicate that dogs are involved in the biological cycle of the organism. Indeed, there has been some thought that dogs only act as mechanical vectors and that eggs passed in feces simply moved passively through the intestinal tract. However, a recent study of dogs in an area in Egypt where outdoor defecation by humans is common reported detection of adult *A. lumbricoides* in 8% of dogs.[14] Furthermore, viable eggs were detected, suggesting that dogs can truly be infected and could potentially play a role in the life cycle of this human parasite. It has also been suggested that the dog's coat could be a source of exposure since the eggs are "sticky" and highly tolerant of environmental effects, and could potentially adhere and mature to the infective stage on the animal.[14]

A study of young Nigerian children indicated that children whose families owned dogs were 3.5 times as likely to be shedding *A. lumbricoides* compared with non-dog-owning families.[15] In contrast, contact with dogs was not a risk factor in a study of adult humans in northern India.[7] Whether there truly is a risk from dogs is unclear, but the limited data indicate that consideration of the role of pets, particularly dogs, in the transmission of this predominantly human-associated parasite is required.

Animals

Clinical presentation

Little is known about *A. lumbricoides* in dogs. While it was previously thought that dogs shedding the parasite represented a mechanical, not biological, vector, there is now evidence that adult worms can grow in the canine intestinal tract. It is not known whether this can result in disease.

Diagnosis

Diagnosis is based on the detection of eggs in feces using fecal flotation and subsequent speciation of the parasite by evaluation of micromorphological features[14] or using molecular methods such as PCR-RFLP.[7]

Management

No specific data are present, but presumably, any prophylactic or therapeutic agent that is used for the treatment of *Toxocara* in dogs would be effective against *A. lumbricoides*. These include milbemycin oxime, moxidectin, fenbendazole, and pyrantel.

Humans

Clinical presentation

Various presentations can occur, but most infections are asymptomatic.[1,2] Large worm burdens can result in malnutrition, nonspecific gastrointestinal signs, or, in rare cases, intestinal obstruction.[2] Obstruction of the bile duct can result in cholangitis, biliary colic, or pancreatitis.[2] Chronic infections can produce insidious disease, with growth retardation and negative effects on cognitive function in children.[5] During larval migration, acute pulmonary signs (Loeffler's syndrome), fever, and marked eosinophilia can occur.[2] There is also increasing concern about the broad effects of ascarid infection on the immune system, something that may be particularly important with concurrent infections such as malaria or for the development of allergic diseases,[16,17] though more research needs to be performed in this area.

Diagnosis

Eggs are usually easily detectable in stool because of the large numbers that are shed by adult worms. Rarely, adult worms will be passed in stool or vomitus.[2] Adult worms may also be identified ultrasonographically as an incidental finding or during investigation of gastrointestinal complaints.

Management

A single dose of albendazole, mebendazole, or pyrantel pamoate has high cure rates (88–95%).[18] Three days of mebendazole or a single dose of ivermectin has also been recommended in people over 2 years of age.[2] Nitazoxanide is also effective.[19] Retesting of stool 2 weeks after treatment has been recommended.[2] Most drugs are only effective against adult parasites, so repeated treatment may be needed.

Prevention

Prevention of zoonotic transmission of *A. lumbricoides*, should it occur, involves basic measures to reduce the incidence of exposure of dogs, to reduce contamination of the environment by dog feces, and to prevent fecal–oral exposure in humans. Evidence-based data are not available for any of these areas, but reasonable recommendations can be made.

Reducing exposure involves decreasing the chance that dogs will ingest infective *A. lumbricoides* eggs, which are predominantly found in human feces. Reducing "promiscuous defecation" by humans, something that is common in some developing regions,[14] is a means of achieving this and involves both education and improved infrastructure.

Reducing contamination of the environment by dogs is as discussed for similar organisms like *Toxocara canis* (e.g., reducing worm burdens, and

therefore shedding levels, by routine antiparasitic chemoprophylaxis). Decreasing the numbers of free-roaming dogs and prompt removal of feces, particularly from public areas such as parks, would presumably help achieve that goal. General hygiene practices are the key to reducing inadvertent ingestion of infective larvae by humans, including good attention to hand hygiene and proper washing of food.

Prophylactic use of albendazole, mebendazole, or pyrantel pamoate in humans can be practical and affordable in endemic areas, particularly in school-age children.[2,20] Based on the commonness of the parasite in humans in some regions and the very rare incidence of patent infections in dogs, prophylactic treatment of dogs directed specifically against *A. lumbricoides* is not indicated. However, routine deworming targeted against other roundworms will be effective against this parasite.

Baylisascaris procyonis

Introduction

B. procyonis is a large nematode that is highly prevalent in healthy raccoons in many regions.[21] Human infections are very rare but can be devastating. Neural larva migrans is the most common form of this rare disease, but visceral (VLM) and ocular larva migrans (OLM) can also develop.

Dogs can shed *B. procyonis* in feces and can also theoretically be a source of human exposure through transporting infective eggs into the household on their hair coat. While objective evidence of a risk from pets is minimal, the severity of disease in humans indicates that basic measures should be taken to reduce the risk of exposure to this parasite.

Etiology

B. procyonis belongs to the order Ascaridida, along with *Toxocora canis* and *T. cati*.[21] The North American raccoon (*Procyon lotor*) is the definitive host, and *B. procyonis* is often termed the "raccoon roundworm." An unusual aspect of *B. procyonis* is its ability to infect a wide range of animal species, causing neural larva migrans in over 100 avian and mammalian species.[21]

Life cycle

Adult worms are found in the small intestine of raccoons. They are large, tan roundworms that can be up to 22 cm long. Female worms are prodigious egg layers, and infected raccoons can pass millions of eggs in feces per day, leading to heavy contamination of the environment. Eggs are not immediately infective, and second-stage larvae must develop in eggs in the environment before infection is possible. This usually requires 2–4 weeks, but may occur as quickly as 11 days in some situations.[21] After ingestion, infective eggs hatch in the small intestine. In intermediate hosts, larvae can penetrate the intestinal mucosa and migrate via portal circulation to the liver, then to the lungs, where they are subsequently distributed throughout the body via the systemic circulation. Larvae that reach the central nervous system (CNS) continue to migrate and grow, causing neurological damage. Migration through other tissues may also occur, and extensive somatic migration is common.[21]

Young raccoons tend to be infected early in life by ingesting infective eggs off their mother's hair coat or in the den environment. Adult raccoons are typically infected by ingestion of third-stage larvae in the tissues of infected intermediate hosts (i.e., rodents). Intermediate hosts (including humans) are infected by ingestion of infective eggs from the environment. Juvenile raccoons tend to have a higher parasite burden than adults.[21]

Geographic distribution/epidemiology

B. procyonis can be found in most places that raccoons can be found. Raccoons are indigenous to North America and B. procyonis can be found widely across the continent, although there appear to be regional variations in prevalence (e.g., this parasite is less common in the southeastern United States). Shedding rates of 13–92% have been reported in North American raccoons.[22–27] During recent years, the parasite has been found, sometimes commonly, in North American regions where it was not previously thought to exist,[21,22] suggesting that its range may be expanding. It is reasonable to assume that B. procyonis is present anywhere raccoons can be found. This includes other continents, since raccoons have been introduced into other regions of the world, and B. procyonis has been found in raccoons in some areas of Europe and Asia.[28,29]

Infected raccoons can shed massive numbers of eggs in feces and lead to marked environmental contamination. This is most pronounced in and around raccoon latrines, areas where raccoons tend to defecate. Raccoon latrines are thought to play a central role in B. procyonis transmission because they are so highly contaminated.[30–32] Other environmental sites, including public parks and playgrounds, can also be contaminated.[33] Infective eggs are highly resistant to environmental effects and can persist in the environment for years,[21,34] long after obvious evidence of raccoon feces has disappeared. The surface of the egg is also rather "sticky," and eggs tend to adhere to animal fur, hands, and other surfaces, which can contribute to exposure of pets and people.

Neural larva migrans and OLM are the main disease concerns associated with this parasite in humans. Neural larva migrans caused by B. procyonis is very rare but has been reported sporadically across North America. Most cases have involved children with developmental delays.[21,35–37] Contact with infected raccoons, their feces, or a contaminated environment, and geophagia or pica are the main risk factors.[21] Young children and developmentally delayed individuals are at increased risk because they are more likely to ingest raccoon feces and contaminated dirt. Children may also be more likely to play outside in or around raccoon latrines. Asymptomatic infections can occur, as evidenced by the presence of B. procyonis antibodies in some healthy individuals.[21] While evidence is sparse, it is suspected that asymptomatic or subclinical infections are the most common form of infection.[2] Asymptomatic infections probably represent infections caused by ingestion of small numbers of B. procyonis, which results in less damage through migration and inflammation. Since the likelihood of clinical infection and severity of neural larva migrans are thought to relate to the number of ingested larvae and the size of the brain (with damage to critical areas more likely in small brains), subclinical infections would be more likely in adults.[21]

The role of dogs in the epidemiology of B. procyonis is poorly understood. They likely play a minimal role in the propagation of this parasite. However, their close contact with humans raises concerns. There are reports of *B. procyonis* infection in dogs, both healthy dogs and dogs with neural larva migrans,[21,38-40] though prevalence data are currently lacking. Even so, compared with raccoons, infections in dogs appear to be uncommon. Dogs can be infected by ingestion of infected small animals.[41] They could also become infected by ingestion of eggs, particularly from raccoon latrines; however, infection following ingestion of eggs is much less likely than infection following ingestion of larvae. Given the ability of eggs to stick to surfaces, pets could theoretically be a source of infection as a mechanical vector, by bringing infective eggs from the environment into the household.

Infections have also been reported in other species, including wild rabbits,[42] captive nonhuman primates,[43] a cockatoo,[44] and a pet guinea pig;[45] however, patent infections have not been reported and the public health consequences are presumably minimal to nonexistent.

Animals

Clinical presentation

The implications of *B. procyonis* infection in dogs have not been well described, and it is likely that subclinical intestinal infection is most common. Neural larva migrans can occur and cause rapidly progressive encephalitis.[38,39]

Diagnosis

Eggs can be identified in feces using routine fecal flotation. Close examination is required to differentiate *B. procyonis* from *Toxocara* or *Toxascaris* spp.[21] PCR may offer another means of directly detecting *B. procyonis* eggs in feces and differentiating them from other ascarids.[46]

Diagnosis of neural larva migrans is as described for humans below, involving clinical signs, peripheral and CSF eosinophilia and seropositivity, and exclusion of other possible causes of disease.[38]

Management

Fenbendazole, milbemycin oxime, moxidectin, and pyrantel are likely to be effective for the elimination of intestinal *B. procyonis*.[47] Milbemycin oxime

was effective at eliminating *B. procyonis* from a small group of naturally infected and experimentally infected dogs.[48] No information is available regarding treatment of larva migrans. Presumably, anthelmintics and corticosteroids are indicated, as is the case in humans, but a grave prognosis would be expected.

Humans

Clinical presentation

Neural larva migrans produces severe and rapidly progressive eosinophilic meningoencephalitis. It is almost exclusively identified in young children or people with developmental delays that make them more likely to ingest dirt or feces. Weakness, lethargy, irritability, behavioral changes, difficulty speaking, headache, and ataxia may be observed, usually with rapid progression.[37]

OLM may occur with neural larva migrans or as a sole entity. Larval migration through the visual cortex or within the eye can lead to visual impairment or blindness.[21] Chorioretinitis and optic neuritis or atrophy may be evident during ophthalmoscopic examination.[21] Occasionally, motile larvae may be observed within the eye. VLM tends to occur most often in the head, neck, and thorax.[21]

Diagnosis

Neural larva migrans is presumptively diagnosed through a combination of clinical signs, cerebrospinal fluid (CSF), and peripheral eosinophilia, and the presence of diffuse white matter disease on CT or MRI, ideally with a history of exposure to raccoons or raccoon feces.[21] Demonstration of antibodies against *B. procyonis* in serum and CSF supports the diagnosis. Definitive diagnosis involves the identification of larvae on brain biopsy specimens.[37] However, it is unlikely that a parasite would be obtained in a biopsy, and biopsy is not recommended if serological tests are available.[21]

Diagnosis of OLM is based on the detection of chorioretinal lesions or larvae on ophthalmoscopic examination.[2] Differentiation of *B. procyonis* from other ocular parasites can be done by measurement of the larvae, with *B. procyonis* larvae being larger (1500–2000 × 60–70 μm) than *Toxocara* (350–445 × 20 μm).[21]

Management

Treatment is difficult because of a lack of objective information regarding different options and the typically advanced nature of disease by the time it is suspected or diagnosed. Currently, treatment involves anthelmintics, corticosteroids, and supportive care. Data regarding the efficacy of different anthelmintics in eliminating intestinal worms in raccoons must be used cautiously when considering the treatment of larva migrans, because drugs that are able to eliminate intestinal parasites in raccoons are typically much less effective in tissues of other hosts[21] and adult worm stages may have different susceptibility to certain drugs compared with larval stages. Albendazole is the most commonly recommended treatment, along with high doses of corticosteroids.[2]

Regardless of treatment, the prognosis is poor. By the time the disease is suspected, patients are usually severely affected and there is little chance of effective treatment. Affected individuals typically die or are left with profound neurological deficits.[37] There is only one report of recovery without residual neurological deficits—a 4-year-old child who had a relatively mild disease.[35] Developmental disabilities, seizures, paralysis, and blindness are common sequelae.[37]

Prevention

Efforts at preventing *B. procyonis* infection in people are best directed against avoiding intentional or inadvertent ingestion of raccoon feces and soil from around raccoon latrines. Raccoons should not be kept as pets or encouraged to live around households. Contact with latrines and adjacent areas should be prevented, particularly by young children or other people at increased risk of geophagia or pica. Raccoon latrines should be cleaned, and contaminated areas should be disinfected.

The risk of human infection from dogs is probably very low, but measures should be taken to reduce the risk of dogs becoming exposed and potentially infected, or from having their hair coats become contaminated. Dogs should not be allowed

to have contact with raccoon latrines. If a dog has been in a raccoon latrine or otherwise may have become contaminated with *B. procyonis* larvae, bathing it with soap and water to remove infective eggs is reasonable measure. Gloves and protective outerwear (i.e., lab coat) should be worn when bathing, and hands should be washed thoroughly in soap and water after contact with a potentially contaminated animal. Ideally, bathing should occur outside. If *B. procyonis* infection is identified during routine fecal examination, treatment is warranted, as described above.

If larva migrans is suspected in a dog or other household pet, the animal should be handled on the assumption that it may also be shedding eggs in feces. Since eggs are not immediately infective, contact with the animal is relatively low risk; however, contamination of the hair coat would be possible. Care should be taken around feces of potentially infected animals. Feces should be promptly removed so that infective eggs are not formed.

Preventive therapy with albendazole is indicated in children that have ingested soil or feces potentially contaminated with *B. procyonis*.[2] Prophylactic treatment of dogs that have ingested raccoon feces could be similarly considered, but the need or usefulness of this is unclear. Routine deworming targeted solely against *B. procyonis* is not indicated because of the apparent rarity of the parasite in dogs. However, most drugs used for routine monthly deworming directed against other helminths should be effective against *B. procyonis*.

Cheyletiella spp.

Introduction

Often referred to as "walking dandruff," cheyletiellosis is a dermatologic disease caused by mites. Different *Cheyletiella* species have different animal hosts, but they can also infest other species, including humans. Cheyletiellosis is a mild zoonotic infection that is most often linked to infested cats.

Etiology

Cheyletiella species are large (350 × 500 μm) mites belonging to the Arachnida class. There are three main species in companion animals: *Cheyletiella yasguri*, *Cheyletiella blakei*, and *Cheyletiella parasitivorax*. Dogs are the host of *C. yasguri*, while *C. blakei* is found on cats and *C. parasitivorax* is found on rabbits.[49–52] *C. parasitivorax* has also been reported in dogs and cats.[53,54] A related genus, *Lynxacarus radovskyi*, can be found on cats in some regions.

Life cycle

Cheyletiella are hair-clasping mites that do not burrow. Rather, they live in the fur of animals and move around freely.[49,50] Periodically, they attach to the epidermis and feed off the keratin layer. Eggs are laid on the host, attached to hairs by fine fibrillar strands.[50] Prelarvae and larvae develop within the egg, and fully developed nymphs emerge.[49] These nymphs develop through two stages and then become adults. The entire life cycle can be completed on a single host and takes approximately 35 days.[50] Adult mites may live off the host for short periods of time, with conflicting data regarding how long this may be. Some authors state that survival is typically for a few days but can be up to 10 days, while others claim that survival for up to 1 month is possible.[49,50] While *Cheyletiella* spp. can accidentally infect humans, they cannot complete their life cycle on human skin.[50,55]

Geographic distribution/epidemiology

Prevalence and incidence data for animals and humans are limited. *C. parasitivorax* was found on 57% of pet rabbits in a South Korean study,[56] but little information has been reported about typical pet dog and cat populations. It has been variably suggested that the disease is uncommon or common but frequently undiagnosed. In dogs, infections appear to occur most often in puppies.[50] No age, breed, or gender associations have been identified in cats. Infestations are most commonly found in animals in kennels or other confined systems.[49] Introduction of new animals into the household may be associated with animal and human infections,[57] although proper risk factor studies are lacking. Infested animals do not necessarily have signs of disease but can still act as a source of infection of people or other animals.[58]

Cheyletiella species appear to be well distributed internationally. *Lynxacarus* has been most commonly reported in Australia, New Zealand, Fiji, Texas, and Hawaii.[59–64]

Transmission is predominantly by direct contact between infected and susceptible individuals. Indirect transmission by the environment and fomites is also possible. Mites have also been found on fleas, lice, and flies, and these could be additional routes of transmission.[50]

Human infestation appears to be relatively common, albeit mild and often undiagnosed.[65,66] One author has reported human infestations associated with 30% of infected cats,[50] but objective data on the incidence of infection are lacking. Infestations are most often associated with *C. blakei* and cats.[67–69] It is unclear if this relates to a higher infectivity of *C. blakei*, greater risk of transmission from cats to humans because of the types of cat–human interaction, or other factors. Human infestations have been associated with *C. yasguri* from dogs,[70–74] but this appears to be rare. Zoonotic *Lynxacarus* infestation has been reported on one occasion.

Animals

Clinical presentation

Infection results in a variably pruritic exfoliative dermatitis with scaling and crusting, most commonly over the dorsum and rump in dogs and around the trunk, face, and tailhead in cats.[49,50] Mites are active, and the associated movement of mites and epidermal debris leads to the appearance of "walking dandruff." The hair coat usually appears dull and dry, and may have a rust-colored tinge. Large numbers of mites and eggs may give the hair coat a granular appearance and feel. There may be excessive hair shedding,[49] and miliary dermatitis may develop in cats.[57]

The distribution is usually different with *L. radovskyic* on cats. Mites are most commonly found on the tailhead, tip of the tail, and the perineum, but can be found over the entire body with severe infestations.

Diagnosis

The presence of dorsal seborrhea sicca (dry white scales) and corresponding "walking dandruff" is highly suggestive of cheyletiellosis.[57] Mites are often visible to the naked eye over the dorsum. Use of magnification will assist in the identification of mites and eggs. Microscopic evaluation of mites allows for confirmation of infection and speciation. Mites may be observed with skin scrapings, not because they reside in the skin but because they are collected during the sampling process. They can also be identified with acetate tape preparations.[50] Occasionally, mites are found in feces of cats after being ingested during grooming. Fecal examination for mites is, however, not a recommended diagnostic test.

Management

Ivermectin, selamectin, imidacloprid/moxidectin, or fipronil is effective.[75–79] Ivermectin is also effective in rabbits.[80] Pyrethrin- or pyrethroid-based shampoos, sprays, or spot-on formulations are effective for dogs,[81] but pyrethroids should not be used on cats.[49] Topical therapies are preferred by some authors because the mites do not live within the skin;[58] however, there is good evidence of efficacy for various systemic treatments. Multiple treatments may be required depending on the potential for reinfection from other animals or the environment.[82] All pets in the household should be treated at the same time. Bedding and grooming equipment should be disinfected or discarded.

Humans

Clinical presentation

Lesions may occur over any part of the body but are more common over the arms, legs, and torso.[50,58,65,66,83,84] The face is rarely affected. Single or multiple macules may be observed initially, and pruritis may be intense. These progress to papules and frequently evolve into vesicles and pustules.[50] There is often an area of central necrosis in older lesions, a finding that is quite suggestive of cheyletiellosis.[65] Multiple people in the household may be affected.[83,84] Systemic manifestations including myalgia, numbness in the fingertips, and poor general health have been reported in association with cheyletiellosis,[65] but this is presumably very rare, if it is even associated with infestation.

Diagnosis

Diagnosis may be difficult if only the human patient is considered, and sometimes the diagnosis is only made after the pet has been diagnosed with cheyletiellosis.[65] Mites may not be observed on the affected person and are rarely identified on skin scrapings.[85] Usually, diagnosis is based on appropriate clinical signs and diagnosis of cheyletiellosis in a pet.[50] Pet contact should be queried in all such cases, and the involvement of the veterinarian may be critical for diagnosis.[70,86] The patient's pet should be referred to his or her veterinarian if cheyletiellosis is suspected. Lack of history of contact with a pet with dermatologic disease does not rule out zoonotic cheyletiellosis as some animals can be infected without clinical signs.[58] Resolution of skin lesions after treatment of the infected pet is further supportive of the diagnosis.

Management

Infection is self-limited since mites cannot complete their life cycle on human skin. Following elimination of infection in the pet, human skin lesions will resolve in approximately 3 weeks.[50,57,83,84,87] Topical therapy with lindane has been used,[65] but there is no evidence that it is required.

Prevention

Human infections are uncommon and mild, and the risk of transmission to other people is low. The mites are more likely to reside on parts of the body normally covered by clothing than on exposed skin. Frequent laundering of clothes and bedding will further help reduce the risk of transmission. The most important elements of prevention of zoonotic transmission from animals are prevention of infestation in pets and prompt diagnosis and treatment of any infestations that do occur.

If cheyletiellosis is diagnosed in a pet, owners should be made aware of the potential for accidental human infection. Pets should be promptly and appropriately treated. All pets should be treated at the same time to prevent cycling of infection in the household. The pet's bedding, as well as other items with which the pet has frequent contact (e.g., bedsheets, sofa cushion covers) should be cleaned thoroughly. Laundering and hot-air drying should be highly effective for this and are likely the best means of decontaminating bedding and similar items. Carpets should be thoroughly vacuumed; steam cleaning may also help eliminate any eggs or mites deep within the carpet pile. Grooming items or other objects that come into regular contact with the pet should be disinfected, or discarded if disinfection is not possible. There is little information regarding optimal cleaning and disinfection techniques. Permethrin sprays can be used to eliminate environmental contamination.[75]

Animals receiving monthly antiparasitic prophylaxis are typically considered to be at low risk because of the high efficacy of most available products against *Cheyletiella*.

Cryptosporidium spp.

Introduction

Cryptosporidiosis is an important and well-recognized zoonotic disease, particularly in people who work with young cattle. It is capable of causing severe diarrhea even in otherwise healthy, immunocompetent hosts, but it can cause life-threatening intestinal and extraintestinal infection in immunocompromised individuals. The relevance of cryptosporidiosis has increased because of its role in disease in HIV/AIDS and other immunosuppressed patients. The role of *Cryptosporidium* in disease in young cattle and humans is well established, but its clinical relevance in companion animals remains unclear. Similarly, the role of pets in human cryptosporidiosis is poorly understood.

Etiology

Cryptosporidium spp. are eukaryotic coccidian parasites of the suborder Eimeria in the phylum Apicomplexa. The taxonomy of the genus *Cryptosporidium*, like many protozoa, is controversial.[88,89] Previously, two species were described, *Cryptosporidium muris* and *Cryptosporidium parvum*, but as many as 23 species have now been described based on various combinations of host predilection,

geographic distribution, genotypic characteristics, and morphology.[88] There is much debate as to which of these species should truly be called species with their own name versus genotypes or subgenotypes of *C. parvum*, of which there are also many.[88] Currently, the more commonly accepted species (and primary hosts) include *Cryptosporidium andersoni* (cattle), *Cryptosporidium baileyi* (chickens and some other birds), *Cryptosporidium canis* (dogs), *Cryptosporidium felis* (cats), *Cryptosporidium galli* (birds), *Cryptosporidium hominis* (humans), *Cryptosporidium meleagridis* (birds and humans), *Cryptosporidium molnari* (fish), *C. muris* (rodents and some other mammals), *C. parvum* (ruminants and humans), *Cryptosporidium wrairi* (guinea pigs), *Cryptosporidium saurophilum* (lizards and snakes), *Cryptosporidium serpentis* (snakes and lizards), and *Cryptosporidium suis* (pigs).[88–90]

Most cryptosporidia that infect reptiles and birds do not appear to infect mammals, except for *C. meleagridis*, which is the third most common type found in humans after *C. hominis* and *C. parvum*. *C. muris* has a limited host range[91] and is not considered a significant concern in humans or companion animals (beyond rodents), although it has been isolated from a cat.[92] *C. felis* can cause diarrhea in humans, although this is rare and may be of greatest concern in immunocompromised individuals. Infection is usually subclinical in cats. *C. canis* is found in dogs, with infection in both dogs and people being generally subclinical. *C. parvum* (also previously known as *C. parvum* genotype 2) has the widest host range, infecting primarily cattle (especially calves) as well as dogs, cats, sheep, goats, horses, laboratory rodents, and humans. *C. hominis* (also previously known as *C. parvum* genotype 1)[89,93] is found primarily in humans and was previously thought to not cause natural infection in other species,[88] but has since been found in a few isolated animal cases.[94] Nonetheless, *C. hominis* is responsible for the majority of human cryptosporidial infections.[88] These various species can only be definitively differentiated based on DNA/genetic testing. The question remains whether or not other strains/species of the parasite are a significant public health threat in general, a threat to only immunocompromised individuals, or not a threat at all,[88] as host adaptation does not necessarily imply host specificity.[88] The five most common species of

Cryptosporidium (*C. hominis*, *C. parvum*, *C. meleagridis*, *C. felis*, and *C. canis*) have been found in both immunocompromised and immunocompetent individuals.[88,95] Case reports of human infection with more uncommon species and genotypes have also been recently published.[96–98]

Geographic distribution/epidemiology

Cryptosporidium infection has a worldwide distribution. The prevalence of oocysts in human feces in North America is thought to be between 0.6% and 4.3%.[99] In the United States, 15–32% of the population may be seropositive for *Cryptosporidium*,[100] while seropositivity in developing countries may be as high as 65%,[99] indicating that exposure is common. Outbreaks of clinical disease in humans have been associated with contaminated food or water, but not household pets. From 1991 to 2000, *Cryptosporidium* was implicated in 40/106 outbreaks of recreational water-associated gastrointestinal disease and 11/130 outbreaks of drinking water-associated gastrointestinal disease.[101–105] However, outbreaks account for less than 10% of diagnoses of *Cryptosporidium* in the United States,[90] and large outbreaks would not be expected to occur from contact with pets. The limited information regarding the role of pets in human cryptosporidiosis must be tempered with an understanding that sporadic cases of cryptosporidiosis, the most likely form of pet-associated disease, would likely be undiagnosed or underreported, if they occur.

Risk factors for human infection include contact with infected farm animals, ingestion of contaminated recreational or drinking water, close contact with infected persons, and travel to high prevalence areas.[93,99] Cryptosporidiosis is more common in immunocompromised individuals as well as in children under 2 years old, livestock handlers (particularly dairy farmers), and men that have sex with men.[99] In most studies, contact with pets is either not associated or negatively associated with the risk of cryptosporidiosis, even among immunocompromised owners.[90,106] Along with the negative association with pets, some studies have found a negative association with consumption of raw vegetables, and it has been hypothesized that these associations may be the result of repeated low-dose exposure to the parasite,

producing better immunity and decreased disease.[90] In contrast, several studies have shown contact with calves or cows[107–109] or farm visits[110] to be significant risk factors for cryptosporidiosis for the general population. Cryptosporidial diarrhea is also common among children in daycare centers, making daycare workers at higher risk for infection.

Some studies have shown a predominance of *C. parvum* among isolates from sporadic cases of cryptosporidiosis, compared with outbreaks in which *C. hominis* is usually implicated.[110,111] These studies and other reports[90] cite this as evidence of zoonotic transmission from livestock (primarily cattle), although given that humans are capable of carrying both species, human-to-human transmission of *C. parvum* must also be considered. Better epidemiological evidence and demonstration of contamination of the water source with infectious effluent from cattle are required to determine the source of the *C. parvum* in these cases.

Exposure to *Cryptosporidium* appears to be common in animals. Reported seroprevalence rates in domestic and feral dogs and cats range from 1.3% to 74%, depending on the region and type of population studied.[112,113] Cats that are allowed outdoors are more likely to be seropositive.[113] Shedding of cryptosporidial oocysts (or the presence of cryptosporidal antigen in feces) is less common, typically ranging from 0% to 8%.[114–119]

In all affected domestic animal species, young unweaned animals are more susceptible to infection and disease from *Cryptosporidium* than adults.[99] In general, kittens less than 6 months of age and cats living in households with more than one cat or with a dog are more likely to be infected.[120]

Cryptosporidium can also be commonly identified in ferrets,[121] but most, if not all, belong to the ferret genotype of *C. parvum*. It is unknown if this genotype can cause disease in humans.[122]

Transmission of the infection occurs through ingestion of oocysts that are shed in the feces of infected humans or animals. As few as 30 oocysts of *C. parvum* can cause subclinical infection in an otherwise healthy person, and as few as 100 oocysts can cause clinical cryptosporidiosis,[100] whereas as few as 10 oocysts of *C. hominis* can cause clinical disease in humans.[123] There are three major routes of transmission in people: person to person, which is particularly important in daycare settings with young children; animal to person, which is sometimes implicated in outbreaks in rural areas although the relative importance of this route remains unclear; and transmission via contaminated water (or food) sources, which is a well-recognized route in outbreaks.[88]

Although owning a dog or a cat has not been identified as a risk factor for cryptosporidiosis in humans, transmission of the parasite from these animals to humans is possible. The most common species of *Cryptosporidium* in dogs, *C. canis*, has only been reported to cause subclinical infection in a few immunocompetent individuals. In contrast, *C. felis* has been reported to cause watery diarrhea in both immunocompetent and immunosuppressed individuals.[124]

Life cycle

Cryptosporidia can undergo their entire life cycle in a single host. Animals or humans are infected by ingesting oocysts from the feces of other infected individuals. In the small intestine, the oocysts release sporozoites that invade the brush border of the epithelium, forming intracellular but extracytoplasmic vacuoles containing trophozoites. The trophozoites replicate asexually to form type I meronts containing merozoites. The released merozoites go on to replicate in other intestinal epithelial cells to form more type I meronts as well as type II meronts. Type II meronts reproduce sexually, producing macrogamonts and microgamonts. Fusing of one of each type of gamont results in the formation of a zygote, which in turn forms an oocyst containing four sporozoites.[125] The oocysts are either thin or thick walled. Thin-walled oocysts rupture within the intestine, and the entire life cycle is repeated (autogenous infection). Thick-walled oocysts are passed in the feces and are immediately infectious to the next host.[125]

Animals

Clinical presentation

Patent infections may be present in cats and dogs with no accompanying clinical signs. It is therefore debated whether or not the organism causes diarrhea in otherwise healthy, immunocompetent cats and dogs, or whether it may be a secondary finding in cases of other gastrointestinal disease. When clinical signs are associated with infection, the primary sign is diarrhea. In both dogs and cats, diarrhea is most severe in immunocompromised animals.

Clinically affected cats typically exhibit high-volume, low-frequency (small bowel type) diarrhea but can chronically develop tenesmus and hematochezia.[126] In puppies experimentally infected with *C. parvum* from calves, the prepatent period was 3–5 days, peak shedding occurred at 7–9 days, and intermittent or low-level shedding continued for at least 80 days.[126]

The parasite may be a primary pathogen in birds in which it can infect both the gastrointestinal and respiratory tracts and bursa of Fabricius. Cryptosporidia tend to infect the stomach of reptiles and therefore cause gastritis and vomiting.[126]

Diagnosis

Although oocysts can be seen on direct fecal smears, concentration techniques using sugar solutions (e.g., Sheather's solution, specific gravity 1.2–1.25) for fecal flotation are preferred.[99,126] The use of phase-contrast or bright-field microscopy is recommended to detect oocysts on unstained preparations. Oocysts are typically slightly smaller than erythrocytes (approximately 2.5–5 μm in diameter) and are refractile (Figure 1.1).[99] They appear as circular or possibly concave disks; dark shadows of four banana-shaped sporozoites can sometimes be seen within them. On wet mounts stained with crystal violet, the oocysts are apparent because

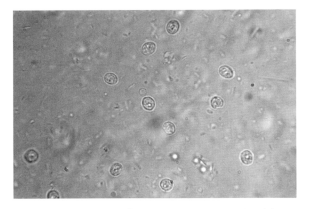

Figure 1.1 *Cryptosporidium parvum* oocysts (4–5 μm) in a stool sample from a person with cryptosporidiosis (public domain, Dr. Peter Drotman, Centers for Disease Control and Prevention).

they do not pick up stain.[126] Of the various species that infect mammals, only *C. muris* and *C. andersoni* oocysts can be differentiated morphologically from the others.[88]

Diagnostic laboratories may use formalin-ethyl acetate sedimentation followed by direct fluorescent antibody staining. The fluorescent antibody test has been used as the reference standard for comparison of other diagnostic tests.[127] Enzyme-linked immunosorbent assays (ELISAs) designed for detection of parasitic antigen in human fecal samples are also available, although it is unknown if these tests can consistently identify certain species such as *C. canis* and *C. felis*. In a comparison of three antigen-based assays on feline fecal samples, the ProSpecT Microplate Assay had the highest sensitivity (71.4%) and specificity (96.7%) for detection of cryptosporidial antigen, compared with a direct fluorescent antibody test.[127] Compared with fluorescent antibody testing of fecal samples from experimentally infected cats, PCR appeared to be more sensitive in another study.[128] Further evaluation of these tests for use in veterinary medicine is warranted.

A serum ELISA for cats is available, but, as in humans, the test only indicates exposure and is not useful for predicting oocyst shedding in individual animals.[129] Intestinal biopsy is an impractical means of diagnosis. Organisms can be found throughout the intestine in animals but are most numerous in the ileum.[126]

Management

Infection in otherwise healthy animals is self-limited. Supportive care including intravenous fluid therapy may be required to prevent or treat dehydration if diarrhea is severe and the animal's fluid intake is inadequate. Specific treatment of coinfections, if possible, should be considered. If no coinfection exists and clinical signs are persistent or severe, specific therapy for *Cryptosporidium* could be considered, although objective information regarding treatment is limited. Currently, there are no drugs that have been shown to be consistently effective and safe for treatment of cryptosporidiosis in companion animals. Paromomycin or azithromycin are the most commonly recommended specific treatments in dogs and cats.[126]

Humans

Clinical presentation

Frequent, watery, and nonbloody diarrhea is the predominant clinical presentation.[2] Nausea, abdominal cramps, low-grade fever, and anorexia may also be present.[130] Fever and vomiting are more likely to occur in children.[2] Diarrhea may be profuse and can result in dehydration, but illness is usually self-limited in immunocompetent individuals. However, cryptosporidiosis can be a serious disease in immunocompromised individuals, with severe diarrhea (over 70 evacuations per day, losing up to 25 L in fluids), dehydration, and a potentially fatal outcome.[99] In HIV/AIDS, disease occurs more frequently and is more severe in patients with lower CD4+ lymphocyte counts, particularly those with CD4+ counts below 200 cells/μL.[89] The incidence of symptomatic infection and severe disease in HIV/AIDS patients has declined with the widespread use of highly active antiretroviral therapy.[90,93] Transplant patients and individuals with IgA deficiency are also at increased risk of severe disease.

Rarely, nonintestinal clinical signs of cryptosporidiosis may occur following acute diarrheal disease, including joint pain, eye pain, recurrent headache, dizzy spells, and fatigue. These signs and symptoms have only been associated with *C. hominis*.[131] Infection of the respiratory and biliary tracts may also occur in immunocompromised individuals.[132,133]

Diagnosis

Infected persons have been reported to shed up to a billion oocysts per day, yet immunocompetent, symptomatic human patients do not always have positive stool samples, and conversely, oocyst shedding may persist for up to 15 days following resolution of clinical disease.[93,134] Evaluation of at least three stool samples collected on different days is recommended.[2] As described above for animals, oocysts can be detected by microscopic examination of stained or unstained fecal preparations. Several antigen-based fecal tests (e.g., fluorescent antibody, ELISA) are also available. PCR-based tests have been developed and appear to have a very low detection threshold (10–100 oocysts/mL compared with 10,000 oocyts/mL for the fluorescent antibody test).[135,136] A nested multiplex PCR has been developed that can differentiate *C. parvum*, *C. hominis*, *C. canis*, and *C. felis* in human fecal samples,[135] something that could be very useful for determining the potential source(s) of infection in sporadic cases and outbreaks.

Serological tests are available with acceptable sensitivity and specificity. However, antibodies usually appear too late to be of use in the diagnosis of acute disease, and may not appear at sufficient levels to be detected in immunocompromised individuals.[99] In addition, they remain high after infection. Serology is most useful for epidemiological studies.

Management

Most infections in immunocompetent persons are self-limited, and individuals ultimately recover completely in 1–20 days (mean 10).[2] In these cases, treatment, if necessary, is limited to supportive care, particularly fluid replacement (either oral or parenteral). A consistently effective anticryptosporidial drug has yet to be found, which leaves individuals with immature or weakened immune systems (including young children and the elderly) at risk of more severe disease.[90,137] In the United States, the only drug approved for the treatment of cryptosporidiosis in people is nitazoxanide.[138,139] Treatment with paromomycin may improve clinical signs and decrease oocyst shedding in people, and has been recommended for the treatment of immunocompromised patients.[140,141] Azithromycin has also been used, but further study is required to determine its true efficacy.[137]

Immune reconstitution in HIV/AIDS patients through administration of highly active antiretroviral therapy will assist with the elimination of *Cryptosporidium*.[2]

Prevention

The key to preventing zoonotic cryptosporidiosis from pets is avoiding inadvertent ingestion of oocysts from the animal, or its environment. In households, diarrheic animals should be handled minimally in case there is fecal staining of the hair coat. Diarrheic animals should be taken outside frequently to reduce the risk of accidental defecation in the house. Ideally, affected dogs should not be walked in public areas. Feces should be promptly removed and hands should be thoroughly washed. If feces are passed in the house, contaminated areas should be promptly cleaned. Thorough cleaning to physically remove oocysts is the key because oocysts are resistant to most disinfectants. Care should be taken to avoid contamination of the environment or hands when cleaning litter boxes, and hands should be thoroughly washed after (even if gloves are used).

Immunocompromised individuals, especially people with HIV/AIDS, should take particular care, especially around diarrheic animals. Careful use of general infection control measures to reduce contact with fecal pathogens is important, regardless of whether the animal has diarrhea or not. Contact with diarrheic animals should be restricted. If possible, immunocompromised individuals should have someone else pick up feces or clean the litter box. If fecal staining of the pet's hair coat occurs, this should be promptly and thoroughly cleaned, ideally not by the immunocompromised person. If contact with feces, litter boxes, or potentially contaminated hair coats is unavoidable, gloves should be used and hands should be washed immediately after glove removal. If there has been potential contamination of clothing, clothes should be promptly removed and laundered, using hot water and a hot-air clothes dryer.

In veterinary clinics, diarrheic animals should be isolated and handled with appropriate contact precautions (e.g., gown, gloves, and designated footwear or shoe covers if there is potential fecal contamination of the floor). Currently, there is insufficient evidence to warrant full isolation of clinically normal pets in which low-level shedding of *Cryptosporidium* is diagnosed as an incidental finding. However, the animal should not be allowed to defecate in common animal areas, feces should be removed and disposed of promptly, and contact with immunocompromised individuals should be avoided.

Cryptosporidium oocysts are highly resistant to routine disinfectants. Oocysts are resistant to routine chlorination of drinking water and are very small ($4.5 \times 5.0\,\mu m$), making them difficult to filter from water.[142] Prolonged contact with high concentrations of chemicals such as formalin (>10%) or ammonia (>50%) can be effective;[141] however, this is typically impractical. Moist heat (e.g., steam, pasteurization), freezing and thawing, or thorough drying are more practical means of disinfection[126] but may not be completely effective. Oocysts survive better in cool water: after 4 weeks in water at 8°C, 75% of oocysts survive, whereas only 50% survive after 4 weeks in water at 25°C.[99] Because oocysts are so resistant to disinfectants, preventing environmental contamination through excellent sanitation (i.e., mechanical cleaning) is critical.

Demodex spp.

Demodex mites are part of the normal microflora of mammals and are not usually associated with disease. However, overgrowth of mites in certain situations can cause alopecia or mild to moderate dermatitis. *Demodex canis* is most common in dogs, although *Demodex injai* or other species may be found rarely.[143–146] In cats, *Demodex cati* predominates, while *Demodex gatoi* can be found in some regions.[147–149] *Demodex folliculorum* and *Demodex brevis* are most commonly reported in humans.[150,151]

In animals, particularly dogs, demodectic mange can be localized or generalized. Either form is more likely to occur in purebred dogs, but any breed or sex can be affected. The localized form is most common in puppies from a few months to 1 year of age, causing alopecia and folliculitis on the head (often around the eyes) and extremities. The vast majority of infected dogs (90%) recover without treatment, but some will progress to the generalized form. Generalized demodecosis typically occurs in young dogs (6–18 months of age) but can also occur in geriatric or immunosuppressed animals. This form of infection is often complicated by secondary bacterial pyoderma, which can be life threatening. Demodecosis is rare in cats.

Demodecosis is not considered transmissible under normal conditions, even from a clinically affected animal to other animals of the same species. Furthermore, *Demodex* mites are host adapted, and there is no convincing evidence of cross-infectivity. There is one report of identification of *D. folliculorum* in a child and his pet dog;[152] however, that is the only report of concurrent detection of the same *Demodex* species in humans and their pet and, being a human *Demodex* species, would possibly indicate human-to-pet transmission. Accordingly, *Demodex* should not be considered a zoonotic risk.

Dipylidium caninum

Introduction

D. caninum is a cyclophyllidean cestode that is also referred to as the common flea tapeworm. Both dogs and cats may be affected. Human infections can occur, particularly in infants and young children, but the clinical consequences are minimal. The greatest problem in most situations is the response of pet owners, patients, or parents to seeing tapeworm segments in feces.

Life cycle

Like other cyclophyllidean tapeworms, *D. caninum* has an indirect life cycle that requires an intermediate host (Figure 1.2). Adult tapeworms attach to the wall of the small intestine by an armed scolex. Gravid proglottids are shed in feces, and eggs are subsequently consumed by intermediate hosts, predominantly *Ctenocephalides felis* (cat flea) and *Ctenocephalides canis* (dog flea). The chewing louse, *Trichodectes canis*, can also act as an intermediate host, but this is rare. Infectious larvae (cysticercoids) develop within the intermediate hosts, and individuals (pet or humans) are usually infected by inadvertent ingestion of infected fleas. After ingestion, the tapeworm completes its life cycle in the small intestine. Proglottids may be visible in feces 2–3 weeks after ingestion of an infected flea.[153]

Geographic distribution/epidemiology

D. caninum is found worldwide. Prevalence data in dogs and cats are highly variable, with most of the variability depending on flea exposure and flea control practices. Shedding rates of 0.3–42% have been reported in dogs, and up to 68% in cats.[154–164] Rates tend to be higher in developing countries and in stray animals, as well as in older reports. More recent studies in developed countries tend to report rates of 0.1–2% in dogs and cats.[154,165–167] Point prevalence studies are presumed to somewhat underestimate the prevalence because proglottids and eggs are unevenly distributed in feces and can be shed intermittently.[153] In addition, fecal tests have a low level of sensitivity.

Dipylidium caninum infection
(Dipylidium caninum)

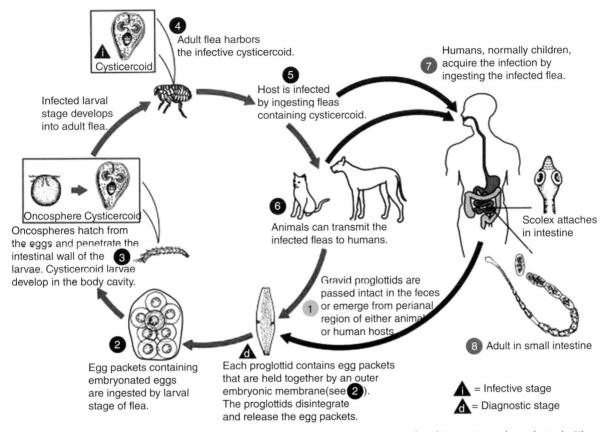

Figure 1.2 *Dipylidium caninum* life cycle (public domain, Centers for Disease Control and Prevention, Alexander J. da Silva, Melanie Moser).

There are numerous reports of *D. caninum* infections in humans,[168–177] all single case reports and almost all involving infants or young children. The incidence of human infection is quite low, and the clinical consequences are minor. This may be considered more of a social disease, with angst surpassing true health risks.

Animals

Clinical presentation

Disease is rare, and the vast majority of infected animals are clinically normal. The most common clinical abnormality is perianal irritation that may be associated with passing proglottids in feces.

Diagnosis

Motile proglottids may be seen exiting the anus or, less commonly, in the pet's environment (i.e., bedding), and this is typically adequate for diagnosis, but these must be differentiated from proglottids of *Taenia* spp. A single fecal negative sample does not rule out the presence of *D. caninum* because of intermittent shedding and nonhomogenous distribution in stool. The eggs themselves (which are released when the proglottids rupture) can be differentiated microscopically from those of *Taenia* spp. and *Echinococcus* spp.

Management

Praziquantel or epsiprantel is effective against *D. caninum*[178] and widely used for the elimination of adult tapeworms in dogs and cats.[153] The commercially available combinations of emodepside and praziquantel, milbemycin and praziquantel, and pyrantel and praziquantel are also effective.[179,180] Treatment of tapeworms alone, however, is not adequate for long-term resolution of the problem if infected fleas are still present on the infected animal, or other animals that it has contact with. To prevent reinfection, all pets in the household should be treated for flea infestation, and measures should be taken to reduce the risk of subsequent flea exposure. This may include management changes (e.g., keeping cats indoors) or prophylactic drug administration, as are discussed in more depth elsewhere.

Humans

Clinical presentation

Infections are usually asymptomatic[174] and only identified because patients or their parents see tapeworm segments in stool.

Diagnosis

Diagnosis is based on the identification of proglottids or eggs in stool.

Management

Praziquantel is the drug of choice. Niclosamide is another option.[2] Pets should be treated concurrently for *D. caninum* and fleas.

Prevention

The main preventive measure is flea control in dogs and cats. Animals that are at risk of flea exposure should be started on an appropriate flea control program.

Dirofilaria immitis

Introduction

D. immitis, the canine and feline heartworm, is predominantly an animal health threat. The greatest impact in humans may be an indirect one since infection can be mistaken for more serious conditions and can necessitate invasive procedures such as thoracotomy.

Etiology

D. immitis is a mosquito-borne nematode parasite that naturally infects canids and can accidentally infect other species such as cats, ferrets, and humans. Many different mosquito species are competent vectors, including various species of *Aedes*, *Anopheles*, *Culex*, and *Psorophora*.[181]

Life cycle

The natural life cycle involves canids and mosquitoes. Microfilaria are present in the blood of infected canids and are ingested by mosquitoes while feeding from infected host. After undergoing two molts, infective L3 larvae reside in the mosquito's mouth parts and are deposited onto the skin during subsequent feeding. Once on the skin, they migrate through the bite wound into the host, where they molt to the L4 stage in subcutaneous tissues. These worms enter the vascular system and are carried to the pulmonary arterial vasculature, where they mature. Microfilaria production is usually detectable 6–7 months after infection.

In animals with extremely heavy worm burdens, the worm mass extends from the pulmonary artery into the right atrium or ventricle. However, in some ways, "heartworm" is a misnomer since the parasite is predominantly a vascular-dwelling organism that is often not present in the heart. Typically, it is found outside of the pulmonary arterial tree only with significant burdens.[182]

While they can be infected, cats, ferrets, and humans tend not to act as biological reservoirs and rarely have detectable microfilaremia.[181]

Geography/epidemiology

The prevalence of *D. immitis* varies geographically, with a high prevalence (up to 70%) in some dog populations.[183–192] In North America, higher rates in dogs tend to be found in the southeastern United States and Mississippi River valley. Human infections follow the same pattern.[193] In Europe, there is a similar distribution with widespread presence in southern countries with few to no cases in northern regions.[194] Italy has the highest number of reported European cases.[194] The geographic variation likely involves the prevalence of mosquito vectors, climate, the size of wild canid populations, and the percentage of pet dogs receiving routine heartworm prophylaxis.

Human infections are uncommon but have been reported internationally.[182,195–205] The incidence of disease is not known, and the available literature consists solely of case reports or small case series.

Animals

Clinical presentation

In dogs, infection may result in pulmonary vasculitis, pulmonary hypertension, right-sided heart failure, and, less commonly, infections of other systems including the CNS. Severe respiratory disease can develop from rapid death of juvenile or adult worms if embolization of dead worms to the lungs occurs. Cats can be similarly infected, but much less often than dogs and tend to have short-term or nondetectable microfilaremia.[206]

Diagnosis

Serum antigen testing is the most sensitive method of diagnosis in dogs; however, infections occurring within the previous 6 months and those involving low worm burdens may be missed.[206] The specificity is very high, but positive tests are usually repeated. Repeated testing of negatives is indicated if there is a clinical suspicion of heartworm disease.

Detection of microfilaria in circulation used to be the standard for diagnosis but is uncommonly used now for either screening or diagnostic purposes because microfilaria are not present in all infected animals at all times, and there are few

advantages over antigen testing. This type of testing is generally good for confirmatory testing in mature infections (those occurring at least 6 months in the past).

Radiography and echocardiography may be used to provide evidence of clinical heartworm infection involving the pulmonary arterial vasculature.

Management

Stabilization of the patient and management of clinical abnormalities that are occurring as a result of infection are important and may include the use of anti-inflammatories, diuretics, intravenous fluids, vasodilators, or positive inotropic agents.

Melarsomine dihydrochloride is the adulticide of choice. It is, however, ineffective against heartworms younger than 4 months of age,[206] which may result in initial treatment failure. Macrocyclic lactones have been used as adulticides but are not recommended.[206] These drugs are effective against microfilaria and migrating L3 and L4 larvae; they will also effectively sterilize adult worms (thus eliminating the risk of transmission to other animals via mosquitoes) and shorten the life span of adult worms. A combination of a macrocyclic lactone and melarsomine has been recommended because of the ability to kill a wider age range of worms and to kill microfilaria, thereby preventing transmission. In cases where clinical signs are not present, administering a macrocyclic lactone for up to 3 months prior to melarsomine therapy is a reasonable option.[207] A combination of ivermectin and doxycycline has been shown to have microfilaricidal and adulticidal activity[208] and may be another option.

Surgical excision of adult worms can be considered with large worm burdens and is required promptly in dogs with caval syndrome and when infections in cats cannot be managed clinically. Melarsomine is contraindicated in cats.

Humans

Clinical presentation

The most common result of *D. immitis* infection in humans is the development of vasculitis in the small to medium branches of the pulmonary tree after the parasite dies. Overt clinical disease is present in less than 50% of patients with pulmonary dirofilariasis at the time the lesion is identified.[182,193] Primary and secondary tumors, cysts, and granulomas can have the same radiological appearance, and because of the concern regarding malignancies, thoracotomy and biopsy are often the approach that is taken for any such lesion.[182] This is compounded by the lack of accurate serological testing for humans to differentiate *D. immitis* from other causes that require invasive surgical procedures. Considering the morbidity and healthcare costs associated with such an aggressive approach, the indirect impact of *D. immitis* infection is apparent.

When clinical signs are present with pulmonary dirofilariasis, cough, chest pain, or hemoptysis may be reported, often associated with pulmonary infarction.[193] Infections of other body sites may occur, including the eye,[200] CNS,[198] adipose tissue,[202] liver,[199] and testicular vasculature.[204]

Diagnosis

The inflammatory response can ultimately lead to development of a granuloma with the radiographic appearance of a "coin lesion."[182] The lesion is a nonspecific finding that simply indicates a discrete pulmonary lesion but cannot be differentiated from malignancy.

Diagnosis is histologically from biopsy samples collected to rule out neoplasia. Dead intact worms are often visible, along with associated vasculitis and infarcted tissue, usually within a granuloma. Eosinophilic inflammation is sometimes present.[193] Serological testing is not currently accurate enough to rely on.[193,194] Microfilaremia does not occur in humans.[194]

Management

Treatment is typically unnecessary since the diagnosis is usually incidental and humans are dead-end hosts for the parasite.[197,209]

Prevention

Humans do not acquire *D. immitis* directly from dogs and cats. However, dogs are likely the primary reservoir hosts and can infect mosquitoes that may subsequently bite and infect humans. Infected cats pose little to no public health risk because they are typically amicrofilaremic. Prevention of human infections involves two main components: decreasing *D. immitis* in dogs and mosquito avoidance.

A variety of routine monthly preventive therapies are available for dogs, including milbemycin oxime, moxidectin, ivermectin, and selamectin. A 6-month injectable moxidectin formulation is available for use in dogs. These drugs should be administered to dogs throughout the transmission season in heartworm-endemic areas. The climate and period of mosquito activity must be considered when deciding the duration of preventive therapy. In some regions, there may be a risk of exposure all year, while in cooler climates, there may only be a risk for a fraction of the year. Annual serological testing of dogs is widely recommended, even in dogs that have received regular prophylactic therapy because of the possibility of treatment failure, missed drug doses, mosquito exposure outside of the treatment period, or other factors that could lead to infection of dogs receiving chemoprophylaxis. Annual testing is less effective in low prevalence areas because of the low predictive value of positive results.

General behavioral practices to avoid exposure to mosquitoes include avoiding areas of mosquito activity (particularly at dusk and dawn), wearing clothing that covers the arms and legs when in areas where mosquitoes may be present, using mosquito repellents, and eliminating standing water and other mosquito breeding grounds.

Echinococcus spp.

Introduction

Echinococcus granulosus and *Echinococcus multilocularis* are two species of cyclophyllidean tapeworms that have dogs (*E. granulosus*) or both dogs and cats (*E. multilocularis*) as their definitive hosts. Humans are intermediate hosts that are inadvertently infected from the feces of infected definitive hosts, with dogs posing the greatest risk. Echinococcosis is a rare but potentially devastating condition caused by the development of larval cysts in the liver, lungs, brain, or other tissues.

Etiology

E. granulosus is maintained in both domestic and sylvatic cycles. The domestic cycle involves dogs that are infected by ingestion of *E. granulosus* cysts in the intestinal viscera of infected ungulates (e.g., sheep) or in the muscle of rabbits. The sylvatic cycle is similar, with wolves and foxes being the main definitive hosts and becoming infected from ingestion of infected ungulates (e.g., moose) or rabbits. Humans can become infected by inadvertently ingesting eggs from canine feces.

E. multilocularis is the most pathogenic *Echinococcus* and is normally transmitted in a cycle involving wild canids such as the red fox, arctic fox, and sylvatic rodent species, along with other wild mammals.[210] Pet dogs and cats can be infected with *E. multilocularis* following ingestion of infected rodents. As with *E. granulosus*, humans are accidental hosts that are infected by ingesting eggs from feces.

Another species, *Echinococcus vogeli*, is found in the South American highlands and is transmitted by wild canids.[211,212] Because this species is rare and not associated with pets, it will not be discussed further here.

Life cycle

Adult worms inhabit the small intestine. The tapeworm consists of a head (scolex), neck, and tail (Figure 1.3). The neck and tail are made up of a chain of independent but connected segments: proglottids. Each proglottid has male and female sexual organs and produces eggs. Egg-laden proglottids break free of the adult worm and are shed in feces.[213] Eggs may be released in stool if the proglottid degenerates, or may be shed still contained within the proglottid. Millions of eggs can be shed daily by an infected definitive host. Eggs are embryonated and immediately infective to the next susceptible host. The prepatent period is 1–2 months.

After ingestion by an intermediate host (including humans), the egg hatches in the small intestine and releases an oncosphere.[213] This penetrates the intestinal mucosa and reaches the systemic circulation, where it can be disseminated to virtually any part of the body. A larval (metacestode) cyst may develop, depending on the tissue/organ that the oncosphere reaches and the *Echinococcus* species. In the viscera, oncospheres encyst.[213]

The life cycle is completed when a definitive host ingests an infected intermediate host, and the cyst develops into an adult tapeworm in the definitive host's small intestine.

Geographic distribution/epidemiology

Animals

E. granulosus is most common in Africa, the Middle East, southern Europe, Latin America, and the southwestern United States.[213] The prevalence of *E. granulosus* infection of dogs also varies greatly within regions. Rates of 5–18% have been reported in stray dogs in endemic regions, with rates of 1.8–51% in pet dogs.[214–224] Reported risk factors include infrequent (>4-month interval) treatment with praziquantel, being allowed to roam, being fed offal from intermediate hosts likely to be infected, and lack of owner knowledge about *Echinococcus*.[216,221,225] The sylvatic life cycle is most important for maintenance of this parasite in most regions. High rates of infection are present in species such as moose in some regions.

E. multilocularis is most common in temperate and holoarctic regions of the Northern Hemisphere, including the northern forest regions of Europe, Switzerland, the midwestern United States, Asia (particularly China and Japan), and the

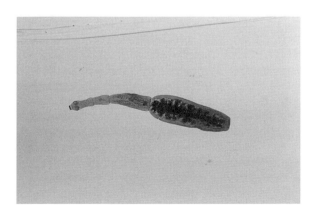

Figure 1.3 *Echinococcus granulosus*, 2–9 mm (public domain, Centers for Disease Control and Prevention, Dr. Peter Schantz).

Arctic.[210,213,226–228] The United Kingdom, Ireland, Sweden, and Malta are considered free of the parasite.[223] As with *E. granulosus*, the prevalence of *E. multilocularis* infection varies greatly between and within regions. Rates of up to 58% have been reported in stray dogs in endemic regions, and 0.2–23% in pet or working dogs.[215,222,229–233] Reported risk factors for fecal shedding by dogs include being fed raw viscera, catching rodents, the density of intermediate hosts in the area, and being allowed to roam.[214,215,229,234] These risk factors are all associated with increased likelihood of ingestion of infected wildlife or being fed potentially infected foods. Limited feline prevalence data are available. While *E. multilocularis* eggs have been found in feline feces in different regions, the prevalence appears to be quite low.[235,236] One study of over 10,000 cats identified *E. multilocularis* eggs in only 0.25% of samples.[235] Experimental studies suggest that cats are poor definitive hosts of this species and are probably less important than dogs in maintenance of infection and transmission to humans.[237]

For both *Echinococcus* species, the prevalence in animals is likely underestimated because of infrequent shedding of proglottids and eggs in the feces of infected animals, and the corresponding potential for false-negative fecal examinations.

Hydatid cyst disease in humans

E. granulosus infection of humans results in hydatid cyst disease (cystic echinococcosis). The main sites of *E. granulosus* hydatid cyst formation are the liver (50–70% of patients), followed by the lungs (20–30%).[213,226,238–240] Other body sites are uncommonly affected, including the brain, heart, kidneys, and bones.[226,238–240] In most (80%) patients, a single cyst is present.[226,241] Hydatid cysts grow relatively slowly but can reach 5–10 cm in diameter over the first year. Cysts are typically filled with clear fluid containing brood capsules and protoscolices.[226] Calcification of cysts is not uncommon.[226] Depending on the location, cysts can reach large sizes over long periods of time (years to decades) before clinical signs are noted.[213] Cysts may undergo asexual budding, resulting in the formation of "daughter" cysts within the main cyst. Proliferation of cysts may also occur following spontaneous or trauma-induced rupture of cysts, with subsequent release of protoscolices into the circulation or local tissues.[226] The space-occupying nature of the hydatid is the reason for most clinical signs, and pressure on adjacent organs can result in impaired function or atrophy.[242]

The incidence of hydatid cyst disease is low, having been estimated or reported at <1–220 per 100,000 persons in endemic regions.[226,241,243,244] Living in a rural area, feeding offal to dogs, and owning a dog are reported risk factors.[241,245,246] Housewives, farmers, and laborers have been reported as overrepresented among the infected population in endemic areas.[241]

Alveolar cyst disease in humans

E. multilocularis infection produces alveolar hydatid disease (alveolar echinococcosis), a particularly serious disease that is characterized by tumorlike infiltration of local tissues.[213,226] Metacestodes of this species almost exclusively develop in the liver (particularly the right lobe),[226] though infections in other organs and tissues are possible. Cysts can range in morphology from collection of a small number of tiny (few millimeters) cysts to infiltration of various tissues with large (15–20 cm or greater) cysts.[226] Lesions may develop granulomatous infiltrates, microcalcifications, and necrotic cavities.[210] Spread to distant parts of the body can also occur through liberation of cystic contents into circulation.

The incidence of alveolar cyst disease is also low, being estimated at 0.03–6.6 per 100,000 persons in endemic regions.[226] Despite the rarity of infection, this is a significant public health concern because of the severity of disease. There is evidence that dogs play a major role in human infection, at least in some regions.[227] Reported risk factors for human infection include dog ownership, total number of dogs owned, cat ownership, and the distribution of small mammals' habitats.[210,246–248]

Animals

Clinical presentation

Clinical disease is rare and abnormalities are not usually identified, even with large worm burdens. Perianal irritation can occur from passage of proglottids, resulting in chewing at the anus or "scooting."

Diagnosis

Occasionally, motile proglottids may be seen exiting the animal's anus. Proglottids may occasionally be identified by pet owners on bedding or other environmental surfaces, or in the animal's feces. Examination of the segment can be performed to differentiate *Echinococcus* spp. from other tapeworms. Proglottids are 1–2 mm in length and may contain 300 (*E. multilocularis*) to 600 (*E. granulosus*) eggs.[242]

Fecal flotation can be used to detect eggs that have been liberated from damaged proglottids; however, the intermittent nature of shedding means that a single negative sample does not rule out *Echinococcus* infection. *Echinococcus* spp. eggs cannot be differentiated from *Taenia* spp. eggs microscopically.[242] To increase the sensitivity of fecal testing, purgation with substances such as arecoline can be used.[249] This is not practical or justifiable in normal clinical settings.

Coproantigen testing is a potentially promising option, considering the limitations of microscopic testing. It has been shown to be able to reliably detect burdens of >50 *Echinococcus* worms in dogs[250] and to be more sensitive than arecoline purgation.[249] PCR may be a good option for identification and speciation in the near future.

Management

Praziquantel is effective against both *E. granulosus* and *E. multilocularis* and is the drug of choice.[242] Epsiprantel is also effective against *E. multilocularis* in dogs and cats, but unlike praziquantel, is not licensed for this purpose.[242,251] Concurrent measures should be taken to reduce the risk of reinfection. If no management changes are made, reinfection is likely.

Humans

Clinical presentation

Hydatid cyst disease
Most infections are asymptomatic, even with large lesions, as long as the cyst is not compromising organ function.[213,226] Often, cysts are only identified as incidental findings on imaging studies.[213] However, disease can occur, ranging from mild to fatal.

Clinical signs usually result from the space occupying nature of the cyst(s) in a confined space. Signs and symptoms relating to hepatic involvement include abdominal pain and a sensation of the presence of an abdominal mass.[241] Cough, dyspnea, chest pain, and hemoptysis may be present with pulmonary involvement.[241,252] Headache, vomiting, hemiparesis, visual deficits, seizures, and diplopia can occur with intracranial cysts.[240]

If hepatic cysts erode into the biliary tract, cyst contents, including daughter cysts, may be released and result in biliary obstruction.[213] Entry of bacteria into cysts can result in abscessation. If cysts leak or rupture, there can be a severe allergic (including anaphylactoid) reaction to cyst contents.[213] Even if there is no severe allergic response to cyst rupture, this event can cause further problems from the dissemination of daughter cysts to other parts of the body. This can result in multiorgan involvement (and failure), with associated high morbidity and mortality.[213]

Alveolar cyst disease
The onset of disease is usually gradual, with progressive signs relating to the organ that is involved. The incubation period is at least 5–15 years. Jaundice and epigastric pain are common signs when there is hepatic involvement.[210,226] Signs such as weight loss, hepatomegaly, and fatigue may also be present.

Diagnosis

Hydatid cyst disease
The main method of diagnosis is the identification of obvious cysts using imaging studies, such as ultrasonography, CT, or MRI.[210,213,226] Serology is a relatively sensitive (80–100%) and specific (88–96%) method for differentiating liver cysts from other cystic structures, but it is less sensitive for the lungs and other organs.[213]

Alveolar cyst disease
Imaging with ultrasonography, CT, or MRI is often suggestive of neoplasia. In those instances, a suspicion of alveolar cyst disease usually arises after biopsy.[213] Serological testing is useful, as described for hydatid cyst disease. Ultrasound-based screening has been used for early diagnosis of infection in some regions.[247]

For both forms, testing of feces is useless because adult tapeworms do not develop in the intestinal tract.

Management

Hydatid cyst disease

Treatment is indicated for cysts that are causing clinical illness. Cysts that are identified incidentally and are not causing clinical problems should be monitored to detect potential complications.[213] Ideally, clinically relevant cysts are surgically removed in toto, taking care not to rupture the cyst during removal.[213,226,253] Rupture of the cyst during surgery can be fatal.[240] Surgery is indicated for large liver cysts with multiple daughter cysts; single liver cysts that are superficially situated and may rupture spontaneously; cysts communicating with the biliary tree; cysts putting pressure on adjacent organs; and cysts in the lungs, brain, kidney, bones, or other organs.[226] Surgical excision is preferred because it is the only approach with a likelihood of complete cure.[226] Because of the potential for dissemination of infection with cyst rupture during removal, a common approach is to expose the cyst surgically, to remove some cystic fluid, and to infuse a cysticidal agent such as hypertonic saline cetrimide or ethanol.[213,226] After approximately 15–30 minutes, surgical removal of the cyst is performed. While commonly used, there is little objective evidence supporting this approach and its use has been questioned. Infusion of cysticidal agents should never be performed when there may be communication with other structures such as the biliary tree.[213] Alternative approaches involve anthelmintic treatment for 4 weeks, followed by a 2-week "rest period" before surgery.[213] Albendazole is the drug of choice.[254]

Surgery may not be an option, depending on patient factors or the presence of multiple cysts, cysts that are difficult to access surgically, cysts that are partially or totally calcified, and very small cysts.[226] Anthelmintic therapy alone is unlikely to be curative but may reduce clinical signs. A cure rate of 30% has been reported for anthelmintic therapy alone, with reduction of cyst size in a further 30–50%.[226] Drug therapy is more effective in young patients and patients with small, thin-walled cysts without secondary infection or communication.[226] Another approach to inoperable cysts is the puncture, aspiration, injection, re-aspiration (PAIR) method.[226] Mortality is uncommon (2–4%) if proper medical care is provided.[226]

Alveolar cyst disease

Treatment of alveolar cyst disease is complicated and best performed by people with previous clinical experience.[226] Early diagnosis is a key factor for successful treatment, but that is often a limiting factor because of the typically advanced state of the disease by the time it is diagnosed.

Surgical resection of the entire cyst is the treatment of choice, and radical excision of the entire lesion that is localized to a liver lobe is often the only potential curative treatment.[210] Wide surgical margins are desired.[213] Unfortunately, complete excision is not always possible. Anthelmintic therapy is indicated after surgery, and long-term treatment is required if there was incomplete resection of the lesion(s).[226] Preoperative albendazole is sometimes used to reduce the risk of dissemination during surgery.[213]

If surgical resection is not possible, treatment with albendazole or mebendazole has been used with some clinical success, although this should be regarded more as parasitostatic than parasitocidal therapy.[210] Frequent monitoring is required, including PET scan and serological testing. Praziquantel has been evaluated, but animal model data indicate that it is much less effective against metacestodes compared with the other drugs.[226] Liver transplantation has been performed in some cases.[255,256] Regrowth of cysts or formation of distant cysts is a concern because of transplant-associated immunosuppressive therapy.[255]

Mortality rates are much higher than in hydatid cyst disease. Seventy percent mortality within 5 years and 94% within 10 years has been reported,[226] although screening to detect earlier infection can significantly reduce mortality.[226,257]

Prevention

The need for, and intensity of, preventive measures depend on the risk in the geographical region. There are two main aspects for prevention of pet-associated zoonotic infection: decreasing the prevalence of *Echinococcus* spp. in pets and decreasing human exposure to *Echinococcus* eggs.

Decreasing *Echinococcus* prevalence in pets involves decreasing exposure and anthelmintic treatment. Since pets can acquire infection by ingestion of wild animals, decreasing roaming and scavenging is important. Keeping animals indoors is most effective, although it is not completely preventive because of the potential for exposure to infected rodents in the household. Accordingly, concurrent rodent control should be used to help reduce exposure to *E. multilocularis*. If animals are allowed outdoors, they should be kept on a leash or in a fenced yard. Offal from sheep or other potential intermediate hosts should never be fed to pets to prevent exposure to *E. granulosus*.[242] Routine prophylaxis could be considered in areas where *Echinococcus* is endemic, particularly when there is reasonable likelihood of wildlife exposure. Deworming every 6 weeks has been shown to be effective in controlling *E. granulosus* in high-risk dogs,[258] and this has been used as a mandatory control measure in some endemic regions.[163] However, a study of rural dogs in Argentina, where such a program was in place, reported an 18% prevalence of cestode shedding, indicating issues with effectiveness of the program.[163] Whether this is due to inadequate treatment of dogs, continued access to infected animals or offal, or some other reason, is unknown. Clearly, focusing on deworming alone may not necessarily have the broad impact that could be expected. Monthly treatment with praziquantel has also been recommended in endemic areas when pets have a reasonable expectation of being exposed,[242] but the efficacy of this approach is unknown.

Decreasing human exposure to *Echinococcus* eggs in feces involves attention to hygiene, including prompt removal of pet feces and routine hand hygiene. Particular care should be taken by people that are in contact with soil in endemic areas with a high likelihood of contamination from foxes or dogs. When infected animals are treated, there is a window of time (~72 hours) where large numbers of eggs may be shed, necessitating extra attention to fecal handling and hygiene during the initial treatment period.[242]

Disinfection of the outdoor environment is impractical so environmental efforts should be directed at decreasing contamination by removing feces, controlling feral animal populations, and decreasing the prevalence of infection in pet dogs.

Multimodal approaches, including controlled slaughtering and meat inspection, as well as routine deworming of pet dogs, have been attributed with controlling human *Echinococcus* infection in some regions,[257] although the true impact of different components is unknown. Monthly baiting with anthelmintics has also been used with success to reduce infection of periurban foxes.[259] *Echinococcus* eradication programs have been successful in Iceland and New Zealand, and similar efforts are under way in other areas.[228]

Early diagnosis of alveolar cyst disease is important, considering the potential severity of disease and treatment difficulties. Active screening programs have been shown to be successful in the reduction of morbidity and mortality in endemic regions.[226]

Praziquantel treatment of imported dogs is mandatory in some *Echinococcus*-free countries.[222] This is to reduce the risk of exposure of people and infection of wildlife, something that could result in endemic infection, and the potential for imported dogs to establish the parasite in the wildlife population is the main concern.

Eucoleus aerophilus

Previously known (and sometimes still referred to) as *Capillaria aerophila*, *E. aerophilus* is a trichurid nematode of the lungs that has been called an emerging zoonotic pathogen,[260] although this designation is rather questionable. It can be found in dogs, cats, and wildlife (particularly foxes) in most, if not all, regions of the world.[260–268] Foxes are thought to be the main reservoirs.[264,269] Generally, low rates (<6%) are found in dogs and cats,[260,263] with higher rates in some wildlife populations.[265,267]

Adult lungworms live within the epithelium of the bronchioles, bronchi, and trachea.[260] Female worms lay eggs that are coughed up and swallowed, and subsequently passed in feces. Eggs are not immediately infective and require 30–45 days in the environment to pose a risk of infection. After ingestion by earthworms, eggs can develop into infective larval stages within the earthworm, although there is some debate as to whether earthworms are required for completion of the lifecycle. Infection of new hosts occurs through ingestion of embryonated eggs or earthworms.[260] Ingested eggs then hatch in the small intestine and larvae migrate to the lungs via the bloodstream.

Infections in dogs and cats are usually mild or subclinical. Coughing, sneezing, and nasal discharge may be observed.[260–262] Occasionally, severe infections can be encountered, including respiratory distress.[260] Diagnosis is based on the identification of eggs in feces or bronchoalveolar lavage fluid. Care must be taken to avoid misdiagnosis as *Trichuris*, since the eggs have a similar appearance, although *Trichuris* eggs are larger.[260] While there are no controlled studies, treatment with ivermectin or fenbendazole appear to be effective.[269]

While publications regarding this organism in dogs and cats have discussed zoonotic concerns, evidence is rather sparse. There are few reports of human infection. One described pulmonary capillariasis in a child in Iran that was *probably* caused by this parasite.[270] Another describes pulmonary disease that mimicked bronchial carcinoma.[271] In neither case was there adequate investigation of possible sources, and pet contact was not reported. Accordingly, there should be minimal concern about zoonotic transmission, particularly in households considering the 30- to 45-day period that is required for eggs to become infective. Proper litter box management should essentially negate the risk of exposure in the household as long as there is no fecal incontinence or long-term fecal staining of the hair coat. The risk of human exposure is presumably greatest from outdoor activities such as gardening that could result in contact with infective eggs from feces or earthworms, and hand hygiene is likely the most important preventive measure.

Fleas

Introduction

Flea infestation is the most common ectoparasitic infection in dogs and cats. The human health implications of flea infestation of pets can be highly variable. Often, no problems are encountered, or the main concern is the emotional response to the presence of fleas, rather than a true health impact. Yet, flea infestation of pets can have human health consequences, including skin irritation from flea bites to the less common but potentially serious transmission of zoonotic pathogens.

Etiology

Fleas are small, wingless insects that are 2–4 mm in length, with laterally compressed bodies. More than 2200 species and subspecies of fleas have been identified,[272] but only a small number infect dogs and cats on a regular basis. Despite the name, dogs are primarily infested with *Ctenocephalides felis* (cat flea).[272–275] *C. canis* can be found in wild and domestic canids but is not commonly found in pet dogs. Other fleas such as the *Pulex irritans* (human flea) and *Echidnophaga gallinacea* (poultry sticktight flea) can also infest dogs. *C. felis* is the predominant flea in cats, although other species like *P. irritans* and *E. gallinacea* may also be encountered. *P. irritans* primarily infests humans but can also infest a wide range of species, including cats, dogs, wild canids, and pigs. *E. gallinacea* is primarily found on poultry but may occasionally infest cats, dogs, and other species. *Pulex simulans* is mainly found on rodents but can also infest dogs, cats, and various mammals. Despite the vast number of flea species and subspecies, and the variety of fleas that can potentially infest dogs and cats, *C. felis* is the most important species in companion animals and their human contacts.

Life cycle

Adult fleas deposit eggs on the hair coat of the host or in the environment; however, eggs on the host quickly fall off and contaminate the environment.[50] Eggs are small (~0.5 mm), oval, and pearly white, and are not easy to identify.

Larvae hatch after 1–12 days,[50,272] depending on the temperature and humidity. Larvae feed on blood from flea feces, organic debris, and flea eggs that are present in their environment. Preferred environments are undisturbed, protected sites that are cool and shady. Larval development does not occur in areas exposed to direct sunlight, and larvae actively avoid light by burrowing deep into carpet fibers or under organic debris.[272] Larvae molt twice then develop into pupae in this protected environment. Moisture is essential for development, and larvae typically fail to develop if the relative humidity is less than 50%.[272]

With optimal environmental conditions (27°C and 80% humidity), adults begin to emerge from pupae in approximately 5 days, although pre-emerged adults may remain quiescent for weeks or months in the absence of suitable stimuli (carbon dioxide, heat, physical pressure) that indicate the presence of a host.[276] After emergence, adults locate hosts using visual and thermal cues, and need to find a host and feed within a few days. Under typical household conditions, this life cycle is completed in 3–8 weeks.[272]

Within 20–24 hours of initial feeding, the females will start to produce eggs, and a female flea may lay several hundred eggs over the course of her approximately 50–100 day life span.[50] Adult fleas can survive off the host for a short period of time. Data regarding survival off the host are somewhat conflicting with some sources indicating all will typically die within 1–2 weeks if a new host is not found and others stating that they can live for 2 months or longer off the host.[50]

Geographic distribution/epidemiology

Flea infestation is very common internationally, and *C. felis* can be found worldwide.[274] There can be a significant variation in the prevalence of fleas and risk of exposure between and within different regions. Fleas are much less common in regions where humidity tends to remain below 50%. In cold and temperate climates, fleas are most common in the summer and fall,[50] and no stage of the life cycle can survive more than 10 days at 3°C or 5 days at 1°C.[277] There is less seasonality in warmer climates, although infestations are still more common or severe in the summer and fall.[50,278] Studies of pet dogs and cats have reported infestation rates of 6.8–17% and 2.5–23%, respectively.[273,275,278,279] Rates of infestation tend to be highest in household pets that have outdoor access, in multipet households, and in households with cats.[273,275]

The environment is the main source of infection of animals.[272] Direct transmission of adult fleas from an infected host can also occur, but this likely accounts for a minority of cases. Animal–animal transmission can occur between pets in the same household, between pets from different households that have transient contact (i.e., parks, boarding kennels, veterinary clinics), between pets and stray animals, and between pets and wildlife. Both the environment and direct contact with infected animals are potential sources of exposure in

humans. The relative importance of each is unknown.

There are two main human health consequences that can arise from exposure to fleas on pets. One is transient or recurrent pruritis from flea bites. This is not a universal response to flea bites and only occurs in sensitized individuals in response to antigenic substances in flea saliva,[50] through type I and type IV hypersensitivity reactions.[50] The other potentially more serious but much less common problem is pathogen transmission. A variety of zoonotic pathogens can be transmitted to people via fleas from pets. These include *Bartonella* spp., *Rickettsia felis*, *Rickettsia typhi*, *Yersinia pestis*, and *D. caninum*.[58,280–282] More information about specific pathogens or diseases can be found in the appropriate sections of this book.

Animals

Clinical presentation

The most common problem with flea infestation is irritation and pruritis that develops as a result of fleas feeding on sensitized animals. This is flea bite allergy. It is rare in dogs and cats under 6 months of age, but beyond that, there are no age, gender, or breed predispositions.[50] The inflammatory response is characterized by pruritic, erythematous, nonfollicular, papular, crusting dermatitis. Clinical signs, when present, may range from simple, uncomplicated pruritis to severe pruritis with significant self-induced trauma from scratching or chewing, along with secondary infections (pyoderma). The severity of response tends to worsen as the animal ages, presumably from increased sensitization with repeated exposure. Moderate to severe peripheral lymphadenopathy may be present in cats.[50] Flea bite allergy is an important predisposing cause of pyoderma in dogs and should be considered in any dog with pyoderma of unknown origin, particularly recurrent infections. Flea bite dermatitis is a separate entity that involves local irritation in response to flea bites and does not necessarily involve an allergic component.[272]

Another potential complication that is largely restricted to young animals with significant flea burdens is anemia, including chronic iron deficiency anemia from blood loss to fleas. This can cause death in severely infested young animals.

Diagnosis

Diagnosis is based on the identification of fleas or flea feces ("flea dirt") on the hair coat of the animal. The hair coat should be closely examined. A flea comb may be helpful to identify fleas and flea dirt. Brushing the animal over a white towel or piece of paper may also be used, particularly in animals with dark hair coats and skin, since flea dirt and fleas may be more easily identifiable on the white surface. Flea dirt can be differentiated from other types of debris by moistening it with water, since true flea dirt will become red from the blood content.[50] Since fleas may spend time off the host, failure to identify adult fleas by no means rules out flea infestation, particularly in highly sensitive animals that may develop severe pruritis with minimal exposure. Finding flea dirt in the absence of adult fleas should be considered a presumptive diagnosis. Intradermal skin testing can be used to confirm flea bite hypersensitivity.[50]

Management

Control of fleas can be challenging. Elimination of fleas requires consideration of different factors: elimination of adult fleas from the animal, elimination of adult fleas from the environment, and prevention of reinfestation. The latter can consist of measures to reduce reexposure and/or routine prophylactic treatment to kill any fleas that are encountered.

Elimination of adult fleas

Various commercial products are available for elimination of adult fleas on dogs and cats (Table 1.1). All pets in the household should be treated at the same time if fleas are identified on any animal.[50,283]

It is important to remember that even if all adult fleas are killed instantly, there will be a period of weeks where new adults may continue to emerge from the environment. Immediate elimination of the problem is therefore impossible.

Table 1.1   Available options for flea treatment and prevention in dogs and cats.[272,287–293]

Drug	Species	Use	Route	Comments
Dinotefuran	Dog/cat	Monthly	Topical	Adulticide; spot on combined with pyriproxyfen for effects on eggs
Fipronil	Dog/cat	Monthly	Topical	Spot-on or spray application; may be combined with methoprene to prevent development of eggs
Imidacloprid	Dog/cat	Monthly	Topical	Adulticide; may have some effect on larvae; may be administered as often as weekly, if needed
Lufenuron	Dog/cat	See "Comments" column	Injectable (cat)	Oral: monthly
			Oral (dog, cat)	Injectable: before flea season then every 6 months
				Does not kill adults; prevents larval development in eggs from exposed females
Metaflumizone	Dog/cat	Monthly	Topical	Available alone for cats and combined with amitraz for dogs (tick control; amitraz has no effect on fleas)
Nitenpyram	Dog/cat	Daily or as needed	Oral	Short-acting adulticide; lasts 24 hours. Not used as a preventive.
Permethrin	Dog	Monthly	Topical	Effective against adults and eggs
Pyrethrins	Dogs/cats	As needed	Topical	
Selamectin	Dog/cat	Monthly	Topical	Kills adults and eggs
Spinosad	Dog	Monthly	Oral	Long-acting oral option

Products are effective against adult fleas unless otherwise noted.

Environmental treatment

Because the environment is an important source of infection, even after successful elimination of adult fleas on pets, environmental treatment may need to be considered in some situations. If there are minimal consequences of flea exposure (e.g., no flea allergy or significant effects on humans), focusing on eliminating adults that reach the pet and/or using medications to prevent successful reproduction may be adequate, and flea infestation of the household should be controlled over time if there is no ongoing external source. If a faster response is required, treatment of the household environment may be indicated.

Treatment of the outdoor environment is unlikely to be an important control measure and issues regarding safety and municipal restrictions on outdoor pesticide application must be considered. There is little indication for outdoor treatment in the control of flea infestation of pets. If this is to be considered, pest control specialists should be consulted.[272]

Prevention of reinfestation: reducing reexposure

Vacuuming of carpets, cushions, and other pet contact areas and washing of pets' bedding can be done to remove many (but not necessarily all) flea eggs and larvae.[272] Removal of pupae is more difficult because they tend to be located deep within the carpets or fabric. Frequent vacuuming may be important, since the physical vibration from vacuuming may stimulate emergence of adult fleas from cocoons and therefore make them accessible during subsequent cleanings.[272] Steam cleaning may help clean the deeper parts of the carpet pile.

Indoor environmental antiflea products (e.g., powders, sprays) may help eliminate certain flea life stages, but they must be used carefully to avoid toxic exposure to pets and children and are ineffective in the absence of proper treatment of the animals. The pupal stage is extremely resistant to pesticides and environmental extremes; therefore, physical removal of the cocoons (through vacuuming or laundering) is most effective, but repeated treatment/cleaning of the environment is required no matter what technique is used.

Restricting contact of pets with potentially infested animals is also important. Preventing roaming or other uncontrolled outdoor access should reduce the risk of acquiring fleas from infested domestic, feral, or wild animals.[272,283] Minimizing the need to board animals at kennels or other similar multiple-animal environments would also presumably help but may not be practical. Use of a kennel that routinely inspects incoming animals for flea infestation (and does not admit infested animals) would be preferred.

The outdoor environment may also be a source of exposure. The risk only involves shaded areas (e.g., under decks or porchs), so eliminating those when practical and reducing the ability of pets to encounter those areas should be considered.

Prevention of reinfestation: prophylactic treatment

A variety of different medications are available for killing adult fleas, either as routine treatment or in response to infestation (Table 1.1). Numerous topical options exist and many have residual activity through the presence of drug residues in the superficial layers of the skin. These can be highly effective, but the potential impact of excessive bathing or other water exposure (i.e., swimming) must be considered.[272] Periodic bathing or swimming should not be a problem, but excessive water exposure, especially if shampoo is used, could reduce efficacy.[272] Water exposure has no impact on the efficacy of orally administered medications, which are also widely available and effective. There is no standard recommendation for a flea control program, and factors such as the presence or absence of flea allergy in the pet(s), whether owners are concurrently affected, the ability of the owner to administer medications, and the potential for excessive bathing or swimming must be considered, as well as whether the program is being implemented for treatment of an existing problem or purely as a preventive measure. If there are significant consequences of flea infestation, such as flea allergy in a pet or bites in an owner, rapid-acting treatments to kill adult fleas along with a plan to address emerging adults from the environment must be developed. If prevention is the key, then approaches directed against either adults or development of immature stages can be considered. While permethrins have been used widely in the past, it is difficult to justify their continued use because of toxicity concerns (particularly in cats)[284,285] and the availability of other effective and safer options.

If routine monthly treatment is considered appropriate, then treatment should be started as soon as indicated by the label on the chosen product. Treatment should be continued throughout the at-risk period, which varies depending on the climate. Year-round treatment is required in some regions.

Alternative approaches such as administration of garlic, brewer's yeast, and thiamine have been tried, but there is currently no objective evidence of efficacy.[286]

Flea-allergic pets should be on a flea-prevention program, which includes prophylactic treatment throughout the at-risk period.

Humans

Clinical presentation

The severity of reaction to flea bites varies between individuals, and both flea bite allergy and flea bite dermatitis can occur. Some people may have no noticeable effects of flea bites, while others have severe hypersensitivity reactions.[50] In adults, there are usually fewer lesions, which often occur in groups of three,[50] sometimes referred to as "breakfast, lunch, and dinner." Extensive lesions are most common in children.[50] Most commonly, urticarial papules are present over the distal extremities, particularly the lower legs.[50,294,295] A hemorrhagic punctum may be present in the center of the lesion, and there may be secondary lesions from self-trauma or secondary bacterial infections.

Diagnosis

Fleas or flea dirt are rarely identified on a person, so diagnosis is made indirectly. Clinical signs and a history of flea infestation of pets or other potential exposure to flea-infested animals or environments provides a high index of suspicion.

Management

Elimination of flea exposure, through control of fleas on pets and in the household, and reduction of contact with potentially contaminated environments are the key aspects of treatment. Topical corticosteroids or oral antihistamines may be required for symptomatic control of pruritis.[50,294] Continuous or repeated exposure to fleas tends to result in desensitization over time.[50]

Prevention

Preventing transmission of fleas from animals to humans involves controlling fleas on pets. The intensity of flea prevention activities should depend on geographic and pet management factors, including the prevalence of fleas, the risk of exposure of the pet, the sensitivity of pets and people to flea bites, and the prevalence of flea-borne zoonotic diseases in the area. Because of marked variation in these factors between and within populations, a standard program applicable to all pets is not reasonable. Individual aspects of flea control in pets are discussed above.

Giardia spp.

Introduction

Giardia is an important cause of diarrhea in humans and animals, and a common cause of waterborne outbreaks in humans in some regions. The most common source of infection of humans is surface water contaminated by human feces (i.e., sewage), and there is very little evidence of direct transmission of *Giardia* infection from companion animals to humans or vice versa. Nonetheless, it is important to be aware of the potential risks of transmission, particularly for high-risk individuals.

Etiology

Giardia spp. are protozoan parasites that can be found in the intestinal tract of virtually all vertebrate species. There are at least 41 species of *Giardia*;[296] however, *Giardia intestinalis* (also known as *Giardia duodenalis* or *Giardia lamblia*) is the most common species involved in infection of wild and domestic animals, and the only species recognized as a cause of infection in humans.

An important aspect with respect to zoonotic disease risk is the *G. intestinalis* assemblage (type).

Table 1.2 Host range of the genetic assemblages of *Giardia intestinalis*.

G. intestinalis assemblage	Host range
A1	Humans, livestock, cats, dogs, beavers, guinea pigs, ferret
A2	Humans
B	Humans, beavers, dogs, chinchillas, rats
C	Dogs
D	Dogs
E	Cattle, goats, pigs, sheep, alpacas
F	Cats
G	Rats

There are various types with different host ranges, and many types are restricted to a single host (Table 1.2). Assemblages A1 and B are potentially zoonotic. Assemblage A2 appears to only infect humans, not animals, so there should be no risk of zoonotic transmission. The other assemblages infect different animal hosts but are of limited to no risk for zoonotic transmission.

Life cycle

Giardia exists in one of two forms: trophozoites or cysts (Figure 1.4). Trophozoites reside primarily in the proximal small intestine and are responsible for causing clinical disease. They have a characteristic appearance that is likened to a smiling face, formed by the appearance of their two nuclei, central axonemes, median bodies, and four pairs of flagellae.[296,297] Typically, as the trophozoites pass down the small intestine, they form a resistant cell wall, ultimately forming ovoid cysts approximately 10μm in length (somewhat smaller than the original trophozoite), which contain four nuclei. Cysts are passed in the feces and are immediately infective to the next susceptible host that ingests them. After ingestion, the organism excysts in the proximal small intestine, releasing two trophozoites that can attach to the mucosal surface but not invade the epithelium. The trophozoites then divide by binary fission, and the cycle continues. In diarrheic

individuals, the trophozoites can cause villous atrophy, crypt hyperplasia, and extensive invasion of the lamina propria by inflammatory cells within the small intestine.

Geographic distribution/epidemiology

Giardiasis is endemic worldwide, but the prevalence and incidence vary considerably between different populations and geographic locations. In industrialized countries, the prevalence of *Giardia* shedding in healthy people is estimated to be between 1% and 7%, and may be higher in some regions.[298–302] In general, all age groups are equally affected during epidemics, but both infection and clinical disease are more common in children in endemic areas.[303–305] Outbreaks occur regularly in childcare facilities.[99] The disease also tends to be seasonal, with the highest incidence over the summer and early fall, especially among hikers and campers.[303,305,306] Chronic disease is more common in people with humoral immunodeficiencies.[2]

Giardia can also be found in healthy and diarrheic animals of various species, particularly young animals. Shedding rates of 1.3–17% (typically ≤7%) have been reported in healthy dogs.[115,119,158,163,307–312] Rates can be higher (21–24%) in dog kennels and shelters.[311,313–315] Despite the fact that *Giardia* is considered an important canine and feline pathogen, no association has been found between diarrhea and the presence of *Giardia* cysts in feces because of the relatively common occurrence of the parasite in healthy animals.[306,315,316] The assemblage is an important consideration in assessing the potential for zoonotic transmission. Dog-specific assemblages C and D predominate in most canine studies;[312,314,317–320] however, zoonotic assemblage A1 can also be found and is occasionally the dominant strain.[321]

The prevalence in cats (5.9–14%)[155,312] is similar but perhaps somewhat lower than in dogs, and infections are also usually subclinical.[117,119,299,306] As in dogs, *Giardia* in cats is more common in high-density populations such as catteries,[306,322] as well as in kittens less than 6 months of age, multi-cat households, and in households that also contain dogs.[120] The feline-specific assemblage F is most common, but zoonotic strains can be found.[312,317,318,323]

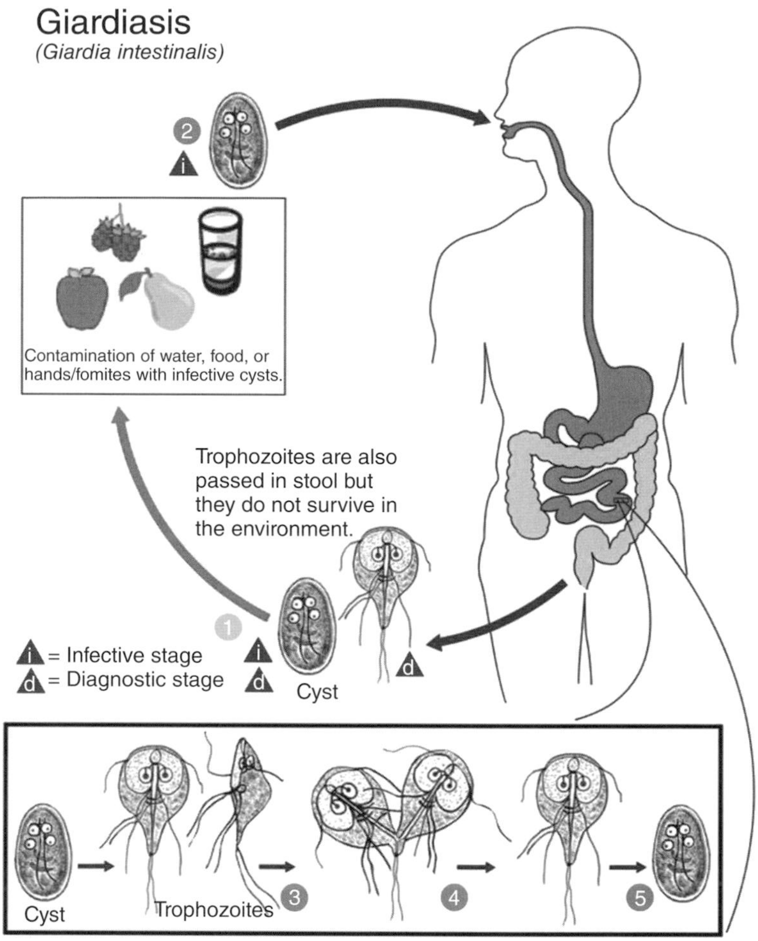

Figure 1.4 *Giardia intestinalis* life cycle (public domain, Centers for Disease Control and Prevention, Alexander J. da Silva, Melanie Moser).

The prevalence of *Giardia* spp. in pocket pets such as mice, rats, gerbils, hamsters, and guinea pigs is variable and typically low, but high rates are sometimes reported, such as the 22% shedding rate in hamsters in a report from China.[324] An important consideration in these animals is the *Giardia* species that is present. *Giardia muris* may be common in rodents, but it does not infect humans and care should be taken in interpreting studies that do not provide information about the *Giardia* spp. The prevalence of *G. intestinalis* is presumably low in these species and they likely represent minimal zoonotic risk, although the potential for transmission cannot be completely excluded since assemblages A1 and B have been found in species such as ferrets and chinchillas.[325]

Giardia is transmitted by ingestion of cysts of an appropriate species and assemblage. As few as 10 cysts can cause infection in a person,[99] while infected individuals may shed up to 900 million cysts per day.[304] Infection most commonly occurs in humans from contamination of drinking water or recreational water such as lakes, ponds, and inadequately treated swimming pools.[99] Hand-to-mouth transmission may occur, especially in child-care facilities. Contamination of food (i.e., vegetables irrigated with contaminated water or handled by infected persons) is also possible.[99,304]

There is currently little convincing evidence that household pets play an important role in human giardiasis. Contact with farm animals or pets was found to be a risk factor for giardiasis.[326] Isolation of the same assemblage of *Giardia* in children and stray dogs that lived in the vicinity has been reported,[327] but clear evidence of pet-to-human transmission is lacking.[296,297] The potential carriage of zoonotic assemblages by dogs and cats cannot be dismissed, however, and one should assume that there is some degree of risk.

Exposure to *Giardia* from canine feces in parks and other public areas has raised concern. The risk of dog–dog transmission may be high, but zoonotic risks are likely minimal. Even though *Giardia* can sometimes be found in canine feces in the environment, zoonotic assemblages are uncommon (0.6% of canine fecal samples in one study of urban green areas) and human exposure is probably rare.[319]

Less information is available regarding the route(s) of infection of animals, but it is reasonable to assume that environmental contamination with feces from infected animals is the main source. Outbreaks of disease can occur, particularly in kennels, but it is impossible to differentiate environmental sources of contamination from direct animal–animal transmission in outbreaks.

Animals

Clinical presentation

The prepatent period is approximately 8 days (range 5–12) in dogs and 10 days (range 5–16) in cats, but clinical signs may develop 1 or 2 days before the organism can be detected in the feces.[306] Infection is usually subclinical, and disease is most common in animals that are young, stressed, immunocompromised, or kept in high-density housing. Acute, intermittent, or chronic small bowel diarrhea may occur in both dogs and cats. Blood or melena should not be present. Fever, vomiting, or inappetance are uncommon, and if these are present, other causes should be considered, and additional diagnostic testing should be performed.

Diagnosis

Diagnosis can be difficult, and *Giardia* spp. have been called "one of the most commonly misdiagnosed, underdiagnosed and overdiagnosed parasites" in veterinary practice.[296] A combination of direct smear, fecal flotation with centrifugation,

and a sensitive and specific fecal ELISA optimized for use in the target animal species is recommended.[297]

Direct smear is mainly used to detect trophozoites. Trophozoites are rarely seen unless very fresh (<30 minutes) diarrheic feces are examined. A drop of fresh, warm feces mixed with a drop of warm (37°C) saline can be examined at 40× magnification for trophozoites exhibiting the characteristic "tumbling leaf" motion of *Giardia*. Care must be taken not to mistake yeasts, plant remnants, and debris as *Giardia*.[296] Lugol's iodine stain may be added to facilitate the identification of trophozoites.[297] In cats, trophozoites must be differentiated from those of *Tritrichomonas foetus*.

Fecal flotation using the zinc sulfate concentration technique (ZSCT) can be used to identify cysts in formed or diarrheic feces. The slides should be examined within 10 minutes or the characteristic internal structures of the cysts may no longer be apparent. *Giardia* cysts will stain with Lugol's iodine, which helps differentiate them from coccidian oocysts and sporocysts.

Immunoassays directed against *Giardia* antigen can be used. Species-specific validation is important, as one cannot assume that a test that performs well on feces from one species will perform similarly when used with feces from other animals.

Shedding of cysts is inconsistent, in terms of number and frequency; therefore, testing of multiple fecal samples may be necessary for diagnosis.[99] Testing of at least three fecal samples over 3–5 days may be optimal; three fecal flotation examinations on samples collected over a 2-week period identified approximately 94% of positive dogs in one investigation.[328]

Duodenal sampling via endoscopy is unnecessarily invasive for diagnosis of giardiasis in dogs, unless endoscopy is being performed for another reason. Duodenal sampling via the peroral string test is insensitive in dogs and carries the risk of intestinal foreign body obstruction.[329] This test has not been evaluated in cats.

PCR has also been used to detect *Giardia* in fecal samples from cats.[330] As with other molecular assays, test development, validation, and quality control affect the usefulness of the tests, and assays that have been specifically validated on feces from dogs and cats should be used.

Identification of the assemblage is important for the determination of the potential for zoonotic transmission. Unfortunately, different assemblages of *G. intestinalis* are morphologically similar and therefore cannot be differentiated microscopically. Molecular-based tests are required to determine the assemblage, and these are now offered by a limited number of veterinary diagnostic laboratories. *G. intestinalis* can be differentiated morphologically from *Giardia agilis* (found in amphibians) and *G. muris* (found in birds, rodents, and reptiles), which are not known to infect humans.[99,331,332]

Management

In most cases, infections are subclinical and treatment is not indicated in nondiarrheic animals, particularly those that are otherwise healthy and from a low-risk environment.[296,297] Treatment might be justifiable in situations where there is particular risk of transmission, although what defines those situations is unclear.

Treatment is usually recommended in diarrheic animals;[296] however, disease is typically self-limited and therefore may require only supportive therapy, which usually consists of oral or parenteral fluids to replace fluid volume lost due to diarrhea. Specific treatment is indicated in moderate to severe cases, or when the risk (or implications) of transmission to humans is high.

Metronidazole has been the mainstay of therapy for *Giardia* infections, in both humans and animals, but it is not universally effective, and there are potential problems with toxicity. Accordingly, fenbendazole is more commonly recommended.[296,297] Combination of fenbendazole and metronidazole can be considered, particularly in refractory cases; however, clear evidence of efficacy is lacking. Albendazole should be avoided because of toxicity concerns.[297,333]

Concurrent bathing of the animal to remove fecal debris and cysts is important and should be performed at the beginning and the end of the treatment period to reduce the risk of reinfection.[296,297]

Retesting of animals after treatment is not required. The aim of treatment is resolution of clinical disease, not necessarily eradication of *Giardia*. If *Giardia* were found in feces after the clinically successful treatment, further treatment would not be recommended, thereby negating any benefit of retesting.

Humans

Clinical presentation

Infection is usually asymptomatic. It has been estimated that of each 100 people that ingest *Giardia* cysts, 5–15 will pass cysts asymptomatically, 25–50 will develop acute diarrhea, and 30–70 will have no trace of infection.[299] When symptoms do occur, there is an incubation period of 1–4 weeks, followed by acute onset of watery (sometimes explosive) nonbloody, foul-smelling diarrhea; bloating; and abdominal pain, which usually lasts for 3–4 days.[2,99] In most individuals, the infection is self-limited; however, duration of diarrhea may be prolonged and chronic infections can develop.[299] Weight loss is common, and decreased growth in children and anemia can develop from anorexia and malabsorption.[2,299] Severe illness requiring hospitalization is most common in children less than 5 years of age, pregnant women, and the immunocompromised.[299]

Chronic disease may be accompanied by malaise, diffuse abdominal discomfort that is exacerbated by eating, greasy and foul-smelling stools, frequent and small-volume diarrhea, and weight loss.[299] Disease may wax and wane over several months.

Diagnosis

Fecal examination can be used for diagnosis in humans, but shedding of cysts may be inconsistent. Cysts may be identified by direct microscopic examination, microscopic examination using specific staining methods (i.e., trichrome direct fluorescent antibody assays), detection of antigen in stool by enzyme immunoassay (ELISA, fluorescent antibody test [FAT]), or by PCR.[2,334,335] Direct examination of stool has a moderately high (75–95%) sensitivity and is more sensitive in diarrheic individuals because of the larger numbers of excreted cysts.[2] Testing of multiple (three or more) samples can improve sensitivity.[2] Immunoassays have a high sensitivity and specificity and are most commonly used. Testing of duodenal contents obtained by direct aspiration or via the peroral string test can be effective, but because of the increased invasiveness, these are typically reserved for situations where giardiasis is suspected but fecal samples have yielded negative results.[2,331]

Management

When clinical disease occurs, it is usually self-limited, and supportive therapy alone may be adequate. When antimicrobial therapy is required, options include nitroimidazoles (metronidazole, tinidazole, ornidazole), nitazoxanide, paromomycin, and albendazole.[2,299] Metronidazole has a cure rate of 80–95%.[2] Tinidazole has a cure rate of 80–100% and may be preferable since single-dose therapy can be used.[2] Other options can be similarly effective and may be preferred in certain situations. Paromomycin is recommended for the treatment of pregnant women in their second and third trimesters.[2] Relapsing disease can be a problem, particularly in immunocompromised individuals.

Treatment of healthy *Giardia* carriers is not generally recommended but could be considered in high-risk households, such as those with people with immunocompromised individuals, especially humoral deficiencies.[2]

Prevention

Giardia can only be transmitted by ingestion of cysts from an infected animal or person, and then only if the species and strain of *Giardia* are compatible with the new host. Because zoonotic and nonzoonotic strains are difficult to differentiate, it is prudent to consider any *Giardia* infection of an animal as potentially transmissible to humans, until proven otherwise. Therefore, control of fecal contamination, both human and animal, is of primary importance. Hand hygiene is an important measure and should be performed after contact with an infected animal or its environment, or contact with feces. Animal feces should be collected and disposed of immediately to prevent environmental contamination with resistant cysts, especially in public areas like parks where other dogs and children may play. Pets should also be prevented from drinking from puddles, ponds, lakes, or other open water sources that may be contaminated with feces from other animals.

An animal with a confirmed or suspected infection should be kept separate from other animals and high-risk individuals including children or immunocompromised persons and sick or immunocompromised animals. Pet areas, particularly runs or kennels, should regularly be thoroughly cleaned to remove all visible fecal material and then disinfected, as discussed below. Bedding and blankets that become soiled with fecal material should be removed and washed.

A *Giardia* vaccine is available for dogs and cats but it has not been shown to prevent infection[336,337] and is not recommended by the American Animal Hospital Association or the American Association of Feline Practitioners vaccination guidelines.[338,339]

There is little indication to test pets after diagnosis of giardiasis in a person since pets are unlikely to be the source of infection. Further, identification of *Giardia* in the pet would not indicate whether the pet was the source of infection, whether the pet was infected by the person, or whether both were infected by the same source. If pets are to be investigated as the potential source of human infection, this is best reserved for situations with recurrent or chronic disease. Concurrent testing of the pet and person, with determination of the assemblage(s) involved, is critical to obtain any useful information.

There is no indication to treat clinically normal animals that are shedding *Giardia* considering the prevalence of *Giardia* shedding by healthy animals, the lack of evidence indicating that shedding predisposes to subsequent disease in the animal, the low risk of transmission of *Giardia* from a healthy pet to an owner (particularly if basic hygiene and infection control measures are used), and the lack of evidence of efficacy of treatment for eradication of shedding in healthy animals. It might be reasonable to consider treatment of healthy animals in very specific circumstances, namely in households where a particularly high-risk person is present and when the animal is known to be shedding a zoonotic assemblage.

Giardia cysts can survive for more than 8 weeks in cool water (8°C), or 4 weeks in warmer water (21°C), but they are killed by freezing, drying, direct sunlight, and certain disinfectants such as accelerated hydrogen peroxide, bleach (1:10 dilution of household bleach), or quaternary ammonium disinfectants.[99,306] Thorough cleaning to remove organic debris is critical for effective disinfection. Cysts may also be able to survive on an animal's hair coat for variable periods of time.[306]

Animals with diarrhea are especially likely to have trace fecal contamination of their coats, even if it is not visible to the naked eye. Therefore, hands should be washed thoroughly after handling any infected pet, even if there is no obvious evidence of fecal contamination.

Hookworms

Introduction

Hookworms are parasitic nematodes that live in the small intestine of their preferred hosts. Intestinal infections are often subclinical or mild in adult dogs and cats, but serious disease can occur in puppies and kittens with large worm burdens. Dog and cat hookworms are the main cause of cutaneous larva migrans in humans, a common condition in some regions that, while uncomfortable, is rarely serious. They can also cause other conditions such as eosinophilic pneumonitis, localized myositis, folliculitis, erythema multiforme, and eosinophilic enteritis in humans.[340]

Etiology

In dogs, *Ancylostoma caninum*, *Ancylostoma braziliense*, and *Uncinaria stenocephala* are the main hookworms, while *Ancylostoma tubaeforme*, *A. braziliense*, and *U. stenocephala* predominate in cats.[340,341] Other species may also be present in some regions, such as *Ancylostoma ceylanicum* in Australasia.[342,343] Infection with more than one hookworm species can occur.

Ancylostoma duodenale and *Necator americanus* are the human equivalents to the dog and cat hookworms. They inhabit the intestinal tract of humans and are not a zoonotic concern.

Life cycle

Adult hookworms live within the small intestine of their host and shed eggs in feces. Eggs are not immediately infective and must larvate, hatch, and develop into infective third-stage larvae before becoming a source of infection. This typically takes 2–9 days and depends on temperature and humidity. Infection occurs when a susceptible host encounters infective third-stage larvae, becomes infected by larvae penetrating the skin, or ingests a prey with infective larvae in its tissues.

Larvae that penetrate the skin migrate through the bloodstream to the lungs. They may then migrate up the respiratory tree and subsequently be coughed up and swallowed, or may migrate through other body tissues. Some may become dormant in tissues. Larvae that reach the small intestinal mucosa mature into adult worms. Some larvae may enter a state of arrested development and be subsequently reactivated after adult worms are removed. With some hookworm species (e.g., *A. caninum*), reactivation can also occur during pregnancy with subsequent transmammary infection. In others (e.g., *A. tuberforme*), young animals are often infected after birth from environmental contamination.[344] The ability of *A. caninum* to be transmitted through the transmammary route is a major factor in the high prevalence in puppies. Even if the mother is regularly dewormed, systemic infection is common, and exposure of young puppies should be assumed.

Larvae that are ingested may penetrate the oral cavity or gastrointestinal mucosa and migrate through tissues as described above, but most remain in the gastrointestinal tract and either mature to adults or enter an arrested state. Similarly, arrested larvae that are ingested from the tissue of prey typically remain in the gastrointestinal tract and mature into adult worms.

In the small intestine, adult worms may live for 4–24 months, attaching to the mucosa and ingesting blood. The worms may move to new attachment sites and leave behind small bleeding ulcers.

Geographic distribution/epidemiology

These parasites are most common in tropical and subtropical countries.[2] There are regional differences in the prevalence of different hookworm species, and *A. braziliense* and *U. stenocephala* have a much narrower range than the other important dog and cat hookworms. In general, *U. stenocephala* (sometimes called the northern hookworm) is found in cooler climates, such as in the northern United States, Canada, and Europe. *A. braziliense* is most common in tropical and subtropical regions such as the Caribbean and in warm coastal regions of the United States.

Hookworms are very common in dogs and cats in some regions, and rare in others. Climate, contact with feral animal populations, access to potentially contaminated environments, and prophylactic anthelmintic use can vary regionally and have profound impacts on the prevalence. Accordingly, reported prevalence rates vary dramatically between studies, ranging from 0.9% to 100% in dogs and 0.2% to 91% in cats.[7,120,158,313,341,342,345-349] In general terms, higher rates are found in tropical and subtropical regions and prevalence rates in cooler developed countries tend to be low. Reported risk factors for hookworm shedding in dogs include living in multi-dog households, being a stray or living in a shelter, age less than 1 year, sampling during hot and humid periods, and a history of no anthelmintic treatment.[158,342,350-352] Similarly, originating in a shelter and not having recent anthelmintic treatment are risk factors for cats.[353] Studies of animals on admission to veterinary hospitals, which are likely more representative of the average, cared-for pet population, typically report shedding rates of 0-4% in dogs and 0-0.5% in cats.[120,308,313,341,353-355]

Care must be taken when interpreting prevalence studies because of the vast differences in prevalence among regions and among different populations (i.e., pet vs. stray) within regions. Extrapolation of data to other regions and populations should be avoided.

Cutaneous larva migrans develops in humans when there is contact of bare skin with infective larvae from the environment. Infections are most common in young children and people that come into contact with soil or sand that might be contaminated with dog and cat feces. Environmental contamination with hookworm larvae can be found in parks and other public areas,[349,356-358] particularly in tropical regions with large feral animal populations.

There is significant variation in the types of disease caused by different species. *A. braziliense* is the most commonly implicated species.[193] In contrast, *A. tubaeforme* and *A. ceylanicum* do not appear to cause cutaneous larva migrans, but *A. ceylanicum* can mature to adults in humans and cause intestinal disease.[340] *A. caninum* can also occasion-

ally cause other conditions such as folliculitis, myositis, and eosinophilic enteritis.[340] The role of *U. stenocephala* in cutaneous larva migrans is unclear.[340]

In the United States, most autochthonous cases originate in the Southeast and Gulf Coast states.[2] In other regions where endogenous cases are rare, most infections are travel associated,[359] particularly in individuals that have spent time on beaches in tropical countries.[360-363] Outbreaks have also been associated with contaminated sandboxes.[361] Any other surfaces contaminated with dog or cat feces could also be a source of infection, such as the outbreak of cutaneous larva migrans associated with the material for dried floral arrangements.[364] Oral infection can also occur in humans, at least experimentally;[365] however, the role of this in natural zoonotic disease is not known.

Eosinophilic enteritis can occur uncommonly from the presence of adult hookworms in the intestinal tract. While the development of adult dog and cat hookworms in the human intestinal tract is rare, there are a few cases of this occurring in association with mild to severe eosinophilic enteritis.[340] There are also reports of identification of adult *A. ceylanicum* in humans.[340,366]

Animals

Clinical presentation

Severe disease is most common in puppies that have been infected through nursing shortly after birth because adult *A. caninum* are voracious feeders. Severe infections may result in anemia, ill thrift, poor weight gain, dehydration, and melena. Death can occur.

In adult dogs, overt signs of infection are uncommon, particularly in dogs that are otherwise healthy and well fed. Anemia, anorexia, weight loss, and weakness may develop in some cases, along with tarry diarrhea. This is more common in feral, stressed, and otherwise ill or malnourished dogs.

Clinical issues are similar in cats. Infections with *A. tubaeforme* tend to be most serious because, like *A. caninum*, it is a voracious feeder.[344] Anemia, weight loss, failure to thrive, diarrhea, and sudden death can occur, mainly in kittens. Infections with *A. braziliense* and *U. stenocephala* tend to be mild

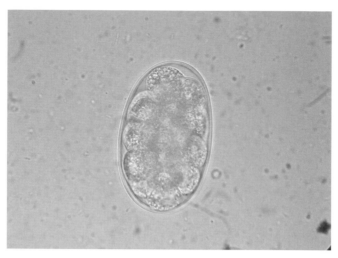

Figure 1.5   *Ancylostoma caninum* egg (public domain, photo credit: Joel Mills).

because they consume much less blood than *A. caninum* and *A. tubaeforme*.[344]

In some situations, cutaneous larva migrans can develop from hookworm larvae penetration of the skin, most commonly on the feet. Erythema, pruritis, and papular rash are common, and *A. braziliense* is usually involved.

Diagnosis

Hookworms are diagnosed by detection of their thin-shelled, morulated eggs in feces using fecal flotation (Figure 1.5). The prepatent period is 2–4 weeks, and worms begin feeding before eggs are passed in feces. With severe burdens in young puppies and kittens, severe disease or death can occur during the prepatent period.[344]

Morphological differentiation of hookworm species is difficult as there is overlap in the egg sizes between different species.[342] Only eggs of some *U. stenocephala* can be reliably distinguished because of their larger size.[340] More recently, molecular methods such as PCR-RFLP have been used for the detection and differentiation of hookworm species.[342,367]

Management

In dogs, fenbendazole, moxidectin, moxidectin/imidacloprid, milbemycin oxime, nitroscanate, and pyrantel pamoate are effective against adult *A. caninum*.[368–370] Moxidectin, pyrantel, fenbendazole,

nitroscanate, and moxidectin/imidacloprid are effective against adult *U. stenocephala*. Limited information about anthelmintic resistance is available, but high-level pyrantel resistance has been reported in *A. caninum*,[371] and monitoring fecal egg counts after deworming is an important means of detecting the emergence of resistance.

In cats, ivermectin, selamectin, moxidectin/imidacloprid, fenbendazole, milbemycin oxime, pyrantel pamoate, and emodepside are effective against adult *A. tubaeforme*, while emodepside and moxidectin are approved for the treatment of fourth-stage and adult *A. tubaeforme*. Fenbendazole is effective against *U. stenocephala*.

Deworming does not kill arrested larvae in tissues. Furthermore, dormant larvae present in the intestinal tract are resistant and can repopulate the intestine with adult worms after existing adults have been successfully eliminated with anthelmintics; therefore, repeated treatment may be necessary to eliminate infection. Detection of hookworm eggs in feces after deworming is most likely a result of this "larval leak" phenomenon, not anthelmintic resistance.

Humans

Clinical presentation

Zoonotic hookworms can cause cutaneous larva migrans. Initially, pruritic, reddish papules develop at the site of infection.[2] As larvae migrate, the characteristic "creeping eruption" develops, with intensely pruritic serpiginous tracks occurring along the path of migration. These may advance several millimeters to a few centimeters per day.[2] In severe infections, hundred of tracks may be present. The infection is ultimately self-limited, but the intense pruritis can lead to excoriation of the skin and secondary infection. In rare cases involving a large number of parasites, pneumonitis (Loeffler's syndrome) can develop, as can myositis.[2] Rarely, larvae can reach the intestine and cause eosinophilic enteritis.

Clinical signs cannot differentiate the hookworm species that is involved, although there are some general differences. *A. braziliense* tends to migrate more extensively in the skin than other hookworms.

Eosinophilic enteritis is an uncommon intestinal manifestation of zoonotic hookworm infection and is mainly associated with unusual situations where *A. ceylanicum* or *A. caninum* mature to adulthood in the human intestine.[340,372] This can produce inapparent infection to severe disease with abdominal pain to the point that exploratory laparotomy is undertaken;[372] however, the incidence of disease appears to be low, and severe disease is quite rare.

Diagnosis

Clinical presentation is usually adequate for diagnosis, especially if in an endemic area or in patients with a history of travel to an endemic area. Creeping eruption with severe pruritis is virtually pathognomonic.[2] Diagnostic tests such as skin biopsy are rarely indicated since clinical signs should suffice and biopsies rarely identify the migrating parasite.[193] In rare cases of pneumonitis, larvae can sometimes be identified in sputum and gastric fluid samples.[2]

Management

Cutaneous larva migrans is typically self-limited; however, several weeks to months may be required for clinical cure. Oral albendazole or ivermectin are most commonly used when treatment is elected and are highly effective.[2,193,363] Topical or oral thiabendazole is also effective.[193]

Prevention

Deworming is the critical component for disease prevention in puppies and kittens and will help decrease environmental contamination. Particular attention should be paid to deworming of puppies and kittens because of the greater likelihood of infection and the potential severity of disease. Puppies and kittens should be treated at 2, 4, 6, and 8 weeks of age.[283,344] New puppies or kittens that are first brought home should receive a minimum of three treatments, 2 weeks apart, then monthly treatment until 6 months of age.[283]

Recommendations for animals over 6 months of age are conflicting and include monthly,[344] once or twice a year,[361] or at least four times a year at intervals not exceeding 3 months.[368] Basing treatment recommendations for adult dogs and cats on fecal examination in low-risk households, with no regular prophylactic treatment has also been recommended.[283] The prevalence of hookworms in the area, management of the pet(s), risk of exposure of the pets, number of pets in the household, and whether there are high-risk humans in the household need to be considered when determining the appropriate strategy. There are concerns about the development of resistance, as has occurred in sheep and horses,[368] and concerns about resistance and prudent anthelmintic use need to be considered when designing deworming regimens.

Pregnant bitches should be treated during pregnancy to prevent transmammary infection, particularly if they have previously had a litter with a hookworm problem. Daily administration of fenbendazole from the fortieth day of gestation to the fourteenth day of lactation or two to four doses of ivermectin during the same time frame have been recommended.[344] A single dose of moxidectin on day 55 of pregnancy or a single dose of moxidectin–imidacloprid on day 56 of gestation was shown to be effective in small clinical trials.[368,373] Nursing animals should be treated concurrently with their offspring.[283]

Regular fecal examination is recommended to monitor worm burdens and efficacy of deworming. It has been recommended that fecal examination should be performed on puppies and kittens two to four times during the first year and one to two times annually thereafter.[344] Centrifugal flotation methods are recommended because of the higher sensitivity compared with other fecal examination methods.

There are currently no proven means for eliminating hookworm larvae in the environment, so decreasing fecal contamination of the environment and the likelihood that feces contain hookworm eggs are the key. Prompt removal and proper disposal of feces will assist in reducing the environmental burden of hookworms attributable to pets.

Regular (every day or two) cleaning of litter boxes will prevent infective third-stage larvae from developing. Preventing predation and scavenging will also reduce the risk of infection from ingestion of infected prey.

While important, measures directed at pet dogs and cats may only have a limited role in the successful prevention of cutaneous larva migrans because much of the environmental contamination, particularly in many tropical and subtropical regions, is from feral animals. If large feral dog and cat populations are present in an area and the prevalence of infection of those animals is high, environmental contamination will continue to be a risk.

Avoiding contact of bare skin with potentially contaminated soil or sand is the key preventive measure, although that can be difficult. Keeping dogs and cats off beaches could be an effective measure but is difficult to achieve, particularly in tropical regions with large feral dog populations. People should avoid contact with potentially contaminated soil, such as through wearing shoes and/or gloves. Similarly, wearing footwear on beaches could reduce the risk of exposure. Sandboxes should be covered when not in use to prevent cats from defecating in them.

Leishmania spp.

Introduction

Leishmaniasis is a wide-ranging spectrum of diseases caused by protozoal parasites of the *Leishmania* genus. There are various *Leishmania* species that can cause human infections, each with different geographic ranges and reservoir hosts. The primary reservoirs are sylvatic mammals such as rodents and wild canids, but pet dogs can be involved. Dogs are the primary reservoir for zoonotic infections in some regions and may also act as a link between sylvatic and domestic cycles of leishmaniasis.[374] Humans are typically accidental hosts but might be reservoir hosts for some species.

The clinical presentation of leishmaniasis can be highly variable, and this variability probably relates to factors such as the individual parasite's invasiveness, tropism, and inherent pathogenicity, plus host factors such as the cell-mediated immune response. Visceral, cutaneous, and mucocutaneous leishmaniasis are the most common forms, and the same *Leishmania* species may cause multiple syndromes. Dogs are most relevant in the transmission of visceral leishmaniasis.

Etiology

Leishmania species are intracellular protozoal parasites. The *Leishmania* genus is divided into two subgenera: *Leishmania* and *Viannia*. Various *Leishmania* species are known to cause disease in humans and animals,[375] but the main companion animal risk comes from *Leishmania infantum* in dogs. *Leishmania chagasi*, the agent implicated in visceral leishmaniasis in South America, is now considered to be the same organism as *L. infantum* based on genetic analyses. *Leishmania braziliensis* and *Leishmania peruviana* can cause cutaneous leishmaniasis in humans and dogs.[376] Less is known about the role of dogs in the transmission of these species, but there is increasing information suggesting dogs may play a role in the transmission of *L. braziliensis*.[377] Dogs are thought to be the reservoir for *L. peruviana*; however, this pathogen is only currently of relevance in the Peruvian Andes.[377] Numerous other *Leishmania* species exist, and pets can sometimes become infected; however, their role as reservoirs of these *Leishmania* species is probably negligible.[377] *Leishmania* spp. can be found in rodents in different regions, but the role of pet rodents in zoonotic disease transmission in unclear.

Life cycle

Leishmania reside in mammalian macrophages as amastigotes. Transmission is via female sand flies

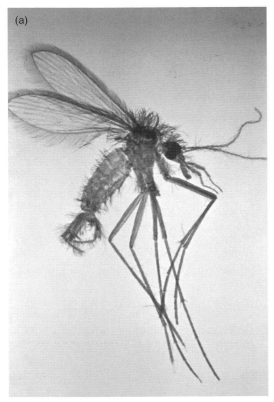

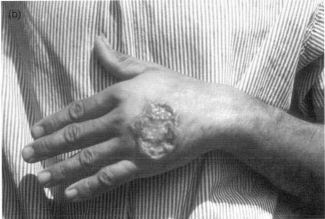

Figure 1.6   (a) *Phlebotomus* species sand fly (public domain, Centers for Disease Control and Prevention). (b) Cutaneous leishmaniasis (public domain, Centers for Disease Control and Prevention, Dr. D.S. Martin).

of the *Lutzomyia* genus in the Americas and *Phlebotomus* genus elsewhere (Figure 1.6a).[375] After a sand fly bites an infected host and acquires *Leishmania*, the parasites develop into extracellular promastigotes in the sand fly gut within approximately 1 week.[375] The transmission cycle is completed when the infected sand fly feeds on another susceptible host, as promastigotes are phagocytosed by macrophages, convert to amastigotes, and multiply. Reservoir hosts may be infected for years, if not lifelong.[378]

Rarely, infection of humans or dogs can occur through other routes such as congenital infection, transfusion of contaminated blood products, needlestick injury, or sharing contaminated needles.[379–384] The potential for dog fleas to transmit *L. infantum* through dogs ingesting infected fleas has been investigated, but it is equivocal whether there is a real risk.[385]

Geographic distribution/epidemiology

Leishmaniasis is an important human health issue in some regions. An estimated 12 million people are affected worldwide,[375] with the vast majority of cases occurring in eastern India and Bangladesh, Sudan, and Brazil.[386,387] The range of the infection depends on both the presence of *Leishmania* in a reservoir population and the presence of the sand fly vector. Dog-associated leishmaniasis is primarily associated with *L. infantum*, which is endemic in the Mediterranean, Middle East, and certain areas of the New World, particularly in Latin America.[375,388] It was previously a problem in southern China but is now rare.[389] Most human *L. infantum* infections occur as sporadic cases in rural areas, but outbreaks can occur and can involve urban and suburban areas.[375] Clustering of cases can occur in households. There are concerns that the range could expand if the insect vector range expands as a result of climate change.[390]

The prevalence of anti-*Leishmania* antibodies in dogs is variable in endemic regions. Rates of 1–81% have been reported in areas of Brazil, Colombia, Italy, Spain, Portugal, and Turkey.[391–398] There is an age-related component; however, different studies have identified different at-risk age groups.[391,392,396] The prevalence of infection has been steadily increasing in some regions, particularly in Europe,[399,400] and leishmaniasis may be an emerging problem in some areas.

The epidemiology of leishmaniasis is different in some regions such as the United States and Canada, where the disease can be found in some populations of animals, but autochthonous vector-borne cases are not recognized.[374] Infected animals belong to two groups: dogs that have been infected while visiting endemic regions[401] and endemic leishmaniasis in select dog breeds that is maintained without vector-borne transmission.[374,402–407] The latter group is the most important and has largely involved foxhounds,[402,405,408] within which leishmaniasis is endemic in at least 18 U.S. states and 2 Canadian provinces.[402] Both dog-to-dog and vertical transmission are suspected.[374,402] Dog-to-dog transmission could include transmission from bites, breeding, or reuse of needles.[402] Vertical transmission is likely as well since transplacental infection has been demonstrated experimentally.[409] There may be some degree of genetic predisposition among, and within, the foxhound breed.[374] Other breeds, particularly breeds that originated in southern Europe like corsicas, Italian spinones, and Neapolitan mastiffs may be similarly overrepresented.[374]

Less information is available regarding cats, although the disease has been recognized in cats for almost 100 years.[410] Cutaneous and visceral leishmaniasis can occur, but cutaneous disease appears to predominate.[376,411] Limited prevalence data are available, but seroprevalence or parasitemia rates of 0.6–59% have been reported.[412–416]

Leishmaniasis is a very important human disease in some regions, where it is the most commonly detected zoonotic disease.[417] Visceral leishmaniasis is mainly caused by *L. infantum* and *Leishmania donovani*, although other species can be involved.[375] Visceral leishmaniasis has traditionally been considered a disease of children; however, adults

with HIV/AIDS, as well as those receiving cytostatic or immunosuppressive therapy are also at increased risk.[418–420] While those groups are at higher risk of infection, disease can occur in anyone.

Dogs are important reservoirs of *L. infantum* but play little to no role in the transmission of other species that cause visceral disease. Dogs are not considered important reservoirs for cutaneous leishmaniasis since they are not natural hosts for the main species that are involved (*Leishmania major*, *Leishmania tropica*, or *Leishmania aethiopica*), except for *L. peruviana*, which is associated with localized ulcerative cutaneous disease in the Peruvian Andes.[377] Transmission of infection from dogs to humans via sand flies is the primary route of transmission of *L. infantum*, but conflicting data are available regarding the risks posed by pet dogs, and there are probably regional differences in risk based on the prevalence of zoonotic *Leishmania* spp. in dogs, the prevalence of vectors, dog density, and dog management (e.g., closeness of contact with humans, time spent outdoors). Village dog density and dog ownership have been identified as risk factors for visceral disease.[421,422] A significant association between the risk of human cutaneous leishmaniasis and the prevalence of corresponding disease in dogs was reported in Peru.[423] Daily contact with animals (but not necessarily dogs) was a risk factor for human disease in an Italian study.[424] Control of leishmaniasis in dogs can decrease human infection rates, providing further evidence of a role of dogs in human infection.[425] Other modes of dog–human transmission have not been proven, such as transmission through contact with infected canine blood or bites. Evidence of a role for cats in human infection is limited.

Animals

Clinical presentation

Only a small percentage of infected animals develop clinical disease.[377,392,397] When disease does occur, the visceral form is most common.

Visceral leishmaniasis
Depression, weight loss (particularly decreased muscle mass over the shoulders, hips, and spine), abdominal distension, splenomegaly, generalized

lymphadenopathy, joint distension, and renal failure are common.[374,402] Vomiting, diarrhea, and melena are less common. Fever may be present but is only identified in approximately one-third of cases.[374] Concurrent cutaneous lesions, including nonpruritic alopecia, hyperkeratosis, epidermal scaling and thickening, and depigmentation may be present.[374]

Cutaneous leishmaniasis

Cutaneous leishmaniasis is most commonly reported in South America, where it causes sporadic disease in dogs and cats, with chronic ulcerative skin lesions, particularly on the ears, mucocutaneous erosions, and lymphadenopathy.[376] Discrete cutaneous nodules may also be present on the skin, particularly in cats.

Diagnosis

Visceral leishmaniasis

Diagnosis is difficult because of limitations in available tests and the fact that only a small percentage of infected animals develop disease. Anemia, thrombocytopenia, hyperproteinemia with hypergammaglobulinemia, hypoalbuminemia, and evidence of renal failure are suggestive in endemic regions but certainly not diagnostic.[374] Elevations in hepatic enzymes may also be noted but are similarly nonspecific. Serological testing is the main component of diagnosis but is complicated by the potentially high baseline seroprevalence in dogs in some endemic areas. Positive serological testing seems to correlate better with disease in foxhounds in the United States than in dogs in endemic areas.[374] Immunofluorescent assay (IFA) testing is more often used in nonendemic areas and is a useful screening test, but it can cross-react with other pathogens like *Trypanosoma cruzi*.[374] A highly specific kinetic ELISA and a K39 antigen-based assay are available in some areas. Quantitative PCR has the potential to be a more sensitive test. Cytological detection or culture of amastigotes in tissues or fluid (i.e., joint fluid) are also diagnostic.[402]

Cutaneous leishmaniasis

Microscopic detection of *Leishmania* in skin lesions is diagnostic, as is culture of the parasite or detection of *Leishmania* DNA in biopsy samples by PCR.

These are more rewarding in cats since dogs tend to have low numbers of parasites in skin. PCR detection of the parasite in blood and bone marrow is possible since hematogenous dissemination is common.[376] Serological testing is suggestive but can be problematic to interpret in areas with a high baseline seroprevalence.

Management

Treatment can be difficult, and dogs seem to respond poorly compared with humans. While treatment can improve clinical signs or produce short- or long-term remission, it is seldom curative.[374] Disease may be advanced by the time leishmaniasis is considered or diagnosed, and the prognosis in emaciated, chronically affected animals is very poor.[374] If treatment is elected, the main goal is clinical improvement, not microbiological cure, and relapse is a common problem. Furthermore, the inability to completely eliminate the parasite means that these animals may pose a risk for further transmission.[374]

There are a limited number of drugs that may be efficacious, and information regarding optimal treatment regimens is limited. Allopurinol has been recommended as the first-choice treatment because it is relatively efficacious and nontoxic.[374] It may be used alone or in combination with pentavalent antimonials such as sodium stibogluconate or meglutamine antimoniate.[374] These may be of limited availability, and sodium stibogluconate, in particular, can be highly toxic. Liposomal or lipid emulsion amphotericin B may also be used, although these are not thought to be superior to allopurinol and are more toxic.[374] Miltefosine and paromomycin have not been adequately studied in dogs. Relapses are common, regardless of the drug(s) used, and may occur months to a year or more after an apparently successful therapy, so regular monitoring is required.

Recently, immunotherapy with a saponin-enriched commercial vaccine was shown to reduce or eliminate clinical signs and latent infection.[426] This may be a critical tool for the management of clinical disease and reducing the zoonotic implications in treated animals. Other aspects of therapy depend on the clinical condition of the animal and may include nutritional support or management of renal disease.

Humans

Clinical presentation

Visceral leishmaniasis

Occasionally, a small papule is noticed at the site of inoculation, but this is not typical.[375] The incubation period is prolonged, typically 3–8 months, although it can be as short as 10 days or longer than a year.[375] It is possible for infection to occur years earlier, only to be expressed when the individual becomes immunocompromised.

The clinical presentation can be highly variable, ranging from inapparent, self-limited infection to classical visceral leishmaniasis with fever, anorexia, weight loss, hepatosplenomegaly, and hyperpigmentation.[375] Onset may be insidious or rapid. Fever may be remittent, intermittent, or, less commonly, continuous, and may mimic malaria.[375] Abdominal enlargement may be present because of massive splenic and hepatic enlargement.

Immunocompromised individuals, such as those with HIV/AIDS or neoplasia, or on immunosuppressive therapy, are at increased risk of developing disseminated visceral disease. In severe cases, death can occur from secondary infections, malnutrition, severe anemia, or hemorrhage.[375]

Cutaneous leishmaniasis

Simple cutaneous leishmaniasis, the typical presentation of infections by dog-associated species, involves the presence of one or more crusting, dry lesions, with occasional large, deep ulcers (Figure 1.6b).[375] They can be found on any part of the body, but are most common at sites of exposed skin. Cutaneous leishmaniasis rarely develops into visceral disease.[2]

Diagnosis

Visceral leishmaniasis

Presumptive diagnosis is often made in endemic areas based on the presence of prolonged fever, weight loss, marked splenomegaly, hepatomegaly, along with normocytic/normochromic anemia, leukopenia, thrombocytopenia, and hypergammaglobulinemia.[375] Demonstration of amastigotes in tissue or isolation of promastigotes in culture is diagnostic. Splenic aspirates are the highest yield material for testing,[2,375] but testing can also be

performed on bone marrow or lymph node aspirates. Liver aspirates are lower in yield. Amastigotes can sometimes be identified or isolated from buffy coat samples or whole blood. Serological testing can be performed, but while sensitive, there may be a lack of specificity from cross-reaction with other organisms.[375] False-negative serological results may be obtained from immunocompromised patients. Leishmanin (Montenegro) skin testing is not useful diagnostically as it is usually negative in people with visceral leishmaniasis, although they typically become positive after spontaneous resolution of infection or successful treatment.[375]

Cutaneous leishmaniasis

Diagnosis of cutaneous leishmaniasis is often presumptive in endemic regions based on the characteristic clinical signs. Definitive diagnosis involves detection of amastigotes in tissue using Wright–Giemsa staining of tissue biopsies or, less commonly, using monoclonal antibodies or molecular methods.[375] Isolation of promastigotes using tissue culture is also diagnostic. Amastigotes may also be seen occasionally on skin scrapings from affected areas. Serological testing is not very useful since antibodies are detected in a minority of infected individuals, and cross-reacting antibodies may be present.[375]

Management

Visceral leishmaniasis

While disease is often self-limited, treatment is indicated in patients diagnosed with visceral leishmaniasis.[2] Liposomal amphotericin B is the drug of choice,[2,375] but cost and availability may be limiting factors in some countries. Conventional amphotericin B is another option. Sodium stibogluconate can be highly effective but carries risks of toxicity, particularly cardiotoxicity.[2] It is avoided in South Asia because of the high prevalence of antimonial resistance, and miltefosine is now widely used in India.[2,375] Supportive therapy may also be required, including nutritional support and treatment of secondary infections.

Cutaneous leishmaniasis

Treatment of cutaneous disease should be considered in all cases, particularly when there is the potential for disfiguring or debilitating injury (i.e., facial lesions, lesions near joints).[2]

Prevention

There are four main approaches to reducing the risk of *Leishmania* transmission: reducing the insect vector, reducing insect bites, reservoir control, and immunoprophylaxis.

Sand flies are weak fliers and tend to stay close to their breeding sites, so elimination of breeding sites in close proximity to humans and susceptible animals is a potential control measure. However, breeding sites are usually difficult to identify, so this is not a highly effective approach.

Bite avoidance includes basic practices (Table 1.3),[2,427] but complete avoidance is difficult to impossible.

The use of insecticides on dogs to repel and kill sand flies has been an effective approach and is important in endemic areas. Deltamethrin- and permethrin-impregnated dog collars can reduce sand fly biting[428–431] and consequently seroconversion in people and dogs.[422,431–433] Collars can provide protection for up to 34 weeks, making them a practical control method.[428,430] Long-acting topical insecticides may also be effective, as application of a deltamethrin-based emulsifiable concentrate had excellent short-term and residual activity, and appears to be suitable for administration every 5–6 months.[434]

Dog culling has also been used to reduce the reservoir population in endemic regions; however, this has been met with little success for various reasons such as the high prevalence of infection (particularly in dogs without clinical signs of disease); the infectiousness of the agent; high replacement rates from migrating strays; high birth rates; test limitations; and time delays between diagnosis and culling.[435,436] A recent report did identify an association between the reduction of human visceral disease and canine euthanasia rates.[437] However, based on the conflicting data and other potential (and more effective) control approaches, it is hard to justify an extreme approach like mass culling.

While transmission through contact with dog blood has not been demonstrated, the fact that this parasite can be transmitted human–human through shared needles indicates that it should be considered a possibility. Accordingly, particular care should be taken by veterinary personnel to avoid needlestick injuries. Direct contact with blood, especially contact with mucous membranes or broken skin, should also be avoided.

A canine vaccine is available in Brazil for the prevention of visceral leishmaniasis.[393,438] Canine vaccination has also been shown to reduce the incidence of human infection[425] and may be a critical control measure.

Recommendations have been developed for infected dogs (predominantly foxhounds) in the United States, including reducing exchange of hounds, segregating infected animals, and banning infected dogs from dog shows or hunts.[402] However, these seem to have been followed only for a short period of time, largely based on the perception that the disease is associated with low illness and death rates and that there are minimal risks to humans.[402] In the absence of more aggressive measures, basic practices such as breeding only known seronegative dogs should be considered.[402]

Euthanasia of infected dogs has been recommended,[402] and in some jurisdictions, positive dogs must be euthanized, treated, or kept under sand fly-proof netting.[399] The aggressive approach to positive dogs in nonendemic regions is designed to reduce the risk of establishment of the disease in the area. This is perhaps most justifiable if sand fly vectors are present in the area, given the low risk of transmission through other means. While euthanasia is a reasonable consideration, the impact of this on overall animal and public health is unclear, and recent evidence of the potential efficacy of vaccination for elimination of *Leishmania*[393]

Table 1.3 Sand fly bite avoidance practices.

Screen windows and doors

Wear long-sleeved clothing and long pants

Avoid areas of sand fly activity, especially at dusk and dawn

Using insect repellent containing DEET or picaridin

Spray clothing with permethrin-containing insecticides

Spray infested living spaces with insecticides

Use a bed net soaked in permethrin when sleeping in nonscreened areas may decrease the pressure and need for automatic euthanasia of infected animals.

Notoedres cati

N. cati is the cause of notoedric mange, a disease that occurs worldwide and often occurs in periodic regional outbreaks. It is most commonly found in domestic cats and has been called the feline counterpart to *Sarcoptes scabiei* in dogs.[439] It can also be found in other felid species such as tigers, cheetahs, leopards, ocelots, and panthers, as well as hamsters, squirrels, civets, raccoons, coatis, and hedgehogs.[440–449] Rarely, it can infect dogs.[450] *N. cati* var. *cuniculi* can be found in rabbits.[451] Transmission is by direct contact with an infected individual.

Adult mites burrow deep within the dermis, where females lay eggs. After hatching, larvae crawl to the surface of the skin, then dig their own burrows to molt. After molting, the first nymphal stage creates a new, superficial burrow where it molts again, at which point the second-stage nymph digs yet another burrow to develop into an adult.

Lesions tend to develop first around the margins of the ears. They are intensely pruritic, and infected animals may have bloody crusts and hair loss from self-mutilation.[452] Weight loss and debilitation may develop in severe cases, particularly when treatment is delayed.

Diagnosis is based on the identification of mites on skin scrapings. Adult mites are almost round and 200–240 μm in diameter (smaller than *S. scabiei*). Mites may also be identified in feces because of ingestion during grooming.

Often, people living with infected cats will develop papular lesions and rashes, usually over the arms and legs.[439] In one study, 63% of human contacts of cats with *N. cati* infection had symptoms of notoedric scabies, with *N. cati* recovered from 50% of skin specimens.[439] Symptoms can develop within hours of contact with an infected cat. Lesions differ from classical scabies since they lack detectable mite burrows and occur over variable sites, including the face.[439] While intensely pruritic and a nuisance, infections are transient and self-limited, typically resolving within 2–3 weeks if contact with infected cats is prevented.[439] Lesions subside when cats are segregated from people.[439] The risk posed by other *Notoedres* species is not known.

Prompt diagnosis and treatment of infected cats with a macrocyclic lactone (ivermectin, moxidectin, doramectin, selamectin) or fipronil is important for both animal welfare and reduction of zoonotic transmission. Restricting contact with infected animals during the initial treatment period may reduce the risk of transmission, but the period of infectivity after treatment has not been described. Keeping cats indoors will reduce the risk of exposure. If cats may have been, or are at risk of being, exposed, prophylactic treatment with selamectin or fipronil may be indicated.

Ornithonyssus bacoti

O. bacoti, the tropical rat mite, is a hematophagous mite that can be found on a variety of wild and captive small mammals and birds worldwide.[453,454] The "tropical" designation is misleading as the mite can be found throughout the world. Pet rodents can be infected, from inapparent to pruritic with excoriation.[453,454] *O. bacoti* will bite humans, resulting in dermatitis.[455] The mite is also the intermediate host for the filarial nematode *Litomosoides carinii*, which can potentially act as a vector of murine typhus, Q fever, Chagas' disease, and Coxsackie virus; however, it is thought that this is of minimal relevance for natural transmission of infection.[454]

Diagnosis is based on the identification of mites on the animal or in its environment.[453] Identification of the mite may be difficult. Unfed mites are gray-white and often very active, while fed mites are darker, red-brown, and sluggish.[453]

Human infections can occur from direct or indirect contact with wild and pet rodents. Cases have been reported in laboratory animal and veterinary personnel, as well as people living or working in rodent-infested areas.[455–460] There are also reports of transmission from pet rodents.[453,454,461,462] In one case report, transmission of *O. bacoti* from a pet hamster was suspected based on the development of infection after contact with the animal.[461] In another, bites developed on members of a family after their pet hamster had been boarded at a pet store.[454] *O. bacoti* mites were identified on the hamster, but there was a concurrent flea infestation in the house so the cause of the skin lesions could not be definitively attributed to *O. bacoti*. In another household, three children developed skin lesions and marked pruritis after contact with infected gerbils, although mites were not observed on the children.[453] As with most animal-associated mites, infestation of humans is expected to be transient and self-limited. Elimination of infestation of the pets is the main component of management of human infections. Topical corticosteroid application may be useful to relieve itching.[453]

While a zoonotic pathogen, the risks associated with *O. bacoti* are limited. Pet rodent contact should be queried in individuals with nonspecific dermatitis, and a veterinarian should examine the animals if it is felt that there is a possibility of zoonotic mite transmission. The animal's environment should also be closely examined since mites are more likely to be found in the environment than on the host itself.[453] New pet rodents should be closely examined for the presence of mites or skin lesions. Rodents with skin lesions (or housed with rodents with skin lesion) should not be purchased. Pet rodents should not be allowed to have contact with wild rodents. Selamectin has been used successfully for the treatment of rodents,[453] along with thorough cleaning and disinfection of cages and other potentially contaminated sites.[453]

Otodectes cynotis

O. cynotis is an ear mite that is commonly found in cats and dogs, along with other species worldwide.[49] It accounts for over 80% of cases of otitis externa in cats and 50% in dogs.[49] Infections are commonly found in strays, shelters and breeding populations,[49,463,464] and in young (3–6 months of age) animals.[465] Transmission is from direct contact with infected animals, including subclinical carriers.

Adult mites typically live deep within the ear canal, where they cause local inflammation and irritation by piercing the skin surface and feeding.[49] This leads to accumulation of dark cerumen, dried blood, and mite feces within the external ear canal.

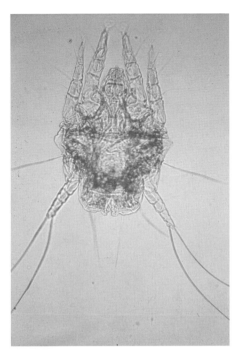

Figure 1.7   Adult *Otodectes cynotis* (public domain, photo credit: Joel Mills, GNU free documentation license).

Affected animals are pruritic and may shake their head or scratch at their ears. Violent scratching and head shaking may lead to further inflammation, excoriations, erythema, and aural hematoma. Uncommonly, lesions may be present on other parts of the body with severe infestations.

The typical "coffee grounds" appearance of the aural exudate provides a high index of suspicion. Mites may be identified directly in the ear canal with an otoscope or via cytological examination of ear swabs (Figure 1.7).

Treatment of *Otodectes* infestation involves cleaning the ear canal and administering parasiticidal drugs. Long-acting compounds or repeated administration is required to kill new mites from hatching eggs and mites acquired from the environment. Milbemycin and ivermectin may be applied directly into the ear canal in cats and dogs.[466] Otic application of fipronil was also reportedly effective in a small study of dogs and cats.[467] Topical selamectin or imidacloprid/moxidectin have also been shown to be efficacious in dogs and cats.[468–471] If multiple pets are in the household, all should be treated concurrently.[49] Grooming equipment and bedding should be discarded or disinfected.[49] Under experimental conditions, mites can survive off the host for 15–17 days at 10°C and 5–6 days at 34°C, while under natural conditions survival should not exceed 12 days.[472] Therefore, new animals should be restricted from entering potentially contaminated areas for 12 days if environmental disinfection is not possible.[472]

O. cynotis is not host specific and can infect humans,[58] although this appears to be rare. This can include ear infestation or more widespread disease including one report of intensely pruritic excoriated papules that began on the torso and spread over the extremities.[473–475] In another report, a child whose two cats had severe O. cynotis infestation developed numerous pruritic papules over the abdomen, and the lesions resolved shortly after the cats were successfully treated.[475] These reports are all somewhat circumstantial, being based on lack of another identifiable cause of the human infection and concurrent diagnosis of O. cynotis infestation in the person's pet. There is one report of identification of O. cynotis from a person with tinnitus.[476] The most convincing evidence of the potential for zoonotic transmission comes from one enterprising veterinarian who, after seeing two suspected cases of O. cynotis infestation in owners of infested pets, intentionally infected himself with an O. cynotis mite from a cat.[475] Intense pruritis developed and persisted for almost a month, but resolved without treatment, leaving behind an ear full of exudate. Rather astoundingly, this person reinfected himself two more times to confirm the findings and to determine whether immunity developed, with milder disease reproduced each time. Clearly, O. cynotis from animals can infect humans and cause self-limited disease.

The risk of zoonotic transmission is quite low given the rarity of reports of human infection and commonness of infection in pets. Good household hygiene practices, particularly hand washing after contact with the ears of infected animals, should reduce any risks. Potentially contaminated fomites (i.e., bedding) should be laundered and dried using high heat in a clothes dryer, and hands should be washed after handling laundry. If human infestation is identified or suspected, treatment of the infested animal is likely to result in clinical resolution of human disease.

Sarcoptes scabiei

Introduction

S. scabiei is a burrowing mite that can cause intensely pruritic skin disease, particularly in dogs, foxes, coyotes, and humans. Infestations of humans and dogs are caused by different varieties of S. scabiei; however, cross-infection can occur.

Etiology

While there is only one species, S. scabiei, mites found on dogs are often referred to as S. scabiei var. canis,[49] while those naturally found on humans are called S. scabiei var. hominis. These designations are more physiological than morphological or genetic, but there is evidence of some degree of genetic variation between S. scabiei var. canis and S. scabiei var. hominis.[477] This genetic variation is best illustrated by a study that showed that mites recovered from people from Australia and North America were more closely related to each other than mites from dogs and humans in the same region (or even in the same household).[477] While this supports strong host adaptation, determination of cross-species infection potential of an individual mite is not straightforward because there are typically few or no morphological differences, and genotyping is not readily available. Further, there is ample evidence that S. scabiei var. canis can infect humans, although disease is usually relatively mild and self-limited.

Life cycle

After exposure, mites burrow into the epidermis where they trigger an intensely pruritic dermatitis, caused by type I and type IV hypersensitivity reaction to the parasite. Female mites lay eggs in the walls of the burrows. Six-legged larvae hatch and molt to become first- and second-stage nymphs, then adults. Adults feed on damaged skin and tissues.[49] After mating, the males die while females migrate to a suitable body site for burrowing. This entire life cycle can be completed in approximately 30 days.

Geographic distribution/epidemiology

S. scabiei can be found worldwide. The prevalence is higher in wild and feral animal populations, with rates of 7–19% being reported for studies of stray dogs.[463,478] Pet dogs that interact with stray animals are presumably at higher risk of infection. Transmission of host-adapted mites to other species can occur but infestations tend to be mild and self-limited.[49] Cats are rarely infected.[479]

Human scabies

Human scabies is endemic in many countries and affects people of all socioeconomic levels,[2] although poverty, poor hygiene, overcrowding, malnutrition, and sexual promiscuity increase the risk of infection.[480] It is a reemerging disease in some areas, particularly in immunocompromised individuals.[481] Transmission is from direct (including sexual) contact with an infected individual or from indirect transmission from the environment or fomites.[480] Mites can live off the host for up to 21 days.[482] Outbreaks of human scabies have been reported in various facilities, particularly schools, hospitals, and nursing homes. These seldom involve animals. Repeated infections tend to be milder than primary infections.[2]

In areas where scabies is endemic in humans, most human cases are from close contact with infected people.[477] Zoonotic transmission is of greater relevance where human scabies is rare, since there is a greater likelihood of having contact with an infected animal (especially a puppy) than an infected person.[483,484] Multiple household members may be infected.[483] A skin rash is usually noted within 24–96 hours of contact with an infected dog.[485] Canine scabies mites can live on humans for up to 6 days and produce ova.[58]

Determination of the role of animals in human disease is not necessarily straightforward. In areas where scabies is rare in humans and an affected individual has had contact with a dog diagnosed with scabies, it is likely that the pet was the source. However, if scabies is endemic in both humans and dogs in an area, determination of the source of infection is difficult since human and canine scabies may be maintained in separate transmission cycles.[477]

Animals

Clinical presentation

Lesions are usually first noted in thinly haired areas such as the ear margins, elbows, stifles, feet, and ventrum.[49,58,486] The ears are almost always involved.[49] Intense pruritis is normal, and infected animals will scratch and chew incessantly, with rapid development of secondary traumatic lesions and alopecia. Papular eruptions may be noted. With time, hair loss along with thickening and hyperpigmentation of the skin will develop.[58] Lesions often spread rapidly and, in severe cases, can cover the entire body.

Diagnosis

Despite the often dramatic nature of the disease, diagnosis can be a challenge. Few mites may be present at the time of examination and only small numbers are required to produce intense disease. Mite burrows may be identified in the skin using magnification. Skin scrapings are more commonly used for diagnosis. Scrapings should be obtained from the edges of the lesion, not excoriated, hyperkeratotic, or otherwise chronically and severely affected areas.[49] Deep scrapings that allow for the examination of the full thickness of the epidermis are required. If blood-tinged scrapings are not obtained, it is likely that the sample is not deep enough. Scrapings are suspended in mineral oil or microscope immersion oil. Multiple (up to 10) scrapings should be evaluated. Adult mites are approximately 0.5 mm long, with a morphology as depicted in Figure 1.8. Eggs, which are approximately 230 μm long, may also be seen.

Failure to identify mites, even with multiple properly collected deep scrapings, does not rule out disease because of the small number of mites that may be present.[49] Consistent clinical signs with no other apparent cause are suggestive of scabies, and response to treatment supports the presumptive diagnosis.

A serum ELISA has been evaluated in dogs;[487] however, it is questionable if it has a useful role in diagnosis. It might be useful in cases where mites cannot be observed on scrapings.[486] The "pinnal–pedal" reflex, hind leg scratching in response to

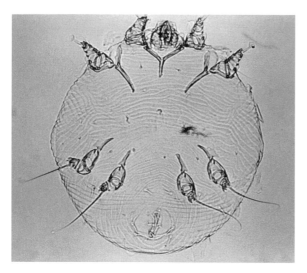

Figure 1.8 *Sarcoptes scabiei*, 350–450 μm (public domain, Centers for Disease Control and Prevention, no specific provider information).

vigorous rubbing of the ear, is used by some as a presumptive diagnosis; however, its positive predictive value is poor (0.57).[488] It is truly just an indicator of ear pruritis, a common sign in scabies, and its main possible role might be to rule out scabies since the negative predictive value is high (0.98).[488]

Management

The coat should be clipped and an antiseborrheic shampoo should be used to remove crusts.[49] Lime sulfur dip, while effective, is not often used because of the foul odor and the potential to stain light-colored hair coats.[467] Amitraz bathing, weekly or every 2 weeks, is another option;[489] however, it should not be used in Chihuahuas, pregnant or nursing bitches, and in puppies less than 3 months of age.[467] Application of 0.25% fipronil as a spray has been used effectively, though this approach may be best with early disease or in patients where other products are contraindicated.[467] Topical or systemic selamectin, ivermectin, milbemycin oxime, moxidectin, and moxidectin/imidacloprid can also be used.[470,486,490–493] Regional availability and label indications affect the options that are available.

Humans

Clinical presentation

Scabies is characterized by an intensely pruritic papular eruption. In adults and older children, the interdigital folds, flexor aspects of the wrists, extensor surfaces of the elbows, anterior axillary folds, waistline, thighs, navel, genitalia, abdomen (especially periumbilical region), intergluteal cleft, and buttocks are most commonly infected.[2,480] In younger children, vesicular lesions are more common and tend to appear on the scalp, face, neck, palms, and soles.[2] Itching is most intense at night, and excoriations are common from scratching. As is the case with dogs, humans will usually only be infected with 10–15 mites.

Scabies may have a different clinical picture in immunocompromised patients, particularly individuals with HIV/AIDS, and the elderly. In those individuals, widespread or localized hyperkeratotic or crusted plaques may be present.[494,495] As opposed to classical scabies, lesions are often non-pruritic because of the altered immune response.[495] This is often termed "Norwegian scabies," and it is highly contagious because of the massive numbers of mites that are usually present.[496] Nosocomial transmission to patients and healthcare workers with subsequent infection of family members can occur, at times causing relatively large outbreaks.[495,497–499]

It is impossible to differentiate zoonotic from human-associated scabies clinically, although *S. scabiei* var. *canis* tends to cause milder and self-limited disease and burrows should not be present.[480,500] Zoonotic scabies lesions are more common on exposed skin areas that have direct contact with the pet, and lesions may be more extensive in people with close, prolonged contact with the pet or when diagnosis of the pet is delayed.[58]

Diagnosis

Definitive diagnosis is based on the identification of mites, mite eggs, or mite feces from skin scrapings. Scrapings should be collected from papules or intact burrows.[2] Scabietic burrows are gray or white tortuous lines, though these can be difficult to identify and may be destroyed by scratching.[2] Burrows are not present in people with *S. scabiei* var. *canis* infestation.[500] Scrapings should be collected and evaluated as described above for animals. Skin scrapings are often negative,[485] so clinical signs and exclusion of other likely causes may be required for presumptive diagnosis. Mite morphology cannot be used to distinguish between human and canine origin *S. scabiei*.[477]

Management

Adults and older children should be treated over the entire body below the head with a scabicide in the form of a lotion or cream.[2] The head and neck should also be treated in younger children. Care should be taken to cover the entire body, including under the fingernails.[2] Five percent permethrin is most commonly used, although it is not approved for children less than 2 months of age.[2] Oral ivermectin and 10% crotamiton cream or lotion are other options. Crotamiton is not approved for use in children, and treatment failures may be common.[2] Oral ivermectin is recommended for treatment of Norwegian scabies[501,502] and is a good option for refractory cases or when topical therapy is not possible.[2] Lindane should not be used because of safety concerns and the availability of other effective options.[2]

All household members should be treated concurrently to prevent cycling of infection. Clothing and bedding should be washed in hot water and dried in a clothes dryer under high heat.

Even with successful elimination of the mites, itching may continue for weeks because of the hypersensitivity reaction.[2] Antihistamines or topical corticosteroids may help decrease itching during this period. If secondary infections of excoriated skin have developed, antimicrobial therapy may be indicated.

In situations where an infected animal is known or highly suspected as being the source, treatment of the animal (and any other in-contact animals) is adequate. Treatment of affected persons is not required because disease will subside naturally.[500]

Prevention

While there are certainly differences in the ability of different *S. scabiei* to infect multiple hosts, it is not possible to differentiate "zoonotic" from "nonzoonotic" types, so infected animals should be managed on the assumption that they can infect humans. When there is endemic or epidemic human scabies in a region that does not appear to be linked to an animal reservoir, control efforts should be directed against human-to-human transmission, not a potential zoonotic source.[477,503] When exposure to infected animals is known or considered likely, measures to reduce the risk of further zoonotic transmission are indicated.

Owners of dogs with sarcoptic mange should restrict contact with the animals until they have been treated. The duration of infectivity after treatment has been started is not known, but animals probably become noninfectious within a few days of treatment. In the interim, attention should be paid to reducing contact with infected dogs, avoiding direct skin-to-dog contact and not permitting the dog to sleep on beds or furniture. As mites can live off the host for a period of time, bedding and other potentially contaminated items should be laundered and dried in a clothes dryer. Steam cleaning of carpets and furniture should help reduce or eliminate mites, though it is unclear whether this is really necessary. Grooming equipment should be disinfected or discarded. All dogs in contact with infected dogs should be treated concurrently.[49,467] Treatment of potentially exposed cats is not required.

Prophylactic treatment of exposed immunocompetent individuals is generally not indicated; however, it is reasonable to consider prophylactic therapy in certain high-risk individuals, particularly those with low CD4+ counts since the likelihood of Norwegian scabies increases as CD4+ count declines.[495]

Routine preventive therapy for *S. scabiei* is not indicated, though routine administration of selamectin or moxidectin/imidacloprid for other purposes will help prevent infection.[504] Efforts should be directed to decreasing the likelihood of exposure, including preventing pet dogs from coming into contact with feral animals or wildlife, prompt treatment of infected animals, quarantine of facilities with ongoing outbreaks, and isolation of infected animals.

Strongyloides stercoralis

Introduction

S. stercoralis is a nematode that is sometimes referred to as the human threadworm. While humans are the principal hosts, dogs and nonhuman primates can also be infected and act as reservoirs for human infection.[2] Cats are rarely infected. As opposed to other causes of larva migrans, *S. stercoralis* can be present in infectious form in fresh feces, something that increases the potential for zoonotic transmission. It is also unique in its ability to complete its entire life cycle in humans. *S. stercoralis* tends to cause inapparent to mild infection in immunocompetent individuals and is of greatest clinical significance as a potential cause of overwhelming infection in immunocompromised persons, especially those on high-dose corticosteroids.[1]

Life cycle

Adult female worms are approximately 2.2 mm in length and reside embedded in the mucosa of the small intestine, where they release eggs. These eggs hatch in the small intestine and become first-stage (rhabditiform) larvae. Most of these noninfectious larvae are subsequently passed in feces, but a small percentage molt to the infective (filariform) stage in the intestinal tract and penetrate the intestinal mucosa or perianal skin, thereby completing the life cycle within a single host. This potential for autoinfection allows for long-term or persistent infection in some individuals.

First-stage larvae that are passed in feces molt in the environment to the filariform stage (Figure 1.9).

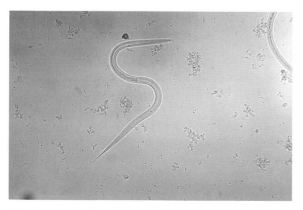

Figure 1.9 Filariform (L3) stage of *Strongyloides stercoralis* (public domain, Centers for Disease Control and Prevention, Dr. Mae Melvin).

Infection can then result from penetration of the skin by these infective larvae in soil. After the penetration of the skin, larvae migrate to the lungs and ascend the tracheobronchial tree. After being swallowed, they mature to adults within the gastrointestinal tract and continue the life cycle. Rarely, infection can occur following ingestion of filariform larvae from inadvertent ingestion of feces. Rarely, in immunocompromised individuals, larvae may migrate throughout the body, including the CNS.

Geographic distribution/epidemiology

There is a sporadic geographic distribution, with *S. stercoralis* being more common in tropical and subtropical regions. Endemic foci can be present in some temperate countries. Highest rates of infection in humans are found in parts of Southeast Asia, Latin America, and the Caribbean. Rates of fecal shedding tend to be low (<3%) in endemic areas[8,9,505–507] but can be very high in some groups, such as alcoholics and people with HIV/AIDS.[508,509] All ages can be affected, but disease is more common in children.

There are numerous reports of *S. stercoralis* in the feces of dogs, most from tropical and subtropical regions, with reported prevalences of larvae in feces ranging from 0% to 1.8%.[6,313,510–513] Infections are more common in young animals, particularly puppies in pet stores and breeding kennels,[313,510,514] because of close mixing of young puppies and greater environmental contamination. It can be a cause of chronic disease in kennels.[515] It is possible that *S. stercoralis* is underdiagnosed because of infrequent and low-level shedding of larvae and the infrequent use of techniques that would detect larvae.[515] Cats are rarely infected, and some studies have failed to find *S. stercoralis*;[516,517] however, there is a report of infection of 18% of stray cats in Qatar.[518]

Human infections usually result from the penetration of infective larvae through the skin, after contact with soil contaminated with human feces. Direct contact with feces containing infectious larvae and fecal–oral infection can also occur. Person-to-person transmission can occur in certain situations, such as day care, mental institutions, and among men that have sex with men.[1,519]

Infections in dogs presumably develop in a similar manner; however, transmammary infection may also be important. The likelihood of transmammary infection depends on the time of the dam's infection. Infection of puppies is almost certain if the dam is infected with L3 larvae during lactation.[520] Unlike *Strongyloides* infections in many other species, there is no hypobiotic state in tissue, and transmammary infection of puppies will only occur during acute infection of the dam.[521]

The role of dogs in human disease is presumed to be minimal. Direct evidence of zoonotic transmission from companion animals is limited. There is a report of *S. stercoralis* infection in a dog colony worker and dogs that he worked with.[522] There is also some evidence that people who work with dogs, such as dog breeding kennel personnel, may be at higher risk of exposure. The seroprevalence in one study of kennel workers in Brazil was 27%,[510] which was higher than the expected community rate, although care must be taken in interpreting results since there was no direct comparison with a control group, and seroprevalence data indicate exposure, not necessarily disease.

Animals

Clinical presentation

Infection is usually inapparent and clinical disease is largely confined to breeding kennels, shelters, and pet stores. Diarrhea, pneumonia, dermatitis, and weight loss can develop but are usually mild in immunocompetent adult dogs.[313] Clinical signs occur most commonly in young dogs. Disseminated disease can occur in immunocompromised dogs and in puppies.[523,524] Disease in cats is rare.

Diagnosis

Diagnosis is based on the detection of larvae in feces. Fecal flotation or Baermann methods are used, but flotation methods are not recommended because of low sensitivity.[510] Zinc sulfate fecal flotation or formalin-ethyl acetate sedimentation techniques can be used to identify larvae.[313] Specimens should be examined promptly because hyperosmotic solutions may make larvae shrink and difficult to detect. Serological testing has been used because of the low recovery rates of other methods, though interpretation of results may be difficult because of the high seroprevalence rates in some groups and the potential that positive results simply indicate historical exposure.

Management

Ivermectin, fenbendazole, or thiabendazole is effective.[521,523] These drugs will not kill migrating larvae. Otherwise healthy dogs are unlikely to have many migrating larvae in their body at any time, but relapse is possible and retreatment may be necessary.[521] Feces should be examined 2–3 weeks after treatment, then monthly for 6 months, to ensure that there is no persistent infection resulting from migrating larvae that escaped initial treatment. All dogs in the household or kennel should be treated concurrently.

Humans

Clinical presentation

Most infections are asymptomatic.[2] Clinical disease, when present, can be the result of cutaneous invasion or systemic migration. Disease in immunocompetent individuals most commonly starts as a localized, pruritic, and erythematous rash at the site of larval penetration. Serpiginous tracks (larva currens) that advance as fast at 10 cm/hour can be observed. After several days, transient pneumonitis can develop as larvae migrate to the lungs. Overt respiratory disease is rare in people without underlying pulmonary disease.[1] Several weeks later, diarrhea and other signs of abdominal disease may develop.[1,2,522] Signs often mimic peptic ulcer pain.[1] Rarely, heavy infestations can result in bowel obstruction from the associated intestinal inflammation. With chronic disease, recurrent larval migration can result in pruritis around the anus, perineum, buttocks, and upper thighs. There may also be intermittent eosinophilia and/or meningitis.

Hyperinfection syndrome occurs as a result of "accelerated autoinfection" from filariform larvae.[1] This is a rare but potentially devastating syndrome that can occur in immunocompromised individuals, particularly people with HIV/AIDS, tuberculosis, neoplasia, and solid organ or stem cell transplantation, as well as people on immuno-suppressive therapy and alcoholics.[509,510,525–527] The most significant risk factor for developing *Strongyloides* hyperinfection syndrome is treatment with high-dose corticosteroids. Hyperinfected individuals have large numbers of *S. stercoralis* in the lungs and intestinal tract, and throughout the body, particularly in the CNS, kidneys, and liver.[1] Wide-ranging and often severe clinical signs may be present. Extensive migration of parasites through the intestinal mucosa can result in translocation of intestinal bacteria, particularly gram-negative organisms, with the potential for sepsis, meningitis, or other sequelae of bacteremia.

Diagnosis

Definitive diagnosis involves detection of *S. stercoralis* larvae in feces by direct smear or culture on agar plates.[1,2] Diagnosis can be difficult because of the typically low worm burden and infrequent excretion of larvae, and at least three serial stool samples should be evaluated.[1,2] Larvae are similar to hookworm larvae but have a shorter buccal cavity. Eggs are rarely, if ever, identified in feces. Collection of duodenal contents by the string test or through endoscopic aspiration may also be used for the detection of larvae. Real-time PCR of feces offers twice the sensitivity of Baermann testing[528] but is not yet available as a routine diagnostic test.

Serological testing is sensitive but nonspecific because of possible cross-reaction with other helminths.[2] Eosinophilia is common and *S. stercoralis* should be considered in all instances of unexplained eosinophilia. Identification of larva currens is considered pathognomonic. Disseminated disease may be diagnosed by the detection of *S. stercoralis* larvae in sputum, bronchoalveolar lavage fluid, or CSF.

Management

Ivermectin is the drug of choice.[1,2,529,530] Albendazole and thiabendazole may also be used but are associated with lower efficacy or poor drug tolerance, respectively.[1,2,529] Prolonged or repeated treatment may be required, particularly with disseminated disease. The prognosis is good in immunocompetent individuals but poor in people with dissemi-

nated disease. Even with appropriate treatment, mortality may exceed 25% in disseminated disease, with rates of 80–100% mortality in untreated individuals.[1]

Prevention

Human feces are the main source of infection, so measures aimed at avoiding environmental contamination with human feces and reducing the risk of contact with contaminated sites are the keys for prevention. Serological testing has been recommended in people in endemic areas that are immunosuppressed or starting immunosuppressive therapy, followed by either fecal examination of seropositive individuals and treatment of people shedding *S. stercoralis* or simply treatment of all seropositive people.[1,531]

Overall, the risk of dog–human transmission of *S. stercoralis* is low, and it is probably only a reasonable consideration in certain tropical or subtropical regions or in people who work closely with young puppies and have a high likelihood of contact with feces (e.g., kennel workers, pet store personnel). Measures to reduce the risk of exposure to *S. stercoralis* from dogs involve basic concepts of avoiding fecal exposure. Particular care should be taken with puppies from breeding kennels or pet stores. Factors such as prompt removal of feces, avoiding direct contact with feces during removal, avoiding contamination of surfaces when handling feces, prompt hand hygiene after handling feces or having contact with a dog with fecal staining of the coat, and proper cleaning of fecal accidents are key points. Because infective larvae can be passed in feces, some degree of risk is present with fresh feces, not just feces that have been in the environment for prolonged periods of time.

Taenia spp.

Introduction

Infections with *Taenia* species tapeworms are a significant risk to humans in some regions. They are typically associated with cattle and pigs, and, more specifically, ingestion of undercooked beef and pork. Human infections with *Taenia* species that infect dogs and cats are rare, and pets play a very minor role in human infection.

Etiology

The most relevant human pathogens are *Taenia saginata*, the beef tapeworm, and *Taenia solium*, the pork tapeworm. Pets are not involved in the transmission of these species. Dogs can occasionally act as intermediate hosts for *T. solium*[532,533] but are not definitive hosts, and therefore do not develop patent intestinal infections and shed eggs.

A variety of *Taenia* species can be found in dogs, including *Taenia crassiceps*, *Taenia hydatigena*, *Taenia multiceps*, *Taenia pisiformis*, and *Taenia serialis*. *Taenia taeniaeformis* is found in cats. Of these, *T. multiceps* is of the greatest relevance in humans.[534]

Life cycle

As with other cyclophyllidean tapeworms, *Taenia* spp. have a life cycle involving definitive and intermediate hosts. Definitive hosts are carnivorous/omnivorous species such as dogs, coyotes, foxes, and humans. Intermediate hosts are species such as cattle, sheep, pigs, hares, rabbits, and various rodents.[534] Humans can be accidental intermediate hosts of many *Taenia* spp.

Adult *Taenia* can be very large, ranging from tens to hundreds of centimeters in length, depending on the species.[535] They live in the small intestine of the definitive host, and gravid proglottids (segments) or eggs are shed in feces. Eggs are released when proglottids are damaged during intestinal passage or in feces as the proglottid degenerates. Eggs are immediately infective and hatch after ingestion by a suitable intermediate host, including humans. Hexacanth embryos then penetrate the intestinal wall and migrate to different sites, such as the liver, skeletal muscle, or heart.[535] There, they mature into second-stage larvae, which are infective to definitive hosts when they ingest infected tissues. Intermediate structures (e.g., coenurus for *T. multiceps*) can develop in tissues, containing the intermediate stage of the parasite. Whether or not disease develops depends on the size and location of the structure.

Geographic distribution/epidemiology

Taenia spp. are commonly found in dogs and cats in some regions, most often in warm climates and in feral populations. In dogs, *Taenia* spp. shedding rates of 1.1–45% in feral and shelter dogs, and 0–4% in household pets may be present.[157,159–161,165,230,235,349,536–541] Shedding rates of 9.1–76% have been reported in studies of *T. taeniaeformis* in stray cats, with lower rates (0–3.5%) reported in household pets.[157,162,235,345,536,542–545]

Human infections with *Taenia* species found in pets are rare. The main concern regarding pet-associated disease is cystic infection caused by *T. multiceps*, *T. crassiceps*, and *T. serialis* from dogs,[213] which can involve formation of unilocular cysts in the CNS, eye, subcutaneous tissues, or within the muscle.[534,546–549]

Disease is rare in humans and is most common in African and South American countries.[550] Only a small number of cases have been reported in North America. Dogs presumably play a minor role in human disease. "Significant" prior exposure to dogs was reported in all six infected people in one report;[534] however, it is uncertain whether that truly represents a causal association in any or all of the cases.

Human infections with *T. taeniaeformis* are exceedingly rare. A larval cyst was identified as an incidental finding in the liver of an elderly man.[551] Adult *T. taeniaeformis* worms were apparently identified in the vomitus of a child in Sri Lanka, although the authors were unclear whether the child may have vomited on a spot on the floor where the child's pet cat had deposited the worms, whether the child may have ingested live worms because of the poor level of hygiene, or whether it was a true infection.[552] If it was a true intestinal infection, however, the source would not have been the cat, since the child would most likely have been infected by ingestion of cysts from an infected intermediate host.

The role of pets in human disease is poorly defined and presumably minimal. The authors are unaware of any studies that have made an objective link between pet ownership or contact and human *Taenia* spp. infection, although the potential certainly exists. The primary concern with intestinal *Taenia* spp. infection in pets is the fact that it cannot be differentiated from infection with

Echinococcus spp. (which is a much more significant zoonotic concern) based on clinical signs or fecal examination.

Systemic *Taenia* infections have been reported in dogs, cats, and rabbits.[553–559] These pose no direct risk to humans, although they indicate that humans could be exposed to the same source as the pet (i.e., undercooked meat).

Animals

Clinical presentation

Disease is rare. Typically, infected animals have no apparent clinical signs. Sometimes, perianal irritation can occur as a result of the passage of proglottids. This may cause "scooting" or chewing at the anus.

Cystic lesions, while exceedingly rare, can cause a wide range of clinical signs in dogs, cats, and rabbits, depending on their location. Progressive and severe neurological disease may be present with CNS lesions.[556] Subcutaneous lesions present as a soft mass, which would be similar to other types of cysts or possibly abscesses.[553,554]

Diagnosis

Diagnosis is based on the identification of tapeworm segments in feces by direct examination or detection of eggs using fecal flotation (Figure 1.10). The individual-sample sensitivity is low because proglottids are not uniformly distributed in feces

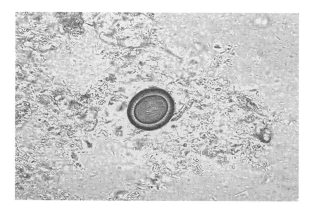

Figure 1.10 *Taenia* spp. egg, 38×32 μm (public domain, Centers for Disease Control and Prevention, Dr. Moore).

nor are they consistently shed in infected animals,[165] and testing of three fecal samples collected over one week is preferred. Purgation with substances such as arecoline can be used to increase recovery,[249] but this is not a practical or justifiable test in routine clinical settings.

Management

Praziquantel and epsiprantel are highly effective for the elimination of intestinal *Taenia*.[180,560] Concurrent measures must be taken to reduce exposure to intermediate hosts.

Treatment of systemic infection depends on the location and severity. CNS infections are typically fatal.[556,558] Surgical removal of cysts is the best option, if they are accessible. The use of anthelmintics alone has not been adequately investigated but probably is of limited efficacy.

Humans

Clinical presentation

Infections with adult *Taenia* spp. are usually asymptomatic. In some cases, there may be mild nonspecific gastrointestinal symptoms such as nausea or abdominal pain. Proglottids may be passed intermittently and noted in the stool.

Cystic disease may occur when a human inadvertently ingests a *Taenia* spp. egg. Clinical manifestations depend on the location and size of cysts. Most commonly, the eye or CNS is involved.[213] CNS disease produces nonspecific signs such as generalized weakness, seizures, inability to walk, and gradual deterioration in neurological status.[534] Hydrocephalus and basal arachnoiditis are common.[213,534] Ocular infections may be associated with vision loss and involvement of vitreous, anterior chamber or subconjunctival tissues.[534,561–563]

Diagnosis

Diagnosis of intestinal disease is made by the identification of eggs in the stool.

Diagnosis of cystic disease is usually made by CT or MRI, which identify the characteristic cysts. Serological testing is available, but it has poor sensitivity when there are single or only a few cysts.

Management

Surgical removal of the cyst is recommended, if feasible.[213,534] Praziquantel is often used as an adjunctive measure to surgery.[534] Information regarding the potential efficacy of praziquantel or other anthelmintics alone is limited. In some cases, treatment with praziquantel has been used as the sole initial approach, and the intermediate stage was apparently killed; however, surgical removal of the mass was still required.[534] Praziquantel has been used for ocular disease, with successful killing of the coenurus but loss of vision.[563] Albendazole may also be used for cystic disease.

Prevention

Efforts for preventing intestinal *Taenia* infection in humans need to involve control of infection in food animal intermediate hosts and avoiding ingestion of undercooked meat. Pets play no role in intestinal *Taenia* infection in humans, and the role of pets in human coenurosis is apparently limited, based both on the rarity of disease and lack of evidence to the contrary. However, considering the potential for transmission and the potential severity of disease, it is still reasonable to consider *Taenia* control in pets to help prevent human infection. Reducing exposure of pets to infected intermediate hosts involves decreasing roaming and scavenging, as well as avoiding feeding raw meat or offal from livestock or wildlife. If owners are determined to feed raw meat, it should be frozen prior to feeding to kill any *Taenia* cysticerci it may contain. *T. solium* cysticerci are effectively killed in 4 days at −5°C, 3 days at −15°C, and 1 day at −24°C.[564] Other *Taenia* species are presumably similarly susceptible, and keeping meat frozen for at least 10 days prior to feeding is a reasonable precaution. If treatment is based on fecal testing, then multiple fecal samples must be examined at each interval due to the low test sensitivity. If tapeworm eggs are identified, treatment should be administered as soon as possible because the eggs cannot be differentiated from those of *Echinococcus* spp.

Taenia spp. eggs can also be found in the soil in various environments.[565] The role of environmental exposure in disease is unclear, but general hygiene measures to avoid inadvertent fecal–oral exposure and controlling roaming of animals may help reduce any risks.

Ticks

Introduction

Ticks are blood-sucking insects that belong to the Arachnida class. There are two main types of ticks: Ixodidae (hard ticks) and Argasidae (soft ticks). Hard ticks include the three most common genera involved in the transmission of zoonotic diseases that can involve both pets and humans: *Ixodes*, *Rhipicephalus*, *Dermacentor*, and *Amblyomma* (Figures 1.11–1.13, Table 1.4).[272,566–571]

There is marked geographic variation in the presence and prevalence of ticks, and an understanding of the regional prevalence, the types of ticks, and the prevalence of tick-borne diseases is important. The simple presence of a tick does not mean that tick-borne infection is likely or even possible, since not all ticks are sources of infection and typically only a minority of ticks are infected.

An important aspect of tick-borne disease is the time required for infection. Infection is transmitted during feeding, something that does not occur

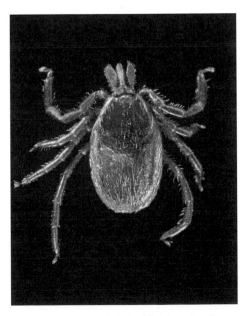

Figure 1.11 *Ixodes scapularis* (public domain, photo credit: James Gathany).

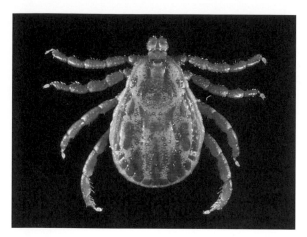

Figure 1.12 *Dermacentor andersoni* (public domain, photo credit: James Gathany).

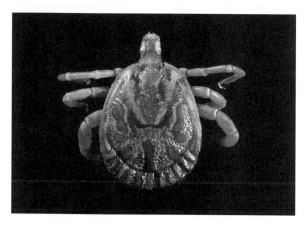

Figure 1.13 *Amblyomma cajennense* (public domain, photo credit: James Gathany).

Table 1.4 Examples of zoonotic pathogens that can be found in ticks from companion animals.

Tick	Pathogen(s)
Rhipicephalus sanguineus (brown dog tick)	*Coxiella burnetii* *Rickettsia rickettsii* *Rickettsia conorii* *Bartonella vinsonii* subsp. *berkhoffii*
Ixodes scapularis (deer tick)	*Anaplasma phagocytophilum* *Ehrlichia chaffeensis* *Ehrlichia ewingii* *Bartonella henselae* (possibly) *Borrelia burgdorferi* *R. rickettsii* *R. conorii*
Ixodes pacificus	*B. burgdorferi*
Ixodes ricinus	*A. phagocytophilum* *C. burnetii* *Borrelia* spp. Tick-borne encephalitis virus
Amblyomma americanum (lone star tick)	*E. chaffeensis* *E. ewingii* *B. burgdorferi* *Francisella tularensis*
Dermacentor variabilis (dog tick)	*R. rickettsii* *F. tularensis*
Dermacentor andersoni (wood tick)	*R. rickettsii* *F. tularensis*

until 24–36 hours after attachment for most tick-borne diseases.[572] This is a critical control point since prompt identification and proper removal of ticks can reduce or negate any risk of pathogen transmission.

Human health relevance of ticks on pets

Finding ticks on pets indicates that ticks are present in the area and that there is the potential for human exposure from the same infected environments. The other concern is the potential that ticks brought into the household could leave the animal and subsequently attach to humans. The incidence of intrahousehold transmission is unknown and is probably low. Pets are probably a better indicator of what ticks are in the environment than a likely source of human infection. An additional but still theoretical risk is the potential for human exposure is contact with infectious fluids from ticks that are crushed during tick removal. Pets could also potentially transport ticks able to cause tick paralysis into the house.

Tick avoidance

One way to reduce the risk of contact is to avoid areas that are likely infested with ticks. If exposure to tick-infested areas is unavoidable, various measures can be taken. These include wearing long-sleeved shirts that seal tightly around the wrists, wearing long pants that are tucked into high socks, and using DEET-containing repellents. Wearing permethrin-treated clothing is also a highly effective measure.[570] Use of DEET on pets is not recommended by the Animal Poison Control Center because of the high sensitivity of dogs and cats.[573]

Identification of ticks

Human and animal bodies should be carefully inspected for ticks after being in potentially tick-infested areas. Careful examination is required, particularly for nymphs that can be the size of a poppy seed.[571] While ticks require 24–36 hours to transmit most relevant diseases, tick inspections should be performed promptly after being in potentially tick-infested environments. In humans, particular attention should be paid to the scalp, pubic, and axillary areas.[574]

Tick removal

Ticks should be carefully removed, to ensure removal of the entire tick and to avoid crushing it and potentially being exposed to infectious fluids. Slow and deliberate movements are required.[272] Constant traction with curved forceps or a tick removal device is ideal. Tweezers are less desirable since they are more likely to result in crushing of the tick. Ticks should be grasped as close to the skin as possible, and twisting should be avoided. Bare fingers should not be used to remove ticks because of the potential for exposure to tick feces or hemolymph, which may be infected with pathogens such as *Rickettsia rickettsii*.[570] Application of substances such as alcohol or the use of direct heat is ineffective at removing ticks and should not be attempted.[272]

Tick control products for pets

Routine use of tick control products (Table 1.5) should be considered in animals at risk of exposure, particularly in areas where ticks are likely to be infected with important pathogens. The use of tick control products should not be relied on as a sole preventive measure, since no product provides 100% protection. Some authors have advocated year-round treatment because of the greater cold tolerance of ticks compared with fleas.[272] This is reasonable in many areas but unlikely to be necessary in regions with long cold periods. The key is to use tick control products during the at-risk period, and that varies between regions.

As all life cycle stages of *Rhipicephalus sanguineus* can use dogs as suitable hosts, infested dogs can be a long-term source of infestation for other dogs. Therefore, treatment of all dogs in a household should be performed if one or more dogs are exposed.[272]

Environmental control

Reducing habitats amenable to intermediate hosts should be performed when possible. This may involve removal of piles of brush or yard waste, or trimming of weeds and plants in areas where the pet has frequent access. Access of wildlife to crawl spaces or similar yard areas should be prevented.

More intensive environmental control is required if *R. sanguineus* is present, since dogs are suitable long-term hosts. The use of environmental acaricides (i.e., synthetic pyrethroids) should be considered in response to finding an infested dog in a household.[272] Methodical treatment of the environment is necessary since these ticks may be found in cracks and crevices, on ceilings, and in other difficult-to-reach areas.[272]

Toxocara and *Toxascaris* spp.

Introduction

T. canis and *T. cati* are dog and cat roundworms (ascarids), respectively. These parasites are commonly found in dogs and cats, and often receive much attention as possible causes of human infection. *Toxascaris leonina* is another roundworm that can infect dogs and cats. Humans are accidental hosts of *T. canis* and *T. cati*, but infections can result in visceral larva migrans (VLM), ocular larva migrans (OLM), and other syndromes, particularly in young children. The relative importance of *T. canis* and *T. cati* is somewhat controversial and difficult to determine because of cross-reactivity of

Table 1.5   Examples of commercial tick preventive formulations for use in dogs and cats.

Active ingredient(s)	Route	Label claims*	Animal species
Amitraz	Collar	Ticks: no specific species claims	Dog
Dinotefuran, pyriproxyfen, permethrin	Topical: spot-on	*Amblyomma maculatum* *D. variabilis* *I. scapularis* *R. sanguineus*	Dog
Fipronil, methoprene	Topical: spot-on	*A. americanum* *D. variabilis* *I. scapularis* *R. sanguineus*	Dog, cat
Fipronil	Topical spot-on or spray	*A. americanum* *D. variabilis* *I. scapularis* *R. sanguineus*	Dog, cat
Imidacloprid-permethrin	Topic: spot-on	*A. americanum* *D. variabilis* *I. scapularis* *R. sanguineus*	Dog
Metaflumizone, amitraz	Topical: spot-on	*A. americanum* *D. variabilis* *I. scapularis* *R. sanguineus*	Dog
Permethrin	Topical: spot-on	*A. americanum* *D. variabilis* *I. scapularis* *R. sanguineus*	Dog
Permethrin, pyriproxyfen	Topical: spray	Ticks: no specific species claims	Dog
Pyrethrins	Topical: dip	Ticks: no specific species claims	Dog, cat
Selamectin	Topical: spot-on	*D. variabilis*	Dog

Adapted from Blagburn and Dryden [272].
* Label claims in the United States.

serological testing. It has classically been assumed that *T. canis* is the main cause of human infection;[575] however, the importance of *T. cati* may be underestimated, especially in ocular disease.[576,577]

Etiology

Ascarids are large, elongated, nonsegmented, cylindrical intestinal nematodes that undergo sexual reproduction in the intestinal tract of their animal hosts, and have a maturation stage outside of the body in soil. *T. canis* is the most common canine roundworm, and *T. cati* is the most common

in cats. *T. canis* is not known to infect cats nor is *T. cati* known to infect dogs. *Toxascaris leonina* can be found in both dogs and cats. Other *Toxocara* species have been identified in cats, such as *Toxocara malaysiensis*.[578] *Toxocara mystax* is a synonym for *T. cati*.[579] The zoonotic significance of these is not known.

Life cycle

The life cycle is shown in Figure 1.14. Adult roundworms inhabit the small intestine of their preferred host. Nonembryonated eggs are passed in feces

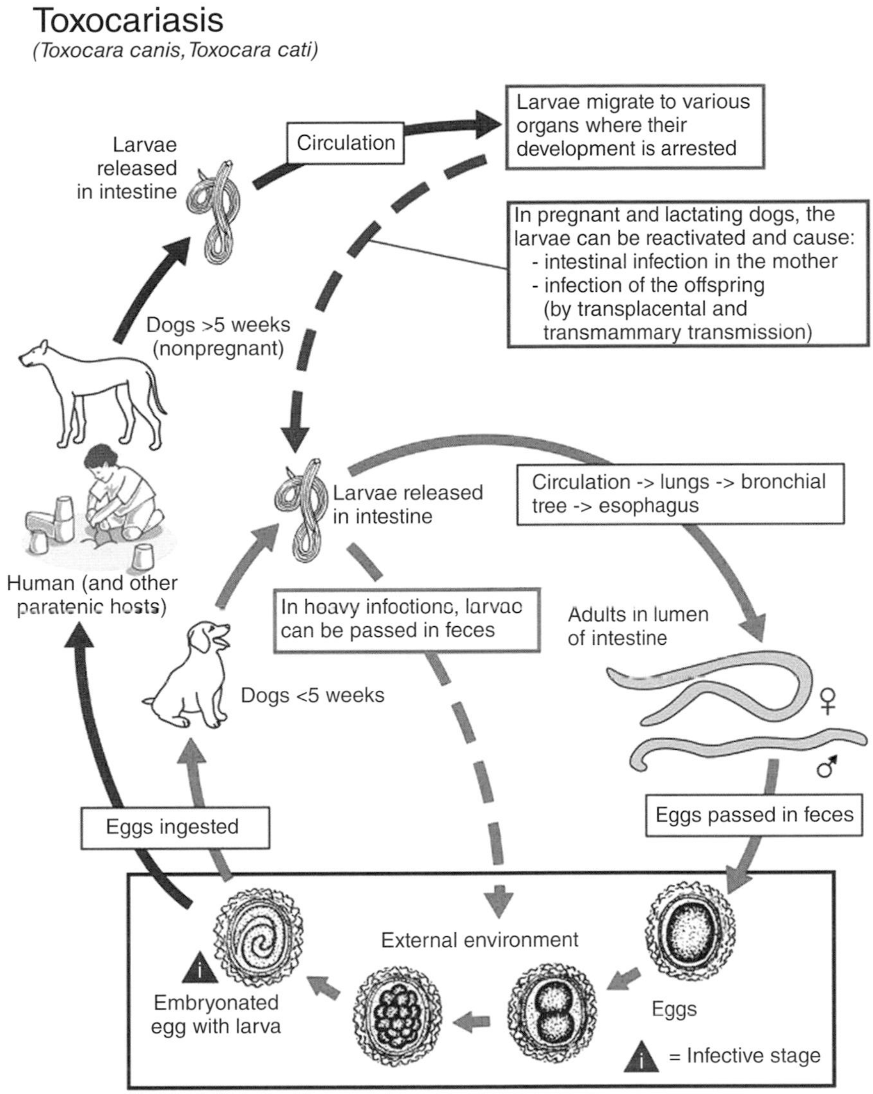

Toxocariasis
(Toxocara canis, Toxocara cati)

Figure 1.14 *Toxocara* life cycle (public domain, Centers for Disease Control and Prevention, Alexander J. da Silva, Melanie Moser).

and mature to the infective third-stage larval form in the environment. Typically, 2–4 weeks are required for *T. canis* and *T. cati* to become infective, although this varies with environmental conditions. Infective larvae can develop in 9–15 days at 25–30°C but require 35 days at 16.5°C.[580] *T. leonina* larvae may become infective in as little as 1 week.[47] Susceptible hosts become infected by ingestion of infective eggs or from ingestion of animals (paratenic hosts) with larvae in tissues. Earthworms

and perhaps other invertebrates can harbor larvae in their intestinal tracts and transmit infection if ingested.

When definitive hosts ingest infective eggs, *T. canis* or *T. cati* migrate through the intestinal wall to the liver and eventually the lungs. After reaching the lungs, larvae are coughed up and swallowed, and mature into adult worms in the small intestine, thereby completing the life cycle. Some larvae remain in tissue in an arrested state. After ingestion of an infected paratenic host, larvae usually do not migrate but mature into adults in the small intestine.[581] The larvae of *T. leonina* do not undergo extraintestinal migration in definitive hosts, regardless of the source of infection.

The prepatent period for *T. canis* is 2–5 weeks, while it is approximately 8 weeks for *T. cati* and 8–11 weeks for *T. leonina*.

In other species (paratenic hosts), after ingestion of infective eggs, the larvae penetrate the intestinal lining and migrate throughout the body. Unlike in definitive hosts, these larvae are unable to mature and complete the life cycle. Migration can continue, usually intermittently, for years, and clinical disease can develop from migration and the associated inflammatory response.

Transplacental infection can occur with *T. canis* in puppies. This may be from acute infection of bitches but is primarily associated reactivation of latent larvae in tissues during late pregnancy, with subsequent in utero infection. There is no evidence of transplacental infection with *T. cati* or *T. leonina*.

Transmammary infection can occur in both puppies and kittens.[47] In cats, while transmammary infection can occur, chronically infected cats tend to harbor few somatic larvae, and transmammary infection only occurs when the female is infected during late gestation.[582] Bitches can be reinfected via ingestion of larvae in the feces of puppies.

Geographic distribution/epidemiology

Dogs and cats

Toxocara species are common internationally, particularly in young kittens and puppies, as well as feral animals and those in shelters. The ability of *T. canis* to be transmitted in utero and both *T. cati* and *T. canis* to be transmitted during nursing, along with the environmental tolerance of larvated eggs, creates an excellent opportunity for high parasite burdens in puppies and kittens. It is often assumed that almost all puppies are born infected with *T. canis*; however, this is based on old data and it is unclear whether this is still true. Reported prevalence rates for dogs and cats vary with age, location (i.e., household, shelter, feral), geography, and the presence or absence of routine deworming. Studies of stray or shelter animals

have reported prevalences of *Toxocara* shedding ranging from 5.3% to 82% in dogs and from 0.8% to 54% in cats.[129,155,158,162,345,536,542,543,583–592] Puppies are more often infected than adult dogs,[158,165,313,351,590,593–596] as are hunting dogs.[597] The prevalence of these parasites in adult cats and dogs in households is lower and is typically 0–4% in developed countries.[115,119,129,154,307,308,312,313,355,541,587,596,598–600] As with *T. canis*, *T. cati* is more common (up to 33%) in kittens versus adults.[117,119,591] Higher rates have also been found in house versus apartment cats,[591] presumably reflecting greater likelihood that cats living in houses are allowed to have outdoor access compared with those living in apartments. *T. leonina* is less common (0–32%) and tends to be focally distributed.[154,160,161,307,536,542,592,593]

Routes of human exposure

Human toxocariasis can be found wherever dogs and cats are found, but the prevalence is highly variable between regions. Since dogs and cats (along with wild canids and felids) are the definitive hosts of these parasites, they clearly play a role in human infection. However, determination of the role of pets versus feral animals, and whether they act as a direct source of infection versus indirect infection from contamination of the outdoor environment can be difficult.

Human infections typically occur following ingestion of infective eggs from contaminated soil, ingestion of larvae in the tissues of infected paratenic hosts (e.g., raw livers of cattle, chickens, ducks, and pigs), or ingestion of inadequately washed or cooked fruits and vegetables.[575,576]

Direct contact with dogs or cats is of limited relevance because of the time required for eggs to become infective, though concerns have been raised about exposure to infective eggs on the hair coats of dogs. Studies have identified *Toxocara* eggs on the hair coats of dogs, including a study of pound dogs from Ireland where 67% of dogs (mainly puppies) were contaminated.[601] Another study reported the presence of *Toxocara* eggs on 22% of (mainly young) dogs in Turkey.[602] In that study, only 8% of eggs were embryonated and therefore potentially infective. Egg counts were relatively low in these studies: 8–12 embryonated eggs per gram of hair. Another study found *Toxocara* eggs on the coats of 12% of dogs, but none were viable,[312] while one other reported the presence of

T. canis eggs on 25% of dogs, with 4.2% embryonated and 24% embryonating.[603] The individual animal does not need to be the source of hair coat contamination, as demonstrated by the presence of eggs from other animal species on the hair coat,[602] indicating that contact with eggs in the outdoor environment may be the source. This has implications for control, since controlling *Toxocara* in pets may not necessarily prevent the risk of exposure from the hair coat of animals that are allowed outside. The true risk of human infection from the hair coat is unclear, particularly considering the small numbers of infective eggs that are typically present. One author used an estimate of 300 eggs per gram of hair and a 4% embryonated egg rate, and determined that someone would have to ingest over 4 g of hair to ingest 50 infective eggs,[312] a level of ingestion that certainly is beyond casual, inadvertent exposure. Hair coat exposure is probably of even less concern in cats because of their fastidious grooming habits, but could be more relevant in debilitated or obese cats that do not groom properly, long-haired cats with a tendency for fecal staining of the perineum, or cats that have close contact with highly infected environmental sites. There is no evidence of transplacental infection in cats.

Contamination of the outdoor environment is common in many areas. Contamination rates of <1–55% of samples from parks, playgrounds, and family gardens have been reported.[33,565,587,604–607] The ability of infective eggs to survive for prolonged periods of time under many climatic conditions allows for accumulation of potentially large egg burdens.

Seroprevalence in humans

Seroconversion is much more common than disease. Seroprevalence rates are variable depending on geographic region and risk factors for exposure. Rates of 1.6–85% have been reported, with the highest rates tending to occur in rural, poor, and/or tropical regions, although conflicting risk factor data are present.[585,597,608–626] The seroprevalence increases with age, and males tend to be more commonly positive than females, perhaps due to differences in outdoor play and work.[611,627]

Dog ownership has been widely reported as a risk factor for seroconversion, despite the fact that the source of infection is probably environmental. Dog ownership, regular contact with dogs, or the presence of dogs in the household have been reported as risk factors for seropositivity in children,[609,610,614,615,618,619,628–630] as well as OLM.[631–633] It is unclear whether the apparent risk of pet ownership is because of household environmental contamination that results from owning a dog or whether there may be other factors involved such as increased exposure to potentially contaminated external environmental sites (i.e., public parks) in dog-owning families. The latter possibility is perhaps supported by a study that reported an association of seroprevalence and pet ownership but not the presence of pets in the household.[611]

The risk of exposure may be higher in dog breeders because of the high prevalence in young puppies and the likelihood of significant environmental contamination.[634] This was demonstrated by a study that found seropositivity in 16% of British dog breeders compared with 2.6% of healthy controls.[635] The likely role of the contaminated canine breeding environment is supported by other studies that did not show increased seroprevalence in other groups with frequent contact with dogs and cats, such as veterinary personnel, kennel workers, and cat breeders compared with the general population.[616,636,637] Other reported risk factors for seroconversion include pica, living in rural areas, visiting a playground frequently, developmental delay in children, reduced IQ scores in children, low socioeconomic status, frequent playing in a sandbox, and frequent contact with soil.[614,615,618,619,628,633,638–641] Most of these are associated with increased likelihood of direct or indirect ingestion of soil and poor hygiene. Not surprisingly, habitual hand washing before eating has been reported as a protective factor in children.[613]

Disease in humans

While seroprevalence data are available, there is little information about the incidence of clinical disease. There is presumably significant variation in the incidence of disease and a parallel between high seroprevalence regions and disease incidence. Risk factors for seroconversion are also presumably risk factors for infection; however, there has been limited objective study. Care must be taken when considering the often high sero-prevalence data (some of which are quite dated) from specific high-risk regions or populations, and extrapolating that to the risk of clinical disease in other areas. Anecdotally, the incidence of infection in many developed regions appears to be low. However, given the relative paucity of data and the potential severity of disease, toxocariasis should be considered a reasonable, if variable, zoonotic disease threat.

The two main human diseases associated with dog and cat ascarids are VLM and OLM, although other syndromes can also occur. Zoonotic disease is most commonly associated with *T. canis*, but *T. cati* can also be involved.[193] VLM occurs most commonly in children less than 4–6 years of age,[2,193] particularly in children with a history of pica or those living in unsanitary conditions.[2,632,642] After ingestion, infective *Toxocara* can migrate throughout the tissues of the body, sometimes entering a dormant state and undergoing further migration later. The potential for dormancy and reactivation means that disease can occur well after infection, and the incubation period range is not known. Infection is most often asymptomatic, with seroconversion being the only detectable change, though fulminant infection and death can occur.[193] Disease manifestations depend on various factors, including the number of larvae and the tissues they are migrating through.

Migration of *Toxocara* larvae into the eye is the cause of OLM. Typically, only one larva is involved, and infection is almost always unilateral.[193,575,631] OLM presumably develops from chance migration of a larva into the eye, where it produces an eosinophilic inflammatory mass. As with VLM, children are most commonly affected, but they tend to be a few years older than those affected with VLM.[193] OLM appears to be quite rare. One large American study estimated the incidence of disease in schoolchildren at 6.6–9.7 cases per 100,000 persons,[631] while an earlier American study estimated an incidence of 1 case per 1000 persons[643] and a study of children in Ireland did not detect any cases of OLM in greater than 2000 children.[644] Concurrent VLM and OLM is very rare but can occur.[193,575]

Other manifestations of *Toxocara* infection and migration depend on the tissues involved and the body's immune response. *Toxocara* infection has been suspected as a cause of a range of allergic or inflammatory diseases. Numerous studies have investigated a possible role of *Toxocara* infection in bronchial asthma in children, with conflicting results.[633,645–648] It has also been implicated as a cause of epilepsy,[649,650] although not all studies have not supported that association.[651] Infection has also been associated with other disorders such as chronic urticaria, chronic pruritis, eczema and allergic rhinitis, and idiopathic eosinophilia.[620,652–658]

Animals

Clinical presentation

Dogs
Infection is usually subclinical, and clinical infections are mainly found in puppies. Puppies with disease attributable to *T. canis* usually have signs such as ill thrift, failure to gain weight, poor hair coat, and a pot-bellied appearance. In rare cases, severe disease or sudden death can occur. Some puppies with significant worm burdens may expel a large number of worms in vomitus.

As larvae migrate through the liver, scarring can develop, but this rarely produces any identifiable signs. In contrast, migration of large numbers of larvae through the lungs can result in respiratory disease from the associated hemorrhage and inflammation. This is usually in young puppies that acquire large numbers of *T. canis* in utero.

Clinical infections in adults are uncommon but can range from mild enteritis to intestinal obstruction from large worm burdens. Vomiting can occur from gastric irritation caused by larvae migrating through the gastric mucosa. Larva migrans has been reported but seems to be very rare.[659,660] It has been suggested that OLM might be a problem in some dogs, such as working sheepdogs,[659] although clear data are lacking.

Clinical disease from *T. leonina* infection is rare and has been poorly described.

Cats
Since in utero infection does not occur in cats, kittens are older at the time of infection and clinical disease does not occur until later, when compared with puppies.[581] Clinical disease in kittens can be similar to that described above for puppies, but the

tendency for kittens to be older age at the time of infection may account for the lower incidence of clinically apparent and severe disease.[581] Mild signs, particularly a pot-bellied appearance, may be all that are evident. Regardless, as far as zoonotic risk is concerned, shedding eggs is more important than clinical disease, and there is clear evidence that kittens can shed eggs by 3 weeks of age.

As with dogs, clinical infections in adult cats are uncommon. Nonspecific signs such as poor hair coat, diarrhea, and a pot-bellied appearance may be present.[581]

Diagnosis

Clinical signs are nonspecific but suggestive in young puppies or kittens, particularly those with no or minimal history of deworming. Identification of worms in vomitus is diagnostic.

Diagnosis is most often based on the detection of eggs in feces using centrifugal flotation. Typically, large numbers of eggs are passed on a regular basis, but detection is not always straightforward. *Toxocara* eggs are difficult to differentiate from *B. procyonis* microscopically; however, *B. procyonis* is very uncommon in dogs and cats. The prepatent period is 2–4 weeks.[47]

Management

Fenbendazole, milbemycin oxime, nitroscanate, moxidectin, febantel, and pyrantel pamoate are effective in dogs and cats.[47,368,560,576,661,662] Piperazine can be used but is less effective than the other options.[47] Emodepside is effective for the treatment of *T. cati* in cats.[47] Most drugs used for monthly heartworm prophylaxis are effective against ascarids. Chemoprophylaxis is discussed below under Prevention. Antihelmintic resistance has not (yet) been identified in *Toxocara* spp.

Humans

Clinical presentation

VLM

Most infections are asymptomatic.[576] Patients with clinical disease can have signs ranging from mild to fulminant to fatal. Mild disease may be charac-terized by nonspecific signs such as cough, fever, wheezing, and hepatomegaly, as a result of migration through the liver and lungs.[193] Anorexia, head-ache, weight loss, fatigue, and abdominal pain may also be present.[576] Radiographic evidence of lung involvement is quite common although severe respiratory disease is rare.[193] Splenomegaly may be present in a small percentage of cases. Myocarditis is another rare manifestation.[2] Concurrent OLM is uncommon but can occur.

Overt neurological disease is uncommon (as opposed to larva migrans caused by *B. procyonis*), but seizures may occur.[193,576] Headache, fever, and other nonspecific neurological or systemic signs may also be noted in patients with neural larva migrans.[576]

OLM

Endophthalmitis and retinitis are most common.[2] Clinical complaints and signs may include loss of visual acuity, leukocoria, strabismus, pars planitis, uveitis, and retinal granuloma or detach-ment.[575,576,663,664] Visual acuity may be maintained in many patients but greatly decreased in others.[665] Blindness is uncommon but can occur. Bilateral disease is rare.[664] Systemic signs such as hepato-megaly and fever are typically absent.

Others

Various other diseases have been associated, with varying strengths of evidence, with zoonotic ascarid infection. Nonspecific eosinophilia may be identified based on the body's response to migrat-ing larvae. Larval migration is a common, but not sole, cause of eosinophilia, and larva migrans should be considered in all cases of unexplained eosinophilia.[193] An association has been made between anti-*Toxocara* antibodies and chronic idio-pathic urticaria.[666]

Diagnosis

VLM

Eosinophilia is a classical sign, and VLM should be considered in any patient (particularly any child) with unexplained eosinophilia.[667] Leukocytosis and hypergammaglobulinemia may also be present.[2,193] Possible exposure risks should be queried, especially pica.

Finding larvae in biopsies of affected tissues (i.e., liver) is diagnostic, but larvae are infrequently found because the inflammatory response often occurs in response to the external coat of the parasite that can be shed frequently during migration, so larvae may not be present at the site of active inflammation.[575,668] Detection of serum antibodies against *Toxocara* is supportive but not definitive because asymptomatic individuals may also be seropositive,[193] and the positive predictive value of serological data depend on the baseline seroprevalence in the population.

OLM

OLM should be considered in any child with vision loss and strabismus.[667] Diagnosis is predominantly based on clinical signs during ophthalmologic examination. Posterior pole granuloma that mimics a retinoblastoma may be observed;[669] B-scan ultrasonography is useful to differentiate those two conditions.[670] Serum antibody levels are not particularly helpful because some people with OLM are seronegative and a variable percentage of healthy individuals may be seropositive.[193,632] Identification of high antibody levels in vitreous fluid versus serum may be useful diagnostically.[665,669,671] Peripheral eosinophilia is rare.

Others

Diagnosis of other manifestations can be difficult because of the often vague nature of the disease. Seropositivity along with the presence of clinical signs potentially attributable to *Toxocara* infection is suggestive but is obviously complicated by the baseline seroprevalence rate in the healthy population.

Management

VLM

Most people have mild disease and recover without therapy.[193] Treatment is provided in people with severe disease, such as neurological disease or severe respiratory disease. Albendazole is the drug of choice.[193] Corticosteroids may be considered in patients with CNS or cardiac involvement.[193]

OLM

There is no standard approach to OLM, and treatment is often unrewarding because of the typically long delay from infection to diagnosis.[2,193]

Albendazole is the anthelmintic of choice,[667] but anthelmintics are often avoided because of concerns about severe, sight-threatening inflammation from dying larvae.[670] Corticosteroid injections may reduce ocular inflammation. Vitrectomy is often required.[667,670]

Others

Treatment depends on the syndrome and severity. Many manifestations are probably self-limited and respond without treatment. Treatment with anti-inflammatories and anthelmintics could be considered.

Prevention

Deworming dogs and cats

Every puppy and kitten should be considered infected, and proper deworming of these animals is critical. All puppies should be dewormed with pyrantel pamoate, fenbendazole, or milbemycin oxime at 2, 4, 6, and 8 weeks of age, then monthly to 6 months of age. Deworming of kittens should start at 3 weeks of age. Nursing dams should be treated at the same time as their offspring. If bitches have previously had a litter with significant *T. canis* burdens, they should be dewormed with daily fenbendazole during pregnancy or two to four times during pregnancy with ivermectin.[47]

Recommendations for animals over 6 months of age are conflicting and include deworming monthly,[344] once or twice a year,[361] or at least four times a year at intervals not exceeding 3 months.[368] Basing treatment recommendations on fecal examination in low-risk households with no regular prophylactic treatment has also been recommended.[283] Factors that need to be considered when developing a roundworm control program include the prevalence of roundworms in the area, the breeding status of the animal, management of the pets, number of pets in the household, and whether there are high-risk people (e.g., children with pica) in the household.

Fecal examinations in dogs and cats

Fecal examinations should be performed periodically to determine the need for deworming and to assess the efficacy of the preventive program.

Varying recommendations have been made, including testing two to four times the first year and one to two times per year thereafter.[47] Centrifugal flotation methods should be used because of their higher sensitivity compared with gravitational flotation techniques.

Reducing exposure of pet dogs and cats

Restricting outdoor exposure, especially uncontrolled outdoor exposure that could be associated with ingestion of feces or killing and eating paratenic hosts, could also help reduce (but not eliminate) the risk of exposure of household pets.

Reducing human exposure

Avoiding contact with feces in the environment is a logical control measure but may be difficult. Because of the time required for eggs to become infective and the tolerance of eggs in the environment, evidence of fecal contamination may not be apparent in environments where infective eggs are present. Prompt removal of feces that are passed outside is therefore an important control measure. Similarly, regular removal of feces from litter boxes will prevent the formation of infective eggs.

Decontamination of the environment is difficult to impossible because of the inherent difficulties in eliminating pathogens from organic-rich sites and the environmental tolerance of the parasite. Application of disinfectants is not a practical method in outdoor environments. Temperature plays an important role in environmental development and persistence of eggs. Larval development ceases at temperatures below 10°C, and larvae die at temperature of −15°C or less.[580] Thorough cleaning is important in areas where puppies or kittens and their dams are housed and after accidental fecal contamination of the environment. Physical removal of eggs from surfaces by thorough cleaning is important because of the resistance of *Toxocara* eggs to most disinfectants.

Ultimately, infection in humans requires ingestion of infective larvae in eggs, so close attention to hand hygiene, particularly after contact with high-risk areas (e.g., puppy/kitten environment) or animals in those environments is important. Close supervision of children should be used to prevent ingestion of soil, sand, feces, or other potentially contaminated items. This is particularly

true for children or other individuals with a tendency toward geophagia or pica. Close attention to hand hygiene after working or playing outside is also important. Sandboxes should be covered to prevent cats from defecating in them, whenever possible. Some cities have removed sandboxes from municipal parks because of the risk of larva migrans.[667] This may be difficult to justify given the low incidence of disease in humans and the ability to reduce the risk with good hygiene practices and child supervision.

There are no specific recommendations for chemoprophylaxis following exposure, such as when a child is observed to ingest potentially contaminated soil.[2]

Education of pet owners and nonpet owners alike is important to increase awareness about the need for proper roundworm control in pets, proper fecal handling, and avoiding inadvertent ingestion of contaminated soil. Understanding of the risks and required infection control measures is poor in the general population. In a British study, pet owners were no more knowledgeable about zoonotic toxocariasis than nonpet owners, and understanding of human or animal *Toxocara* infection was poor.[672]

Toxoplasma gondii

Introduction

This intracellular protozoal parasite is a significant zoonotic pathogen and receives ample attention with respect to risks of infection of immunologically naive pregnant women. It is also of particular importance in immunocompromised individuals. Cats and wild felids are the only known definitive hosts of *T. gondii*, but other sources of transmission, including consumption of tissue cysts in undercooked meat and fecal–oral transmission from contaminated soil or water, are equally, if not more, responsible for human infection. The incidence of toxoplasmosis in humans in the United States has declined despite increases in cat ownership.[673]

Etiology

T. gondii is an apicomplexan protozoal parasite capable of infecting almost any warm-blooded species, including humans. There are three major genotypes of *T. gondii* that can be differentiated for epidemiological purposes, but clinically, they are not significantly different.[674]

Life cycle

As with all coccidian parasites, *T. gondii* has both sexual and asexual stages (Figure 1.15). Both cycles occur in the definitive host, the cat, while only the asexual stage occurs in nonfeline (intermediate) hosts.[675] Unlike most other coccidians, *T. gondii* can be transmitted in multiple ways, including fecal–oral, carnivorism, and transplacental infection.[675]

Cats, the definitive hosts (along with wild felids), are thought to be infected mainly through ingestion of tissue cysts in infected intermediate hosts.[675] After ingestion of tissue cysts, bradyzoites are released in the intestinal tract and invade the epi-

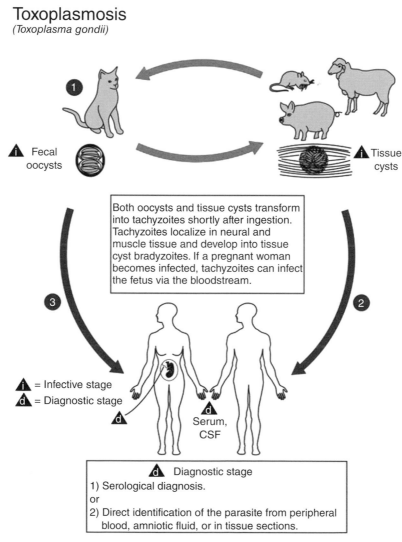

Figure 1.15   *Toxoplasma gondii* life cycle (public domain, Centers for Disease Control and Prevention, Alexander J. da Silva, Melanie Moser).

thelial cells. Schizonts are formed, followed by the development and release of merozoites, which invade other epithelial cells and form either male or female gamonts. The male gamonts (microgamonts) divide to form numerous flagellated, motile microgametes, which penetrate and fertilize the female gamont (the macrogamont). The macrogamont then forms a wall and becomes an unsporulated oocyst, which is passed in the feces of the cat in its noninfective state. Approximately 97% of naive cats fed tissue cysts will shed oocysts in their feces, usually within 3–10 days (the prepatent period). Patency may last up to 20 days, with the majority of oocysts being shed over only 1–2 days.[676] In contrast, only ~20% of previously exposed cats fed oocysts will develop a patent infection, and the prepatent period for cats fed oocysts may be 18 days or longer.[675] Immunosuppression may increase the likelihood of a previously infected cat shedding oocysts. Other circumstances under which reshedding may occur remain undefined.[675,676] Regardless, further shedding is likely an uncommon event, meaning that there is only a very small window in an infected cat's life when it is shedding oocysts.

Unsporulated oocysts passed in the feces of cats must sporulate in the environment to become infective. This occurs most efficiently in warm (20°C) and moist conditions, and typically takes between 1 and 5 days at room temperature.[675] This results in the formation of two sporocysts, each containing four infective, banana-shaped sporozoites. Sporozoites, within the oocyst, are infective and can survive in the environment for prolonged periods of time, waiting to be ingested by a susceptible warm-blooded host. After ingestion by nonfelid species, the sporozoites excyst in the small intestine, invading intestinal cells and dividing asexually to produce two lunate-shaped tachyzoites. The tachyzoites migrate throughout the body, invading cells in various tissues and multiplying until the cells rupture. Clinical signs of toxoplasmosis, including fetal injury, are caused by cellular destruction due to this migration and multiplication of tachyzoites. The most commonly affected tissues are the brain, liver, lungs, skeletal muscle, and eyes.[675] The process remains subclinical in the majority of cases.

If an infected cell fails to rupture, the tachyzoites eventually cease multiplying and encyst, becoming bradyzoites and remaining within the cell. A cyst may ultimately grow to 15–60 µm but remain separated from the cytoplasm of the host cell by a very thin elastic wall. Cysts can form in the CNS, muscles, and other internal organs, and, in most cases, likely persist until the death of the host, usually without causing any clinical signs. Reactivation of latent infections is an important process in immunocompromised individuals.

Geographic distribution/epidemiology

Toxoplasmosis is present worldwide. Seroprevalence rates in cats are high (9.3–40%) and can be influenced by their diet and whether they are allowed outside.[116,675–678] Seroprevalence is also related to age, with older animals more likely to be seropositive.[673]

While cats are the definitive host and the seroprevalence is high, the likelihood that any given cat is shedding T. gondii is very low, with the prevalence of oocyst shedding often ranging from 0% to 1%.[116,312,679–682] Higher rates of shedding may be present in some animal populations, such as was reported in a study of an Australian aboriginal community where 18% of cats were shedding oocysts.[517] It is reasonable to assume that the likelihood of shedding is higher in cats that are allowed outdoors and hunt.

Less information is available for other companion animal species. Seroprevalence rates of 11–89% have been reported in dogs.[683–688] Higher rates are usually present in studies from developing countries and those evaluating stray versus pet dogs. Shedding of oocysts is very rare; one study only found T. gondii oocysts in 2/24,089 fecal samples from German dogs.[689]

Human exposure is common. Seropositivity indicates previous exposure and likely latent infection, and is relatively common with reported rates of 12–97%.[687,690–694] Higher rates are present in older individuals.[695] While exposure is clearly a relatively common event, disease is much less common. Because toxoplasmosis is not a reportable disease in most regions, it is difficult to estimate the prevalence of disease in humans. An average of 15,000 human cases of clinical toxoplasmosis are reported annually in the United States, but it has been estimated that the actual number of cases that occur is likely closer to 225,000, of which 50% of cases are thought to be the result of food-borne transmission.[695]

Because cats are the definitive host for *T. gondii*, investigations have not surprisingly investigated the impact of cat ownership or contact on seroconversion or disease. Cleaning a cat litter box was found to be a strong risk factor for *T. gondii* infection in pregnant women in one study.[696] However, the same study and others have reported no association between *T. gondii* seropositivity and just owning or living with a cat.[692,696] Other studies have found associations between *T. gondii* exposure and owning three or more kittens,[697] and cat ownership in children in rural (but not urban) areas.[698] Studies that only look at cat ownership, however, provide only partial information, considering the studies that have implicated fecal exposure, not cohabitation, as the risk factor. Several studies have identified consumption of undercooked meat as the principle risk factor for *T. gondii* infection.[676,697] There is also evidence that people who handle raw meat (such as abattoir workers) may be more commonly exposed to the parasite.[99] Contamination of water sources and soil with the feces of wild or domestic cats is an important source of exposure as well. Infection may occur following ingestion of oocysts on unwashed, uncooked vegetables or in contaminated water.[696,699,700] Geophagia, contact with soil or sand (e.g., from a children's sandbox or gardening), and poor hand hygiene have also been associated with toxoplasmosis.[676,701,702] Dogs could also act as mechanical vectors if their hair coat becomes contaminated with sporulated oocysts.[703]

T. gondii is transmitted through ingestion of sporozoites in sporulated oocysts in feline feces or the environment, bradyzoites within cysts in the tissues of latently infected individuals, and trophozoites in the tissues of acutely infected individuals.[676,704] Oocysts are shed only in the feces of cats. Epidemiologically, oocysts are an extremely important means of transmission because, when sporulated, they are the most environmentally resistant life stage of the parasite. At that stage, as few as 10 cysts may infect an intermediate host such as a pig,[704] while 100 or more cysts can cause a patent infection in a cat, which may ultimately shed tens to hundreds of millions of oocysts.[675,676]

Ingestion of oocysts from cat feces can occur; however, because of the time required for oocysts to become infective after defecation, fresh feces pose no risk. Risk of exposure is from old cat feces in litter boxes, in the outdoor environment (especially gardens and sandboxes), and potentially on the hair coat of debilitated or long-haired cats that have difficulty properly grooming themselves.

Carnivorous or omnivorous animals (and people) are often infected through ingestion of encysted bradyzoites in the tissues of their prey. Tachyzoites can be shed in the milk of acutely infected animals.

Vertical transmission of *T. gondii* is a particular concern in humans but may also occur in dogs and cats.[704,705] In humans, the main concern is exposure of immunologically naive women during pregnancy. Previous exposure is adequate to protect against subsequent infection in immunocompetent individuals. Under normal circumstances, a naive female that has been exposed to *Toxoplasma* 4–6 months prior to pregnancy will develop sufficient immunity to protect herself and the fetus for the rest of her life.[676] In naive individuals, parasitemia with tachyzoites results in placentitis and subsequent infection of the fetus. In humans, the risk of the infection being passed on to the fetus is lower in the first trimester (10–25%) than during the third trimester (60–90%), though the consequences and potential congenital defects are more severe with earlier infections.[706]

While previous infection is typically considered to be protective in humans, there may be situations where reinfection is possible. If the immune response is suppressed by drug therapy or disease such as HIV/AIDS in humans, both the mother and the fetus become susceptible to infection once again. Additionally, transplacental infection with subsequent fetal deaths has been reported in experimentally infected dogs that had previous *Toxoplasma* exposure.[707] Care should be taken in extrapolating this study to natural infection and infection in other species, but it does raise concerns that prior infection may not be completely protective, at least in dogs. Infection through milk has been documented in kittens.[708,709] Transmission to bitches has also been reported via semen of experimentally infected dogs;[710] however, the clinical relevance of this is likely minimal. In humans, *T. gondii* has also been transmitted by organ transplants and blood transfusions, but this is uncommon.[676]

Animals

Clinical presentation

In healthy, immunologically naive cats, primary infection with *T. gondii* is typically either subclinical or causes mild diarrhea that persists for up to 10 days.[704] Though severe disease may occur in healthy, naive cats, it is most common in immunosuppressed cats, as well as in transplacentally or lactationally infected kittens.[704] Reactivation of chronic encysted infection can also occur in older cats that become immunosuppressed.[704] Signs of systemic disease may include fever, lethargy, anorexia, pneumonia, hepatitis, stiff gait with shifting lameness, or neurological signs from encephalitis.[675] Pancreatic, cardiac, and ocular tissues are also commonly affected. Dermatitis, vomiting, and diarrhea have been reported.[675] Kittens may exhibit fever, cough, dyspnea, icterus, and leukopenia. Chronic infection may result in diarrhea, emaciation, nausea, ataxia, and ocular lesions. The onset of signs may be slow, though the disease may be rapidly fatal, particularly with lung or brain involvement. Neurological and ocular signs without systemic illness occur more commonly with reactivated infections than with primary infection.[675]

Congenitally or lactationally infected kittens are often severely affected due to uncontrolled replication of tachyzoites and subsequent tissue damage. Kittens may be stillborn or die before weaning, typically with signs related to pulmonary or hepatic disease, or encephalitis.[704,708,709,711] However, in some cases, the only signs of disease may be chorioretinitis and, occasionally, concurrent anterior uveitis.[712]

Clinical signs and tissue involvement can be similar in dogs, with respiratory, neurological, gastrointestinal, or generalized infection.[704] Generalized disease is mainly seen in young (<1 year) dogs.[704] The most apparent clinical signs in older dogs are associated with encephalitis and myositis, and appear very similar to *Neospora caninum* infection,[713] which is more common than toxoplasmosis.

Because of *Toxoplasma*'s opportunistic nature, infection may be associated with other diseases such as distemper or ehrlichiosis in dogs, hemotrophic mycoplasma infection, FIV or feline infectious peritonitis (FIP) in cats, or immunosuppressive therapy in any species.

Diagnosis

Definitive antemorten diagnosis of clinical toxoplasmosis is difficult. The diagnosis should be made based on a fourfold or greater change in antibody titer or high IgM titer, response to anti-*Toxoplasma* therapy, and exclusion of other diagnoses. *Toxoplasma*-specific antibody may also be detected in the aqueous humor or CSF of cats with ocular or neurological signs, respectively, but the titer must be compared with that of a non-ocular or non-neurological pathogen to determine if the antibody was produced locally, as opposed to leakage of antibodies through a compromised blood-ocular barrier or blood-brain barrier.[714] Changes in the CSF of encephalitic cats are inconsistent but may include increased protein and lymphocytic or mixed inflammatory cells.[715]

In acute infection, tachyzoites may rarely be seen in peripheral blood, CSF, or lung or tracheal wash fluid, but are more commonly found in thoracic or abdominal effusions.[704] Detection of the organism in tissues or body fluids can be done using either PCR or bioassays in mice. Due to the potentially high sensitivity of PCR, the test may be positive in both healthy (i.e., latently infected) and diseased cats, and therefore cannot be used to distinguish acute from chronic infection.[704]

Serological testing is commonly used for diagnosis, but there is currently no test that can definitively diagnose toxoplasmosis. An IgM titer of >1:64 by indirect FAT or ELISA, with or without concurrent IgG, or demonstration of seroconversion (fourfold or higher increase IgG as determined by indirect FAT, ELISA, or modified agglutination test), is supportive of active infection.[704]

Serological testing is not useful for determining whether there is a risk of *T. gondii* shedding. Most cats are seronegative during the short period of time they are shedding *T. gondii*. A cat that is seronegative is unlikely to be shedding oocysts at any given time, but poses the most significant public health risk because it is most likely to develop a patent infection and shed large numbers of oocysts over a short period of time if it is exposed to *T.*

gondii. A cat that is IgG seropositive was presumably infected some time in the past and is unlikely to be actively shedding oocysts. If reexposed to the parasite, seropositive cats may shed some oocysts, albeit in low numbers, and thus they remain a potential risk for human exposure.[704] Fecal examination is unreliable because a single negative sample cannot rule out the possibility that the cat is shedding[716] or will do so in the near future.

Fecal examination for oocysts is of limited use since shedding tends to occur for only 1–2 weeks after exposure, and usually occurs in the absence of clinical signs.[704] If present, the oocysts are best detected using a centrifugal fecal flotation technique with Sheather's sugar solution (500 g sugar, 300 mL water, 6.5 g melted phenol crystals).[675] The oocysts are unsporulated with no distinct internal structures and approximately 10 μm in diameter (one-fourth the size of *Isospora* cysts and one-eighth the size of *T. cati* eggs). They are indistinguishable from the oocysts of some species of *Hammondia* and *Besnoitia*, which also occur in cats. Any identified oocysts should be considered *Toxoplasma* until proven otherwise.[675]

Management

Clindamycin is the drug of choice for the treatment of clinical toxoplasmosis in dogs and cats. The dose is higher than is used for treatment of anaerobic bacterial infections and can cause anorexia, vomiting, and diarrhea. A response should be seen within 48 hours, but feline immunodeficiency virus (FIV)-infected cats may be more difficult to treat. Cats with ocular inflammation should be treated either topically (ideally) or systemically with anti-inflammatory doses of glucocorticoids as well. The second-choice treatment for toxoplasmosis is a combination of pyrimethamine and a sulfonamide. Newer macrolides such as azithromycin and clarithromycin also have efficacy against *Toxoplasma*, but their role in treatment is unclear. Doxycycline or minocycline could be considered if there is concurrent infection with an agent susceptible to tetracyclines.[704]

Oocyst shedding in cats is reduced by use of the therapeutic dose of clindamycin,[717] or high doses of a sulfonamide/pyrimethamine combination.[675] Other anticoccidials that can be used for this purpose include monensin and toltrazuril, if given within 1–2 days of exposure or administration of immunosuppressive therapy to the animal (which could cause recrudescence of infection).[704] Routine use of these is not recommended because of the short duration of shedding and the ability to use basic infection control and hygiene measures to reduce the risk of human exposure. An oral vaccine to reduce oocyst shedding in cats has been developed but is not currently commercially available.[705,718,719]

Humans

Clinical presentation

Only 10–15% of human cases of toxoplasmosis are associated with clinical signs.[695,720,721] These are typically mild and include fever, malaise, sore throat, myalgia, and lymphadenopathy.[2,695,721] In some cases, disease may mimic mononucleosis, with macular rash and hepatosplenomegaly.[2] Signs may persist for 1–12 weeks, but the clinical course is typically mild and self-limited. Severe manifestations are very rare in immunocompetent individuals that acquire the infection postnatally, but potential problems include myocarditis, pericarditis, and pneumonitis.[2,676]

Ocular toxoplasmosis can occur with acute infection or reactivation of latent infection. Chorioretinitis is uncommon following clinical toxoplasmosis, occurring in 0.2–0.7% of infections,[695] but this small percentage is not insignificant considering the high rate of infection.[2]

Severe toxoplasmosis is a serious problem in immunocompromised persons, particularly those with AIDS. It is estimated that 4000 AIDS patients develop *Toxoplasma* encephalitis each year in the United States,[695] although this number is decreasing because of highly active antiretroviral therapy.[676] In the past, the condition was estimated to affect up to 40% of AIDS patients worldwide.[676] Most cases are thought to develop from reactivation of latent infections, not new infections,[722] so zoonotic infection from pets is of limited relevance in this population. Individuals with low CD4+ counts (<100 cells/mm^3) and high *Toxoplasma* titers may be treated prophylactically for the disease with trimethoprim–sulfamethoxazole.[722–724]

Clinical signs in congenitally infected neonates are not apparent at birth in the majority of cases

(67–90%), but eye (e.g., blindness, retinochoroiditis), ear (e.g., deafness), and CNS (e.g., mental retardation, learning difficulties, psychomotor deficiencies) problems can develop later.[2,676,706] Approximately 10% of cases result in abortion or neonatal death.[676] If signs of toxoplasmosis are apparent at birth (10–23% of cases), they may include generalized lymphadenopathy, maculopapular rash, hydrocephalus, chorioretinitis, intracranial calcifications (which can also be detected on prenatal ultrasonography), hepatosplenomegaly, thrombocytopenia, microcephaly, convulsions, fever, and small size for gestational age.[2,676,706] Ocular toxoplasmosis may occur in up to one-third of children who survive congenital infection and is the most common manifestation of the disease in these individuals.[676] It is possible for a person to develop clinical toxoplasmosis from a congenital infection up to 20–30 years of age.[706] Congenital toxoplasmosis has been estimated to occur in 1:1000 to 1:10,000 live births in the United States.[2]

Diagnosis

Once infected with *T. gondii*, people usually develop an antibody titer that lasts indefinitely,[721] possibly because the tissue cysts that form also persist for the lifetime of the host. Therefore, serological testing is a reliable indicator of previous exposure. Severely immunocompromised individuals may be unable to mount or sustain an appropriate humoral immune response, and serological testing is less reliable in this subgroup.

Serological testing is the main component of diagnosis, but results must be interpreted carefully because of the high seroprevalence in the population. Serum IgG titers typically indicate previous infection and therefore are of limited use for diagnosis of acute infection or reactivation of latent infection. Serum IgM titers are an important component of diagnosis since they indicate more recent, acute infection. Both types of antibodies are usually detectable within 1–2 weeks of infection.[706] If IgG is present without IgM, then infection likely took place 6–12 months earlier.[2,706] The avidity of the IgG can also be measured, and this is used in situations where the determination of the timing of infection is critical (e.g., infection of a pregnant woman). The presence of high avidity IgG indicates that the infection likely took place 3–4 months

prior to testing.[2,706] Further identification of timing can sometimes be accomplished by testing for IgE and IgA, both of which decline faster than IgM.[2]

Diagnosis of in utero infection is most commonly accomplished by testing amniotic fluid for the presence of *T. gondii* DNA by PCR or by isolation of the parasite by mouse inoculation or tissue culture.[2,706] Testing of fetal blood (by cordocentesis) is less sensitive and a higher-risk procedure.[706] If test results are positive, ultrasonography should be used to check the fetus for abnormalities such as intracerebral calcifications, microcephaly, hydrocephalus, or excessively small size, which are consistent with toxoplasmosis.[706]

Congenital toxoplasmosis can present in several ways: severe neonatal disease, disease presenting over the first few months of life, disease (either as the sequelae of infection or relapse) presenting in later childhood or adolescence, and subclinical disease. The challenge is recognizing subclinical disease in infants as toxoplasmosis can cause later, potentially devastating, sequelae including CNS abnormalities and eye lesions. Diagnosis is confirmed by the isolation of *T. gondii* in blood (from the infant or cord blood) or tissue, including the placenta. PCR of peripheral white blood cells, CSF, or placenta is also an option. It should be noted that PCR testing for *T. gondii* has not been standardized. There is no universal protocol regarding when, or whether, to screen pregnant women or women considering becoming pregnant. In some countries, pregnant women are regularly screened during gestation to detect infection and allow for early intervention.[706,725] In others, screening may be sporadic or rare. Regardless of the approach to screening, general preventive measures outlined below are the key for reducing the risk of infection during pregnancy.

Management

Most clinical infections in immunocompetent persons are mild and self-limited, and do not require treatment.[2] Treatment is most often considered in pregnant women or immunocompromised individuals. Antimicrobials, if used, are directed against tachyzoites and do not eradicate encysted bradyzoites.[725] Pyrimethamine is considered to be the most effective agent and should be included as part of the treatment in adults,[725] usually in combination with sulfadiazine and folinic acid.[706,721] Combination of pyrimethamine and clindamycin is another option.[725] Other drugs such as azithromycin, clarithromycin, atovaquone, dapsone, and trimethoprim–sulfamethoxazole can be considered, but their role in treatment is unclear.[725,726]

Spiramycin is one of the current drugs of choice for treatment of pregnant women with toxoplasmosis to reduce the risk of transmission to the fetus.[706,721] It is ineffective for acute therapy, maintenance therapy, or prevention of *Toxoplasma* encephalitis in AIDS patients.[725] It has been suggested that such treatment decreases the severity of congenital toxoplasmosis, but not the risk of transmission,[727] yet there is evidence to support both possibilities.[676,728] It remains unknown if treatment of a pregnant woman reduces transmission, reduces congenital disease, or reduces long-term sequelae in vertically infected children; the cost-effectiveness of such therapy is often debated. Early treatment of prenatally infected children has been shown to reduce or prevent long-term sequelae later in life.[676]

Prevention

In the majority of studies, no direct association has been found between cat ownership and clinical toxoplasmosis. However, cats are the primary definitive host for this organism, serious disease can occur in humans, and some studies have implicated contact with cats as a risk factor for exposure, so consideration of the possible risks is warranted. Given the emotional benefits associated with owning a cat, and the minimal risk of transmission if appropriate hygiene is practiced, even pregnant and immunocompromised individuals do not need to give up their cats. If a cat in a household with a naive pregnant woman or other high-risk individual is found to be shedding oocysts, it could be removed from the premises temporarily and either treated to eliminate shedding or monitored to determine when shedding ceases naturally.[675] As cats are usually meticulous groomers, it is very unlikely that oocysts will be found on their fur, so regular handling is not a significant risk.[675] Care should be taken with debilitated cats that are unable to groom themselves adequately and long-haired cats that might be more prone to fecal staining of perineal hair.

Measures should be taken to reduce the risk of exposure of cats to *T. gondii* and thus decrease the risk that they become infected and shed oocysts. The two main measures that can be used are keeping cats inside so they do not ingest infected small prey and not feeding them raw meat.[675,729]

Avoiding contact with old (as opposed to fresh) cat feces that may contain sporulated oocysts is critical. Oocysts take longer to sporulate under cooler conditions. At room temperature, sporulation may occur within 1–3 days, but this can take 3 weeks at 11°C.[675] Litter box management is a critical component of avoiding exposure to *T. gondii* from pet cats. Ideally, feces should be removed from litter boxes on a daily basis to prevent sporulation of oocysts. This is particularly true in households with seronegative women (or women of unknown serological status) who are pregnant or may become pregnant, as well as households with immunocompromised individuals. Litter boxes should not be cleaned by high-risk people if possible, but the lack of someone else to clean the litter box should not be taken as an indication that cat ownership is inappropriate. If a high-risk person must handle used litter or feces, gloves should be worn and hands should be washed thoroughly immediately after completing the task.[729] Litter boxes, scoops, and any other objects or surfaces that have come in contact with cat feces should, on a regular basis, be thoroughly cleaned and immersed in hot water (>70°C).[676] This must not be done in kitchen or washroom sinks. Chemical disinfection can be achieved but requires high concentrations of chemicals such as ammonia (5% ammonia for at least 1 hour or 10% ammonia for at least 10 minutes)[675] and may not be practical.

Cat feces or contaminated cat litter should not be composted because backyard composting may not produce sufficient heat to destroy oocysts.

Other measures to reduce the risk of *T. gondii* exposure include proper cooking of meat, use of appropriate food handling procedures, washing vegetables thoroughly, restricting cats from having access to sandboxes by keeping sandboxes covered when not in use, and good attention to hand hygiene after working in gardens or flower beds.[675,676,729]

Once sporulated, oocysts can survive in the environment for prolonged periods of time and are highly resistant to environmental effects and disinfectants.[675] Sporulated oocysts can survive up to 4.5 years in water at 4°C, up to 18 months in moist soil or sand, and at least 200 days in water at 10–25°C.[676]

In any species other than cats, *T. gondii* infection is not patent. However, it is possible for sporulated oocysts from cat feces to survive passage through the intestine of a dog. Dogs that eat cat feces could therefore have infective oocysts in their feces,[730] but given the extremely low incidence of *Toxoplasma* oocysts in dog feces,[689] the risk is probably inconsequential.

There is a small risk of oocyst shedding in any cat that may be immunosuppressed due to illness or medication, and greater care should perhaps be taken with this group. Keeping the cat inside, not feeding it raw meat, and proper litter box management largely negate the potential added risks.

Trichuris vulpis

The canine whipworm, *T. vulpis*, is a nematode that is found in dogs, foxes, and coyotes, where it can cause disease ranging from inapparent to severe bloody diarrhea. Whipworm eggs can be found in the feces of 0–23% of healthy dogs.[157,158,537,634]

Adult whipworms live mainly in the cecum, but may also be present in the distal small intestine or colon. Unembryonated eggs are laid and passed with feces. Eggs embryonate and become infective in 1–2 months. After ingestion by a susceptible host, larvae hatch in the small intestine, migrate further along the intestinal tract, and mature, thereby completing the life cycle.

There are few reports of human infections with *T. vulpis*.[731–736] One report described infection of 19 individuals, all of whom had mental illness or physical disabilities.[733] Another described detection of *T. vulpis* from two children from urban slums in India.[736] Both had abdominal pain and one had diarrhea. Severe diarrhea and detection of *T. vulpis* eggs were reported in a woman who owned multiple dogs, though apparently, her dogs were not tested for whipworms to determine if they may have been the source of infection.[731] Adult *T. vulpis* were identified incidentally in the cecum of a person in a postmortem examination.[735] *T. vulpis* eggs were also identified in 6.1% of healthy individuals in an Indian ethnic group.[737] There are also rare reports of VLM attributed to *T. vulpis*.[738,739] However, in one of these reports, the two individuals had "almost asymptomatic" infections, and diagnosis was based on immunoelectrophoretic studies[739] with the accuracy of diagnosis having been challenged.[740]

In none of these reports was the source of the infection clearly identified. Given the time required for eggs to become infective, inadvertent ingestion of eggs from contaminated environmental surfaces is most likely. *T. vulpis* eggs can be found in the soil in various environmental sites, including playgrounds.[10,356]

Diagnosis is based on the identification of characteristic eggs in feces by centrifugal fecal flotation.[731] Eggs must be measured when evaluating human specimens, since eggs from the human whipworm, *Trichuris trichiura*, have a similar appearance to *T. vulpis*, but are smaller (50–56 by 21–26 μm for *T. trichiura* compared with 72–89 by 37–40 μm for *T. vulpis*) (Figure 1.16).[731] Misidentification of *T. vulpis* as *T. trichiura* in human feces is possible if adequate care is not taken by the microscopist.[731]

Care should be taken in extrapolating the limited reports of human infections in specific populations (e.g., slum residents, institutionalized individuals, certain ethnic groups) to the broader population. *T. vulpis* is likely of limited zoonotic risk given the small number of reports and the rarity of clinical infections. Nevertheless, these

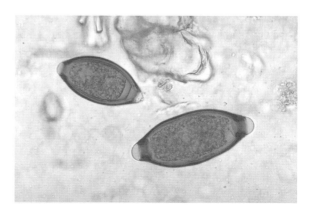

Figure 1.16 Eggs of *Trichuris trichiura* (left) and *T. vulpis* (right) (public domain, Centers for Disease Control and Prevention).

reports indicate that some thought should be given to this parasite as a potential cause of human infection. Measures taken to avoid infection from other, more relevant gastrointestinal parasites, particularly avoiding contact with feces and hand hygiene, would be effective at reducing any risk that might be present from *Trichuris* spp. Routine deworming with milbemycin, milbemycin/lufenuron, or fenbendazole, febantel, or oxantel is effective at controlling *T. vulpis* in dogs. Prompt removal of feces will help reduce the prevalence of infective eggs in the environment.

Tritrichomonas foetus

Introduction/life cycle

T. foetus is a trichomonad parasite that is an emerging cause of enteric disease in cats.[741] It is characterized morphologically by three anterior flagella and a single recurrent flagellum that acts as an undulating membrane.[296,742] Reproduction occurs in the intestinal tract by binary fission, and there is no cyst stage.[296] In addition to cats and cattle, *T. foetus* can be found in many other animal species, including pigs and rarely dogs.[743,744]

Geographic distribution/epidemiology

T. foetus shedding and disease can be common in cats in breeding colonies and shelters, with reported prevalences of 0–31%.[322,745,746] Dense housing is likely the most important risk factor.[296,322] Purebred cats are often overrepresented,[296,747] but this is more likely a function of housing and management rather than a true breed predisposition. Colonization is rare in nondiarrheic household cats.[746,748] Transmission is via the fecal–oral route, with the litter box a prime source of infection of cats.[741]

Animals

Clinical presentation

Diarrhea is more common in younger (<1 year of age) cats,[749–751] and is mainly large bowel in character, with occasional blood and mucus.[749] Chronic diarrhea is common.

Diagnosis

Diagnosis requires specialized methods. Routine fecal flotation is not adequate for diagnosis. Microscopic evaluation of fecal wet mounts in saline has a poor sensitivity and can also result in misdiagnosis of *Giardia* as *T. foetus*. Culture of feces in specialized media followed by microscopic evaluation of the sample can be a sensitive and specific test if performed properly and is commonly used.[752] PCR has excellent sensitivity and specificity with a lower detection threshold than culture.[322] Cost and availability are the main current limitations.

Management

While up to 90% of cats with *T. foetus* diarrhea will resolve without treatment, they may continue to shed the organism for prolonged periods of time, potentially for life.[741] Ronidazole is the drug of choice and is usually administered because, while spontaneous resolution of clinical signs is common, it may take up to 2 years.[753] Care must be taken since ronidazole administration can be associated with adverse neurological effects.[296] Even with clinically successful treatment, persistent shedding of *T. foetus* is common[753] with one study reporting a median posttreatment shedding duration of 39 months.[753]

Humans

The broad range of animal species that *T. foetus* can infect and the close association between people and pet cats has raised questions about the potential for zoonotic transmission.[741,754] However, the risk of transmission of *T. foetus* from cats to humans (or at least transmission with the development of clinical disease) is presumably very low because of the apparent rarity of human infections and lack of reported cases of transmission of *T. foetus* from a cat to a person. There is a report of detection of "*T. foetus*-like organisms" from a bronchoalveolar lavage sample of a person with AIDS and *Pneumocystis* pneumonia.[754] The role of the *T. foetus*-like organism in disease was unclear, and there was no reported link to animals. While the potential for zoonotic transmission should not be dismissed, there is limited evidence indicating any risk.

Prevention

Routine screening of cats for *T. foetus* shedding is difficult to justify from a zoonotic disease prevention standpoint considering the extremely low incidence of human disease and the low prevalence of shedding by healthy pet cats. Detection of *T. foetus* in nondiarrheic animals is also challenging, and optimal recovery is obtained by inducing diarrhea in the cat by pretreating with lactulose.[741] Given the low likelihood of zoonotic risk and the potential for environmental or hair coat contamination with various pathogens from induced diarrhea, this is not recommended. Even if a cat was shedding *T. foetus* and if a susceptible person was in the household, the main recommendation would be to avoid direct and indirect contact with feces through proper litter box management and other general infection control measures, the same approach that should be taken in any household. There is no evidence that treatment of carriers is indicated. Even in a household with an immunocompromised owner, the need for treatment of a nondiarrheic cat is debatable, as many other potentially zoonotic pathogens could still be shed in feces and the approach to management of the cat in the household would not change. Because *T. foetus* does not have a cyst stage, it is very susceptible to environmental conditions, particularly drying. Therefore, the highest risk in terms of feces containing *T. foetus* is wet diarrheic stool or fresh, wet feces.

Trypanosoma cruzi

Introduction

T. cruzi is a protozoal parasite and the cause of Chagas' disease (also known as American trypanosomiasis). Humans and dogs are accidental hosts and are not required for maintenance of the transmission cycle, but infections in both are common. It is a leading cause of cardiomyopathy in humans and has a greater disease burden than any other parasite in the New World.[755] It is also a cause of cardiomyopathy in dogs.[756] The overwhelming majority of human infections are not associated with dogs; however, dogs can be part of the transmission cycle.

Etiology

There are approximately 20 different *Trypanosoma* species, all of which are flagellated protozoa that pass through different morphological stages in their vertebrate and insect hosts.[757] *T. cruzi* is adapted to infect a wild range of hosts, including more than 150 wild and domestic mammal species.[757] This, combined with the ability to produce long-term (including lifelong) parasitemia, creates the opportunity for the development of a large reservoir.

Life cycle

There are three morphological forms. The trypomastigote is found in circulation in the host. It is 15–20 μm long, with a flattened, spindle-shaped body (Figure 1.17). The amastigote form is the intracellular form. It is smaller (1.5–4.0 μm) and roughly spheroid.[756] The epimastigote is the third form and is found in the reduviid insect vector (subfamily Tritominae).[756] These large (up to 2.5 cm in length) insects, commonly known as "kissing bugs" or "assassin bugs" in South America, become infected by ingesting circulating trypomastigotes from infected humans or animals. In the insect, trypomastigotes transform to epimastigotes and multiply by binary fission before transforming back into metacyclic trypomastigotes in the insect's hindgut.[756] In humans, infection typically occurs

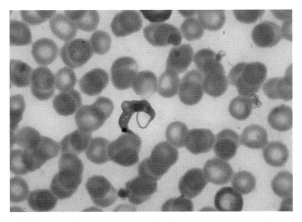

Figure 1.17 *Trypanosoma cruzi* (public domain, Centers for Disease Control and Prevention).

when the insect vector deposits feces containing trypomastigotes at the bite site.[756] The individual becomes infected by rubbing contaminated insect feces into the bite wound or by transferring it to the mucous membranes of the eyes or mouth.[2] Transfusion of infected blood is another possible route, as is organ transplantation.[2,757] Transplacental infection occurs in approximately 5% of infants born to infected mothers.[757] Laboratory-acquired infections can also occur from needlestick injuries involving blood from an infected subject.[758,759] Outbreaks have also been described in association with the consumption of sugarcane juice and the consumption of Acai palm fruit juice or paste. The presumption is that infected insect vectors were inadvertently crushed and mixed into the juice during production.[760]

Dogs can be infected similarly, including by ingestion of infected vectors, with release of the parasite in the mouth.[756] Infection from ingestion of infected meat has been considered, but evidence from raccoons fed infected meat suggests that this route is unimportant.[761] The greater role of ingestion of insects in canine infections compared with human infections means that there can be disproportionate prevalences of infection in humans and dogs in certain regions. Specifically, in areas where insect vectors tend not to defecate shortly after feeding and are therefore at lower risk of causing bite-associated infections, canine infections (from ingesting insects) may be much more common than human infections.

Regardless of the route of entry, trypomastigotes either enter macrophages where they transform to amastigotes and multiply by binary fission, or remain free in circulation.[756] Circulating trypomastigotes may infect myocardial cells, where they transform into amastigotes, multiply, transform back to trypomastigotes, and are released back into circulation following myocardial cell rupture.[756]

Geographic distribution/epidemiology

This parasite is endemic in many regions in South and Central America, and appears to be increasing in Mexico.[756,762] It is estimated that 8 million people are infected in the Americas.[763] Large numbers of infected people have been identified in the United States, but the overwhelming majority is associated with travel to or immigration from endemic regions

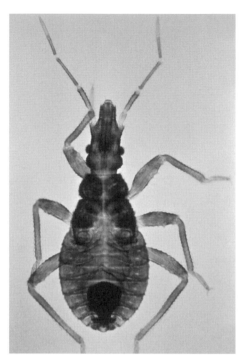

Figure 1.18   *Triatoma infestans*, a vector for *Trypanosoma cruzi* (public domain, Centers for Disease Control and Prevention, and World Health Organization, Geneva, Switzerland).

(or previously via transfusion of contaminated blood). It has been estimated that over 300,000 people with *T. cruzi* infection live in the United States, with 30,000–450,000 cases of cardiomyopathy and 63–315 congenital infections occurring annually.[763] Only a small number of autochthonous infections have been identified in the United States, such as a case that occurred in New Orleans in 2006 after an influx of vectors following hurricane Katrina.[764] There is a similar distribution of canine cases, with endemic infection in regions of Central and South America, increasing reports in Mexico,[762,765] and sporadic cases in the United States, most often in southeastern Texas.[766–770] Infected dogs have been identified in other parts of the United States,[771,772] including as far north as Virginia.[773]

The geographic distribution is largely related to the presence of competent insect vectors and susceptible hosts in close proximity. Social aspects also play a role, particularly keeping animals in houses. Three insect species, *Triatoma infestans* (Figure 1.18), *Triatoma dimidiata*, and *Rhodnius prolixus*, are the main vectors based on their propensity to feed off both animals and people, live in close proximity to humans, defecate soon after taking a meal, and reproduce prolifically.[756,774] There are a few probable reasons why autochthonous transmission is rare in most of the United States. The two main potential vectors, *Triatoma protracta* and *Triatoma sanguisuga*, have lower infection rates than corresponding vectors in other regions, and they tend to defecate 20 minutes after feeding, by which time they have left the animal host.[756,775] Differences in housing, with less cohabitation of people with multiple animal species, and routine use of measures to avoid insect bites also play a role.[756] Climate is also important, because insect activity decreases at cooler temperatures, and the vectors cease developing and feeding below 16–18°C.[776]

Seroprevalence or parasitemia rates are highly variable (0–83%) in dogs in endemic regions,[404,762,765,777–782] although disease rates are low since most infected dogs do not develop clinical disease.[783] Studies of pet and stray dogs from southern U.S. states have reported seropositivity in 2–4.7%,[784,785] more often in dogs with known contact with wild mammalian hosts.[784] Coinfection with other vector-borne pathogens such as *D. immitis* can occur.[786] Less information is available regarding cats, in part because cats are less commonly present in households in endemic regions. Cats can become infected, and feline seroprevalence rates of up to 42% have been reported.[777,778,787] Little information about clinical disease is available.

The role of dogs in human infection is poorly quantified, and identification of the risks posed by one species in a pathogen with a complex cycle involving many potential reservoir hosts is difficult. Regardless, it is suspected that domestic animals, including dogs, play a crucial role in *T. cruzi* transmission in developing countries, particularly in rural regions with poor housing standards and cohabitation with other species like chickens.[779,780,788,789] Chickens, while not susceptible to infection themselves, can encourage the presence of the insect vector. The presence of infected dogs has been associated with a much greater likelihood that infected insect vectors are also present in the household.[779,780,788] As well, a correlation between the presence of infected dogs and infected humans has been reported.[762] The risks are probably highly variable geographically even within endemic regions, and dogs probably play a limited role in human infection in some endemic areas, particularly urban areas.[782]

The risks associated with pet dogs in developed countries are probably minimal because of housing and hygiene standards. Risks may be greater in areas with less insect control, where many dogs live closely with people and where other animals are also living in the house. The potential role of dogs in *T. cruzi* transmission has been modeled using households in rural Argentina, in households where people, dogs, and chickens cohabitated and where people slept outdoors during a part of the year.[789] This model indicated that keeping two infected domestic dogs was the worst thing people could do in terms of promoting the prevalence of *T. cruzi*. It also reported that eliminating infected dogs from the household was nearly sufficient for eliminating *T. cruzi* transmission, in the absence of reintroduction of infected dogs, children, or insects. Similar data are not available for other household situations, and the risk of dog–human transmission is presumably lower in the absence of conditions such as those that were modeled. The serious nature of the infection and difficulty of treating infected individuals means that the potential for transmission from dogs should not be ignored, even if the risk is low.

Animals

Clinical presentation

The acute phase of infection is characterized by vague signs such as lethargy, lymphadenopathy and weakness, or overt signs of right-sided heart failure.[790] Sudden death may be the only sign in some cases, particularly in dogs less than 1 year of age.[768,790] Neurological abnormalities, including ataxia, profound weakness, and hyperreflexia, have been found in natural and experimental infections.

The acute stage may not be identified and an unknown percentage of dogs surviving acute infection will progress to the chronic stage, which progresses over 1 or more years.[756] Cardiomyopathy with associated lethargy, ascites, arrhythmias, and heart failure may develop in chronic cases.[768,769] Sudden death may occur.[790]

Diagnosis

Diagnosis is difficult and may be missed if trypanosomiasis is not considered. This disease should be considered in any dog that has ever lived in or near an endemic region.[756] During acute infection trypomastigotes may be seen on blood smears. Parasitemia levels are often low, and the the parasite may not be seen without careful observation or the use of special techniques. Examination of the buffy coat stained with Wright's or Giemsa's stain is more sensitive than blood smear examination.[756] There are also techniques for centrifugation of plasma that can concentrate trypomastigotes. PCR, best done on concentrated samples, is available. Occasionally, trypomastigotes can be seen on lymph node aspirates or from abdominal effusion.

Serology is useful and, in combination with appropriate clinical signs, is considered the gold standard.[790] However, cross-reaction with *Leishmania* is a problem in areas that these two pathogens overlap, and further exploration in positive cases is required to interpret seropositive results. Xenodiagnosis, testing of insect vectors that have fed from the animal's blood for the presence of trypomastigotes, can also be performed.[777]

Management

Treatment of the acute phase is difficult, and little objective information is available, partly because this stage is uncommonly recognized. A combination of corticosteroids and benznidazole can be used.[756] Most cases are identified in the chronic stage, but treatment of this stage is rarely successful. Supportive therapy for heart failure and arrhythmia is the mainstay of treatment. Euthanasia is often elected because of the poor prognosis and advanced state of disease by the time a diagnosis is made.

Humans

Clinical presentation

Acute and chronic forms of disease may be present, with the acute form often not being recognized. In acute infection, a red nodule (chagoma) that becomes indurated and later, hypopigmented, may develop at the site of infection, usually on the face or arms.[2,757] If the conjunctiva is the site of inoculation, firm eyelid edema (Romana's sign) may be present. Fever, malaise, and generalized lymphadenopathy may then occur. Muscles, including myocardial muscle, are the most heavily parasitized tissues.[757] Rarely, myocarditis, hepatosplenomegaly, or meningoencephalitis is seen. In most patients, the acute phase of the disease resolves in 1–3 months and an asymptomatic (indeterminate) period follows.[2] In 10–30% of cases, chronic disease develops over the course of years to decades, most often presenting with cardiomyopathy, megaesophagus, or megacolon.[2,757] There seems to be a wide variation in the incidence and types of severe sequelae among different regions.[757] Cardiomyopathy is the most common and concerning sequela and may lead to embolic disease, intractable congestive heart failure, complete heart block, and other arrhythmias including ventricular arrhythmias leading to sudden death. Congenital infections are usually asymptomatic but can result in low birth weight, hepatosplenomegaly, and/or meningitis.[2] Reactivation of latent infection can occur in people that become immunosuppressed, and the disease may be more severe than is typically encountered otherwise.[2,757] The incidence of this is unknown.[757]

Diagnosis

During the acute phase of infection, *T. cruzi* may be detected using Giemsa staining of blood smears, buffy coat preparation, or after a concentration technique.[2] The indeterminate and chronic phases have low-level parasitemia and detection requires the use of special media, with negative results being common. Isolation of *T. cruzi* from a triatomine insect that has been allowed to feed on patient blood (xenodiagnosis) is sometimes performed in South and Central America.[2] Because of the low level of sensitivity of these procedures, serological testing is the primary test for chronic disease.

Management

Current treatment options are far from ideal. Nifurtimox can reduce the duration and severity of disease and decrease mortality, but it only results in parasitological cure (complete elimination of *T. cruzi*) in approximately 70% of cases and can have severe adverse effects.[757] Benznidazole has similar efficacy and is viewed as the drug of choice in some Latin American countries.[757]

Treatment of acute infections should be initiated as soon as possible, including prophylactically, following needlestick injury or laboratory exposure that has a reasonable likelihood of having transmitted *T. cruzi*.[757] There has been considerable debate as to whether to treat chronic or indeterminate asymptomatic infections. Current expert consensus now is to treat, despite no clear evidence that outcomes are improved.[757]

Prevention

There are two main considerations for reducing the risk of dogs as sources of human infection. One is the role of dogs as a reservoir for *T. cruzi* and attractor of insect vectors. Keeping dogs out of the house has been recommended as an important human disease control measure, as dogs can both act as a reservoir of infection and attract the insects.[789] It is important to recognize that modeling data that have identified this as a control measure used the scenario of rural households in developing countries with people, dogs, and chickens living in the house,[789] so extrapolation to having pets in households under different circumstances should be done with caution.

The other main consideration is the potential for occupational infection in veterinary or laboratory personnel handling blood from infected dogs.[2,756,785] Sharps handling practices are often lax in veterinary medicine,[791] and while transmission via needlestick injuries involving dog blood have not been reported, there is no reason to suspect that those would be different from needlesticks involving humans or laboratory animals, both of which are known to be able to transmit *T. cruzi*.[2,758,759] Good sharps handling practices must be used at all times but with particular care in areas where *T. cruzi* is endemic and where infection is suspected. Other general measures to reduce the risk of exposure to blood, such as the use of appropriate contact precautions when dealing with bleeding animals or procedures that might result in blood, should also be used. Any needlestick injury that might have resulted in inoculation of blood from an infected dog should result in prompt consultation with an infectious disease physician.

Other measures for the reduction of *T. cruzi* transmission include control of insect vector populations (e.g., insecticide spraying), measures to exclude insects from the house (e.g., screens), and screening blood donors from endemic areas.[777,789] Insect control has been shown to have a dramatic impact on the incidence of disease in dogs in endemic areas.[777,779]

References

1. Maguire JH. Intestinal nematodes. In: Mandell GL, Bennett JE, Dolin R, eds. *Principles and Practice of Infectious Diseases*. Philadelphia: Elsevier, 2005, pp. 3260–3267.
2. American Academy of Pediatrics. *Red Book: 2009 Report of the Committee on Infectious Diseases*, 28th ed. Elk Grove Village, IL: American Academy of Pediatrics, 2009.
3. Crompton DWT. Ascaris lumbricoides. In: Scott ME, Smith GA, eds. *Parasitic and Infectious Diseases*. London: Academic, 1994, pp. 175–196.
4. Okaeme AN. Canine and human gastrointestinal helminthiasis of the Kainji Lake area, Nigeria. *Int J Zoonoses* 1985;12:241–246.
5. Holland CV. Predisposition to ascariasis: patterns, mechanisms and implications. *Parasitology* 2009;136: 1537–1547.
6. Roldán WH, Espinoza YA, Huapaya PE, et al. Frequency of human toxocariasis in a rural population from Cajamarca, Peru determined by DOT-ELISA test. *Rev Inst Med Trop Sao Paulo* 2009;51: 67–71.
7. Traub RJ, Robertson ID, Irwin P, et al. The role of dogs in transmission of gastrointestinal parasites in a remote tea-growing community in northeastern India. *Am J Trop Med Hyg* 2002;67:539–545.
8. Jacobsen KH, Ribeiro PS, Quist BK, et al. Prevalence of intestinal parasites in young Quichua children in the highlands of rural Ecuador. *J Health Popul Nutr* 2007;25:399–405.
9. Knopp S, Mohammed KA, Simba Khamis I, et al. Spatial distribution of soil-transmitted helminths, including *Strongyloides stercoralis*, among children in Zanzibar. *Geospatial Health* 2008;3:47–56.
10. Umeche N. Helminth ova in soil from children's playgrounds in Calabar, Nigeria. *Cent Afr J Med* 1989;35:432–434.
11. Motazedian H, Mehrabani D, Tabatabaee SH, et al. Prevalence of helminth ova in soil samples from

public places in Shiraz. *East Mediterr Health J* 2006;12: 562–565.

12. Seah SK, Hucal G, Law C. Dogs and intestinal parasites: a public health problem. *CMAJ* 1975;112: 1191–1194.

13. Joshi BN, Sabne SS, Kalkadkar RK. Intestinal helminthic infections in stray dogs: a public health problem. *Indian J Public Health* 1977;21:34–37.

14. Shalaby HA, Abdel-Shafy S, Derbala AA. The role of dogs in transmission of *Ascaris lumbricoides* for humans. *Parasitol Res* 2010;106:1021–1026.

15. Kirwan P, Asaolu SO, Abiona TC, et al. Soil-transmitted helminth infections in Nigerian children aged 0–25 months. *J Helminthol* 2009;83: 261–266.

16. Mwangi TW, Bethony JM, Brooker S. Malaria and helminth interactions in humans: an epidemiological viewpoint. *Ann Trop Med Parasitol* 2006;100: 551–570.

17. Maizels RM, Yazdanbakhsh M. Immune regulation by helminth parasites: cellular and molecular mechanisms. *Nat Rev Immunol* 2003;3:733–744.

18. Keiser J, Utzinger J. Efficacy of current drugs against soil-transmitted helminth infections: systematic review and meta-analysis. *JAMA* 2008;299: 1937–1948.

19. Galvan-Ramirez ML, Rivera N, Loeza ME, et al. Nitazoxanide in the treatment of *Ascaris lumbricoides* in a rural zone of Colima, Mexico. *J Helminthol* 2007;81:255–259.

20. St Georgiev V. Pharmacotherapy of ascariasis. *Expert Opin Pharmacother* 2001;2:223–239.

21. Gavin PJ, Kazacos KR, Shulman ST. Baylisascariasis. *Clin Microbiol Rev* 2005;18:703–718.

22. Eberhard ML, Nace EK, Won KY, et al. *Baylisascaris procyonis* in the metropolitan Atlanta area. *Emerg Infect Dis* 2003;9:1636–1637.

23. Moore L, Ash L, Sorvillo F, et al. *Baylisascaris procyonis* in California. *Emerg Infect Dis* 2004;10: 1693–1694.

24. Sexsmith JL, Whiting TL, Green C, et al. Prevalence and distribution of *Baylisascaris procyonis* in urban raccoons (*Procyon lotor*) in Winnipeg, Manitoba. *Can Vet J* 2009;50:846–850.

25. Souza MJ, Ramsay EC, Patton S, et al. *Baylisascaris procyonis* in raccoons (*Procyon lotor*) in eastern Tennessee. *J Wildl Dis* 2009;45:1231–1234.

26. Yeitz JL, Gillin CM, Bildfell RJ, et al. Prevalence of *Baylisascaris procyonis* in raccoons (*Procyon lotor*) in Portland, Oregon, USA. *J Wildl Dis* 2009;45:14–18.

27. Ching HL, Leighton BJ, Stephen C. Intestinal parasites of raccoons (*Procyon lotor*) from southwest British Columbia. *Can J Vet Res* 2000;64:107–111.

28. Bauer C, Gey A. Efficacy of six anthelmintics against luminal stages of *Baylisascaris procyonis* in naturally

infected raccoons (*Procyon lotor*). *Vet Parasitol* 1995;60:155–159.

29. Sato H, Kamiya H, Furuoka H. Epidemiological aspects of the first outbreak of *Baylisascaris procyonis* larva migrans in rabbits in Japan. *J Vet Med Sci* 2003;65:453–457.

30. Evans RH. *Baylisascaris procyonis* (Nematoda: Ascaridoidea) eggs in raccoon (*Procyon lotor*) latrine scats in Orange County, California. *J Parasitol* 2002;88:189–190.

31. Page LK, Anchor C, Luy E, et al. Backyard raccoon latrines and risk for *Baylisascaris procyonis* transmission to humans. *Emerg Infect Dis* 2009;15:1530–1531.

32. Roussere GP, Murray WJ, Raudenbush CB, et al. Raccoon roundworm eggs near homes and risk for larva migrans disease, California communities. *Emerg Infect Dis* 2003;9:1516–1522.

33. Chorazy ML, Richardson DJ. A survey of environmental contamination with ascarid ova, Wallingford, Connecticut. *Vector Borne Zoonotic Dis* 2005;5:33–39.

34. Sorvillo F, Ash LR, Berlin OG, et al. *Baylisascaris procyonis*: an emerging helminthic zoonosis. *Emerg Infect Dis* 2002;8:355–359.

35. Pai PJ, Blackburn BG, Kazacos KR, et al. Full recovery from *Baylisascaris procyonis* eosinophilic meningitis. *Emerg Infect Dis* 2007;13:928–930.

36. Park SY, Glaser C, Murray WJ, et al. Raccoon roundworm (*Baylisascaris procyonis*) encephalitis: case report and field investigation. *Pediatrics* 2000;106:E56.

37. Wise ME, Sorvillo FJ, Shafir SC, et al. Severe and fatal central nervous system disease in humans caused by *Baylisascaris procyonis*, the common roundworm of raccoons: a review of current literature. *Microbes Infect* 2005;7:317–323.

38. Rudmann DG, Kazacos KR, Storandt ST, et al. *Baylisascaris procyonis* larva migrans in a puppy: a case report and update for the veterinarian. *J Am Anim Hosp Assoc* 1996;32:73–76.

39. Thomas JS. Encephalomyelitis in a dog caused by *Baylisascaris* infection. *Vet Pathol* 1988;25:94–95.

40. Windsor RC, Sturges BK, Vernau KM, et al. Cerebrospinal fluid eosinophilia in dogs. *J Vet Intern Med* 2009;23:275–281.

41. Murray WJ, Kazacos KR. Raccoon roundworm encephalitis. *Clin Infect Dis* 2004;39:1484–1492.

42. Sato H, Furuoka H, Kamiya H. First outbreak of *Baylisascaris procyonis* larva migrans in rabbits in Japan. *Parasitol Int* 2002;51:105–108.

43. Sato H, Une Y, Kawakami S, et al. Fatal *Baylisascaris* larva migrans in a colony of Japanese macaques kept by a safari-style zoo in Japan. *J Parasitol* 2005;91:716–719.

44. Wolf KN, Lock B, Carpenter JW, et al. *Baylisascaris procyonis* infection in a Moluccan cockatoo (*Cacatua moluccensis*). *J Avian Med Surg* 2007;21:220–225.

45. Craig SJ, Conboy GA, Hanna PE. *Baylisascaris* sp. infection in a guinea pig. *Lab Anim Sci* 1995; 45:312–314.

46. Dangoudoubiyam S, Vemulapalli R, Kazacos KR. PCR assays for detection of *Baylisascaris procyonis* eggs and larvae. *J Parasitol* 2009;95:571–577.

47. Companion Animal Parasite Council. *Roundworm (Ascarid)*. Bel Air, MD: Companion Animal Parasite Council, 2009.

48. Bowman DD, Ulrich MA, Gregory DE, et al. Treatment of *Baylisascaris procyonis* infections in dogs with milbemycin oxime. *Vet Parasitol* 2005;129:285–290.

49. Arther RG. Mites and lice: biology and control. *Vet Clin North Am Small Anim Pract* 2009;39:1159–1171, vii.

50. Scott DW, Horn RT. Zoonotic dermatoses of dogs and cats. *Vet Clin North Am Small Anim Pract* 1987;17:117–144.

51. Davis GB, Kyle MG. *Cheyletiella yasguri* infestation of a dog. *N Z Vet J* 1969;17:136.

52. Dodd K. *Cheyletiella yasguri*: widespread infestation in a breeding kennel. *Vet Rec* 1970;86:346–347.

53. Du Plessis RS. A review of the parasitic status of *Cheyletiella parasitivorax* (Acarina: Trombidoidea) with special reference to cases in dogs and man in South Africa. *J S Afr Vet Med Assoc* 1972;43: 305–308.

54. Skirnisson K, Olafsson JH, Finnsdottir H. Dermatitis in cats and humans caused by *Cheyletiella* mites reported in Iceland. *Laeknabladid* 1997;83:30–34.

55. Thomsett LR. Mite infestations of man contracted from dogs and cats. *Br Med J* 1968;3:93–95.

56. Kim SH, Jun HK, Song KH, et al. Prevalence of fur mites in pet rabbits in South Korea. *Vet Dermatol* 2008;19:189–190.

57. Wagner R, Stallmeister N. *Cheyletiella* dermatitis in humans, dogs and cats. *Br J Dermatol* 2000;143: 1110–1112.

58. Moriello KA. Zoonotic skin diseases of dogs and cats. *Anim Health Res Rev* 2003;4:157–168.

59. Bowman WL, Domrow R. The cat fur-mite (*Lynxacarus radovskyi*) in Australia. *Aust Vet J* 1978; 54:403–404.

60. Craig TM, Teel PD, Dubuisson LM, et al. *Lynxacarus radovskyi* infestation in a cat. *J Am Vet Med Assoc* 1993;202:613–614.

61. Heath AC, Mariadass B. A New Zealand record for the cat fur-mite, *Lynxacarus* (*Felistrophorus*) *radovskyi* Tenorio (Acarina: Astigmata: Listrophoridae). *N Z Vet J* 1999;47:211–212.

62. Jones DL. The finding of the cat fur-mite *Lynxacarus radovskyi* in New Zealand. *N Z Vet J* 2000;48:88.

63. Munro R, Munro HM. *Lynxacarus* on cats in Fiji. *Aust Vet J* 1979;55:90.

64. Tenorio JM. A new species of *Lynxacarus* (Acarina: Astigmata: Listrophoridae) from *Felis catus* in the Hawaiian islands. *J Med Entomol* 1974;11:599–604.

65. Dobrosavljevic DD, Popovic ND, Radovanovic SS. Systemic manifestations of *Cheyletiella* infestation in man. *Int J Dermatol* 2007;46:397–399.

66. Lee BW. *Cheyletiella dermatitis*: a report of fourteen cases. *Cutis* 1991;47:111–114.

67. Keh B, Lane RS, Shachter SP. *Cheyletiella blakei*, an ectoparasite of cats, as cause of cryptic arthropod infestations affecting humans. *West J Med* 1987; 146:192–194.

68. Paradis M. Mite dermatitis caused by *Cheyletiella blakei*. *J Am Acad Dermatol* 1998;38:1014–1015.

69. Tsianakas P, Polack B, Pinquier L, et al. *Cheyletiella* dermatitis: an uncommon cause of vesiculobullous eruption. *Ann Dermatol Venereol* 2000;127: 826–829.

70. Shelley ED, Shelley WB, Pula JF, et al. The diagnostic challenge of nonburrowing mite bites. *Cheyletiella yasguri*. *JAMA* 1984;251:2690–2691.

71. Brandrup F, Andersen KE, Kristensen S. Infestations in human and dogs with the mite *Cheyletiella yasguri* Smiley. *Ugeskr Laeg* 1979;141:1015–1017.

72. Brandrup F, Andersen KE, Kristensen S. Infection in man and dog with the mite, *Cheyletiella yasguri* Smiley. *Hautarzt* 1979;30:497–500.

73. Fain A, Scheepers L, De Groot W. Long-lasting pruriginous dermatitis in a woman caused by an acarian dog parasite, *Cheyletiella yasguri* Smiley. *Rev Med Liege* 1982;37:623–625.

74. Powell RF, Palmer SM, Palmer CH, et al. *Cheyletiella* dermatitis. *Int J Dermatol* 1977;16:679–682.

75. Chadwick AJ. Use of a 0.25 per cent fipronil pump spray formulation to treat canine cheyletiellosis. *J Small Anim Pract* 1997;38:261–262.

76. Chailleux N, Paradis M. Efficacy of selamectin in the treatment of naturally acquired cheyletiellosis in cats. *Can Vet J* 2002;43:767–770.

77. Dourmishev AL, Dourmishev LA, Schwartz RA. Ivermectin: pharmacology and application in dermatology. *Int J Dermatol* 2005;44:981–988.

78. Fisher MA, Shanks DJ. A review of the off-label use of selamectin (Stronghold/Revolution) in dogs and cats. *Acta Vet Scand* 2008;50:46.

79. Scarampella F, Pollmeier M, Visser M, et al. Efficacy of fipronil in the treatment of feline cheyletiellosis. *Vet Parasitol* 2005;129:333–339.

80. Mellgren M, Bergvall K. Treatment of rabbit cheyletiellosis with selamectin or ivermectin: a retrospective case study. *Acta Vet Scand* 2008;50:1.

81. Endris RG, Reuter VE, Nelson JD, et al. Efficacy of 65% permethrin applied as a topical spot-on against walking dandruff caused by the mite, *Cheyletiella yasguri* in dogs. *Vet Ther* 2000;1:273–279.

82. White SD, Rosychuk RA, Fieseler KV. Clinicopathologic findings, sensitivity to house dust mites and efficacy of milbemycin oxime treatment of dogs with *Cheyletiella* sp. infestation. *Vet Dermatol* 2001;12:13–18.

83. Cohen SR. *Cheyletiella* dermatitis. A mite infestation of rabbit, cat, dog, and man. *Arch Dermatol* 1980; 116:435–437.

84. Lee BW. *Cheyletiella* dermatitis. *Arch Dermatol* 1981;117:677–678.

85. Hewitt M, Walton GS, Waterhouse M. Pet animal infestations and human skin lesions. *Br J Dermatol* 1971;85:215–225.

86. Rivers JK, Martin J, Pukay B. Walking dandruff and *Cheyletiella* dermatitis. *J Am Acad Dermatol* 1986;15:1130–1133.

87. Kunkle GA, Miller WH. *Cheyletiella* infestation in humans. *Arch Dermatol* 1980;116:1345.

88. Xiao L, Fayer R. Molecular characterisation of species and genotypes of *Cryptosporidium* and *Giardia* and assessment of zoonotic transmission. *Int J Parasitol* 2008;38:1239–1255.

89. Xiao L, Fayer R, Ryan U, et al. *Cryptosporidium* taxonomy: recent advances and implications for public health. *Clin Microbiol Rev* 2004;17:72–97.

90. Hunter PR, Thompson RC. The zoonotic transmission of *Giardia* and *Cryptosporidium*. *Int J Parasitol* 2005;35:1181–1190.

91. Aydin Y, Ozkul IA. Infectivity of *Cryptosporidium muris* directly isolated from the murine stomach for various laboratory animals. *Vet Parasitol* 1996;66: 257–262.

92. Pavlasek I, Ryan U. The first finding of a natural infection of *Cryptosporidium muris* in a cat. *Vet Parasitol* 2007;144:349–352.

93. Hlavsa MC, Watson JC, Beach MJ. Cryptosporidiosis surveillance—United States 1999–2002. *MMWR Surveill Summ* 2005;54:1–8.

94. Giles M, Chalmers R, Pritchard G, et al. *Cryptosporidium hominis* in a goat and a sheep in the UK. *Vet Rec* 2009;164:24–25.

95. Gatei W, Suputtamongkol Y, Waywa D, et al. Zoonotic species of *Cryptosporidium* are as prevalent as the anthroponotic in HIV-infected patients in Thailand. *Ann Trop Med Parasitol* 2002;96:797–802.

96. Robinson RA, Pugh RN. Dogs, zoonoses and immunosuppression. *J R Soc Promot Health* 2002; 122:95–98.

97. Chalmers RM, Robinson G, Elwin K, et al. *Cryptosporidium* sp. rabbit genotype, a newly identified human pathogen. *Emerg Infect Dis* 2009;15: 829–830.

98. Kvác M, Kvetonová D, Sak B, et al. *Cryptosporidium* pig genotype II in immunocompetent man. *Emerg Infect Dis* 2009;15:982–983.

99. Acha PN, Szyfres B. *Zoonoses and Communicable Diseases Common to Man and Animals*. Washington, DC: Pan American Health Organization, Pan American Sanitary Bureau, Regional Office of the World Health Organization, 2003.

100. Dupont HL, Chappell CL, Sterling CR, et al. The infectivity of *Cryptosporidium parvum* in healthy volunteers. *N Engl J Med* 1995;332:855–859.

101. Barwick RS, Levy DA, Craun GF, et al. Surveillance for waterborne-disease outbreaks—United States, 1997–1998. *MMWR CDC Surveill Summ* 2000;49: 1–21.

102. Kramer MH, Herwaldt BL, Craun GF, et al. Surveillance for waterborne-disease outbreaks—United States, 1993–1994. *MMWR CDC Surveill Summ* 1996;45:1–33.

103. Lee SH, Levy DA, Craun GF, et al. Surveillance for waterborne-disease outbreaks—United States, 1999–2000. *MMWR Surveill Summ* 2002;51:1–47.

104. Levy DA, Bens MS, Craun GF, et al. Surveillance for waterborne-disease outbreaks—United States, 1995–1996. *MMWR CDC Surveill Summ* 1998;47:1–34.

105. Moore AC, Herwaldt BL, Craun GF, et al. Surveillance for waterborne disease outbreaks—United States, 1991–1992. *MMWR CDC Surveill Summ* 1993;42:1–22.

106. Glaser CA, Safrin S, Reingold A, et al. Association between *Cryptosporidium* infection and animal exposure in HIV-infected individuals. *J Acquir Immune Defic Syndr Hum Retrovirol* 1998;17:79–82.

107. Hunter PR, Hughes S, Woodhouse S, et al. Sporadic cryptosporidiosis case-control study with genotyping. *Emerg Infect Dis* 2004;10:1241–1249.

108. Robertson B, Sinclair MI, Forbes AB, et al. Case-control studies of sporadic cryptosporidiosis in Melbourne and Adelaide, Australia. *Epidemiol Infect* 2002;128:419–431.

109. Roy SL, Delong SM, Stenzel SA, et al. Risk factors for sporadic cryptosporidiosis among immunocompetent persons in the United States from 1999 to 2001. *J Clin Microbiol* 2004;42:2944–2951.

110. Goh S, Reacher M, Casemore DP, et al. Sporadic cryptosporidiosis, North Cumbria, England, 1996–2000. *Emerg Infect Dis* 2004;10:1007–1015.

111. Feltus DC, Giddings CW, Schneck BL, et al. Evidence supporting zoonotic transmission of *Cryptosporidium* spp. in Wisconsin. *J Clin Microbiol* 2006;44: 4303–4308.

112. Mtambo MM, Nash AS, Wright SE, et al. Prevalence of specific anti-*Cryptosporidium* IgG, IgM and IgA antibodies in cat sera using an indirect immunofluorescence antibody test. *Vet Parasitol* 1995; 60:37–43.

113. McReynolds CA, Lappin MR, Ungar B, et al. Regional seroprevalence of *Cryptosporidium parvum*-

specific IgG of cats in the United States. *Vet Parasitol* 1999;80:187–195.

114. Mtambo MM, Nash AS, Blewett DA, et al. *Cryptosporidium* infection in cats: prevalence of infection in domestic and feral cats in the Glasgow area. *Vet Rec* 1991;129:502–504.

115. Lefebvre S, Waltner-Toews D, Peregrine A, et al. Prevalence of zoonotic agents in dogs visiting hospitalized people in Ontario: implications for infection control. *J Hosp Infect* 2006;62:458–466.

116. Hill SL, Cheney JM, Taton-Allen GF, et al. Prevalence of enteric zoonotic organisms in cats. *J Am Vet Med Assoc* 2000;216:687–692.

117. Spain CV, Scarlett JM, Wade SE, et al. Prevalence of enteric zoonotic agents in cats less than 1 year old in central New York State. *J Vet Intern Med* 2001;15:33–38.

118. el-Ahraf A, Tacal JV, Sobih M, et al. Prevalence of cryptosporidiosis in dogs and human beings in San Bernardino County, California. *J Am Vet Med Assoc* 1991;198:631–634.

119. Shukla R, Giraldo P, Kraliz A, et al. *Cryptosporidium* spp. and other zoonotic enteric parasites in a sample of domestic dogs and cats in the Niagara region of Ontario. *Can Vet J* 2006;47:1179–1184.

120. McGlade TR, Robertson ID, Elliot AD, et al. Gastrointestinal parasites of domestic cats in Perth, Western Australia. *Vet Parasitol* 2003;117:251–262.

121. Rehg JE, Gigliotti F, Stokes DC. Cryptosporidiosis in ferrets. *Lab Anim Sci* 1988;38:155–158.

122. Abe N, Iseki M. Identification of genotypes of *Cryptosporidium parvum* isolates from ferrets in Japan. *Parasitol Res* 2003;89:422–424.

123. Chappell CL, Okhuysen PC, Langer-Curry R, et al. *Cryptosporidium hominis*: experimental challenge of healthy adults. *Am J Trop Med Hyg* 2006;75:851–857.

124. Cacciò S, Pinter E, Fantini R, et al. Human infection with *Cryptosporidium felis*: case report and literature review. *Emerg Infect Dis* 2002;8:85–86.

125. Gookin JL, Nordone SK, Argenzio RA. Host responses to *Cryptosporidium* infection. *J Vet Intern Med* 2002;16:12–21.

126. Barr CS. Cryptosporidiosis and cyclosporiasis. In: Greene CE, ed. *Infectious Diseases of the Dog and Cat*. Philadelphia: Saunders Elsevier, 2006, pp. 785–793.

127. Mekaru SR, Marks SL, Felley AJ, et al. Comparison of direct immunofluorescence, immunoassays, and fecal flotation for detection of *Cryptosporidium* spp. and *Giardia* spp. in naturally exposed cats in 4 Northern California animal shelters. *J Vet Intern Med* 2007;21:959–965.

128. Scorza AV, Brewer MM, Lappin MR. Polymerase chain reaction for the detection of *Cryptosporidium* spp. in cat feces. *J Parasitol* 2003;89:423–426.

129. Lappin MR, Ungar B, Brown-Hahn B, et al. Enzyme-linked immunosorbent assay for the detection of *Cryptosporidium parvum* IgG in the serum of cats. *J Parasitol* 1997;83:957–960.

130. Chen XM, Keithly JS, Paya CV, et al. Cryptosporidiosis. *N Engl J Med* 2002;346:1723–1731.

131. Hunter PR, Hughes S, Woodhouse S, et al. Health sequelae of human cryptosporidiosis in immunocompetent patients. *Clin Infect Dis* 2004;39:504–510.

132. Chen XM, LaRusso NF. Cryptosporidiosis and the pathogenesis of AIDS-cholangiopathy. *Semin Liver Dis* 2002;22:277–289.

133. Clavel A, Arnal AC, Sánchez EC, et al. Respiratory cryptosporidiosis: case series and review of the literature. *Infection* 1996;24:341–346.

134. Jokipii L, Jokipii AM. Timing of symptoms and oocyst excretion in human cryptosporidiosis. *N Engl J Med* 1986;315:1643–1647.

135. Lindergard G, Nydam DV, Wade SE, et al. A novel multiplex polymerase chain reaction approach for detection of four human infective *Cryptosporidium* isolates: *Cryptosporidium parvum*, types H and C, *Cryptosporidium canis*, and *Cryptosporidium felis* in fecal and soil samples. *J Vet Diagn Invest* 2003;15:262–267.

136. Weber R, Bryan RT, Bishop HS, et al. Threshold of detection of *Cryptosporidium* oocysts in human stool specimens: evidence for low sensitivity of current diagnostic methods. *J Clin Microbiol* 1991;29:1323–1327.

137. Gargala G. Drug treatment and novel drug target against *Cryptosporidium*. *Parasite* 2008;15:275–281.

138. Rossignol JF, Ayoub A, Ayers MS. Treatment of diarrhea caused by *Cryptosporidium parvum*: a prospective randomized, double-blind, placebo-controlled study of Nitazoxanide. *J Infect Dis* 2001;184:103–106.

139. White AC. Nitazoxanide: an important advance in anti-parasitic therapy. *Am J Trop Med Hyg* 2003;68:382–383.

140. Hewitt RG, Yiannoutsos CT, Higgs ES, et al. Paromomycin: no more effective than placebo for treatment of cryptosporidiosis in patients with advanced human immunodeficiency virus infection. AIDS Clinical Trial Group. *Clin Infect Dis* 2000;31:1084–1092.

141. Hoepelman AI. Current therapeutic approaches to cryptosporidiosis in immunocompromised patients. *J Antimicrob Chemother* 1996;37:871–880.

142. Betancourt WQ, Rose JB. Drinking water treatment processes for removal of *Cryptosporidium* and *Giardia*. *Vet Parasitol* 2004;126:219–234.

143. Desch CE, Hillier A. *Demodex injai*: a new species of hair follicle mite (Acari: Demodecidae) from the

domestic dog (Canidae). *J Med Entomol* 2003;40: 146–149.

144. Ordeix L, Bardagí M, Scarampella F, et al. *Demodex injai* infestation and dorsal greasy skin and hair in eight wirehaired fox terrier dogs. *Vet Dermatol* 2009;20:267–272.

145. Ugbomoiko US, Ariza L, Heukelbach J. Parasites of importance for human health in Nigerian dogs: high prevalence and limited knowledge of pet owners. *BMC Vet Res* 2008;4:49.

146. Xhaxhiu D, Kusi I, Rapti D, et al. Ectoparasites of dogs and cats in Albania. *Parasitol Res* 2009; 105:1577–1587.

147. Desch CE, Stewart TB. *Demodex gatoi*: new species of hair follicle mite (Acari: Demodecidae) from the domestic cat (Carnivora: Felidae). *J Med Entomol* 1999;36:167–170.

148. Löwenstein C, Beck W, Bessmann K, et al. Feline demodicosis caused by concurrent infestation with *Demodex cati* and an unnamed species of mite. *Vet Rec* 2005;157:290–292.

149. Neel JA, Tarigo J, Tater KC, et al. Deep and superficial skin scrapings from a feline immunodeficiency virus-positive cat. *Vet Clin Pathol* 2007; 36:101–104.

150. Castanet J, Monpoux F, Mariani R, et al. Demodicidosis in an immunodeficient child. *Pediatr Dermatol* 1997;14:219–220.

151. Czepita D, Kuzna-Grygiel W, Czepita M, et al. *Demodex folliculorum* and *Demodex brevis* as a cause of chronic marginal blepharitis. *Ann Acad Med Stetin* 2007;53:63–67, discussion 67.

152. Morsy TA, el Okbi MM, el-Said AM, et al. *Demodex* (follicular mite) infesting a boy and his pet dog. *J Egypt Soc Parasitol* 1995;25:509–512.

153. Companion Animal Parasite Council. *Tapeworm (Cyclophyllidean Cestodes)*. Bel Air, MD: Companion Animal Parasite Council, 2006.

154. Barutzki D, Schaper R. Endoparasites in dogs and cats in Germany 1999–2002. *Parasitol Res* 2003;90 (Suppl. 3):S148–S150.

155. Coelho WM, do Amarante AF, de Soutello RV, et al. Occurrence of gastrointestinal parasites in fecal samples of cats in Andradina City, São Paulo. *Rev Bras Parasitol Vet* 2009;18:46–49.

156. Dai RS, Li ZY, Li F, et al. Severe infection of adult dogs with helminths in Hunan Province, China poses significant public health concerns. *Vet Parasitol* 2009;160:348–350.

157. Fok E, Szatmári V, Busák K, et al. Prevalence of intestinal parasites in dogs in some urban and rural areas of Hungary. *Vet Q* 2001;23:96–98.

158. Katagiri S, Oliveira-Sequeira TC. Prevalence of dog intestinal parasites and risk perception of zoonotic infection by dog owners in São Paulo State, Brazil. *Zoonoses Public Health* 2008;55:406–413.

159. Kazacos KR. Gastrointestinal helminths in dogs from a humane shelter in Indiana. *J Am Vet Med Assoc* 1978;173:995–997.

160. Minnaar WN, Krecek RC. Helminths in dogs belonging to people in a resource-limited urban community in Gauteng, South Africa. *Onderstepoort J Vet Res* 2001;68:111–117.

161. Minnaar WN, Krecek RC, Fourie LJ. Helminths in dogs from a peri-urban resource-limited community in Free State Province, South Africa. *Vet Parasitol* 2002;107:343–349.

162. Mohsen A, Hossein H. Gastrointestinal parasites of stray cats in Kashan, Iran. *Trop Biomed* 2009;26:16–22.

163. Soriano SV, Pierangeli NB, Roccia I, et al. A wide diversity of zoonotic intestinal parasites infects urban and rural dogs in Neuquén, Patagonia, Argentina. *Vet Parasitol* 2010;167:81–85.

164. Sowemimo OA. The prevalence and intensity of gastrointestinal parasites of dogs in Ile-Ife, Nigeria. *J Helminthol* 2009;83:27–31.

165. Martínez-Carrasco C, Berriatua E, Garijo M, et al. Epidemiological study of non-systemic parasitism in dogs in southeast Mediterranean Spain assessed by coprological and post-mortem examination. *Zoonoses Public Health* 2007;54:195–203.

166. Pomroy WE. A survey of helminth parasites of cats from Saskatoon. *Can Vet J* 1999;40:339–340.

167. Yamamoto N, Kon M, Saito T, et al. Prevalence of intestinal canine and feline parasites in Saitama Prefecture, Japan. *Kansenshōgaku Zasshi* 2009;83: 223–228.

168. Anderson OW. *Dipylidium caninum* infestation. *Am J Dis Child* 1968;116:328–330.

169. Brandstetter W, Auer H. *Dipylidium caninum*, a rare parasite in man. *Wien Klin Wochenschr* 1994; 106:115–116.

170. Currier RW, Kinzer GM, DeShields E. *Dipylidium caninum* infection in a 14-month-old child. *South Med J* 1973;66:1060–1062.

171. Ferraris S, Reverso E, Parravicini LP, et al. *Dipylidium caninum* in an infant. *Eur J Pediatr* 1993;152:702.

172. Jackson D, Crozier WJ, Andersen SE, et al. Dipylidiasis in a 57-year-old woman. *Med J Aust* 1977;2:740–741.

173. Molina CP, Ogburn J, Adegboyega P. Infection by *Dipylidium caninum* in an infant. *Arch Pathol Lab Med* 2003;127:e157–e159.

174. Neafie RC, Marty AM. Unusual infections in humans. *Clin Microbiol Rev* 1993;6:34–56.

175. Raitiere CR. Dog tapeworm (*Dipylidium caninum*) infestation in a 6-month-old infant. *J Fam Pract* 1992;34:101–102.

176. Reddy SB. Infestation of a five-month-old infant with *Dipylidium caninum*. *Del Med J* 1982;54: 455–456.

177. Reid CJ, Perry FM, Evans N. *Dipylidium caninum* in an infant. *Eur J Pediatr* 1992;151:502–503.

178. Thomas H, Gönnert R. The efficacy of praziquantel against cestodes in cats, dogs and sheep. *Res Vet Sci* 1978;24:20–25.

179. Altreuther G, Radeloff I, LeSueur C, et al. Field evaluation of the efficacy and safety of emodepside plus praziquantel tablets (Profender tablets for dogs) against naturally acquired nematode and cestode infections in dogs. *Parasitol Res* 2009; 105(Suppl. 1):S23–S29.

180. Schroeder I, Altreuther G, Schimmel A, et al. Efficacy of emodepside plus praziquantel tablets (Profender tablets for dogs) against mature and immature cestode infections in dogs. *Parasitol Res* 2009;105(Suppl. 1):S31–S38.

181. Bowman DD, Atkins CE. Heartworm biology, treatment, and control. *Vet Clin North Am Small Anim Pract* 2009;39:1127–1158, vii.

182. Theis JH. Public health aspects of dirofilariasis in the United States. *Vet Parasitol* 2005;133:157–180.

183. Bolio-Gonzalez ME, Rodriguez-Vivas RI, Sauri-Arceo CH, et al. Prevalence of the *Dirofilaria immitis* infection in dogs from Merida, Yucatan, Mexico. *Vet Parasitol* 2007;148:166–169.

184. Bowman D, Little SE, Lorentzen L, et al. Prevalence and geographic distribution of *Dirofilaria immitis*, *Borrelia burgdorferi*, *Ehrlichia canis*, and *Anaplasma phagocytophilum* in dogs in the United States: results of a national clinic-based serologic survey. *Vet Parasitol* 2009;160:138–148.

185. Duran-Struuck R, Jost C, Hernandez AH. *Dirofilaria immitis* prevalence in a canine population in the Samana Peninsula (Dominican Republic)—June 2001. *Vet Parasitol* 2005;133:323–327.

186. Klotins KC, Martin SW, Bonnett BN, et al. Canine heartworm testing in Canada: are we being effective? *Can Vet J* 2000;41:929–937.

187. Levy JK, Edinboro CH, Glotfelty CS, et al. Seroprevalence of *Dirofilaria immitis*, feline leukemia virus, and feline immunodeficiency virus infection among dogs and cats exported from the 2005 Gulf Coast hurricane disaster area. *J Am Vet Med Assoc* 2007;231:218–225.

188. Miterpáková M, Antolová D, Hurníková Z, et al. *Dirofilaria* infections in working dogs in Slovakia. *J Helminthol* 2009;84:173–176.

189. Montoya JA, Morales M, Juste MC, et al. Seroprevalence of canine heartworm disease (*Dirofilaria immitis*) on Tenerife Island: an epidemiological update. *Parasitol Res* 2006;100:103–105.

190. Morchón R, Moya I, González-Miguel J, et al. Zoonotic *Dirofilaria immitis* infections in a province of Northern Spain. *Epidemiol Infect* 2010;138: 380–383.

191. Pantchev N, Norden N, Lorentzen L, et al. Current surveys on the prevalence and distribution of *Dirofilaria* spp. in dogs in Germany. *Parasitol Res* 2009;105(Suppl. 1):S63–S74.

192. Slocombe JO, Villeneuve A. Heartworm in dogs in Canada in 1991. *Can Vet J* 1993;34:630–633.

193. Nash TE. Visceral larva migrans and other unusual helminth infections. In: Mandell GL, Bennett JE, Dolin R, eds. *Principles and Practice of Infectious Diseases*. Philadelphia: Elsevier, 2005, pp. 3293–3299.

194. Muro A, Genchi C, Cordero M, et al. Human dirofilariasis in the European Union. *Parasitol Today (Regul Ed)* 1999;15:386–389.

195. Abadie SH, Swartzwelder JC, Holman RL. A human case of *Dirofilaria immitis* infection. *Am J Trop Med Hyg* 1965;14:117–118.

196. Beskin CA, Colvin SH, Beaver PC. Pulmonary dirofilariasis. Cause of pulmonary nodular disease. *JAMA* 1966;198:665–667.

197. Bielawski BC, Harrington D, Joseph E. A solitary pulmonary nodule with zoonotic implications. *Chest* 2001;119:1250–1252.

198. Dobson C, Welch JS. Dirofilariasis as a cause of eosinophilic meningitis in man diagnosed by immunofluorescence and Arthus hypersensitivity. *Trans R Soc Trop Med Hyg* 1974;68:223–228.

199. Kim MK, Kim CH, Yeom BW, et al. The first human case of hepatic dirofilariasis. *J Korean Med Sci* 2002;17:686–690.

200. Moorehouse DE. *Dirofilaria immitis*: a cause of human intra-ocular infection. *Infection* 1978;6: 192–193.

201. Navarrette AR. Pulmonary dirofilariasis. *Chest* 1972;61:51–55.

202. Tada I, Sakaguchi Y, Eto K. *Dirofilaria* in the abdominal cavity of a man in Japan. *Am J Trop Med Hyg* 1979;28:988–990.

203. Tannehill AW, Hatch HB. Coin lesions of the lung due to *Dirofilaria immitis*. Report of a case. *Dis Chest* 1968;53:369–371.

204. Theis JH, Gilson A, Simon GE, et al. Case report: Unusual location of *Dirofilaria immitis* in a 28-year-old man necessitates orchiectomy. *Am J Trop Med Hyg* 2001;64:317–322.

205. Tuazon RA, Firestone F, Blaustein AU. Human pulmonary dirofilariasis manifesting as a "coin" lesion. A case report. *JAMA* 1967;199:45–46.

206. Companion Animal Parasite Council. *Heartworm (Dirofilaria immitis)*. Bel Air, MD: Companion Animal Parasite Council, 2010.

207. Society AH. *Canine Guidelines*. Wilmington, DE: American Heartworm Society, 2010.
208. Bazzocchi C, Mortarino M, Grandi G, et al. Combined ivermectin and doxycycline treatment has microfilaricidal and adulticidal activity against *Dirofilaria immitis* in experimentally infected dogs. *Int J Parasitol* 2008;38:1401–1410.
209. Miyoshi T, Tsubouchi H, Iwasaki A, et al. Human pulmonary dirofilariasis: a case report and review of the recent Japanese literature. *Respirology* 2006;11:343–347.
210. Craig P. Echinococcus multilocularis. *Curr Opin Infect Dis* 2003;16:437–444.
211. D'Alessandro A, Rausch RL. New aspects of neotropical polycystic (*Echinococcus vogeli*) and unicystic (*Echinococcus oligarthrus*) echinococcosis. *Clin Microbiol Rev* 2008;21:380–401, table of contents.
212. Somocurcio JR, Sánchez EL, Náquira C, et al. First report of a human case of polycystic echinococcosis due to *Echinococcus vogeli* from neotropical area of Peru, South America. *Rev Inst Med Trop Sao Paulo* 2004;46:41–42.
213. King CH. Cestodes (tapeworms). In: Mandell GL, Bennett JE, Dolin R, eds. *Principles and Practice of Infectious Diseases*. Philadelphia: Saunders, 2005, pp. 3290–3293.
214. Acosta-Jamett G, Cleaveland S, Bronsvoort BM, et al. *Echinococcus granulosus* infection in domestic dogs in urban and rural areas of the Coquimbo region, north-central Chile. *Vet Parasitol* 2009; 169:117–122.
215. Budke CM, Campos-Ponce M, Qian W, et al. A canine purgation study and risk factor analysis for echinococcosis in a high endemic region of the Tibetan plateau. *Vet Parasitol* 2005;127: 43–49.
216. Buishi I, Walters T, Guildea Z, et al. Reemergence of canine *Echinococcus granulosus* infection, Wales. *Emerg Infect Dis* 2005;11:568–571.
217. El Shazly AM, Awad SE, Nagaty IM, et al. Echinococcosis in dogs in urban and rural areas in Dakahlia Governorate, Egypt. *J Egypt Soc Parasitol* 2007;37:483–492.
218. Elshazly AM, Awad SE, Abdel Tawab AH, et al. Echinococcosis (zoonotic hydatidosis) in street dogs in urban and rural areas, Dakahlia Governorate, Egypt. *J Egypt Soc Parasitol* 2007;37:287–298.
219. Haridy FM, Holw SA, Hassan AA, et al. Cystic hydatidosis: a zoonotic silent health problem. *J Egypt Soc Parasitol* 2008;38:635–644.
220. Lahmar S, Boufana BS, Lahmar S, et al. *Echinococcus* in the wild carnivores and stray dogs of northern Tunisia: the results of a pilot survey. *Ann Trop Med Parasitol* 2009;103:323–331.
221. Moro PL, Lopera L, Bonifacio N, et al. Risk factors for canine echinococcosis in an endemic area of Peru. *Vet Parasitol* 2005;130:99–104.
222. Torgerson PR, Craig PS. Risk assessment of importation of dogs infected with *Echinococcus multilocularis* into the UK. *Vet Rec* 2009;165:366–368.
223. Torgerson PR, Rosenheim K, Tanner I, et al. Echinococcosis, toxocarosis and toxoplasmosis screening in a rural community in eastern Kazakhstan. *Trop Med Int Health* 2009;14:341–348.
224. Wachira TM, Sattran M, Zeyhle E, et al. Intestinal helminths of public health importance in dogs in Nairobi. *East Afr Med J* 1993;70:617–619.
225. Buishi I, Njoroge E, Zeyhle E, et al. Canine echinococcosis in Turkana (north-western Kenya): a coproantigen survey in the previous hydatid-control area and an analysis of risk factors. *Ann Trop Med Parasitol* 2006;100:601–610.
226. Guidelines for treatment of cystic and alveolar echinococcosis in humans. WHO Informal Working Group on Echinococcosis. *Bull World Health Organ* 1996;74:231–242.
227. Craig PS, Echinococcosis Working Group in China. Epidemiology of human alveolar echinococcosis in China. *Parasitol Int* 2006;55(Suppl.):S221–S225.
228. Craig PS, Larrieu E. Control of cystic echinococcosis/hydatidosis: 1863–2002. *Adv Parasitol* 2006;61: 443–508.
229. Antolová D, Reiterová K, Miterpáková M, et al. The first finding of *Echinococcus multilocularis* in dogs in Slovakia: an emerging risk for spreading of infection. *Zoonoses Public Health* 2009;56:53–58.
230. Ben Musa NA, Sadek GS. Prevalence of echinococcosis in street dogs in Tripole District, Libya. *J Egypt Soc Parasitol* 2007;37:793–800.
231. Deplazes P, Alther P, Tanner I, et al. *Echinococcus multilocularis* coproantigen detection by enzyme-linked immunosorbent assay in fox, dog, and cat populations. *J Parasitol* 1999;85:115–121.
232. Nonaka N, Kamiya M, Kobayashi F, et al. *Echinococcus multilocularis* infection in pet dogs in Japan. *Vector Borne Zoonotic Dis* 2009;9: 201–206.
233. Shaikenov BS, Torgerson PR, Usenbayev AE, et al. The changing epidemiology of echinococcosis in Kazakhstan due to transformation of farming practices. *Acta Trop* 2003;85:287–293.
234. Wang Q, Raoul F, Budke C, et al. Grass height and transmission ecology of *Echinococcus multilocularis* in Tibetan communities, China. *Chin Med J* 2010; 123:61–67.
235. Dyachenko V, Pantchev N, Gawlowska S, et al. *Echinococcus multilocularis* infections in domestic dogs and cats from Germany and other European countries. *Vet Parasitol* 2008;157:244–253.

236. Nonaka N, Hirokawa H, Inoue T, et al. The first instance of a cat excreting *Echinococcus multilocularis* eggs in Japan. *Parasitol Int* 2008;57:519–520.

237. Kapel CM, Torgerson PR, Thompson RC, et al. Reproductive potential of *Echinococcus multilocularis* in experimentally infected foxes, dogs, raccoon dogs and cats. *Int J Parasitol* 2006;36:79–86.

238. Altay M, Unverdi S, Altay FA, et al. Renal injury due to hepatic hydatid disease. *Nephrol Dial Transplant* 2010;25:2611–2615.

239. Krasniqi A, Limani D, Gashi-Luci L, et al. Primary hydatid cyst of the gallbladder: a case report. *J Med Case Reports* 2010;4:29.

240. Duishanbai S, Jiafu D, Guo H, et al. Intracranial hydatid cyst in children: report of 30 cases. *Childs Nerv Syst* 2009;26:821–827.

241. Ahmadi NA, Hamidi M. A retrospective analysis of human cystic echinococcosis in Hamedan province, an endemic region of Iran. *Ann Trop Med Parasitol* 2008;102:603–609.

242. Conboy G. Cestodes of dogs and cats in North America. *Vet Clin North Am Small Anim Pract* 2009;39:1075–1090, vi.

243. Altintas N. Past to present: echinococcosis in Turkey. *Acta Trop* 2003;85:105 112.

244. Torgerson PR, Karaeva RR, Corkeri N, et al. Human cystic echinococcosis in Kyrgystan: an epidemiological study. *Acta Trop* 2003;85:51–61.

245. Carmona C, Perdomo R, Carbo A, et al. Risk factors associated with human cystic echinococcosis in Florida, Uruguay: results of a mass screening study using ultrasound and serology. *Am J Trop Med Hyg* 1998;58:599–605.

246. Yang YR, Sun T, Li Z, et al. Community surveys and risk factor analysis of human alveolar and cystic echinococcosis in Ningxia Hui Autonomous Region, China. *Bull World Health Organ* 2006;84:714–721.

247. Craig PS, Giraudoux P, Shi D, et al. An epidemiological and ecological study of human alveolar echinococcosis transmission in south Gansu, China. *Acta Trop* 2000;77:167–177.

248. Kreidl P, Allerberger F, Judmaier G, et al. Domestic pets as risk factors for alveolar hydatid disease in Austria. *Am J Epidemiol* 1998;147:978–981.

249. Lahmar S, Lahmar S, Boufana B, et al. Screening for *Echinococcus granulosus* in dogs: comparison between arecoline purgation, coproELISA and coproPCR with necropsy in pre-patent infections. *Vet Parasitol* 2007;144:287–292.

250. Allan JC, Craig PS. Coproantigens in taeniasis and echinococcosis. *Parasitol Int* 2006;55(Suppl.):S75–S80.

251. Thompson RC, Reynoldson JA, Manger BR. In vitro and in vivo efficacy of epsiprantel against *Echinococcus granulosus*. *Res Vet Sci* 1991;51:332–334.

252. Arinc S, Kosif A, Ertugrul M, et al. Evaluation of pulmonary hydatid cyst cases. *Int J Surg* 2009;7:192–195.

253. Sall I, Ali AA, El Kaoui H, et al. Primary hydatid cyst of the retroperitoneum. *Am J Surg* 2010;199:e25–e26.

254. Horton J. Albendazole for the treatment of echinococcosis. *Fundam Clin Pharmacol* 2003;17:205–212.

255. Bresson-Hadni S, Franza A, Miguet JP, et al. Orthotopic liver transplantation for incurable alveolar echinococcosis of the liver: report of 17 cases. *Hepatology* 1991;13:1061–1070.

256. Xia D, Yan LN, Li B, et al. Orthotopic liver transplantation for incurable alveolar echinococcosis: report of five cases from west China. *Transplant Proc* 2005;37:2181–2184.

257. Richter J, Orhun A, Grüner B, et al. Autochthonous cystic echinococcosis in patients who grew up in Germany. *Euro Surveill* 2009;14:pii.19229.

258. Cabrera PA, Lloyd S, Haran G, et al. Control of *Echinococcus granulosus* in Uruguay: evaluation of different treatment intervals for dogs. *Vet Parasitol* 2002;103:333–340.

259. Hegglin D, Deplazes P. Control strategy for *Echinococcus multilocularis*. *Emerg Infect Dis* 2008;14:1626–1628.

260. Traversa D, Di Cesare A, Milillo P, et al. Infection by *Eucoleus aerophilus* in dogs and cats: is another extra-intestinal parasitic nematode of pets emerging in Italy? *Res Vet Sci* 2009;87:270–272.

261. Burgess H, Ruotsalo K, Peregrine AS, et al. *Eucoleus aerophilus* respiratory infection in a dog with Addison's disease. *Can Vet J* 2008;49:389–392.

262. Foster SF, Martin P, Allan GS, et al. Lower respiratory tract infections in cats: 21 cases (1995–2000). *J Feline Med Surg* 2004;6:167–180.

263. Foster SF, Martin P, Braddock JA, et al. A retrospective analysis of feline bronchoalveolar lavage cytology and microbiology (1995–2000). *J Feline Med Surg* 2004;6:189–198.

264. Morgan ER, Tomlinson A, Hunter S, et al. *Angiostrongylus vasorum* and *Eucoleus aerophilus* in foxes (*Vulpes vulpes*) in Great Britain. *Vet Parasitol* 2008;154:48–57.

265. Popiołek M, Szczesnaa J, Nowaka S, et al. Helminth infections in faecal samples of wolves *Canis lupus* L. from the western Beskidy Mountains in southern Poland. *J Helminthol* 2007;81:339–344.

266. Sato H, Inaba T, Ihama Y, et al. Parasitological survey on wild carnivora in north-western Tohoku, Japan. *J Vet Med Sci* 1999;61:1023–1026.

267. Sréter T, Széll Z, Marucci G, et al. Extraintestinal nematode infections of red foxes (*Vulpes vulpes*) in Hungary. *Vet Parasitol* 2003;115:329–334.

268. Holmes PR, Kelly JD. *Capillaria aerophila* in the domestic cat in Australia. *Aust Vet J* 1973;49:472–473.

269. Companion Animal Parasite Council. *Lungworm.* Bel Air, MD: Companion Animal Parasite Council, 2007.

270. Aftandelians R, Raafat F, Taffazoli M, et al. Pulmonary capillariasis in a child in Iran. *Am J Trop Med Hyg* 1977;26:64–71.

271. Lalosević D, Lalosević V, Klem I, et al. Pulmonary capillariasis miming bronchial carcinoma. *Am J Trop Med Hyg* 2008;78:14–16.

272. Blagburn BL, Dryden MW. Biology, treatment, and control of flea and tick infestations. *Vet Clin North Am Small Anim Pract* 2009;39:1173–1200, viii.

273. Bond R, Riddle A, Mottram L, et al. Survey of flea infestation in dogs and cats in the United Kingdom during 2005. *Vet Rec* 2007;160:503–506.

274. Marchiondo AA, Holdsworth PA, Green P, et al. World Association for the Advancement of Veterinary Parasitology (W.A.A.V.P.) guidelines for evaluating the efficacy of parasiticides for the treatment, prevention and control of flea and tick infestation on dogs and cats. *Vet Parasitol* 2007;145:332–344.

275. Rinaldi L, Spera G, Musella V, et al. A survey of fleas on dogs in southern Italy. *Vet Parasitol* 2007;148:375–378.

276. Silverman J, Rust MK. Extended longevity of the pre-emerged adult cat flea (Siphonaptera: Pulicidae) and factors stimulating emergence from the pupal cocoon. *Ann Entemol Soc Am* 1985;78:763–768.

277. Hudson BW, Prince FM. A method for large scale rearing of the cat flea, *Ctenocephalides felis felis. Bull World Health Organ* 1958;19:1126–1129.

278. Farkas R, Gyurkovszky M, Solymosi N, et al. Prevalence of flea infestation in dogs and cats in Hungary combined with a survey of owner awareness. *Med Vet Entomol* 2009;23:187–194.

279. Glickman L, Moore G, Glickman N, et al. Purdue University-Banfield National Companion Animal Surveillance Program for emerging and zoonotic diseases. *Vector Borne Zoonotic Dis* 2006;6:14–23.

280. Beugnet F, Marié JL. Emerging arthropod-borne diseases of companion animals in Europe. *Vet Parasitol* 2009;163:298–305.

281. Eisen RJ, Borchert JN, Holmes JL, et al. Early-phase transmission of *Yersinia pestis* by cat fleas (*Ctenocephalides felis*) and their potential role as vectors in a plague-endemic region of Uganda. *Am J Trop Med Hyg* 2008;78:949–956.

282. McElroy KM, Blagburn BL, Breitschwerdt EB, et al. Flea-associated zoonotic diseases of cats in the USA: bartonellosis, flea-borne rickettsioses, and plague. *Trends Parasitol* 2010;26:197–204.

283. Beck K, Conboy G, Gilleard J, et al. Canadian Guidelines for the Treatment of Parasites in Dogs and Cats, 2009.

284. Malik R, Ward MP, Seavers A, et al. Permethrin spot-on intoxication of cats: literature review and survey of veterinary practitioners in Australia. *J Feline Med Surg* 2010;12:5–14.

285. Boland LA, Angles JM. Feline permethrin toxicity: retrospective study of 42 cases. *J Feline Med Surg* 2010;12:61–71.

286. Baker NF, Farver TB. Failure of brewer's yeast as a repellent to fleas on dogs. *J Am Vet Med Assoc* 1983;183:212–214.

287. Blagburn BL, Hendrix CM, Vaughan JL, et al. Efficacy of lufenuron against developmental stages of fleas (*Ctenocephalides felis felis*) in dogs housed in simulated home environments. *Am J Vet Res* 1995;56:464–467.

288. Blagburn BL, Young DR, Moran C, et al. Effects of orally administered spinosad (Comfortis) in dogs on adult and immature stages of the cat flea (*Ctenocephalides felis*). *Vet Parasitol* 2010;168:312–317.

289. Franc M, Bouhsira E. Evaluation of speed and duration of efficacy of spinosad tablets for treatment and control of *Ctenocephalides canis* (Siphonaptera: Pulicidae) infestations in dogs. *Parasite* 2009;16:125–128.

290. Heaney K, Lindahl RG. Safety of a topically applied spot-on formulation of metaflumizone plus amitraz for flea and tick control in dogs. *Vet Parasitol* 2007;150:225–232.

291. Holzmer S, Hair JA, Dryden MW, et al. Efficacy of a novel formulation of metaflumizone for the control of fleas (*Ctenocephalides felis*) on cats. *Vet Parasitol* 2007;150:219–224.

292. McTier TL, Shanks DJ, Jernigan AD, et al. Evaluation of the effects of selamectin against adult and immature stages of fleas (*Ctenocephalides felis felis*) on dogs and cats. *Vet Parasitol* 2000;91:201–212.

293. Schnieder T, Wolken S, Mencke N. Comparative efficacy of imidacloprid, selamectin, fipronil-(S)-methoprene, and metaflumizone against cats experimentally infested with *Ctenocephalides felis. Vet Ther* 2008;9:176–183.

294. Naimer SA, Cohen AD, Mumcuoglu KY, et al. Household papular urticaria. *Isr Med Assoc J* 2002;4:911–913.

295. Thieu KP, Lio PA. Recurrent papular urticaria in a 6-year-old girl. *Arch Dis Child* 2008;93:750.

296. Payne PA, Artzer M. The biology and control of *Giardia* spp and *Tritrichomonas foetus*. *Vet Clin North Am Small Anim Pract* 2009;39:993–1007.

297. Companion Animal Parasite Council. *Giardiasis*. Bel Air, MD: Companion Animal Parasite Council, 2007.

298. Haque R, Mondal D, Karim A, et al. Prospective case-control study of the association between common enteric protozoal parasites and diarrhea in Bangladesh. *Clin Infect Dis* 2009;48:1191–1197.

299. Hill DR. Giardia lamblia. In: Mandell GL, Bennett JE, Dolin R, eds. *Principles and Practice of Infectious Diseases*. Philadelphia: Elsevier, 2005, pp. 3198–3205.

300. Robinson RD, Murphy EL, Wilks RJ, et al. Gastrointestinal parasitic infection in healthy Jamaican carriers of HTLV-I. *J Trop Med Hyg* 1991;94:411–415.

301. Spinelli R, Brandonisio O, Serio G, et al. Intestinal parasites in healthy subjects in Albania. *Eur J Epidemiol* 2006;21:161–166.

302. Svenungsson B, Lagergren A, Ekwall E, et al. Enteropathogens in adult patients with diarrhea and healthy control subjects: a 1-year prospective study in a Swedish clinic for infectious diseases. *Clin Infect Dis* 2000;30:770–778.

303. Greig JD, Michel P, Wilson JB, et al. A descriptive analysis of giardiasis cases reported in Ontario, 1990–1998. *Can J Public Health* 2001;92:361–365.

304. Knight R. Epidemiology and transmission of giardiasis. *Trans R Soc Trop Med Hyg* 1980;74:433–436.

305. Yoder JS, Beach MJ. (CDC) CfDCaP. Giardiasis surveillance—United States, 2003–2005. *MMWR Surveill Summ* 2007;56:11–18.

306. Barr CS. Giardiasis. In: Greene CE, ed. *Infectious Diseases of the Dog and Cat*. Philadelphia: Saunders Elsevier, 2006, pp. 736–742.

307. Batchelor DJ, Tzannes S, Graham PA, et al. Detection of endoparasites with zoonotic potential in dogs with gastrointestinal disease in the UK. *Transbound Emerg Dis* 2008;55:99–104.

308. Hackett T, Lappin MR. Prevalence of enteric pathogens in dogs of north-central Colorado. *J Am Anim Hosp Assoc* 2003;39:52–56.

309. Itoh N, Muraoka N, Aoki M, et al. Prevalence of *Giardia lamblia* infection in household dogs. *Kansenshōgaku Zasshi* 2001;75:671–677.

310. Little SE, Johnson EM, Lewis D, et al. Prevalence of intestinal parasites in pet dogs in the United States. *Vet Parasitol* 2009;166:144–152.

311. Meireles P, Montiani-Ferreira F, Thomaz-Soccol V. Survey of giardiosis in household and shelter dogs from metropolitan areas of Curitiba, Paraná state, Southern Brazil. *Vet Parasitol* 2008;152:242–248.

312. Overgaauw PA, van Zutphen L, Hoek D, et al. Zoonotic parasites in fecal samples and fur from dogs and cats in The Netherlands. *Vet Parasitol* 2009;

313. Itoh N, Kanai K, Hori Y, et al. Prevalence of *Giardia intestinalis* and other zoonotic intestinal parasites in private household dogs of the Hachinohe area in Aomori prefecture, Japan in 1997, 2002 and 2007. *J Vet Sci* 2009;10:305–308.

314. Scaramozzino P, Di Cave D, Berrilli F, et al. A study of the prevalence and genotypes of *Giardia duodenalis* infecting kennelled dogs. *Vet J* 2009;182: 231–234.

315. Papini R, Gorini G, Spaziani A, et al. Survey on giardiosis in shelter dog populations. *Vet Parasitol* 2005;128:333–339.

316. Jacobs SR, Forrester CP, Yang J. A survey of the prevalence of Giardia in dogs presented to Canadian veterinary practices. *Can Vet J* 2001;42:45–46.

317. Lebbad M, Mattsson JG, Christensson B, et al. From mouse to moose: Multilocus genotyping of *Giardia* isolates from various animal species. *Vet Parasitol* 2009;168:231–239.

318. Palmer CS, Traub RJ, Robertson ID, et al. Determining the zoonotic significance of *Giardia* and *Cryptosporidium* in Australian dogs and cats. *Vet Parasitol* 2008;154:142–147.

319. Papini R, Marangi M, Mancianti F, et al. Occurrence and cyst burden of *Giardia duodenalis* in dog faecal deposits from urban green areas: implications for environmental contamination and related risks. *Prev Vet Med* 2009;92:158–162.

320. Solarczyk P, Majewska AC. A survey of the prevalence and genotypes of *Giardia duodenalis* infecting household and sheltered dogs. *Parasitol Res* 2010; 106:1015–1019.

321. Leonhard S, Pfister K, Beelitz P, et al. The molecular characterisation of Giardia from dogs in southern Germany. *Vet Parasitol* 2007;150:33–38.

322. Gookin JL, Stebbins ME, Hunt E, et al. Prevalence of and risk factors for feline *Tritrichomonas foetus* and *Giardia* infection. *J Clin Microbiol* 2004;42:2707–2710.

323. Vasilopulos RJ, Rickard LG, Mackin AJ, et al. Genotypic analysis of *Giardia duodenalis* in domestic cats. *J Vet Intern Med* 2007;21:352–355.

324. Lv CC, Feng C, Qi M, et al. Investigation on the prevalence of gastrointestinal parasites in pet hamsters. *Zhongguo Ji Sheng Chong Xue Yu Ji Sheng Chong Bing Za Zhi* 2009;27:279–280.

325. Abe N, Read C, Thompson RC, et al. Zoonotic genotype of *Giardia intestinalis* detected in a ferret. *J Parasitol* 2005;91:179–182.

326. Warburton AR, Jones PH, Bruce J. Zoonotic transmission of giardiasis: a case control study. *Commun Dis Rep CDR Rev* 1994;4:R32–R36.

327. Marangi M, Berrilli F, Otranto D, et al. Genotyping of *Giardia duodenalis* among children and dogs in a closed socially deprived community from Italy. *Zoonoses Public Health* 2009. Epub ahead of print.

328. Zimmer JF, Burrington DB. Comparison of four techniques of fecal examination for detecting canine giardiasis. *J Am Anim Hosp Assoc* 1986;22:161–167.

329. Barr SC, Bowman DD, Erb HN. Evaluation of two test procedures for diagnosis of giardiasis in dogs. *Am J Vet Res* 1992;53:2028–2031.

330. McGlade TR, Robertson ID, Elliot AD, et al. High prevalence of *Giardia* detected in cats by PCR. *Vet Parasitol* 2003;110:197–205.

331. Wolfe MS. Giardiasis. *Clin Microbiol Rev* 1992;5: 93–100.

332. Thompson RC. The zoonotic significance and molecular epidemiology of *Giardia* and giardiasis. *Vet Parasitol* 2004;126:15–35.

333. Stokol T, Randolph JF, Nachbar S, et al. Development of bone marrow toxicosis after albendazole administration in a dog and cat. *J Am Vet Med Assoc* 1997;210:1753–1756.

334. Zimmerman SK, Needham CA. Comparison of conventional stool concentration and preserved-smear methods with Merifluor *Cryptosporidium/Giardia* Direct Immunofluorescence Assay and ProSpecT *Giardia* EZ Microplate Assay for detection of *Giardia lamblia*. *J Clin Microbiol* 1995;33:1942–1943.

335. Rosoff JD, Sanders CA, Sonnad SS, et al. Stool diagnosis of giardiasis using a commercially available enzyme immunoassay to detect *Giardia*-specific antigen 65 (GSA 65). *J Clin Microbiol* 1989;27: 1997–2002.

336. Anderson KA, Brooks AS, Morrison AL, et al. Impact of *Giardia* vaccination on asymptomatic *Giardia* infections in dogs at a research facility. *Can Vet J* 2004;45:924–930.

337. Stein JE, Radecki SV, Lappin MR. Efficacy of *Giardia* vaccination in the treatment of giardiasis in cats. *J Am Vet Med Assoc* 2003;222:1548–1551.

338. American Animal Hospital Association (AAHA) Canine Vaccine Task Force, Paul MA, Carmichael LE, et al. 2006 AAHA canine vaccine guidelines. *J Am Anim Hosp Assoc* 2006;42:80–89.

339. American Association of Feline Practitioners. *2006 Feline Practice Guidelines*. Hillsborough, NJ: American Association of Feline Practitioners, 2006.

340. Bowman DD, Montgomery SP, Zajac AM, et al. Hookworms of dogs and cats as agents of cutaneous larva migrans. *Trends Parasitol* 2010;26:162–167.

341. Gates MC, Nolan TJ. Endoparasite prevalence and recurrence across different age groups of dogs and cats. *Vet Parasitol* 2009;166:153–158.

342. Palmer CS, Traub RJ, Robertson ID, et al. The veterinary and public health significance of hookworm

343. Traub RJ, Inpankaew T, Sutthikornchai C, et al. PCR-based coprodiagnostic tools reveal dogs as reservoirs of zoonotic ancylostomiasis caused by *Ancylostoma ceylanicum* in temple communities in Bangkok. *Vet Parasitol* 2008;155:67–73.

344. Companion Animal Parasite Council. *Hookworms.* Bel Air, MD: Companion Animal Parasite Council, 2009.

345. Millán J, Casanova JC. High prevalence of helminth parasites in feral cats in Majorca Island (Spain). *Parasitol Res* 2009;106:183–188.

346. Kelly JD, Ng BKY. Helminth parasites of dogs and cats II, prevalence in urban environments in Australasia. *Aust Vet Pract* 1975;6:89–100.

347. Blake RT, Overend DJ. The prevalence of *Dirofilaria immitis* and other parasites in urban pound dogs in north-eastern Victoria. *Aust Vet J* 1982;58:111–114.

348. Prescott CW. *Parasitic Diseases of the Cat in Australia.* Sydney, Australia: The University of Sydney, 1984.

349. Azian MY, Sakhone L, Hakim SL, et al. Detection of helminth infections in dogs and soil contamination in rural and urban areas. *Southeast Asian J Trop Med Public Health* 2008;39:205–212.

350. Nikolić A, Dimitrijević S, Katić-Radivojević S, et al. High prevalence of intestinal zoonotic parasites in dogs from Belgrade, Serbia—short communication. *Acta Vet Hung* 2008;56:335–340.

351. Ponce-Macotela M, Peralta-Abarca GE, Martínez-Gordillo MN. *Giardia intestinalis* and other zoonotic parasites: prevalence in adult dogs from the southern part of Mexico City. *Vet Parasitol* 2005;131: 1–4.

352. Sager H, Moret CS, Grimm F, et al. Coprological study on intestinal helminths in Swiss dogs: temporal aspects of anthelminthic treatment. *Parasitol Res* 2006;98:333–338.

353. Palmer CS, Thompson RC, Traub RJ, et al. National study of the gastrointestinal parasites of dogs and cats in Australia. *Vet Parasitol* 2008;151:181–190.

354. Wright I, Wolfe A. Prevalence of zoonotic nematode species in dogs in Lancashire. *Vet Rec* 2007; 161:790.

355. Guest CM, Stephen JM, Price CJ. Prevalence of *Campylobacter* and four endoparasites in dog populations associated with hearing dogs. *J Small Anim Pract* 2007;48:632–637.

356. Rinaldi L, Biggeri A, Carbone S, et al. Canine faecal contamination and parasitic risk in the city of Naples (southern Italy). *BMC Vet Res* 2006;2:29.

357. Tiyo R, Guedes TA, Falavigna DL, et al. Seasonal contamination of public squares and lawns by parasites with zoonotic potential in southern Brazil. *J Helminthol* 2008;82:1–6.

358. Veneziano V, Rinaldi L, Carbone S, et al. Geographical Information Systems and canine faecal contamination: the experience in the city of Naples (southern Italy). *Parassitologia* 2006;48:125–128.

359. Nakamura-Uchiyama F, Yamasaki E, Nawa Y. One confirmed and six suspected cases of cutaneous larva migrans caused by overseas infection with dog hookworm larvae. *J Dermatol* 2002;29: 104–111.

360. Green AD, Mason C, Spragg PM. Outbreak of cutaneous larva migrans among British military personnel in Belize. *J Travel Med* 2001;8:267–269.

361. Centers for Disease. Control and Prevention (CDC). Outbreak of cutaneous larva migrans at a children's camp—Miami, Florida, 2006. *MMWR Morb Mortal Wkly Rep* 2007;56:1285–1287.

362. Hochedez P, Caumes E. Hookworm-related cutaneous larva migrans. *J Travel Med* 2007;14:326–333.

363. Bouchaud O, Houzé S, Schiemann R, et al. Cutaneous larva migrans in travelers: a prospective study, with assessment of therapy with ivermectin. *Clin Infect Dis* 2000;31:493–498.

364. Galanti B, Fusco FM, Nardiello S. Outbreak of cutaneous larva migrans in Naples, southern Italy. *Trans R Soc Trop Med Hyg* 2002;96:491–492.

365. Landmann JK, Prociv P. Experimental human infection with the dog hookworm, *Ancylostoma caninum*. *Med J Aust* 2003;178:69–71.

366. Tu CH, Liao WC, Chiang TH, et al. Pet parasites infesting the human colon. *Gastrointest Endosc* 2008;67:159–160, commentary 160.

367. Traub RJ, Robertson ID, Irwin P, et al. Application of a species-specific PCR-RFLP to identify *Ancylostoma* eggs directly from canine faeces. *Vet Parasitol* 2004;123:245–255.

368. Epe C. Intestinal nematodes: biology and control. *Vet Clin North Am Small Anim Pract* 2009;39:1091–1107, vi–vii.

369. Schimmel A, Altreuther G, Schroeder I, et al. Efficacy of emodepside plus praziquantel tablets (Profender tablets for dogs) against mature and immature adult *Ancylostoma caninum* and *Uncinaria stenocephala* infections in dogs. *Parasitol Res* 2009;105(Suppl. 1): S9–S16.

370. von Samson-Himmelstjerna G, Epe C, Schimmel A, et al. Larvicidal and persistent efficacy of an imidacloprid and moxidectin topical formulation against endoparasites in cats and dogs. *Parasitol Res* 2003; 90(Suppl. 3):S114–S115.

371. Kopp SR, Kotze AC, McCarthy JS, et al. High-level pyrantel resistance in the hookworm *Ancylostoma caninum*. *Vet Parasitol* 2007;143:299–304.

372. Croese J, Loukas A, Opdebeeck J, et al. Human enteric infection with canine hookworms. *Ann Intern Med* 1994;120:369–374.

373. Krämer F, Epe C, Mencke N. Investigations into the prevention of neonatal *Ancylostoma caninum* infections in puppies by application of imidacloprid 10% plus moxidectin 2.5% topical solution to the pregnant dog. *Zoonoses Public Health* 2009;56: 34–40.

374. Petersen CA, Barr SC. Canine leishmaniasis in North America: emerging or newly recognized? *Vet Clin North Am Small Anim Pract* 2009;39:1065–1074, vi.

375. Jeronimo SMB, de Quiroz Sousa A, Pearson RD. *Leishmania* species: visceral (Kala-Azar), cutaneous and mucocutaneous leishmaniasis. In: Mandell GL, Bennett JE, Dolin R, eds. *Principles and Practice of Infectious Diseases*. Philadelphia: Elsevier, 2005, pp. 3145–3156.

376. Baneth G. Canine and feline integumentary leishmaniasis. In: Greene CE, ed. *Infectious Diseases of the Dog and Cat*. Philadelphia: Saunders Elsevier, 2006, pp. 695–698.

377. Dantas-Torres F. The role of dogs as reservoirs of *Leishmania* parasites, with emphasis on *Leishmania* (*Leishmania*) *infantum* and *Leishmania* (*Viannia*) *braziliensis*. *Vet Parasitol* 2007;149:139–146.

378. Moreno J, Alvar J. Canine leishmaniasis: epidemiological risk and the experimental model. *Trends Parasitol* 2002;18:399–405.

379. Chicharro C, Morales MA, Serra T, et al. Molecular epidemiology of *Leishmania infantum* on the island of Majorca: a comparison of phenotypic and genotypic tools. *Trans R Soc Trop Med Hyg* 2002;96 (Suppl. 1):S93–S99.

380. Cruz I, Morales MA, Noguer I, et al. *Leishmania* in discarded syringes from intravenous drug users. *Lancet* 2002;359:1124–1125.

381. Eltoum IA, Zijlstra EE, Ali MS, et al. Congenital kala-azar and leishmaniasis in the placenta. *Am J Trop Med Hyg* 1992;46:57–62.

382. Herwaldt BL, Juranek DD. Laboratory-acquired malaria, leishmaniasis, trypanosomiasis, and toxoplasmosis. *Am J Trop Med Hyg* 1993;48:313–323.

383. Owens SD, Oakley DA, Marryott K, et al. Transmission of visceral leishmaniasis through blood transfusions from infected English foxhounds to anemic dogs. *J Am Vet Med Assoc* 2001;219: 1076–1083.

384. Shulman IA. Parasitic infections and their impact on blood donor selection and testing. *Arch Pathol Lab Med* 1994;118:366–370.

385. Coutinho MT, Linardi PM. Can fleas from dogs infected with canine visceral leishmaniasis transfer the infection to other mammals? *Vet Parasitol* 2007;147:320–325.

386. Bryceson A. Visceral leishmaniasis in India. *Lancet* 2000;356:1933.

387. Elias M, Rahman AJ, Khan NI. Visceral leishmaniasis and its control in Bangladesh. *Bull World Health Organ* 1989;67:43–49.

388. Morsy TA, el Shazly AM, el Kady GA, et al. Natural *Leishmania* infections in two stray dogs and two *Gerbillus pyramidum* in Dakahlia Governorate, Egypt. *J Egypt Soc Parasitol* 1994;24:383–394.

389. Desjeux P. *Programme for the Surveillance and Control of Leishmaniasis*. Geneva: World Health Organization, 2001.

390. Shaw SE, Langton DA, Hillman TJ. Canine leishmaniasis in the United Kingdom: a zoonotic disease waiting for a vector? *Vet Parasitol* 2009;163: 281–285.

391. Amela C, Mendez I, Torcal JM, et al. Epidemiology of canine leishmaniasis in the Madrid region, Spain. *Eur J Epidemiol* 1995;11:157–161.

392. Cardoso L, Rodrigues M, Santos H, et al. Seroepidemiological study of canine *Leishmania* spp. infection in the municipality of Alijó (Alto Douro, Portugal). *Vet Parasitol* 2004;121:21–32.

393. Dantas-Torres F. Leishmune vaccine: the newest tool for prevention and control of canine visceral leishmaniasis and its potential as a transmission-blocking vaccine. *Vet Parasitol* 2006;141:1–8.

394. de Paiva Diniz PP, Schwartz DS, de Morais HS, et al. Surveillance for zoonotic vector-borne infections using sick dogs from southeastern Brazil. *Vector Borne Zoonotic Dis* 2007;7:689–697.

395. Evans TG, Teixeira MJ, McAuliffe IT, et al. Epidemiology of visceral leishmaniasis in northeast Brazil. *J Infect Dis* 1992;166:1124–1132.

396. Maresca C, Scoccia E, Barizzone F, et al. A survey on canine leishmaniasis and phlebotomine sand flies in central Italy. *Res Vet Sci* 2009;87:36–38.

397. Miró G, Montoya A, Mateo M, et al. A leishmaniosis surveillance system among stray dogs in the region of Madrid: ten years of serodiagnosis (1996–2006). *Parasitol Res* 2007;101:253–257.

398. Ozensoy Töz S, Sakru N, Ertabaklar H, et al. Serological and entomological survey of zoonotic visceral leishmaniasis in Denizli Province, Aegean Region, Turkey. *New Microbiol* 2009;32:93–100.

399. Antoniou M, Messaritakis I, Christodoulou V, et al. Increasing incidence of zoonotic visceral leishmaniasis on Crete, Greece. *Emerg Infect Dis* 2009;15: 932–934.

400. Martín-Sánchez J, Morales-Yuste M, Acedo-Sánchez C, et al. Canine leishmaniasis in southeastern Spain. *Emerg Infect Dis* 2009;15:795–798.

401. Binhazim AA, Chapman WL, Latimer KS, et al. Canine leishmaniasis caused by *Leishmania leishmania infantum* in two Labrador retrievers. *J Vet Diagn Invest* 1992;4:299–305.

402. Duprey ZH, Steurer FJ, Rooney JA, et al. Canine visceral leishmaniasis, United States and Canada, 2000–2003. *Emerg Infect Dis* 2006;12:440–446.

403. Gaskin AA, Schantz P, Jackson J, et al. Visceral leishmaniasis in a New York foxhound kennel. *J Vet Intern Med* 2002;16:34–44.

404. Rosypal AC, Tidwell RR, Lindsay DS. Prevalence of antibodies to *Leishmania infantum* and *Trypanosoma cruzi* in wild canids from South Carolina. *J Parasitol* 2007;93:955–957.

405. Rosypal AC, Troy GC, Zajac AM, et al. Emergence of zoonotic canine leishmaniasis in the United States: isolation and immunohistochemical detection of *Leishmania infantum* from foxhounds from Virginia. *J Eukaryot Microbiol* 2003;50(Suppl.): 691–693.

406. Schantz PM, Steurer FJ, Duprey ZH, et al. Autochthonous visceral leishmaniasis in dogs in North America. *J Am Vet Med Assoc* 2005;226: 1316–1322.

407. Sellon RK, Menard MM, Meuten DJ, et al. Endemic visceral leishmaniasis in a dog from Texas. *J Vet Intern Med* 1993;7:16–19.

408. Rosypal AC, Zajac AM, Lindsay DS. Canine visceral leishmaniasis and its emergence in the United States. *Vet Clin North Am Small Anim Pract* 2003; 33:921–937.

409. Rosypal AC, Troy GC, Zajac AM, et al. Transplacental transmission of a North American isolate of *Leishmania infantum* in an experimentally infected beagle. *J Parasitol* 2005;91:970–972.

410. Sergent E, Sergent E, Lonbard J, et al. La leishmaniose a Alger. Infection simultanee d'un enfant, d'un chien et d'un chat dans la meme habitation. *Bull Soc Path Exot* 1912;5:93–98.

411. Morsy TA, Abou el Seoud SM. Natural infection in two pet cats in a house of a zoonotic cutaneous leishmaniasis patient in Imbaba area, Giza Governorate, Egypt. *J Egypt Soc Parasitol* 1994;24: 199–204.

412. Gramiccia M, Gradoni L. The current status of zoonotic leishmaniases and approaches to disease control. *Int J Parasitol* 2005;35:1169–1180.

413. Martín-Sánchez J, Acedo C, Muñoz-Pérez M, et al. Infection by *Leishmania infantum* in cats: epidemiological study in Spain. *Vet Parasitol* 2007;145: 267–273.

414. Vita S, Santori D, Aguzzi I, et al. Feline leishmaniasis and ehrlichiosis: serological investigation in Abruzzo region. *Vet Res Commun* 2005;29(Suppl. 2):319–321.

415. Mancianti F. Feline leishmaniasis: what's the epidemiological role of the cat? *Parassitologia* 2004;46: 203–206.

416. Maia C, Nunes M, Campino L. Importance of cats in zoonotic leishmaniasis in Portugal. *Vector Borne Zoonotic Dis* 2008;8:555–559.

417. Benitez JA, Rodriguez-Morales AJ, Vivas P, et al. Burden of zoonotic diseases in Venezuela during 2004 and 2005. *Ann N Y Acad Sci* 2008;1149:315–317.

418. Alvar J, Cañavate C, Gutiérrez-Solar B, et al. *Leishmania* and human immunodeficiency virus coinfection: the first 10 years. *Clin Microbiol Rev* 1997;10:298–319.

419. de La Rosa R, Pineda JA, Delgado J, et al. Incidence of and risk factors for symptomatic visceral leishmaniasis among human immunodeficiency virus type 1-infected patients from Spain in the era of highly active antiretroviral therapy. *J Clin Microbiol* 2002;40:762–767.

420. Montalban C, Calleja JL, Erice A, et al. Visceral leishmaniasis in patients infected with human immunodeficiency virus. Co-operative Group for the Study of Leishmaniasis in AIDS. *J Infect* 1990; 21:261–270.

421. Bashaye S, Nombela N, Argaw D, et al. Risk factors for visceral leishmaniasis in a new epidemic site in Amhara Region, Ethiopia. *Am J Trop Med Hyg* 2009;81:34–39.

422. Gavgani AS, Hodjati MH, Mohite H, et al. Effect of insecticide-impregnated dog collars on incidence of zoonotic visceral leishmaniasis in Iranian children: a matched-cluster randomised trial. *Lancet* 2002; 360:374–379.

423. Reithinger R, Canales Espinoza J, Llanos-Cuentas A, et al. Domestic dog ownership: a risk factor for human infection with *Leishmania* (*Viannia*) species. *Trans R Soc Trop Med Hyg* 2003;97:141–145.

424. Biglino A, Bolla C, Concialdi E, et al. Asymptomatic *Leishmania infantum* infection in an area of northwestern Italy (Piedmont region) where such infections are traditionally nonendemic. *J Clin Microbiol* 2010;48:131–136.

425. Palatnik-de-Sousa CB, Silva-Antunes I, AdeA M, et al. Decrease of the incidence of human and canine visceral leishmaniasis after dog vaccination with Leishmune in Brazilian endemic areas. *Vaccine* 2009;27:3505–3512.

426. Borja-Cabrera GP, Santos FN, Santos FB, et al. Immunotherapy with the saponin enriched-Leishmune vaccine versus immunochemotherapy in dogs with natural canine visceral leishmaniasis. *Vaccine* 2010;28:597–603.

427. Alexander B, Maroli M. Control of phlebotomine sandflies. *Med Vet Entomol* 2003;17:1–18.

428. David JR, Stamm LM, Bezerra HS, et al. Deltamethrin-impregnated dog collars have a potent anti-feeding and insecticidal effect on *Lutzomyia longipalpis* and *Lutzomyia migonei*. *Mem Inst Oswaldo Cruz* 2001; 96:839–847.

429. Halbig P, Hodjati MH, Mazloumi-Gavgani AS, et al. Further evidence that deltamethrin-impregnated collars protect domestic dogs from sandfly bites. *Med Vet Entomol* 2000;14:223–226.

430. Killick-Kendrick R, Killick-Kendrick M, Focheux C, et al. Protection of dogs from bites of phlebotomine sandflies by deltamethrin collars for control of canine leishmaniasis. *Med Vet Entomol* 1997;11: 105–111.

431. Maroli M, Mizzon V, Siragusa C, et al. Evidence for an impact on the incidence of canine leishmaniasis by the mass use of deltamethrin-impregnated dog collars in southern Italy. *Med Vet Entomol* 2001; 15:358–363.

432. Ferroglio E, Poggi M, Trisciuoglio A. Evaluation of 65% permethrin spot-on and deltamethrin-impregnated collars for canine *Leishmania infantum* infection prevention. *Zoonoses Public Health* 2008; 55:145–148.

433. Reithinger R, Coleman PG, Alexander B, et al. Are insecticide-impregnated dog collars a feasible alternative to dog culling as a strategy for controlling canine visceral leishmaniasis in Brazil? *Int J Parasitol* 2004;34:55–62.

434. Courtenay O, Kovacic V, Gomes PA, et al. A long-lasting topical deltamethrin treatment to protect dogs against visceral leishmaniasis. *Med Vet Entomol* 2009;23:245–256.

435. Courtenay O, Quinnell RJ, Garcez LM, et al. Infectiousness in a cohort of Brazilian dogs: why culling fails to control visceral leishmaniasis in areas of high transmission. *J Infect Dis* 2002;186: 1314–1320.

436. Moreira ED, Mendes de Souza VM, Sreenivasan M, et al. Assessment of an optimized dog-culling program in the dynamics of canine *Leishmania* transmission. *Vet Parasitol* 2004;122:245–252.

437. Nunes CM, Pires MM, da Silva KM, et al. Relationship between dog culling and incidence of human visceral leishmaniasis in an endemic area. *Vet Parasitol* 2010;170:131–133.

438. Borja-Cabrera GP, Correia Pontes NN, da Silva VO, et al. Long lasting protection against canine kala-azar using the FML-QuilA saponin vaccine in an endemic area of Brazil (São Gonçalo do Amarante, RN). *Vaccine* 2002;20:3277–3284.

439. Chakrabarti A. Human notoedric scabies from contact with cats infested with *Notoedres cati*. *Int J Dermatol* 1986;25:646–648.

440. Maehr DS, Greiner EC, Lanier JE, et al. Notoedric mange in the Florida panther (*Felis concolor coryi*). *J Wildl Dis* 1995;31:251–254.

441. Ninomiya H, Ogata M. Notoedric mange in two free-ranging North American racoons (*Procyon lotor*) in Japan. *Vet Dermatol* 2002;13:119–121.

442. Ninomiya H, Ogata M, Makino T. Notoedric mange in free-ranging masked palm civets (*Paguma larvata*) in Japan. *Vet Dermatol* 2003;14:339–344.

443. Pantchev N, Hofmann T. Notoedric mange caused by *Notoedres cati* in a pet African pygmy hedgehog (*Atelerix albiventris*). *Vet Rec* 2006;158:59–60.

444. Pence DB, Tewes ME, Shindle DB, et al. Notoedric mange in an ocelot (*Felis pardalis*) from southern Texas. *J Wildl Dis* 1995;31:558–561.

445. Ryser-Degiorgis MP, Ryser A, Bacciarini LN, et al. Notoedric and sarcoptic mange in free-ranging lynx from Switzerland. *J Wildl Dis* 2002;38:228–232.

446. Uzal FA, Houston RS, Riley SP, et al. Notoedric mange in two free-ranging mountain lions (*Puma concolor*). *J Wildl Dis* 2007;43:274–278.

447. Valenzuela D, Ceballos G, García A. Mange epizootic in white-nosed coatis in western Mexico. *J Wildl Dis* 2000;36:56–63.

448. Beco L, Petite A, Olivry T. Comparison of subcutaneous ivermectin and oral moxidectin for the treatment of notoedric acariasis in hamsters. *Vet Rec* 2001;149:324–327.

449. Cornis TE, Linders MJ, Little SE, et al. Notoedric mange in western gray squirrels from Washington. *J Wildl Dis* 2001;37:630–633.

450. Leone F. Canine notoedric mange: a case report. *Vet Dermatol* 2007;18:127–129.

451. Isingla LD, Juyal PD, Gupta PP. Therapeutic trial of ivermectin against *Notoedres cati* var. *cuniculi* infection in rabbits. *Parasite* 1996;3:87–89.

452. Delucchi L, Castro E. Use of doramectin for treatment of notoedric mange in five cats. *J Am Vet Med Assoc* 2000;216:215–216, 193–214.

453. Beck W. Occurrence of a house-infesting tropical rat mite (*Ornithonyssus bacoti*) on murides and human beings. *Travel Med Infect Dis* 2008;6:245–249.

454. Fox MT, Baker AS, Farquhar R, et al. First record of *Ornithonyssus bacoti* from a domestic pet in the United Kingdom. *Vet Rec* 2004;154:437–438.

455. Chung SL, Hwang SJ, Kwon SB, et al. Outbreak of rat mite dermatitis in medical students. *Int J Dermatol* 1998;37:591–594.

456. Baumstark J, Beck W, Hofmann H. Outbreak of tropical rat mite (*Ornithonyssus bacoti*) dermatitis in a home for disabled persons. *Dermatology* 2007;215:66–68.

457. Engel PM, Welzel J, Maass M, et al. Tropical rat mite dermatitis: case report and review. *Clin Infect Dis* 1998;27:1465–1469.

458. Fox JG. Outbreak of tropical rat mite dermatitis in laboratory personnel. *Arch Dermatol* 1982;118:676–678.

459. Kelaher J, Jogi R, Katta R. An outbreak of rat mite dermatitis in an animal research facility. *Cutis* 2005;75:282–286.

460. Ram SM, Satija KC, Kaushik RK. *Ornithonyssus bacoti* infestation in laboratory personnel and veterinary students. *Int J Zoonoses* 1986;13:138–140.

461. Creel NB, Crowe MA, Mullen GR. Pet hamsters as a source of rat mite dermatitis. *Cutis* 2003;71:457–461.

462. Skírnisson K. The tropical rat mite *Ornithonyssus bacoti* attacks humans in Iceland. *Laeknabladid* 2001;87:991–993.

463. Chee JH, Kwon JK, Cho HS, et al. A survey of ectoparasite infestations in stray dogs of Gwang-ju City, Republic of Korea. *Korean J Parasitol* 2008;46:23–27.

464. Akucewich LH, Philman K, Clark A, et al. Prevalence of ectoparasites in a population of feral cats from north central Florida during the summer. *Vet Parasitol* 2002;109:129–139.

465. Lefkaditis MA, Koukeri SE, Mihalca AD. Prevalence and intensity of *Otodectes cynotis* in kittens from Thessaloniki area, Greece. *Vet Parasitol* 2009;163:374–375.

466. Bowman DD, Kato S, Fogarty EA. Effects of an ivermectin otic suspension on egg hatching of the cat ear mite, *Otodectes cynotis*, in vitro. *Vet Ther* 2001;2:311–316.

467. Curtis CF. Current trends in the treatment of *Sarcoptes*, *Cheyletiella* and *Otodectes* mite infestations in dogs and cats. *Vet Dermatol* 2004;15:108–114.

468. Blot C, Kodjo A, Reynaud MC, et al. Efficacy of selamectin administered topically in the treatment of feline otoacariosis. *Vet Parasitol* 2003;112:241–247.

469. Fourie LJ, Kok DJ, Heine J. Evaluation of the efficacy of an imidacloprid 10%/moxidectin 1% spot-on against *Otodectes cynotis* in cats. *Parasitol Res* 2003;90(Suppl. 3):S112–S113.

470. Krieger K, Heine J, Dumont P, et al. Efficacy and safety of imidacloprid 10% plus moxidectin 2.5% spot-on in the treatment of sarcoptic mange and otoacariosis in dogs: results of a European field study. *Parasitol Res* 2005;97(Suppl. 1):S81–S88.

471. Shanks DJ, McTier TL, Rowan TG, et al. The efficacy of selamectin in the treatment of naturally acquired aural infestations of *Otodectes cynotis* on dogs and cats. *Vet Parasitol* 2000;91:283–290.

472. Otranto D, Milillo P, Mesto P, et al. *Otodectes cynotis* (Acari: Psoroptidae): examination of survival off-the-host under natural and laboratory conditions. *Exp Appl Acarol* 2004;32:171–179.

473. Van de Heyning J, Thienpont D. Otitis externa in man caused by the mite *Otodectes cynotis*. *Laryngoscope* 1977;87:1938–1941.

474. Herwick RP. Lesions caused by canine ear mites. *Arch Dermatol* 1978;114:130.

475. Lopez RA. Of mites and man. *J Am Vet Med Assoc* 1993;203:606–607.

476. Suetake M, Yuasa R, Saijo S. Canine ear mites *Otodectes cynotis* found on both tympanic membranes of adult woman causing tinnitus. *Tohoku Rosai Hosp Pract Otol Kyoto* 1991;84:38–42.

477. Walton SF, Choy JL, Bonson A, et al. Genetically distinct dog-derived and human-derived *Sarcoptes scabiei* in scabies-endemic communities in northern Australia. *Am J Trop Med Hyg* 1999;61:542–547.

478. Rodriguez-Vivas RI, Ortega-Pacheco A, Rosado-Aguilar JA, et al. Factors affecting the prevalence of mange-mite infestations in stray dogs of Yucatán, Mexico. *Vet Parasitol* 2003;115:61–65.

479. Malik R, McKellar Stewart K, Sousa CA, et al. Crusted scabies (sarcoptic mange) in four cats due to *Sarcoptes scabiei* infestation. *J Feline Med Surg* 2006;8:327–339.

480. Mathieu ME, Wilson BB. Scabies. In: Mandell GL, Bennett JE, Dolin R, eds. *Principles and Practice of Infectious Diseases*. Philadelphia: Elsevier, 2005, pp. 3305–3307.

481. Ambroise-Thomas P. Emerging parasite zoonoses: the role of host-parasite relationship. *Int J Parasitol* 2000;30:1361–1367.

482. Arlian LG, Vyszenski-Moher DL, Pole MJ. Survival of adults and development stages of *Sarcoptes scabiei* var. *canis* when off the host. *Exp Appl Acarol* 1989;6:181–187.

483. Meijer P, van Voorst Vader PC. Canine scabies in man. *Ned Tijdschr Geneeskd* 1990;134:2491–2493.

484. Morsy TA, Bakr ME, Ahmed MM, et al. Human scabies acquired from a pet puppy. *J Egypt Soc Parasitol* 1994;24:305–308.

485. Burroughs RF, Elston DM. What's eating you? Canine scabies. *Cutis* 2003;72:107–109.

486. Pin D, Bensignor E, Carlotti DN, et al. Localised sarcoptic mange in dogs: a retrospective study of 10 cases. *J Small Anim Pract* 2006;47:611–614.

487. Curtis CF. Evaluation of a commercially available enzyme-linked immunosorbent assay for the diagnosis of canine sarcoptic mange. *Vet Rec* 2001;148:238–239.

488. Mueller RS, Bettenay SV, Shipstone M. Value of the pinnal-pedal reflex in the diagnosis of canine scabies. *Vet Rec* 2001;148:621–623.

489. Hugnet C, Bruchon-Hugnet C, Royer H, et al. Efficacy of 1.25% amitraz solution in the treatment of generalized demodicosis (eight cases) and sarcoptic mange (five cases) in dogs. *Vet Dermatol* 2001;12:89–92.

490. Fourie LJ, Heine J, Horak IG. The efficacy of an imidacloprid/moxidectin combination against naturally acquired *Sarcoptes scabiei* infestations on dogs. *Aust Vet J* 2006;84:17–21.

491. Paradis M, de Jaham C, Pagé N. Topical (pour-on) ivermectin in the treatment of canine scabies. *Can Vet J* 1997;38:379–382.

492. Wagner R, Wendlberger U. Field efficacy of moxidectin in dogs and rabbits naturally infested with *Sarcoptes* spp., *Demodex* spp. and *Psoroptes* spp. mites. *Vet Parasitol* 2000;93:149–158.

493. Six RH, Clemence RG, Thomas CA, et al. Efficacy and safety of selamectin against *Sarcoptes scabiei* on dogs and *Otodectes cynotis* on dogs and cats presented as veterinary patients. *Vet Parasitol* 2000;91:291–309.

494. Ambroise-Thomas P. Parasitic diseases and immunodeficiencies. *Parasitology* 2001;122(Suppl.):S65–S71.

495. Zafar AB, Beidas SO, Sylvester LK. Control of transmission of Norwegian scabies. *Infect Control Hosp Epidemiol* 2002;23:278–279.

496. Ruiz-Maldonado R, Tamayo L, Dominguez J. Norwegian scabies due to *Sarcoptes scabiei* var *canis*. *Arch Dermatol* 1977;113:1733.

497. Clark J, Friesen DL, Williams WA. Management of an outbreak of Norwegian scabies. *Am J Infect Control* 1992;20:217–220.

498. Corbett EL, Crossley I, Holton J, et al. Crusted ("Norwegian") scabies in a specialist HIV unit: successful use of ivermectin and failure to prevent nosocomial transmission. *Genitourin Med* 1996;72:115–117.

499. Guggisberg D, de Viragh PA, Constantin C, et al. Norwegian scabies in a patient with acquired immunodeficiency syndrome. *Dermatology (Basel)* 1998;197:306–308.

500. Emde RN. Sarcoptic mange in the human. A report of an epidemic of 10 cases of infection by *Sarcoptes scabiei*, variety *canis*. *Arch Dermatol* 1961;84:633–636.

501. Huffam SE, Currie BJ. Ivermectin for *Sarcoptes scabiei* hyperinfestation. *Int J Infect Dis* 1998;2:152–154.

502. Scheinfeld N. Controlling scabies in institutional settings: a review of medications, treatment models, and implementation. *Am J Clin Dermatol* 2004;5:31–37.

503. Walton SF, Dougall A, Pizzutto S, et al. Genetic epidemiology of *Sarcoptes scabiei* (Acari: Sarcoptidae) in northern Australia. *Int J Parasitol* 2004;34:839–849.

504. Companion Animal Parasite Council. *Mites Other Than Demodex*. Bel Air, MD: Companion Animal Parasite Council, 2007.

505. Kitvatanachai S, Boonslip S, Watanasatitarpa S. Intestinal parasitic infections in Srimum suburban area of Nakhon Ratchasima Province, Thailand. *Trop Biomed* 2008;25:237–242.

506. Nasiri V, Esmailnia K, Karim G, et al. Intestinal parasitic infections among inhabitants of Karaj City, Tehran province, Iran in 2006–2008. *Korean J Parasitol* 2009;47:265–268.

507. Warunee N, Choomanee L, Sataporn P, et al. Intestinal parasitic infections among school children in Thailand. *Trop Biomed* 2007;24:83–88.

508. Mariam ZT, Abebe G, Mulu A. Opportunistic and other intestinal parasitic infections in AIDS patients, HIV seropositive healthy carriers and HIV seronegative individuals in southwest Ethiopia. *East Afr J Public Health* 2008;5:169–173.

509. de Oliveira LC, Ribeiro CT, Mendes DM, et al. Frequency of *Strongyloides stercoralis* infection in alcoholics. *Mem Inst Oswaldo Cruz* 2002;97:119–121.

510. Gonçalves AL, Machado GA, Gonçalves-Pires MR, et al. Evaluation of strongyloidiasis in kennel dogs and keepers by parasitological and serological assays. *Vet Parasitol* 2007;147:132–139.

511. Júnior AF, Gonçalves-Pires MR, Silva DA, et al. Parasitological and serological diagnosis of *Strongyloides stercoralis* in domesticated dogs from southeastern Brazil. *Vet Parasitol* 2006;136:137–145.

512. Mercado R, Ueta MT, Castillo D, et al. Exposure to larva migrans syndromes in squares and public parks of cities in Chile. *Revista de saúde pública* 2004;38:729–731.

513. Papazahariadou M, Founta A, Papadopoulos E, et al. Gastrointestinal parasites of shepherd and hunting dogs in the Serres Prefecture, Northern Greece. *Vet Parasitol* 2007;148:170–173.

514. Itoh N, Muraoka N, Aoki M, et al. Prevalence of *Strongyloides* spp. infection in household dogs. *Kansenshōgaku Zasshi* 2003;77:430–435.

515. Dillard KJ, Saari SA, Anttila M. *Strongyloides stercoralis* infection in a Finnish kennel. *Acta Vet Scand* 2007;49:37.

516. Epe C, Ising-Volmer S, Stoye M. Parasitological fecal studies of equids, dogs, cats and hedgehogs during the years 1984–1991. *Dtsch Tierarztl Wochenschr* 1993;100:426–428.

517. Meloni BP, Thompson RC, Hopkins RM, et al. The prevalence of *Giardia* and other intestinal parasites in children, dogs and cats from aboriginal communities in the Kimberley. *Med J Aust* 1993;158:157–159.

518. Abu-Madi MA, Al-Ahbabi DA, Al-Mashhadani MM, et al. Patterns of parasitic infections in faecal samples from stray cat populations in Qatar. *J Helminthol* 2007;81:281–286.

519. Gatti S, Lopes R, Cevini C, et al. Intestinal parasitic infections in an institution for the mentally retarded. *Ann Trop Med Parasitol* 2000;94:453–460.

520. Shoop WL, Michael BF, Eary CH, et al. Transmammary transmission of *Strongyloides stercoralis* in dogs. *J Parasitol* 2002;88:536–539.

521. Mansfield LS, Schad GA. Ivermectin treatment of naturally acquired and experimentally induced *Strongyloides stercoralis* infections in dogs. *J Am Vet Med Assoc* 1992;201:726–730.

522. Georgi JR, Sprinkle CL. A case of human strongyloidosis apparently contracted from asymptomatic colony dogs. *Am J Trop Med Hyg* 1974;23:899–901.

523. Itoh N, Kanai K, Hori Y, et al. Fenbendazole treatment of dogs with naturally acquired *Strongyloides stercoralis* infection. *Vet Rec* 2009;164:559–560.

524. Snook ER, Baker DG, Bauer RW. Verminous myelitis in a pit bull puppy. *J Vet Diagn Invest* 2009;21:400–402.

525. Dulley FL, Costa S, Cosentino R, et al. *Strongyloides stercoralis* hyperinfection after allogeneic stem cell transplantation. *Bone Marrow Transplant* 2009;43:741–742.

526. Keiser PB, Nutman TB. *Strongyloides stercoralis* in the immunocompromised population. *Clin Microbiol Rev* 2004;17:208–217.

527. Roxby AC, Gottlieb GS, Limaye AP. Strongyloidiasis in transplant patients. *Clin Infect Dis* 2009;49:1411–1423.

528. Verweij JJ, Canales M, Polman K, et al. Molecular diagnosis of *Strongyloides stercoralis* in faecal samples using real-time PCR. *Trans R Soc Trop Med Hyg* 2009;103:342–346.

529. Zaha O, Hirata T, Kinjo F, et al. Strongyloidiasis—progress in diagnosis and treatment. *Intern Med* 2000;39:695–700.

530. Zaha O, Hirata T, Uchima N, et al. Comparison of anthelmintic effects of two doses of ivermectin on intestinal strongyloidiasis in patients negative or positive for anti-HTLV-1 antibody. *J Infect Chemother* 2004;10:348–351.

531. Siddiqui AA, Berk SL. Diagnosis of *Strongyloides stercoralis* infection. *Clin Infect Dis* 2001;33:1040–1047.

532. Fan PC, Chung WC, Wu JC. Experimental infection of an isolate of *Taenia solium* from Hainan in domestic animals. *J Helminthol* 1994;68:265–266.

533. Ito A, Putra MI, Subahar R, et al. Dogs as alternative intermediate hosts of *Taenia solium* in Papua (Irian Jaya), Indonesia confirmed by highly specific ELISA and immunoblot using native and recombinant antigens and mitochondrial DNA analysis. *J Helminthol* 2002;76:311–314.

534. Ing MB, Schantz PM, Turner JA. Human coenurosis in North America: case reports and review. *Clin Infect Dis* 1998;27:519–523.

535. Georgi JR, Georgi ME. *Parasitology for Veterinarians.* Philadelphia: W.B. Saunders, 1990.

536. Dubná S, Langrová I, Nápravník J, et al. The prevalence of intestinal parasites in dogs from Prague, rural areas, and shelters of the Czech Republic. *Vet Parasitol* 2007;145:120–128.

537. Martínez-Moreno FJ, Hernández S, López-Cobos E, et al. Estimation of canine intestinal parasites in Córdoba (Spain) and their risk to public health. *Vet Parasitol* 2007;143:7–13.

538. Schantz PM, Alstine CV, Blacksheep A, et al. Prevalence of *Echinococcus granulosus* and other cestodes in dogs on the Navajo reservation in Arizona and New Mexico. *Am J Vet Res* 1977;38:669–670.

539. Streitel RH, Dubey JP. Prevalence of *Sarcocystis* infection and other intestinal parasitisms in dogs from a humane shelter in Ohio. *J Am Vet Med Assoc* 1976;168:423–424.

540. Wang CR, Qiu JH, Zhao JP, et al. Prevalence of helminthes in adult dogs in Heilongjiang Province, the People's Republic of China. *Parasitol Res* 2006;99:627–630.

541. Claerebout E, Casaert S, Dalemans AC, et al. *Giardia* and other intestinal parasites in different dog populations in Northern Belgium. *Vet Parasitol* 2009; 161:41–46.

542. Abu-Madi MA, Behnke JM, Prabhaker KS, et al. Intestinal helminths of feral cat populations from urban and suburban districts of Qatar. *Vet Parasitol* 2010;168:284–292.

543. Abu-Madi MA, Pal P, Al-Thani A, et al. Descriptive epidemiology of intestinal helminth parasites from stray cat populations in Qatar. *J Helminthol* 2008;82:59–68.

544. Umeche N, Ima AE. Intestinal helminthic infections of cats in Calabar, Nigeria. *Folia Parasitol* 1988;35: 165–168.

545. Zibaei M, Sadjjadi SM, Sarkari B. Prevalence of *Toxocara cati* and other intestinal helminths in stray cats in Shiraz, Iran. *Trop Biomed* 2007;24:39–43.

546. Benger A, Rennie RP, Roberts JT, et al. A human coenurus infection in Canada. *Am J Trop Med Hyg* 1981;30:638–644.

547. Johnstone HG, Jones OW. Cerebral coenurosis in an infant. *Am J Trop Med Hyg* 1950;30:431–441.

548. Orihel TC, Gonzalez F, Beaver PC. Coenurus from neck of Texas woman. *Am J Trop Med Hyg* 1970; 19:255–257.

549. Hermos JA, Healy GR, Schultz MG, et al. Fatal human cerebral coenurosis. *JAMA* 1970;213: 1461–1464.

550. Pau A, Perria C, Turtas S, et al. Long-term follow-up of the surgical treatment of intracranial coenurosis. *Br J Neurosurg* 1990;4:39–43.

551. Stěrba J, Barus V. First record of *Strobilocercus fasciolaris* (Taenidae-larvae) in man. *Folia Parasitol* 1976;23:221–226.

552. Ekanayake S, Warnasuriya ND, Samarakoon PS, et al. An unusual "infection" of a child in Sri Lanka, with *Taenia taeniaeformis* of the cat. *Ann Trop Med Parasitol* 1999;93:869–873.

553. Ballweber LR. *Taenia crassiceps* subcutaneous cysticercosis in an adult dog. *Vet Rec* 2009;165: 693–694.

554. Bethell F, Truszkowska A. *Taenia serialis* in a domestic rabbit. *Vet Rec* 2010;166:282.

555. Hoberg EP, Ebinger W, Render JA. Fatal cysticercosis by *Taenia crassiceps* (Cyclophyllidea: Taeniidae) in a presumed immunocompromised canine host. *J Parasitol* 1999;85:1174–1178.

556. Huss BT, Miller MA, Corwin RM, et al. Fatal cerebral coenurosis in a cat. *J Am Vet Med Assoc* 1994; 205:69–71.

557. Ivens V, Conroy JD, Levine ND. *Taenia pisiformis* cysticerci in a dog in Illinois. *Am J Vet Res* 1969; 30:2017–2020.

558. Smith MC, Bailey CS, Baker N, et al. Cerebral coenurosis in a cat. *J Am Vet Med Assoc* 1988;192: 82–84.

559. Wills J. Coenurosis in a pet rabbit. *Vet Rec* 2001; 148:188.

560. Grandemange E, Claerebout E, Genchi C, et al. Field evaluation of the efficacy and the safety of a combination of oxantel/pyrantel/praziquantel in the treatment of naturally acquired gastrointestinal nematode and/or cestode infestations in dogs in Europe. *Vet Parasitol* 2007;145:94–99.

561. Manschot WA. Coenurus infestation of eye and orbit. *Arch Ophthalmol* 1976;94:961–964.

562. Templeton AC. Anatomical and geographical location of human coenurus infection. *Trop Geogr Med* 1971;23:105–108.

563. Ibechukwu BI, Onwukeme KE. Intraocular coenurosis: a case report. *Br J Ophthalmol* 1991;75:430–431.

564. Sotelo J, Rosas N, Palencia G. Freezing of infested pork muscle kills cysticerci. *JAMA* 1986;256: 893–894.

565. Maikai BV, Umoh JU, Ajanusi OJ, et al. Public health implications of soil contaminated with helminth eggs in the metropolis of Kaduna, Nigeria. *J Helminthol* 2008;82:113–118.

566. Dantas-Torres F. Biology and ecology of the brown dog tick, *Rhipicephalus sanguineus*. *Parasit Vectors* 2010;3:26.

567. Otranto D, Dantas-Torres F. Canine and feline vector-borne diseases in Italy: current situation and perspectives. *Parasit Vectors* 2010;3:2.

568. Spitalská E, Kocianová E. Detection of *Coxiella burnetii* in ticks collected in Slovakia and Hungary. *Eur J Epidemiol* 2003;18:263–266.

569. Toledo A, Jado I, Olmeda AS, et al. Detection of *Coxiella burnetii* in ticks collected from Central Spain. *Vector Borne Zoonotic Dis* 2009;9:465–468.

570. Greene CE, Breitschwerdt E. Rocky mountain spotted fever, murine typhuslike disease, rickettsialpox, typhus and Q fever. In: Greene CE, ed. *Infectious Diseases of the Dog and Cat*. Philadelphia: Saunders Elsevier, 2006, pp. 232–245.

571. Mathieu ME, Wilson BB. Ticks (including tick paralysis). In: Mandell GL, Bennett JE, Dolin P, eds. *Principles and Practice of Infectious Diseases*. Philadelphia: Elsevier, 2005, pp. 3312–3315.

572. Greene CE. Environmental factors in infectious disease. In: Greene CE, ed. *Infectious Diseases of the Dog and Cat*. Philadelphia: Saunders Elsevier, 2006, pp. 991–1013.

573. Animal Poison Control Center. The ASPCA Animal Poison Control Center alerts dog owners to important information regarding West Nile virus, 2002. http://www2.aspca.org/site/News2?page=NewsArticle&ID=10900. Accessed October 14, 2010.

574. Walker DH, Raoult D. *Rickettsia rickettsii* and other spotted fever group Rickettsiae. In: Mandell GL, Bennett JE, Dolin P, eds. *Principles and Practice of Infectious Diseases*. Philadelphia: Elsevier, 2005, pp. 2287–2295.

575. Overgaauw PA. Aspects of *Toxocara* epidemiology: human toxocarosis. *Crit Rev Microbiol* 1997;23:215–231.

576. Lee AC, Schantz PM, Kazacos KR, et al. Epidemiologic and zoonotic aspects of ascarid infections in dogs and cats. *Trends Parasitol* 2010;26:155–161.

577. Fisher M. *Toxocara cati*: an underestimated zoonotic agent. *Trends Parasitol* 2003;19:167–170.

578. Li MW, Zhu XQ, Gasser RB, et al. The occurrence of *Toxocara malaysiensis* in cats in China, confirmed by sequence-based analyses of ribosomal DNA. *Parasitol Res* 2006;99:554–557.

579. Schuster RK, Thomas K, Sivakumar S, et al. The parasite fauna of stray domestic cats (*Felis catus*) in Dubai, United Arab Emirates. *Parasitol Res* 2009;105:125–134.

580. Parsons JC. Ascarid infections of cats and dogs. *Vet Clin North Am Small Anim Pract* 1987;17:1307–1339.

581. Overgaauw PA. Aspects of *Toxocara* epidemiology: toxocarosis in dogs and cats. *Crit Rev Microbiol* 1997;23:233–251.

582. Coati N, Schnieder T, Epe C. Vertical transmission of *Toxocara cati* Schrank 1788 (Anisakidae) in the cat. *Parasitol Res* 2004;92:142–146.

583. Agudelo C, Villareal E, Cáceres E, et al. Human and dogs *Toxocara canis* infection in a poor neighborhood in Bogota. *Mem Inst Oswaldo Cruz* 1990;85:75–78.

584. Bridger KE, Whitney H. Gastrointestinal parasites in dogs from the Island of St. Pierre off the south coast of Newfoundland. *Vet Parasitol* 2009;162:167–170.

585. Cancrini G, Bartoloni A, Zaffaroni E, et al. Seroprevalence of *Toxocara canis*-IgG antibodies in two rural Bolivian communities. *Parassitologia* 1998;40:473–475.

586. Gingrich EN, Scorza AV, Clifford EL, et al. Intestinal parasites of dogs on the Galapagos Islands. *Vet Parasitol* 2010;169:404–407.

587. Holland C, O'Connor P, Taylor MR, et al. Families, parks, gardens and toxocariasis. *Scand J Infect Dis* 1991;23:225–231.

588. Inpankaew T, Traub R, Thompson RC, et al. Canine parasitic zoonoses in Bangkok temples. *Southeast Asian J Trop Med Public Health* 2007;38:247–255.

589. Adams PJ, Elliot AD, Algar D, et al. Gastrointestinal parasites of feral cats from Christmas Island. *Aust Vet J* 2008;86:60–63.

590. Daryani A, Sharif M, Amouei A, et al. Prevalence of *Toxocara canis* in stray dogs, northern Iran. *Pak J Biol Sci* 2009;12:1031–1035.

591. Martínez-Barbabosa I, Vázquez Tsuji O, Cabello RR, et al. The prevalence of *Toxocara cati* in domestic cats in Mexico City. *Vet Parasitol* 2003;114:43–49.

592. Sommerfelt IE, Cardillo N, López C, et al. Prevalence of *Toxocara cati* and other parasites in cats' faeces collected from the open spaces of public institutions: Buenos Aires, Argentina. *Vet Parasitol* 2006;140:296–301.

593. Fontanarrosa MF, Vezzani D, Basabe J, et al. An epidemiological study of gastrointestinal parasites of dogs from Southern Greater Buenos Aires (Argentina): age, gender, breed, mixed infections, and seasonal and spatial patterns. *Vet Parasitol* 2006;136:283–295.

594. Itoh N, Muraoka N, Aoki M, et al. Prevalence of *Toxocara canis* infection in household dogs. *Kansenshōgaku Zasshi* 2004;78:114–119.

595. López J, Abarca K, Paredes P, et al. Intestinal parasites in dogs and cats with gastrointestinal symptoms in Santiago, Chile. *Rev Med Chil* 2006;134:193–200.

596. Mohamed AS, Moore GE, Glickman LT. Prevalence of intestinal nematode parasitism among pet dogs in the United States (2003–2006). *J Am Vet Med Assoc* 2009;234:631–637.

597. Habluetzel A, Traldi G, Ruggieri S, et al. An estimation of *Toxocara canis* prevalence in dogs, environmental egg contamination and risk of human infection in the Marche region of Italy. *Vet Parasitol* 2003;113:243–252.

598. Haridy FM, Hassan AA, Hafez AO, et al. External and intestinal parasites of pet dogs with reference to zoonotic toxocariasis. *J Egypt Soc Parasitol* 2009; 39:321–326.

599. Ho SY, Watanabe Y, Lee YC, et al. Survey of gastro-intestinal parasitic infections in quarantine dogs in Taiwan. *J Vet Med Sci* 2006;68:69–70.

600. Pullola T, Vierimaa J, Saari S, et al. Canine intestinal helminths in Finland: prevalence, risk factors and endoparasite control practices. *Vet Parasitol* 2006;140:321–326.

601. Roddie G, Stafford P, Holland C, et al. Contamination of dog hair with eggs of *Toxocara canis*. *Vet Parasitol* 2008;152:85–93.

602. Aydenizöz-Ozkayhan M, Yağci BB, Erat S. The investigation of *Toxocara canis* eggs in coats of different dog breeds as a potential transmission route in human toxocariasis. *Vet Parasitol* 2008;152: 94–100.

603. Wolfe A, Wright IP. Human toxocariasis and direct contact with dogs. *Vet Rec* 2003;152:419–422.

604. Avcioglu H, Burgu A. Seasonal prevalence of *Toxocara* ova in soil samples from public parks in Ankara, Turkey. *Vector Borne Zoonotic Dis* 2008; 8:345–350.

605. Campos Filho PC, Barros LM, Campos JO, et al. Zoonotic parasites in dog feces at public squares in the municipality of Itabuna, Bahia, Brazil. *Rev Bras Parasitol Vet* 2008;17:206–209.

606. Devera R, Blanco Y, Hernández H, et al. *Toxocara* spp. and other helminths in squares and parks of Ciudad Bolívar, Bolivar State (Venezuela). *Enferm Infecc Microbiol Clin* 2008;26:23–26.

607. Paquet-Durand I, Hernández J, Dolz G, et al. Prevalence of *Toxocara* spp., *Toxascaris leonina* and ancylostomidae in public parks and beaches in different climate zones of Costa Rica. *Acta Trop* 2007;104:30–37.

608. Chomel BB, Kasten R, Adams C, et al. Serosurvey of some major zoonotic infections in children and teenagers in Bali, Indonesia. *Southeast Asian J Trop Med Public Health* 1993;24:321–326.

609. Doğan N, Dinleyici EC, Bor O, et al. Seroepidemiological survey for *Toxocara canis* infection in the northwestern part of Turkey. *Turkiye Parazitol Derg* 2007;31:288–291.

610. Ellis GS, Pakalnis VA, Worley G, et al. *Toxocara canis* infestation. Clinical and epidemiological associations with seropositivity in kindergarten children. *Ophthalmology* 1986;93:1032–1037.

611. Espinoza YA, Huapaya PH, Roldán WH, et al. Clinical and serological evidence of *Toxocara* infection in school children from Morrope district, Lambayeque, Peru. *Rev Inst Med Trop Sao Paulo* 2008;50:101–105.

612. Fallah M, Azimi A, Taherkhani H. Seroprevalence of toxocariasis in children aged 1–9 years in western Islamic Republic of Iran, 2003. *East Mediterr Health J* 2007;13:1073–1077.

613. Fan CK, Hung CC, Du WY, et al. Seroepidemiology of *Toxocara canis* infection among mountain aboriginal schoolchildren living in contaminated districts in eastern Taiwan. *Trop Med Int Health* 2004; 9:1312–1318.

614. Fan CK, Liao CW, Kao TC, et al. Sero-epidemiology of *Toxocara canis* infection among aboriginal schoolchildren in the mountainous areas of north-eastern Taiwan. *Ann Trop Med Parasitol* 2005;99:593–600.

615. Fernando SD, Wickramasinghe VP, Kapilananda GM, et al. Epidemiological aspects and risk factors of toxocariasis in a pediatric population in Sri Lanka. *Southeast Asian J Trop Med Public Health* 2007;38:983–990.

616. Glickman LT, Cypess RH. *Toxocara* infection in animal hospital employees. *Am J Public Health* 1977;67:1193–1195.

617. Hayashi E, Tuda J, Imada M, et al. The high prevalence of asymptomatic *Toxocara* infection among schoolchildren in Manado, Indonesia. *Southeast Asian J Trop Med Public Health* 2005;36:1399–1406.

618. Herrmann N, Glickman LT, Schantz PM, et al. Seroprevalence of zoonotic toxocariasis in the United States: 1971–1973. *Am J Epidemiol* 1985; 122:890–896.

619. Iddawela DR, Kumarasiri PV, de Wijesundera MS. A seroepidemiological study of toxocariasis and risk factors for infection in children in Sri Lanka. *Southeast Asian J Trop Med Public Health* 2003; 34:7–15.

620. Kim YH, Huh S, Chung YB. Seroprevalence of toxocariasis among healthy people with eosinophilia. *Korean J Parasitol* 2008;46:29–32.

621. Lévesque B, Messier V, Bonnier-Viger Y, et al. Seroprevalence of zoonoses in a Cree community (Canada). *Diagn Microbiol Infect Dis* 2007;59: 283–286.

622. Muradian V, Gennari SM, Glickman LT, et al. Epidemiological aspects of visceral larva migrans in children living at São Remo Community, São Paulo (SP), Brazil. *Vet Parasitol* 2005;134:93–97.

623. Nourian AA, Amiri M, Ataeian A, et al. Seroepidemiological study for toxocariasis among children in Zanjan-northwest of Iran. *Pak J Biol Sci* 2008;11:1844–1847.

624. Prestes-Carneiro LE, Santarém V, Zago SC, et al. Sero-epidemiology of toxocariasis in a rural settlement in São Paulo state, Brazil. *Ann Trop Med Parasitol* 2008;102:347–356.

625. Rubinsky-Elefant G, da Silva-Nunes M, Malafronte RS, et al. Human toxocariasis in rural Brazilian

Amazonia: seroprevalence, risk factors, and spatial distribution. *Am J Trop Med Hyg* 2008;79:93–98.

626. Stensvold CR, Skov J, Møller LN, et al. Seroprevalence of human toxocariasis in Denmark. *Clin Vaccine Immunol* 2009;16:1372–1373.

627. Antonios SN, Eid MM, Khalifa EA, et al. Seroprevalence study of *Toxocara canis* in selected Egyptian patients. *J Egypt Soc Parasitol* 2008;38: 313–318.

628. Worley G, Green JA, Frothingham TE, et al. *Toxocara canis* infection: clinical and epidemiological associations with seropositivity in kindergarten children. *J Infect Dis* 1984;149:591–597.

629. Won KY, Kruszon-Moran D, Schantz PM, et al. National seroprevalence and risk factors for Zoonotic *Toxocara* spp. infection. *Am J Trop Med Hyg* 2008;79:552–557.

630. Zarnowska H, Borecka A, Gawor J, et al. A serological and epidemiological evaluation of risk factors for toxocariasis in children in central Poland. *J Helminthol* 2008;82:123–127.

631. Good B, Holland CV, Taylor MR, et al. Ocular toxocariasis in schoolchildren. *Clin Infect Dis* 2004; 39:173–178.

632. Schantz PM, Meyer D, Glickman LT. Clinical, serologic, and epidemiologic characteristics of ocular toxocariasis. *Am J Trop Med Hyg* 1979;28:24–28.

633. El-Shazly AM, Abdel Baset SM, Kamal A, et al. Seroprevalence of human toxocariasis (visceral larva migrans). *J Egypt Soc Parasitol* 2009;39: 731–744.

634. Overgaauw PA, Boersema JH. Nematode infections in dog breeding kennels in The Netherlands, with special reference to *Toxocara*. *Vet Q* 1998;20:12–15.

635. Woodruff AW, de Savigny D, Jacobs DE. Study of toxocaral infection in dog breeders. *Br Med J* 1978;2:1747–1748.

636. Woodruff AW, de Savigny DH, Hendy-Ibbs PM. Toxocaral and toxoplasmal antibodies in cat breeders and in Icelanders exposed to cats but not to dogs. *Br Med J (Clin Res Ed)* 1982;284:309–310.

637. Jacobs DE, Woodruff AW, Shah AI, et al. *Toxocara* infections and kennel workers. *Br Med J* 1977;1:51.

638. Glickman LT, Chaudry IU, Costantino J, et al. Pica patterns, toxocariasis, and elevated blood lead in children. *Am J Trop Med Hyg* 1981;30:77–80.

639. Kaplan M, Kalkan A, Hosoglu S, et al. The frequency of *Toxocara* infection in mental retarded children. *Mem Inst Oswaldo Cruz* 2004;99:121–125.

640. Nelson S, Greene T, Ernhart CB. *Toxocara canis* infection in preschool age children: risk factors and the cognitive development of preschool children. *Neurotoxicol Teratol* 1996;18:167–174.

641. Paludo ML, Falavigna DL, Elefant GR, et al. Frequency of *Toxocara* infection in children attended by the health public service of Maringá, south Brazil. *Rev Inst Med Trop Sao Paulo* 2007;49:343–348.

642. Bratt DE, Tikasingh ES. Visceral larva migrans in seven members of one family in Trinidad. *Trop Geogr Med* 1992;44:109–112.

643. Maetz HM, Kleinstein RN, Federico D, et al. Estimated prevalence of ocular toxoplasmosis and toxocariasis in Alabama. *J Infect Dis* 1987;156:414.

644. Holland CV, O'Lorcain P, Taylor MR, et al. Seroepidemiology of toxocariasis in school children. *Parasitology* 1995;110(Pt. 5):535–545.

645. Buijs J, Borsboom G, Renting M, et al. Relationship between allergic manifestations and *Toxocara* seropositivity: a cross-sectional study among elementary school children. *Eur Respir J* 1997;10: 1467–1475.

646. Fernando D, Wickramasinghe P, Kapilananda G, et al. *Toxocara* seropositivity in Sri Lankan children with asthma. *Pediatr Int* 2009;51:241–245.

647. Kustimur S, Dogruman Al F, Oguzulgen K, et al. *Toxocara* seroprevalence in adults with bronchial asthma. *Trans R Soc Trop Med Hyg* 2007;101: 270–274.

648. Sharghi N, Schantz PM, Caramico L, et al. Environmental exposure to *Toxocara* as a possible risk factor for asthma: a clinic-based case-control study. *Clin Infect Dis* 2001;32:E111–E116.

649. Nicoletti A, Bartoloni A, Sofia V, et al. Epilepsy and toxocariasis: a case-control study in Burundi. *Epilepsia* 2007;48:894–899.

650. Nicoletti A, Sofia V, Mantella A, et al. Epilepsy and toxocariasis: a case-control study in Italy. *Epilepsia* 2008;49:594–599.

651. Akyol A, Bicerol B, Ertug S, et al. Epilepsy and seropositivity rates of *Toxocara canis* and *Toxoplasma gondii*. *Seizure* 2007;16:233–237.

652. Kwon NH, Oh MJ, Lee SP, et al. The prevalence and diagnostic value of toxocariasis in unknown eosinophilia. *Ann Hematol* 2006;85:233–238.

653. Roldán WH, Espinoza YA, Atúncar A, et al. Frequency of eosinophilia and risk factors and their association with *Toxocara* infection in schoolchildren during a health survey in the north of Lima, Peru. *Rev Inst Med Trop Sao Paulo* 2008; 50:273–278.

654. Sviben M, Cavlek TV, Missoni EM, et al. Seroprevalence of *Toxocara canis* infection among asymptomatic children with eosinophilia in Croatia. *J Helminthol* 2009;83:369–371.

655. Yariktas M, Demirci M, Aynali G, et al. Relationship between *Toxocara* seropositivity and allergic rhinitis. *Am J Rhinol* 2007;21:248–250.

656. Gavignet B, Piarroux R, Aubin F, et al. Cutaneous manifestations of human toxocariasis. *J Am Acad Dermatol* 2008;59:1031–1042.

657. Humbert P, Niezborala M, Salembier R, et al. Skin manifestations associated with toxocariasis: a case-control study. *Dermatology (Basel)* 2000;201:230–234.

658. Ismail MA, Khalafallah O. *Toxocara canis* and chronic urticaria in Egyptian patients. *J Egypt Soc Parasitol* 2005;35:833–840.

659. Hughes PL, Dubielzig RR, Kazacos KR. Multifocal retinitis in New Zealand sheep dogs. *Vet Pathol* 1987;24:22–27.

660. Johnson BW, Kirkpatrick CE, Whiteley HE, et al. Retinitis and intraocular larval migration in a group of Border Collies. *J Am Anim Hosp Assoc* 1989; 25:623–629.

661. Bowman DD, Parsons JC, Grieve RB, et al. Effects of milbemycin on adult *Toxocara canis* in dogs with experimentally induced infection. *Am J Vet Res* 1988;49:1986–1989.

662. Schenker R, Cody R, Strehlau G, et al. Comparative effects of milbemycin oxime-based and febantel-pyrantel embonate-based anthelmintic tablets on *Toxocara canis* egg shedding in naturally infected pups. *Vet Parasitol* 2006;137:369–373.

663. Holland CV, Smith HV. *Toxocara: The Enigmatic Parasite*. Oxfordshire, UK: CABI Publishing, 2006.

664. Stewart JM, Cubillan LD, Cunningham ET. Prevalence, clinical features, and causes of vision loss among patients with ocular toxocariasis. *Retina* 2005;25:1005–1013.

665. Yokoi K, Goto H, Sakai J, et al. Clinical features of ocular toxocariasis in Japan. *Ocul Immunol Inflamm* 2003;11:269–275.

666. Wolfrom E, Chêne G, Boisseau H, et al. Chronic urticaria and *Toxocara canis*. *Lancet* 1995;345:196.

667. Despommier D. Toxocariasis: clinical aspects, epidemiology, medical ecology, and molecular aspects. *Clin Microbiol Rev* 2003;16:265–272.

668. Smith HV, Quinn R, Kusel JR, et al. The effect of temperature and antimetabolites on antibody binding to the outer surface of second stage *Toxocara canis* larvae. *Mol Biochem Parasitol* 1981;4:183–193.

669. Fomda BA, Ahmad Z, Khan NN, et al. Ocular toxocariasis in a child: a case report from Kashmir, north India. *Indian J Med Microbiol* 2007;25:411–412.

670. Frazier M, Anderson ML, Sophocleous S. Treatment of ocular toxocariasis with albendazole: a case report. *Optometry* 2009;80:175–180.

671. Biglan AW, Glickman LT, Lobes LA. Serum and vitreous *Toxocara* antibody in nematode endophthalmitis. *Am J Ophthalmol* 1979;88:898–901.

672. Wells DL. Public understanding of toxocariasis. *Public Health* 2007;121:187–188.

673. Jones JL, Kruszon-Moran D, Wilson M, et al. *Toxoplasma gondii* infection in the United States: seroprevalence and risk factors. *Am J Epidemiol* 2001;154:357–365.

674. Su C, Evans D, Cole RH, et al. Recent expansion of *Toxoplasma* through enhanced oral transmission. *Science* 2003;299:414–416.

675. Dubey JP, Lindsay DS, Lappin MR. Toxoplasmosis and other intestinal coccidial infections in cats and dogs. *Vet Clin North Am Small Anim Pract* 2009;39:1009–1034, v.

676. Tenter AM, Heckeroth AR, Weiss LM. *Toxoplasma gondii*: from animals to humans. *Int J Parasitol* 2000;30:1217–1258.

677. Dubey JP, Bhatia C, Lappin M, et al. Seroprevalence of *Toxoplasma gondii* and *Bartonella* spp. antibodies in cats from Pennsylvania. *J Parasitol* 2008;95: 578–580.

678. Vollaire MR, Radecki SV, Lappin MR. Seroprevalence of *Toxoplasma gondii* antibodies in clinically ill cats in the United States. *Am J Vet Res* 2005; 66:874–877.

679. Dabritz HA, Miller MA, Atwill ER, et al. Detection of *Toxoplasma gondii*-like oocysts in cat feces and estimates of the environmental oocyst burden. *J Am Vet Med Assoc* 2007;231:1676–1684.

680. Herrmann DC, Pantchev N, Vrhovec MG, et al. Atypical *Toxoplasma gondii* genotypes identified in oocysts shed by cats in Germany. *Int J Parasitol* 2010;40:285–292.

681. Mancianti F, Nardoni S, Ariti G, et al. Cross-sectional survey of *Toxoplasma gondii* infection in colony cats from urban Florence (Italy). *J Feline Med Surg* 2009;12:351–354.

682. Schares G, Vrhovec MG, Pantchev N, et al. Occurrence of *Toxoplasma gondii* and *Hammondia hammondi* oocysts in the faeces of cats from Germany and other European countries. *Vet Parasitol* 2008;152:34–45.

683. Dubey JP, Cortés-Vecino JA, Vargas-Duarte JJ, et al. Prevalence of *Toxoplasma gondii* in dogs from Colombia, South America and genetic characterization of *T. gondii* isolates. *Vet Parasitol* 2007;145: 45–50.

684. Dubey JP, Lappin M, Mofya S, et al. Seroprevalence of *Toxoplasma gondii* and concurrent *Bartonella* spp., feline immunodeficiency virus, and feline leukemia infections in cats from Grenada, West Indies. *J Parasitol* 2009;95:1129–1133.

685. Dubey JP, Rajapakse RP, Wijesundera RR, et al. Prevalence of *Toxoplasma gondii* in dogs from Sri Lanka and genetic characterization of the parasite isolates. *Vet Parasitol* 2007;146:341–346.

686. Figueredo LA, Dantas-Torres F, de Faria EB, et al. Occurrence of antibodies to *Neospora caninum* and *Toxoplasma gondii* in dogs from Pernambuco, Northeast Brazil. *Vet Parasitol* 2008;157:9–13.

687. Santos TR, Costa AJ, Toniollo GH, et al. Prevalence of anti-*Toxoplasma gondii* antibodies in dairy cattle,

dogs, and humans from the Jauru micro-region, Mato Grosso state, Brazil. *Vet Parasitol* 2009;161: 324–326.

688. Tsai YJ, Chung WC, Fei AC, et al. Prevalence of *Toxoplasma gondii* antibodies in stray dogs in Taipei, Taiwan. *J Parasitol* 2008;94:1437.

689. Schares G, Pantchev N, Barutzki D, et al. Oocysts of *Neospora caninum, Hammondia heydorni, Toxoplasma gondii* and *Hammondia hammondi* in faeces collected from dogs in Germany. *Int J Parasitol* 2005;35: 1525–1537.

690. Antoniou M, Economou I, Wang X, et al. Fourteen-year seroepidemiological study of zoonoses in a Greek village. *Am J Trop Med Hyg* 2002;66:80–85.

691. Juncker-Voss M, Prosl H, Lussy H, et al. Screening for antibodies against zoonotic agents among employees of the Zoological Garden of Vienna, Schönbrunn, Austria. *Berl Munch Tierarztl Wochenschr* 2004;117:404–409.

692. Kamani J, Mani AU, Egwu GO, et al. Seroprevalence of human infection with *Toxoplasma gondii* and the associated risk factors, in Maiduguri, Borno state, Nigeria. *Ann Trop Med Parasitol* 2009;103: 317–321.

693. Messier V, Lévesque B, Proulx JF, et al. Seroprevalence of *Toxoplasma gondii* among Nunavik Inuit (Canada). *Zoonoses Public Health* 2009;56:188–197.

694. Xiao Y, Yin J, Jiang N, et al. Seroepidemiology of human *Toxoplasma gondii* infection in China. *BMC Infect Dis* 2010;10:4.

695. Mead PS, Slutsker L, Dietz V, et al. Food-related illness and death in the United States. *Emerg Infect Dis* 1999;5:607–625.

696. Kapperud G, Jenum PA, Stray-Pedersen B, et al. Risk factors for *Toxoplasma gondii* infection in pregnancy. Results of a prospective case-control study in Norway. *Am J Epidemiol* 1996;144: 405–412.

697. Jones JL, Dargelas V, Roberts J, et al. Risk factors for *Toxoplasma gondii* infection in the United States. *Clin Infect Dis* 2009;49:878–884.

698. Pereira LH, Staudt M, Tanner CE, et al. Exposure to *Toxoplasma gondii* and cat ownership in Nova Scotia. *Pediatrics* 1992;89:1169–1172.

699. Bowie WR, King AS, Werker DH, et al. Outbreak of toxoplasmosis associated with municipal drinking water. The BC *Toxoplasma* Investigation Team. *Lancet* 1997;350:173–177.

700. Roghmann MC, Faulkner CT, Lefkowitz A, et al. Decreased seroprevalence for *Toxoplasma gondii* in Seventh Day Adventists in Maryland. *Am J Trop Med Hyg* 1999;60:790–792.

701. Stagno S, Dykes AC, Amos CS, et al. An outbreak of toxoplasmosis linked to cats. *Pediatrics* 1980;65:706–712.

702. Weigel RM, Dubey JP, Dyer D, et al. Risk factors for infection with *Toxoplasma gondii* for residents and workers on swine farms in Illinois. *Am J Trop Med Hyg* 1999;60:793–798.

703. Frenkel JK, Lindsay DS, Parker BB, et al. Dogs as possible mechanical carriers of *Toxoplasma*, and their fur as a source of infection of young children. *Int J Infect Dis* 2003;7:292–293.

704. Dubey JP, Lappin MR. Toxoplasmosis and neosporosis. In: Greene CE, ed. *Infectious Diseases of the Dog and Cat*. Philadelphia: Saunders Elsevier, 2006, pp. 754–775.

705. Al-Qassab S, Reichel MP, Su C, et al. Isolation of *Toxoplasma gondii* from the brain of a dog in Australia and its biological and molecular characterization. *Vet Parasitol* 2009;164:335–339.

706. Many A, Koren G. Toxoplasmosis during pregnancy. *Can Fam Physician* 2006;52:29–30, 32.

707. Bresciani KD, Costa AJ, Toniollo GH, et al. Transplacental transmission of *Toxoplasma gondii* in reinfected pregnant female canines. *Parasitol Res* 2009;104:1213–1217.

708. Dubey JP, Carpenter JL. Neonatal toxoplasmosis in littermate cats. *J Am Vet Med Assoc* 1993;203: 1546–1549.

709. Dubey JP, Lappin MR, Thulliez P. Diagnosis of induced toxoplasmosis in neonatal cats. *J Am Vet Med Assoc* 1995;207:179–185.

710. Arantes TP, Lopes WD, Ferreira RM, et al. *Toxoplasma gondii*: evidence for the transmission by semen in dogs. *Exp Parasitol* 2009;123:190–194.

711. Dubey JP, Carpenter JL. Histologically confirmed clinical toxoplasmosis in cats: 100 cases (1952–1990). *J Am Vet Med Assoc* 1993;203:1556–1566.

712. Powell CC, Lappin MR. Clinical ocular toxoplasmosis in neonatal kittens. *Vet Ophthalmol* 2001;4: 87–92.

713. Patitucci AN, Alley MR, Jones BR, et al. Protozoal encephalomyelitis of dogs involving *Neospora caninum* and *Toxoplasma gondii* in New Zealand. *N Z Vet J* 1997;45:231–235.

714. Hill SL, Lappin MR, Carman J, et al. Comparison of methods for estimation of *Toxoplasma gondii*-specific antibody production in the aqueous humor of cats. *Am J Vet Res* 1995;56:1181–1187.

715. Lappin MR, Greene CE, Winston S, et al. Clinical feline toxoplasmosis. Serologic diagnosis and therapeutic management of 15 cases. *J Vet Intern Med* 1989;3:139–143.

716. Brodie S, Biley F. An exploration of the potential benefits of pet-facilitated therapy. *J Clin Nurs* 1999;8:329–337.

717. Malmasi A, Mosallanejad B, Mohebali M, et al. Prevention of shedding and re-shedding of *Toxoplasma gondii* oocysts in experimentally infected

cats treated with oral clindamycin: a preliminary study. *Zoonoses Public Health* 2009;56:102–104.

718. Frenkel JK, Pfefferkorn ER, Smith DD, et al. Prospective vaccine prepared from a new mutant of *Toxoplasma gondii* for use in cats. *Am J Vet Res* 1991;52:759–763.

719. Freyre A, Choromanski L, Fishback JL, et al. Immunization of cats with tissue cysts, bradyzoites, and tachyzoites of the T-263 strain of *Toxoplasma gondii*. *J Parasitol* 1993;79:716–719.

720. Kravetz JD, Federman DG. Cat-associated zoonoses. *Arch Intern Med* 2002;162:1945–1952.

721. Montoya JG, Liesenfeld O. Toxoplasmosis. *Lancet* 2004;363:1965–1976.

722. Belanger F, Derouin F, Grangeot-Keros L, et al. Incidence and risk factors of toxoplasmosis in a cohort of human immunodeficiency virus-infected patients: 1988–1995. HEMOCO and SEROCO Study Groups. *Clin Infect Dis* 1999;28:575–581.

723. Ribera E, Fernandez-Sola A, Juste C, et al. Comparison of high and low doses of trimethoprim-sulfamethoxazole for primary prevention of toxoplasmic encephalitis in human immunodeficiency virus-infected patients. *Clin Infect Dis* 1999;29:1461–1466.

724. Aberg J, Gallant J, Anderson J, et al. Primary care guidelines for the management of persons infected with human immunodeficiency virus: recommendations of the HIV Medicine Association of the Infectious Diseases Society of America. *Clin Infect Dis* 2004;39:609–629.

725. Montoya JG, Kovacs JA, Remington JS. Toxoplasma gondii. In: Mandell GL, Bennett JE, Dolin R, eds. *Principles and Practice of Infectious Diseases.* Philadelphia: Elsevier, 2005, pp. 3170–3198.

726. Tunkel A, Glaser C, Bloch K, et al. The management of encephalitis: clinical practice guidelines by the Infectious Diseases Society of America. *Clin Infect Dis* 2008;47:303–327.

727. Foulon W, Villena I, Stray-Pedersen B, et al. Treatment of toxoplasmosis during pregnancy: a multicenter study of impact on fetal transmission and children's sequelae at age 1 year. *Am J Obstet Gynecol* 1999;180:410–415.

728. Montoya JG, Remington JS. Management of *Toxoplasma gondii* infection during pregnancy. *Clin Infect Dis* 2008;47:554–566.

729. Lopez A, Dietz VJ, Wilson M, et al. Preventing congenital toxoplasmosis. *MMWR Recomm Rep* 2000;49:59–68.

730. Lindsay DS, Dubey JP, Butler JM, et al. Mechanical transmission of *Toxoplasma gondii* oocysts by dogs. *Vet Parasitol* 1997;73:27–33.

731. Dunn JJ, Columbus ST, Aldeen WE, et al. *Trichuris vulpis* recovered from a patient with chronic diar-

rhea and five dogs. *J Clin Microbiol* 2002;40:2703–2704.

732. Hall JE, Sonnenberg B. An apparent case of human infection with the whipworm of dogs, *Trichuris vulpis* (Froelich, 1789). *J Parasitol* 1956;42:197–199.

733. Kagei N, Hayashi S, Kato K. Human cases of infection with canine whipworms, *Trichuris vulpis* (Froelich, 1789), in Japan. *Jpn J Med Sci Biol* 1986;39:177–184.

734. Kenney M, Eveland LK. Infection of man with *Trichuris vulpis*, the whipworm of dogs. *Am J Clin Pathol* 1978;69:199.

735. Kenney M, Yermakov V. Infection of man with *Trichuris vulpis*, the whipworm of dogs. *Am J Trop Med Hyg* 1980;29:1205–1208.

736. Mirdha BR, Singh YG, Samantray JC, et al. *Trichuris vulpis* infection in slum children. *Indian J Gastroenterol* 1998;17:154.

737. Singh S, Samantaray JC, Singh N, et al. *Trichuris vulpis* infection in an Indian tribal population. *J Parasitol* 1993;79:457–458.

738. Masuda Y, Kishimoto T, Ito H, et al. Visceral larva migrans caused by *Trichuris vulpis* presenting as a pulmonary mass. *Thorax* 1987;42:990–991.

739. Sakano T, Hamamoto K, Kobayashi Y, et al. Visceral larva migrans caused by *Trichuris vulpis*. *Arch Dis Child* 1980;55:631–633.

740. Coulter JB, Jewsbury JM, Beesley WN, et al. Visceral larva migrans and *Trichuris vulpis*. *Arch Dis Child* 1981;56:406.

741. Gookin JL, Dybas D. *An Owner's Guide to Diagnosis and Treatment of Cats Infected with Tritrichomonas foetus*, 4th ed. Raleigh, NC, 2009.

742. Gookin JL, Stauffer SH, Coccaro MR, et al. Efficacy of tinidazole for treatment of cats experimentally infected with *Tritrichomonas foetus*. *Am J Vet Res* 2007;68:1085–1088.

743. Gookin JL, Birkenheuer AJ, St John V, et al. Molecular characterization of trichomonads from feces of dogs with diarrhea. *J Parasitol* 2005;91:939–943.

744. Tachezy J, Tachezy R, Hampl V, et al. Cattle pathogen *Tritrichomonas foetus* (Riedmüller, 1928) and pig commensal *Tritrichomonas suis* (Gruby & Delafond, 1843) belong to the same species. *J Eukaryot Microbiol* 2002;49:154–163.

745. Bissett SA, Stone ML, Malik R, et al. Observed occurrence of *Tritrichomonas foetus* and other enteric parasites in Australian cattery and shelter cats. *J Feline Med Surg* 2009;11:803–807.

746. van Doorn DC, de Bruin MJ, Jorritsma RA, et al. Prevalence of *Tritrichomonas foetus* among Dutch cats. *Tijdschr Diergeneeskd* 2009;134:698–700.

747. Gunn-Moore DA, McCann TM, Reed N, et al. Prevalence of *Tritrichomonas foetus* infection in cats

with diarrhoea in the UK. *J Feline Med Surg* 2007;9:214–218.

748. Stockdale HD, Givens MD, Dykstra CC, et al. *Tritrichomonas foetus* infections in surveyed pet cats. *Vet Parasitol* 2009;160:13–17.

749. Burgener I, Frey C, Kook P, et al. *Tritrichomonas fetus*: a new intestinal parasite in Swiss cats. *Schweiz Arch Tierheilkd* 2009;151:383–389.

750. Bissett SA, Gowan RA, O'Brien CR, et al. Feline diarrhoea associated with *Tritrichomonas cf. foetus* and *Giardia* co-infection in an Australian cattery. *Aust Vet J* 2008;86:440–443.

751. Gunn-Moore D, Tennant B. *Tritrichomonas foetus* diarrhoea in cats. *Vet Rec* 2007;160:850–851.

752. Gookin JL, Foster DM, Poore MF, et al. Use of a commercially available culture system for diagnosis of *Tritrichomonas foetus* infection in cats. *J Am Vet Med Assoc* 2003;222:1376–1379.

753. Foster DM, Gookin JL, Poore MF, et al. Outcome of cats with diarrhea and *Tritrichomonas foetus* infection. *J Am Vet Med Assoc* 2004;225:888–892.

754. Duboucher C, Caby S, Dufernez F, et al. Molecular identification of *Tritrichomonas foetus*-like organisms as coinfecting agents of human *Pneumocystis* pneumonia. *J Clin Microbiol* 2006;44:1165–1168.

755. World Health Organization. *Global Burden of Disease Estimates: 2004 Update*. Geneva, Switzerland: WHO, 2008.

756. Barr SC. Canine Chagas' disease (American trypanosomiasis) in North America. *Vet Clin North Am Small Anim Pract* 2009;39:1055–1064, v–vi.

757. Kirchhoff LV. *Trypanosoma* species (American trypanosomiasis, Chagas' disease): biology of trypanosomes. In: Mandell GL, Bennett JE, Dolin R, eds. *Principles and Practice of Infectious Diseases*. Philadelphia: Elsevier, 2005, pp. 3156–3154.

758. Hofflin JM, Sadler RH, Araujo FG, et al. Laboratory-acquired Chagas disease. *Trans R Soc Trop Med Hyg* 1987;81:437–440.

759. Kinoshita-Yanaga AT, Toledo MJ, Araújo SM, et al. Accidental infection by *Trypanosoma cruzi* follow-up by the polymerase chain reaction: case report. *Rev Inst Med Trop Sao Paulo* 2009;51:295–298.

760. Nóbrega AA, Garcia MH, Tatto E, et al. Oral transmission of Chagas disease by consumption of açaí palm fruit, Brazil. *Emerg Infect Dis* 2009;15:653–655.

761. Roellig DM, Ellis AE, Yabsley MJ. Oral transmission of *Trypanosoma cruzi* with opposing evidence for the theory of carnivory. *J Parasitol* 2009;95:360–364.

762. Estrada-Franco JG, Bhatia V, Diaz-Albiter H, et al. Human *Trypanosoma cruzi* infection and seropositivity in dogs, Mexico. *Emerg Infect Dis* 2006;12:624–630.

763. Bern C, Montgomery SP. An estimate of the burden of Chagas disease in the United States. *Clin Infect Dis* 2009;49:e52–e54.

764. Dorn PL, Perniciaro L, Yabsley MJ, et al. Autochthonous transmission of *Trypanosoma cruzi*, Louisiana. *Emerg Infect Dis* 2007;13:605–607.

765. Jimenez-Coello M, Poot-Cob M, Ortega-Pacheco A, et al. American trypanosomiasis in dogs from an urban and rural area of Yucatan, Mexico. *Vector Borne Zoonotic Dis* 2008;8:755–761.

766. Barr SC. Canine American trypanosomiasis. *Compend Cont Educ Pract Vet* 1991;13:745–755.

767. Beard CB, Pye G, Steurer FJ, et al. Chagas disease in a domestic transmission cycle, southern Texas, USA. *Emerg Infect Dis* 2003;9:103–105.

768. Kjos SA, Snowden KF, Craig TM, et al. Distribution and characterization of canine Chagas disease in Texas. *Vet Parasitol* 2008;152:249–256.

769. Meurs KM, Anthony MA, Slater M, et al. Chronic *Trypanosoma cruzi* infection in dogs: 11 cases (1987–1996). *J Am Vet Med Assoc* 1998;213:497–500.

770. Nabity MB, Barnhart K, Logan KS, et al. An atypical case of *Trypanosoma cruzi* infection in a young English Mastiff. *Vet Parasitol* 2006;140:356–361.

771. Fox JC, Ewing SA, Buckner RG, et al. *Trypanosoma cruzi* infection in a dog from Oklahoma. *J Am Vet Med Assoc* 1986;189:1583–1584.

772. Snider TG, Yaeger RG, Dellucky J. Myocarditis caused by *Trypanosoma cruzi* in a native Louisiana dog. *J Am Vet Med Assoc* 1980;177:247–249.

773. Barr SC, Van Beek O, Carlisle-Nowak MS, et al. *Trypanosoma cruzi* infection in Walker hounds from Virginia. *Am J Vet Res* 1995;56:1037–1044.

774. Carcavallo RU. The subfamily Triatominae (Hemiptera, Reduviidae): systematics and ecological factors. In: Brenner RR, Stoke A, eds. *Chagas' Disease Vectors*. Boca Raton, FL: CRC Press, 1987, pp. 13–18.

775. Yaeger RG. The present status of Chagas' disease in the United States. *Bull Tulane Univ Med Fac* 1961;21:9–13.

776. Catalá S. The biting rate of *Triatoma infestans* in Argentina. *Med Vet Entomol* 1991;5:325–333.

777. Cardinal MV, Castañera MB, Lauricella MA, et al. A prospective study of the effects of sustained vector surveillance following community-wide insecticide application on *Trypanosoma cruzi* infection of dogs and cats in rural Northwestern Argentina. *Am J Trop Med Hyg* 2006;75:753–761.

778. Gürtler RE, Cecere MC, Lauricella MA, et al. Domestic dogs and cats as sources of *Trypanosoma cruzi* infection in rural northwestern Argentina. *Parasitology* 2007;134:69–82.

779. Gürtler RE, Cécere MC, Rubel DN, et al. Chagas disease in north-west Argentina: infected dogs as a risk factor for the domestic transmission of *Trypanosoma cruzi*. *Trans R Soc Trop Med Hyg* 1991;85:741–745.

780. Gurtler RE, Cohen JE, Cecere MC, et al. Influence of humans and domestic animals on the household prevalence of *Trypanosoma cruzi* in *Triatoma infestans* populations in northwest Argentina. *Am J Trop Med Hyg* 1998;58:748–758.

781. Jimenez-Coello M, Ortega-Pacheco A, Guzman-Marin E, et al. Stray dogs as reservoirs of the zoonotic agents *Leptospira interrogans*, *Trypanosoma cruzi*, and *Aspergillus* spp. in an urban area of Chiapas in Southern Mexico. *Vector Borne Zoonotic Dis* 2009;

782. Rosypal AC, Cortés-Vecino JA, Gennari SM, et al. Serological survey of *Leishmania infantum* and *Trypanosoma cruzi* in dogs from urban areas of Brazil and Colombia. *Vet Parasitol* 2007;149:172–177.

783. Dantas-Torres F. Canine vector-borne diseases in Brazil. *Parasit Vectors* 2008;1:25.

784. Barr SC, Dennis VA, Klei TR. Serologic and blood culture survey of *Trypanosoma cruzi* infection in four canine populations of southern Louisiana. *Am J Vet Res* 1991;52:570–573.

785. Bradley KK, Bergman DK, Woods JP, et al. Prevalence of American trypanosomiasis (Chagas disease) among dogs in Oklahoma. *J Am Vet Med Assoc* 2000;217:1853–1857.

786. Cruz-Chan JV, Quijano-Hernandez I, Ramirez-Sierra MJ, et al. *Dirofilaria immitis* and *Trypanosoma cruzi* natural co-infection in dogs. *Vet J* 2009. Epub ahead of print.

787. Fujita O, Sanabria L, Inchaustti A, et al. Animal reservoirs for *Trypanosoma cruzi* infection in an endemic area in Paraguay. *J Vet Med Sci* 1994;56:305–308.

788. Barr S, Baker D, Markovits J. Trypanosomiasis and laryngeal paralysis in a dog. *J Am Vet Med Assoc* 1986;188:1307–1309.

789. Cohen JE, Gürtler RE. Modeling household transmission of American trypanosomiasis. *Science* 2001;293:694–698.

790. Barr SC. American trypanosomiasis. In: Greene CE, ed. *Infectious Diseases of the Dog and Cat*. Philadelphia: Saunders Elsevier, 2006, pp. 676–685.

791. Weese JS, Faires M. A survey of needle handling practices and needlestick injuries in veterinary technicians. *Can Vet J* 2009;50:1278–1282.

2 Bacterial Diseases

J. Scott Weese and Martha B. Fulford

Introduction

All companion animals have a remarkably large and diverse bacterial microflora that may be comprised of harmless commensals, opportunistic pathogens, and primary pathogens. Some bacteria are among the least host-adapted pathogens and can infect numerous animals and humans, with resultant disease ranging from mild to rapidly and typically fatal. Other bacteria are almost exclusively found in a single host species and seldom cause cross-species infection or disease.

An additional aspect of bacterial diseases requiring consideration is antimicrobial resistance. Companion animals are not immune to the epidemic of antimicrobial resistance that is sweeping developed and developing countries alike. Antimicrobial use in both animals and humans is driving the development of some multidrug-resistant (MDR) pathogens in companion animals, and the spread of certain MDR bacteria from people to their pets is a remarkable illustration of the "one medicine" concept and the potential influence of people and animals on each other's microflora.

The diversity of potential zoonotic bacteria is impressive, yet a large percentage of potential

pathogens are quite rare causes of disease, and the overall burden of human illness is caused by a small percentage of the bacterial pathogens discussed below.

Anaerobiospirillum spp.

Anaerobiospirillum is a genus of anaerobic gram-negative spiral organisms that can cause diarrhea and septicemia in humans.[1–3] A morphologically similar organism was isolated from the healthy dog of a child with *Anaerobiospirillum* diarrhea; however, the isolate was lost on subculture.[4] In another case, a "similar" organism was isolated from a healthy pet dog in the same household as a baby with *Anaerobiospirillum* diarrhea.[5] These circumstantial reports, along with the isolation of *Anaerobiospirillum* spp. from healthy cats and dogs[2,6] raise concern that this may be a zoonotic pathogen. It is presumably a minimally important zoonotic disease, although it is possible that it is underdiagnosed in humans.

Anaplasma phagocytophilum

A. phagocytophilum (also referred to as *Anaplasma phagocytophila*) is the cause of granulocytic anaplasmosis in humans, dogs, cats, horses, and probably

Companion Animal Zoonoses. Edited by J. Scott Weese and Martha B. Fulford. © 2011 Blackwell Publishing Ltd.

other animal species. This bacterium has a wide natural host range, including humans, dogs, cats, horses, sheep, cats, deer, and various rodents, and is transmitted by several tick species, particularly *Ixodes scapularis*, *Ixodes pacificus*, *Ixodes ricinus*, and *Ixodes persulcatus*.[7] It cannot be transmitted directly between animals (or between animals and humans). It is possible that animals could be mechanical vectors by bringing infected ticks into contact with humans; however, if this occurs, it is probably uncommon. Diagnosis of granulocytic anaplasmosis in one species indicates risk to other species if they are also exposed to ticks.

Arcobacter spp.

Arcobacter is a genus consisting of four main pathogenic species, *Arcobacter butzleri*, *Arcobacter cryaerophilus*, *Arcobacter cibarius*, and *Arcobacter skirrowii*,[8–10] that can cause a variety of diseases in humans and animals. Other *Arcobacter* spp. have also been described, but pathogenicity to animals or humans has not been described. These gram-negative spiral-shaped bacteria are similar in many respects to *Campylobacter* but are able to grow in aerobic conditions and at low temperatures.[9]

Most reports of *Arcobacter* in animals have involved farm animals such as cattle, pigs, sheep, horses, and chickens, in both healthy animals and as causes of abortion, mastitis, and enteritis, as well as being found in meat.[11,12] In humans, *Arcobacter* has been identified primarily as a cause of enteritis.[10,13–15] Fecal–oral infection is the presumed route of transmission, with water and food being the most commonly implicated sources of infection.[16]

There have been few reported investigations of *Arcobacter* spp. in companion animals, with conflicting results. *A. butzleri* and *A. cryaerophilus* were detected in the oral cavity of 77% of healthy pet cats in one study[8] and 50% of dogs and 25% of cats in another study.[17] In contrast, *Arcobacter* spp. were not found in the oral cavity or feces of any cats, and only in feces and oral cavity samples of 1.9% and 0.7% of dogs, respectively, in another.[18] Studies reporting a high detection rate in cats relied on molecular methods versus culture in the low prevalence studies. It is possible that *Arcobacter* is commonly present in very low numbers that are more readily detectable with polymerase chain reaction (PCR) versus culture.

The public health implications of *Arcobacter* colonization in pets are completely unclear at this point. *Arcobacter* may be a relatively ubiquitous organism, being found in animals, food, water, and the environment;[8] however, given its close relationship to *Campylobacter*, which can clearly be transmitted from pets to people, its potential as a zoonosis should not be dismissed. Good general hygiene measures to avoid ingestion of *Arcobacter* from the oral cavity or feces should be standard practices, and the risk to humans from regular contact with household pets is probably quite low.

Bacillus anthracis

Introduction

As the cause of anthrax, *B. anthracis* has been an important public and animal health concern for centuries. It is predominantly a disease of herbivores, with humans and other species such as dogs and cats infected incidentally. Human infections are predominantly associated with contact with infected herbivores or animal products. Anthrax is a significant bioterrorism concern.

Etiology

B. anthracis is a gram-positive spore-forming bacterium. As a spore former, it can exist in both vegetative and spore forms. Vegetative cells have a characteristic polypeptide capsule that is visible with methylene blue or Giemsa stains. Spores are dormant forms that are highly resistant to environmental effects and disinfectants.

Geographic distribution/epidemiology

Anthrax is present worldwide but there is significant regional variability. The spore-forming nature of *B. anthracis* allows it to persist in areas for prolonged periods of time. It is more common in warm, moist climates and in soils that are alkaline and with a high nitrogen content. It is most commonly encountered in agricultural regions of South and Central America, sub-Saharan Africa, central and southwestern Asia, and southern and eastern Europe.[19] In North America, it is most commonly reported in the central and Mississippi delta regions.[20] Livestock epizootics tend to occur in summer or fall, particularly after heavy rainfall or flooding that follows drought conditions. Livestock are most commonly infected through ingestion of *B. anthracis* spores, which can survive in soil for decades.

Cases of anthrax in humans typically occur following contact with infected animals, animal tissues, or products from infected animals.[19] Agriculture-associated exposure is common, from contact with sick or dead livestock or handling carcasses and infected tissues.[21,22] Ingestion of meat from animals that have died of anthrax can result in gastrointestinal anthrax, while inhalation of anthrax spores can cause inhalation anthrax, which is often fatal. Veterinary-associated infections can be associated with performing necropsies on animals that have died of anthrax.[19] Industrial exposure can result in cutaneous or inhalation exposure to spores from hides, hair, or wool. Historically, woolsorters were a high-risk group for anthrax.[22]

Dogs and cats are considered at low risk for development of disease following exposure to *B. anthracis*.[23] There are few reports of anthrax in dogs and cats, but isolated infections may occur during livestock epizootics.[20] Most infections occur as a result of ingestion of meat from animals that have died of anthrax. Pets are a minor source of anthrax in humans. The relative resistance of pets to anthrax limits their use as sentinels of human exposure, either in natural circumstances or bioterrorist attacks. The risk of zoonotic infection is likely greatest in veterinary personnel who might handle infected animals or high-risk diagnostic specimens. Regardless, animals with anthrax should be considered possible sources of infection. Further, anthrax is a reportable disease in most regions, and prompt diagnosis and reporting is important.

Animals

Clinical presentation

In pets, infection almost always originates from oral exposure. Early signs tend to consist of fever, anorexia, and inflammation of regional lymph nodes of the head, neck, and mediastinum.[20,23] Local and systemic spread can result in infection of deeper lymph nodes, the spleen, and liver. Severe lymph node enlargement can cause asphyxiation, although toxemia and shock are more common causes of death. Hemorrhagic gastroenteritis can develop, particularly in younger animals, and can be fatal.[20] Fulminant septicemia can occur but is uncommon.[20] Infection by inhalation is rare to nonexistent.[20] Cutaneous anthrax has not been reported.

Diagnosis

A history of potential exposure greatly facilitates diagnosis, both in terms of making the correct diagnosis and safety of the diagnostician. Classical clinical signs in an animal with known exposure should be treated as presumptive anthrax. Aspirates of blood, lymph nodes, other affected tissues, or pharyngeal swabs can be collected for cytological examination and culture.[23] Methylene blue or Giemsa stains should be used on aspirates to look for the characteristic encapsulated organism. Culture is the definitive diagnostic test but should only be attempted by facilities with proper containment. Shipping of specimens for culture should only be done after contacting both the shipping company and diagnostic laboratory to determine whether testing can be done and to obtain guidelines for safe shipping. Serological testing using enzyme-linked immunosorbent assay (ELISA) can be performed to detect antibodies against *B. anthracis* protective antigen.[20] Identification of a fourfold increase in antibody titer is diagnostic. Simple assessment of seropositivity is not diagnostic because of the potential for antibodies from prior exposure. PCR might be a rapid means of diagnosis, but its use has not been reported in dogs and cats.

Animals that have died of anthrax typically display little or no rigor mortis and often have dark blood oozing from various orifices. Necropsy should not be performed because it will permit the formation of highly resistant *B. anthracis* spores.

Management

B. anthracis tends to have a predictable and stable antimicrobial susceptibility pattern. There are concerns about engineering of resistant strains for bioterrorism purposes. This would be more of a concern in anthrax cases occurring in low-risk (especially urban) areas that might be prone to bioterrorist attacks. In the absence of other information, empirical treatment with potassium or sodium penicillin is recommended.[20] Oxytetracycline and enrofloxacin have also been recommended.[23] Other antimicrobials such as chloramphenicol, erythromycin, and aminoglycosides might be effective based on *in vitro* testing, but *in vivo* data are lacking.[20] Potentiated sulfonamides and cephalosporins are generally ineffective and should be avoided. Prompt therapy is required because of the often rapid clinical progression. Supportive care is important, the nature of which depends on the clinical presentation and severity of disease.

Humans

Clinical presentation

Anthrax is typically classified by route of exposure (inhalation, cutaneous, gastrointestinal) and rate of progression (peracute, acute, subacute/chronic).

Cutaneous anthrax (Figure 2.1) is most common, accounting for approximately 95% of infections.[21] It is characterized by a pruritic papule or vesicle at the site of inoculation that may resemble a spider bite.[21,24] The lesion enlarges and ulcerates over 1–2 days, forming a central black eschar. Nonpitting edema and hyperemia develop locally,

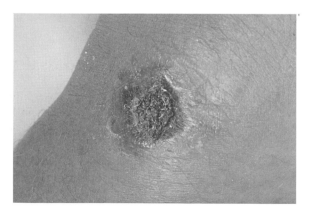

Figure 2.1   Cutaneous anthrax in a person (public domain, James H. Steele, Center for Disease Control and Prevention).

along with regional lymphadenopathy. The lesion is typically painless, in contrast to lesions caused by spider bites, *Staphylococcus aureus*, or most other infections.[21,24] There may be concurrent systemic signs and symptoms such as fever, malaise, and headache. Usually, the eschar falls off and clinical signs resolve in 1–2 weeks.

Inhalation, or pulmonary, anthrax is an often dramatic manifestation of infection. After an initial flu-like phase with nonspecific signs that might include fever, chills, fatigue, sweating, nonproductive cough, headache, myalgia, chest pain, nausea, and vomiting, fulminant respiratory disease may develop.[25] This is often rapidly followed by very severe disease with pronounced hypotension, dyspnea, hypoxia, cyanosis, and shock.[24]

Gastrointestinal anthrax is uncommon, accounting for less than 5% of cases.[21] It can involve the intestinal tract or oropharynx, but intestinal disease is more common. Patients with oropharyngeal disease have posterior oropharyngeal ulcers, pronounced swelling of the neck, regional lymphadenopathy, and fever, and may be septic.[21,24] Intestinal anthrax results in nonspecific abnormalities like diarrhea, nausea, vomiting, and fever, with a progression to more serious disease including severe abdominal pain, hematemesis, bloody diarrhea, and ascites.[24]

In uncommon situations, infection of other body systems, such as the central nervous system (CNS), may occur without apparent cutaneous, gastrointestinal, or respiratory involvement.[24]

Diagnosis

Identification of encapsulated gram-positive bacteria on blood smears or sputum is suggestive.[24] Bacterial culture of appropriate specimens (i.e., blood, tissue biopsies, cerebrospinal fluid (CSF), pleural fluid) is the standard for diagnosis. Culture performed after the initiation of antimicrobial therapy is unlikely to be successful, so cultures should be collected as soon as possible.[24] Anthrax is a biosafety level 3 organism, and culture should only be attempted in appropriate facilities. Rapid, culture-independent methods are useful because of faster turnaround time and no need for advanced biocontainment laboratories. These include tissue immunohistochemistry, ELISA, and PCR. Thoracic radiographs or CT should be performed in patients with suspected inhalation anthrax, since a widened mediastinum, mediastinal lymphadenopathy, and pleural effusion are classical imaging findings.[25,26]

Management

Prompt initiation of appropriate therapy is critical, particularly for inhalation and gastrointestinal anthrax. Consideration of risk factors for exposure is critical to identify potentially infected individuals given the rarity and severity of disease.

Controlled trials are lacking, but clinical observation indicates that penicillins and tetracyclines can be effective for the treatment of uncomplicated cutaneous anthrax.[24] In general, either doxycycline or ciprofloxacin are recommended as first-line treatment.[26]

Ciprofloxacin or doxycycline should be used initially for inhalation anthrax, gastrointestinal anthrax, anthrax meningitis, or cutaneous anthrax with systemic signs, in combination with one or more other antimicrobials such as vancomycin, imipenem, ampicillin, chloramphenicol, clindamycin, clarithromycin, penicillin, or rifampin.[24,26] Treatment should be modified as needed based on culture and susceptibility results. Anthrax-specific hyperimmune globulin should be considered in severe cases.[27] Resection of affected intestine may be required in gastrointestinal anthrax that has not responded quickly to medical treatment.[21] Supportive therapy is indicated, based on the type and severity of disease.

Ciprofloxacin is the most commonly recommended drug for postexposure prophylaxis in bioterrorism-related exposure[24,26] and is reasonable for any postexposure treatment. Vaccination is recommended in conjunction with antimicrobial prophylaxis as a means of preventing inhalation anthrax.[24]

Prognosis varies with the type of disease and how quickly proper treatment is initiated. With proper treatment, the mortality rate for cutaneous anthrax is less than 1%; however, it can approach 20% without treatment.[21] Mortality rates are higher for other forms of anthrax, even with proper treatment. Gastrointestinal anthrax has a 25–60% mortality rate,[21] while inhalation anthrax has a mortality rate of 45–85%.[21,25,26] Anthrax meningitis is fatal in approximately 95% of cases.[21]

Prevention

The risk of anthrax exposure from companion animals, either in households or in veterinary clinics, is very low in most areas. An understanding of the risk of anthrax in the local area (and areas when animals may visit) is critical for determining the risk of exposure. Anthrax should be considered in endemic areas, particularly in animals that have uncontrolled outdoor access and which may encounter affected wildlife or livestock. Reducing roaming of dogs and cats should greatly reduce the risk of anthrax exposure and infection.

In veterinary clinics, care should be taken to reduce the risk of environmental contamination or personnel exposure. Animals with anthrax should be considered infectious and isolated. Barrier precautions (gown, gloves) should be used for any contact with the animal. Particular care should be taken by individuals with skin lesions because of the potential for cutaneous infection from contact with the animal or contaminated environment. If skin or wound infections are present in an animal, they should be covered with an impermeable dressing if at all possible. Bandage materials should be disposed of as biohazardous waste. Sporulation requires an aerobic environment and does not occur in unopened carcasses. Therefore, it is critical that necropsy not be performed on anthrax suspects outside of proper biocontainment facilities. Animals that have died of anthrax should be incinerated or deeply buried, using a covering of anhydrous calcium oxide (quicklime).

Good information regarding disinfection practices for veterinary clinics and households is lacking. Information is available for households and other public areas in response to potential bioterrorism-associated contamination, but the relevance of that for animal-associated contamination is unclear. Bioterrorism response tends to focus on widespread and large-scale contamination with spores. In contrast, infected animals in a household would presumably result in minimal to moderate contamination, depending on the type of disease and duration. Despite the lack of objective information, attention should be paid to the potential for household contamination and the response. Relevant public health authorities may be able to provide guidance about disinfection practices; however, most are unlikely to have additional information pertaining to household pets. If there has been potential contamination of households, contaminated areas and objects should be disinfected or discarded. Potentially contaminated areas should be thoroughly cleaned and disinfected. Bleach (1:10 dilution of household bleach) should be used where possible, making sure that organic debris has been removed and a 60-minute contact time is provided.[23] Most routine disinfectants are not sporidical. Carpets or other areas not amenable to bleach disinfection are hard to thoroughly disinfect. Removal of carpets seems drastic in most circumstances but is a reasonable consideration when there has been high-risk contamination, such as blood contamination from an animal with systemic anthrax. Protective outerwear and gloves should be worn during environmental cleaning. Respiratory and face protection may be warranted. Vacuuming should be avoided unless a properly functional HEPA filter is present in the vacuum because of the potential for aerosolization of spores.

Prophylactic treatment with doxycycline is recommended for pets with potential exposure.[23] Amoxicillin can be used in animals that cannot be treated with doxycycline. Careful decontamination of the hair coat is also recommended.[23] Since sporicidal treatment of the hair coat is impractical, repeated bathing is recommended to mechanically remove the organism.[23] Infection control practices for bathing potentially contaminated animals have not been described, but the use of gloves, gowns, and either full face or eye and respiratory protection should be considered. Hands should be washed thoroughly after bathing the animal and the area disinfected. Because of the potential for inadvertent contamination of the body during bathing, it is prudent for people to change all items of clothing and shower promptly after bathing the animal.

Since ingestion is the most common route of exposure, care should be taken to reduce the risk of animals ingesting spore-contaminated meat. Animals should not be allowed to ingest dead animals, particularly in endemic regions. Animals should never be fed meat from animals that have died of unknown causes, particularly ones that have signs suggestive of anthrax. Vaccination of livestock is useful in endemic areas and could help reduce the risk of incidental infection of pets. There is no vaccine for dogs and cats.

A vaccine is available for humans and is useful in high-risk situations. Occupational or recreational contact with pets, even in endemic areas, is not an indication for human vaccination.

Bartonella species

Bartonella spp. are hemotropic gram-negative alphaproteobacteria that are distantly related to Rickettsiaceae. At least 20 species and subspecies are currently recognized,[28] all of which are highly adapted to survive long term in selected mammalian hosts. Many of these can cause disease in humans. The three most common human pathogens are *Bartonella henselae*, *Bartonella bacilliformis*, and *Bartonella quintana*. Of these, *B. hensalae* is the main pathogen associated with companion animals. *B. bacilliformis* is limited to a narrow range in the Andes Mountains in South America and is not associated with companion animals. In contrast, *B. quintana* can be found worldwide as the cause of trench fever. The human louse transmits this species, and no other vertebrate reservoirs are known. *Bartonella clarridgeiae* and *Bartonella vinsonii* subsp. *berkhoffii* are less common in humans but may be transmissible from pets. *Bartonella koehlerae* has been found in the blood of healthy cats[29] and may be a rare cause of endocarditis in people.[30] *Bartonella elizabethae* has been isolated from dogs[31,32] and has been rarely implicated in human disease.[33] The relevance of this species is currently unclear. Based on recent advances in the field of *Bartonella* research, particularly improved molecular methods to detect and characterize *Bartonella*, it is likely that other potentially zoonotic *Bartonella* will be identified.

Bartonella henselae

Introduction

B. henselae is a predominantly cat-associated pathogen and the cause of cat scratch disease (CSD). Less commonly, it can cause bacillary angiomatosis, bacillary peliosis, and various other syndromes. Human disease is strongly associated with cat contact.

Etiology

B. henselae is a fastidious, hemotropic, slow-growing gram-negative bacterium. Domestic cats are the natural reservoir. Various genotypes are present, and it appears that only a limited number of these genotypes are associated with human infection.[34]

Geographic distribution/epidemiology

Animals

B. henselae is endemic in domestic cats worldwide.[28,35] Seropositivity is very common in healthy cats, with reports ranging from 1% to 81%.[29,36–39] Regional differences in seroprevalence are present, with higher rates tending to occur in warmer, more humid regions.[40] Reported bacteremia rates are variable and can be quite high, ranging from 3% to 68%.[37,39,41–45] In general, seroprevalence is higher in older animals, while bacteremia is most common in younger animals.[46,47] Flea infested and stray or former stray cats are also more likely to be bacteremic or seropositive.[39,47–49]

The bacterium primarily resides within erythrocytes, but may also be detected in vascular endothelial cells. In either event, clinical signs are typically absent, and this bacterium can be present in variable levels in the blood for prolonged periods of time. After experimental infection, most cats resolve bacteremia spontaneously after 22–33 weeks;[50,51] however, long-term or cyclic bacteremia can develop, and some cats may be bacteremic for greater than 1 year.[52] Recurrent bacteremia does not always indicate long-term shedding since reinfection with distinct strains can occur.[53] Regardless, the end result is that a substantial percentage of healthy cats can have *B. henselae* in circulation at any given time.

The cat flea, *Ctenocephalides felis*, is the main source of transmission, and experimental infection of cats by intradermal inoculation of flea feces has been documented.[54] Exposure of cats to infected fleas in capsules that prevented contamination of the cat with flea feces did not reproduce disease, suggesting that flea feces, not saliva, are the route of transmission.[54] The critical role of fleas is further

supported by studies indicating that *B. henselae* transmission does not occur in cohabitating cats in the absence of fleas, nor between cats through bites, scratches, grooming, or other contacts in flea-free environments.[50,52,55] Blood transfusion can be a route of iatrogenic transmission.

While mainly associated with cats, *B. henselae* can also be found in healthy dogs. Prevalence data are limited and are compromised by potential cross-reaction with other *Bartonella* spp. Most studies have reported relatively low (0–8%) seroprevalence rates in healthy dogs,[38,56–59] but 24% of dogs from the southeastern United States were seropositive in one study.[60] Bacteremia rates are also low, typically ≤1%.[61,62] *B. henselae* has been isolated from saliva of dogs,[63] suggesting that zoonotic transmission could occur through dog bites, although this has not been proven. Coinfection with other *Bartonella* species can occur.[57]

Human exposure

Human exposure to *B. henselae* may be common in some regions and some groups. Seroprevalence rates are rather low in the general population, such as the 2–6% seroprevalence rates reported for blood donors.[45,64,65] Contact with cats or having a cat in the household is a risk factor for seropositivity.[66] Quite high (7–51%) seroprevalence rates have been reported for veterinary personnel,[64,67] perhaps not surprisingly given the high contact with cats and fleas. However, this can be variable because only 1.7% of veterinary personnel in Taiwan were seropositive.[41] *B. henselae* bacteremia can be identified in healthy, immunocompetent people, especially those with animal contact,[68] although bacteremia rates in healthy individuals are poorly understood.

As with cat–cat transmission, cat–human transmission involves the presence of fleas. It is believed that zoonotic infection occurs most commonly through inoculation of contaminated flea feces into the body through scratches. Transmission via bites could also occur if infected flea feces were present at the site of the bite or in the mouth of the animal. Inoculation of infected feline blood via a bite could also be a source of infection.[40]

Despite the clear role of cats in *B. henselae* transmission, CSD (and *B. henselae* infection of any type) is not strictly associated with cats or scratches. *B. henselae* has been identified in ticks, including ticks attached to people or animals,[69] and ticks (particularly *Rhipicephalus sanguineus*, *Ixodes scapularis*, and *I. ricinus*) could be vectors.[40,70,71] However, this has not been proven, and the role of ticks in transmission is still unclear.[72] Dogs have been implicated in the transmission of *B. henselae* through scratches,[73] and *B. henselae* can be found in canine saliva, suggesting a potential role of bites in transmission.[63] Dogs are probably more commonly accidental hosts and a minor source of human infection compared with cats.[40] Infections have also been diagnosed in people without a history of animal contact, but this accounts for a very small percentage of CSD cases,[74] and it is always difficult to determine whether there was truly no form of animal contact. It is even more difficult to rule out the possibility of contact with fleas. Transfusion-associated infection has been reported.[75,76]

Human disease

CSD is the most common manifestation of *B. henselae* infection. It is estimated to affect 22,000 people in the United States every year[77] and is probably a common (but often undiagnosed) problem.[24] The other classical manifestations of *B. henselae* infection are bacillary angiomatosis and bacillary peliosis (both of which occur most often in patients with HIV/AIDS).[24] Advances in identification of *B. henselae* have demonstrated that our understanding of the role of *B. henselae* in various diseases is quite superficial and evolving, and there is emerging evidence that this microorganism may cause a wide range of diseases, including vague chronic neurological or neurocognitive disorders.[78]

CSD can occur in people of all ages; however, children less than 10 years of age are overrepresented.[79] It is clear that *B. henselae* can be transmitted from cats to humans, and *B. henselae* can commonly be isolated from cats of CSD patients.[28,68] Reported risk factors for CSD include contact with cats 12 months of age or younger, a history of a cat scratch or bite and contact with fleas.[28,80] Contact with cats has also been identified as a risk factor for *B. henselae* endocarditis and bacillary angiomatosis in immunocompromised patients.[81]

Animals

Clinical presentation

B. henselae infection in cats is almost always subclinical. Typically, subclinical bacteremia waxes and wanes without any detectable clinical abnormalities. Recurrent bacteremia can persist for years. Experimentally infected cats have no or mild and transient signs such as induration or abscess at experimental inoculation sites, lymphadenopathy, anorexia, or lethargy.[50] Similar transient and mild signs can be observed in some infected cats following surgery or trauma,[28] perhaps as a result of stress and being immunocompromised. Limited reports have also implicated *B. henselae* as a cause of endocarditis in cats.[82,83] It has been suggested that coinfection with feline immunodeficiency virus (FIV) or feline leukemia virus (FeLV) and *B. henselae* could be associated with increased pathogenicity and signs such as gingivitis, lymphadenopathy, stomatitis, and urinary tract disease.[28]

As opposed to the situation in cats, *B. henselae* is clearly a pathogen in dogs, with endocarditis being the most common manifestation.[82]

Diagnosis

Culture of *B. henselae* from blood or infected tissues (i.e., lymph node, heart vale) or detection of *Bartonella* species DNA by PCR is the standard for diagnosis. Culture can be difficult, and *B. henselae* will not be recovered using routine blood culture methods because of the fastidious, slow-growing nature of the organism. Ten to fifty-six days may be required before visible colonies are identified.[28] Prolonged culture using selective media is required for adequate sensitivity. Care must be taken when collecting blood samples for culture to avoid contamination, since low levels of skin contaminants can overwhelm *B. henselae* during the prolonged culture period. Combination of culture and PCR, where PCR testing is performed on samples enriched in *Bartonella* alphaproteobacteria growth medium (BAPGM), may provide optimal sensitivity.[84] Successful isolation of *B. henselae* from dogs may be more difficult than from cats because of the typically lower level of bacteremia.[28]

Serological testing is available, but determining the clinical relevance of serology can be difficult considering the seroprevalence in healthy animals in many regions. Cytological identification of *B. henselae* in erythrocytes is rare and not useful clinically.

Management

There is little objective information regarding treatment. Elimination of *Bartonella* bacteremia may be difficult, if not impossible. There is little indication for treatment in cats considering the minimally pathogenic nature of infection and lack of evidence of efficacy. Treatment is indicated in dogs when *Bartonella* is suspected to be involved with disease. Administration of macrolides (erythromycin, azithromycin) or a combination of a penicillin and a fluoroquinolone for a minimum of 6 weeks has been recommended for chronic disease.[85] For severe, life-threatening infection, initial treatment with ampicillin or amoxicillin plus amikacin is recommended.[85]

Humans

Clinical presentation

CSD is the most common clinical manifestation of *B. henselae* infection. Approximately 7–12 days after inoculation (primarily from a scratch or bite), a papule or pustule develops.[24] This may persist for 1–3 weeks. Regional lymphadenopathy is the most common sign, being present in >90% of cases,[35] and is often pronounced. A small lesion is usually present at the site of inoculation when lymphadenopathy develops; however, it may have healed by then in some people. Thirty to sixty percent of patients report a low-grade fever that can last several days. Malaise, arthalgia, arthritis, fatigue, headache, and sore throat are also occasionally reported.[35,86] Lymph node suppuration develops in 16–25% of patients.[24,35] Lymphadenopathy often persists for 2–4 months, if not longer. Approximately 10% of patients develop extranodal manifestations.[74,87] The most common is Parinaud's oculoglandular syndrome, characterized by conjunctivitis, and local lymphadenitis.[74] Other uncommon manifestations include aseptic meningitis, granulomatous hepatitis/splenitis, encephalopathy, chorioretinitis, neuroretinitis, pneumonitis,

osteitis, and myocarditis.[78,87–94] Disseminated infections have been reported in transplant patients.[95]

Bacteremia is more common in immunocompromised hosts, particularly HIV/AIDS patients, and is characterized by weight loss, malaise, aches, fatigue, recurrent fever, and sometimes headache.[35] As opposed to most other causes of bacteremia, *B. henselae* bacteremia in immunocompromised individuals often has an insidious onset. Signs, therefore, are rather nonspecific. In immunocompetent individuals, onset is often abrupt, with fever that may be relapsing or persistent.[35]

B. henselae is increasingly being identified as a cause of "blood culture negative" endocarditis in both immunocompetent and immunocompromised adults.[96,97] While children are overrepresented in CSD, endocarditis is rare.[35]

Bacillary angiomatosis (Figure 2.2) is characterized by neovascular proliferation in the skin and regional lymph nodes, sometimes with involvement of other organs such as the spleen, liver, lungs, bone, brain, intestinal tract, and cervix.[35] It is most commonly described in immunocompromised patients,[81] particularly individuals with HIV/AIDS, but can affect immunocompetent individuals. Skin lesions, which may be solitary or number in the hundreds, are subcutaneous nodules/papules that can be fixed or freely mobile.

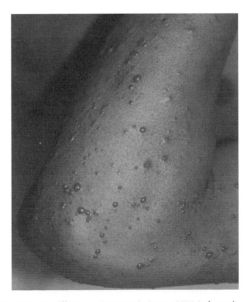

Figure 2.2 Bacillary angiomatosis in an HIV-infected patient (open source, Anisa Mosam, www.IDimages.org).

They may range from a few millimeters to centimeters in diameter, and be skin colored, red, or purple. Ulceration can occur. Internal lesions can be present without skin lesions, which complicates diagnosis.

Bacillary peliosis involves the presence of blood-filled cystic structures, predominantly in the liver, spleen, or lymph nodes. Inflammatory reactions in organs, such as the liver, spleen, lymph nodes, heart, lungs, and bone marrow, can also occur in immunocompromised hosts in the absence of angiomatosis or peliosis.[98]

Recent research has suggested a role of B. henselae in chronic neurological or neurocognitive disease, based on the isolation of the organism from patients with chronic symptoms such as fatigue, headaches, blurred vision, ataxia, memory loss, and tremors.[78] Some individuals improved following doxycycline treatment, although this was an uncontrolled case series and the true effect of treatment (and role of B. henselae) is unconfirmed. B. henselae infection should perhaps be considered in people with vague neurological and neurocognitive symptoms; however, interpretation of this potential link is currently difficult.

Diagnosis

Because of the nonspecific nature and often insidious onset of disease, diagnosis can be delayed, particularly if a history of cat exposure (especially a bite or scratch) is not obtained. Clinical pathology results are nonspecific and consistent with an infectious inflammatory process, with a transient mild leukocytosis, neutrophilia, and elevated erythrocyte sedimentation rate.[35] Specific diagnosis can involve testing of blood or affected tissues. B. henselae is a slow-growing fastidious organism that is rarely detected using routine culture methods. Selective culture media or a combination of selective culture and PCR has higher yield. Recently, commercial testing using PCR from BAPGM-enriched samples has become available commercially, and this may greatly improve the diagnosis of B. henselae infections.

Serological testing is available and is relatively sensitive but marginally specific. IgG immunoblot assay, immunofluoresence assays, enzyme immunoassay (EIA), and radioimmunoprecipitation have all been used. An indirect fluorescent assay is likely the most commonly used test.[35] This test, as with most others, has significant cross-reaction with B. quintana. Histological examination of lymph nodes indicates nonspecific inflammation. Bartonella spp. may be identified in lymph node aspirates or biopsies using silver staining (Dieterle, Warthin–Starry, or Steiner stains), but this is not specific for B. henselae.[35]

The increasing availability of molecular diagnostic tests has greatly improved the ability to diagnose B. henselae infection, although this testing is currently of variable availability. PCR-based diagnostic testing will likely become the standard for diagnosis.

Bacillar angiomatosis and bacillary peliosis are usually diagnosed by histological examination of skin or internal lesions. Bacteria may be identified using silver staining early in disease, but organisms are usually not apparent during the later granulomatous stage.[35]

Management

CSD is often self-limited, and it is questionable whether all cases require treatment.[99] Mild to moderate disease in low-risk individuals is often not treated, though it may be reasonable to treat to accelerate response and decrease the chance of complications or persistent infection. Severe or complicated disease and disease in immunocompromised individuals is treated. Susceptibility testing is rarely available and does not necessarily predict response to treatment,[35] so empirical therapy is the norm. Azithromycin is the only antimicrobial that has been shown to be effective for accelerating clinical response.[100] Needle aspiration can be performed for symptomatic relief of painful nodules, but incision and drainage should be avoided.[24]

Erythromycin or doxycycline is most commonly used for uncomplicated bacteremia, bacillary angiomatosis, and bacillary peliosis.[35] Azithromycin may also be used. At least 4 weeks of treatment is indicated, with a longer time (8–12 weeks) required for HIV/AIDS patients or patients with persistent fever or bacteremia.

In patients with endocarditis, addition of an aminoglycoside for the first 2 weeks may be useful. Eight to twelve weeks of antimicrobial therapy is indicated, and valvular resection is often required.

An adequate duration of therapy is important, as relapsing or persistent infection can develop with premature termination of treatment.[35]

Prevention

The main preventive measures are proper training and handling of cats to avoid bites, scratches, and licks, and flea control. Particular care should be taken around cats at higher risk of being infected: kittens, feral cats, outdoor cats, and cats with fleas. Keeping cats indoors at all times is recommended to reduce the chance of infection and flea infestation. Any bites or scratches should be promptly and carefully cleaned. There is no evidence that declawing will reduce the risk of *B. henselae* transmission, and this is not recommended as a control measure. Routine flea control measures are indicated. The role of ticks is also unclear, but general tick avoidance practices should be used.

Extra care should be taken in households with immunocompromised individuals. Despite the potential for severe disease in this population, removal of cats for fear of *B. henselae* infection is not indicated.[35] As part of the guidelines for preventing opportunistic infections in HIV-infected persons, the United States Public Health Service/Infectious Diseases Society of America has recommended that people in high-risk households only adopt cats greater than 1 year of age that are in good health, avoid rough play with cats, maintain flea control, wash any bites or scratches promptly, and prevent cats from licking skin wounds or abrasions.[101] Routine testing of cats for *B. henselae* infection is not indicated.[24,102] Positive serological tests do not indicate that the animal is currently infected nor do they indicate the potential pathogenicity to humans, while negative serological tests can be obtained from some bacteremic cats.[28] Serological tests can also cross-react with other *Bartonella* species,[28] some of which are not of zoonotic concern. Negative culture or PCR does not mean that the animal is truly negative, based on periodic or low-level shedding. Furthermore, animals that are negative could be exposed any time thereafter, so a negative result cannot be taken as indication of an absence of the risk of *B. henselae* exposure. Similarly, routine treatment of healthy animals to eliminate *Bartonella* is not indicated. Even in situations where

a cat has been implicated in a case of CSD, there is no indication that treatment is an effective or necessary preventive measure.

Screening of feline blood donors for *B. henselae* has been recommended because of the ability to transmit infection through contaminated blood. There was mixed opinion of an expert panel on the subject because of the high prevalence and low pathogenicity of the organism.[103]

While dogs are infrequently associated with the transmission of *B. henselae*, bites and scratches are presumably the main route of transmission, and recommendations pertaining to cats largely apply to dogs.

Bartonella clarridgeiae

Similar to *B. henselae*, cats are the natural reservoir of *B. clarridgeiae*.[40] This *Bartonella* species can be found in 0–31% of healthy cats.[41,104–106] Bacteremia rates of 0–42% have been reported,[29,37,38,42,107,108] and coinfection with *B. henselae* can occur.[29,41] Feral cats or cats with outdoor access may be predisposed to *B. clarridgeiae* bacteremia, with one study reporting a 0% prevalence in indoor cats versus 2.9% in stray cats. A French study reported bacteremia rates of 21–25% in pet cats versus 30–42% in stray cats.[37,40] This may be related to increased flea exposure in outdoor or stray cats, since the cat flea (*C. felis*) is the vector.[40] Variations in reported prevalence rates may be, in part, due to uneven distribution of the organism worldwide. There has been less investigation of dogs, but bacteremia rates of 0.3–5.6% have been reported.[38,43,59] Infection in cats is mild to subclinical,[40] but endocarditis has been reported in infected dogs.[82,109]

The role of this *Bartonella* species in CSD is currently unclear, although *B. clarridgeiae* seropositivity has been identified in people with typical signs of the disease.[110,111] It is likely an uncommon, but potential, cause of CSD, with the vast majority of cases caused by *B. henselae*. Management and preventive measures are presumably the same as for *B. henselae*.

Bartonella vinsonii subsp. berkhoffii

This *Bartonella* species appears to be an emerging canine pathogen with unknown zoonotic implications. The geographic range is unclear, but it may be present throughout most tropical and subtropical regions on the world and much of the United States.[112] The natural cycle of *B. vinsonii* subsp. *berkhoffii* is only superficially understood. Coyotes are thought to be the main reservoir,[113] but it can be found in healthy and ill dogs. Studies from various regions have reported seroprevalence rates of 0–38%,[57–59,114–118] with most studies reporting less than 5% prevalence. Coinfection with *Ehrlichia canis* or *Babesia canis* can occur, as highlighted by a 36% seropositivity of dogs with *E. canis* infection compared with just 3.6% overall.[119] Heavy tick exposure, cattle exposure, heavy flea burden, and rural origin were associated with seropositivity in one study.[119] Coinfection with *B. henselae* can occur.[57]

It is suspected that natural transmission involves ticks such as *R. sanguineus*, *Amblyomma americanum*, and *Dermacentor* spp.[120,121]

B. vinsonii subsp. *berkhoffii* has been implicated in a variety of clinical syndromes in dogs, including endocarditis, lymphadenitis, pleural and abdominal effusion, multifocal granulomatous disease, immune-mediated thrombocytopenia, neurological disease, and polyarthritis.[109,122,123] Chronic infections can occur. Isolation of *B. vinsonii* subsp. *berkhoffii* is very difficult, and a combination of selective enrichment culture followed by PCR may have the optimal sensitivity.

Reports of *B. vinsonii* subsp. *berkhoffii* infections in humans are limited. It was isolated from a person with endocarditis[124] and a boy with epithelioid hemangioendothelioma.[125] Coinfection of *B. henselae* and *B. vinsonii* subsp. *berkhoffii* was also identified in a patient with chronic fatigue, headaches, and blurred vision.[78] It was also isolated alone or in combination with *B. henselae* from eight individuals with intermittent or chronic symptoms such as fatigue, myalgia, arthralgia, headache, memory loss, ataxia, or paresthesia, all of which had frequent animal and/or arthropod contact.[68]

This bacterium is probably of limited zoonotic concern, and objective recommendations for prevention are lacking. The role of companion animals in human infection is unclear. Based on the presumed routes of transmission, tick avoidance and tick control for dogs are probably the most impor-

tant and practical measures. Routine testing or treatment of dogs is not indicated.

Bergeyella zoohelcum

This gram-negative rod-shaped aerobic bacterium, formerly termed *Weeksella zoohelcum*, is an upper respiratory tract commensal in dogs and cats.[126] It is an uncommonly reported cause of dog and cat bite-associated infections, including cellulitis, abscessation, tenosynovitis, septicemia, pneumonia, and meningitis.[126–128] Rarely, infections without history of a bite can be encountered.[126] Presumably, these are from other routes of direct or indirect transmission from animals, as is discussed in more detail under *Pasteurella multocida*. It has been stated that *B. zoohelcum* grows readily on routine culture media;[129] however, there is a report of detection of a fastidious strain of this bacterium from a cat-bite infection,[128] suggesting that infections caused by this bacterium could be underdiagnosed. Documented infections in humans are rare. This organism is likely of minimal zoonotic relevance, but bite avoidance is a prudent measure to reduce any risks associated with this pathogen.

Bordetella bronchiseptica

Introduction

B. bronchiseptica is an opportunistic upper respiratory tract pathogen in dogs, cats, and other animal species, and a rare cause of infection in humans. It is most common as part of the "kennel cough" syndrome (infectious tracheobronchitis) in dogs. Human infections occur most commonly in immunocompromised individuals.

Etiology

B. bronchiseptica is a gram-negative coccobacillus that is closely related to *Bordetella pertussis* and *Bordetella parapertussis*. While *B. pertussis* and *B. parapertussis* are primarily human pathogens, *B. bronchiseptica* does not have the same degree of host restriction and can colonize and infect various animal species, including dogs, cats, rabbits, mice, and rats.[130–134]

Geographic distribution/epidemiology

This bacterium can be found worldwide. Reports of seroprevalence have ranged from 24% to 79% in cats and 22% in dogs.[135,136] Shedding rates are highly variable, depending on the population that is studied, and can range from 1.3% to 47%.[137,138] Shedding rates are very low in healthy animals in households, with 0% of household cats identified as colonized in one study.[137] Higher prevalences have been reported in more concentrated environments or with higher risk animals such as shelters, research colonies, or in dogs with signs of respiratory tract infection.[132,137] Transmission can occur between dogs and cats.[136] The colloquial name "kennel cough" is a testament to its predilection for high-density situations such as kennels and shelters.

Pathophysiology

B. bronchiseptica is shed in oral and nasal secretions of infected or colonized animals. Exposure of the oral and nasal cavities is the most likely route of exposure. Both direct and indirect transmission is plausible. After the bacterium comes into contact with the respiratory epithelium, it attaches to cilia, resulting in ciliostasis, destruction of cilia, and impairment of mucociliary clearance. This facilitates further infection with B. bronchiseptica as well as other potential pathogens. Local and systemic inflammation can develop from release of bacterial toxins as well as the body's immune response. Upper respiratory tract infection, tracheobronchitis, or pneumonia may develop, and can be complicated by secondary bacterial infections.

Most reported human infections have occurred in immunocompromised or elderly individuals,[139–143] although infections in immunocompetent individuals have been reported.[144–147] People with underlying respiratory tract disease may also be at higher risk.[148] It is possible that infections are underreported because of a low index of suspicion

among clinicians and the potential for cross-reaction with B. pertussis immunofluorescence testing and subsequent misdiagnosis.[145]

Infection of a transplant patient following exposure to a modified live intranasal canine vaccine has also been reported.[140,141] This was a solid organ transplant recipient who developed B. bronchiseptica pneumonia. It was suspected that the person's dogs, who had been vaccinated recently, were the source, but the time frame from vaccination to human exposure and infection was not reported, nor was there confirmation that the vaccine strain was the cause of disease. In another reported case, a 14-year-old boy developed respiratory tract disease after being inadvertently sprayed in the face with modified live vaccine; however, cultures were not obtained to confirm B. bronchiseptica infection.[149]

Animals

Clinical presentation

Respiratory tract disease is the most common manifestation. Tracheobronchitis (kennel cough) is most common in dogs and often involves coinfection with other respiratory pathogens such as canine parainfluenza virus, canine adenovirus-2, canine distemper virus, and canine herpesvirus; none of which are zoonotic. An acute onset of severe paroxysmal coughing episodes is common. Fever and anorexia are typically present. Expectoration of mucus may be misinterpreted as vomiting by owners. In cats, upper respiratory tract signs including sneezing, ocular discharge, and nasal discharge are more common, but lower respiratory tract disease may also develop. Severe pneumonia, both primary and secondary, can develop. In rabbits, the classical presentation is "snuffles," an upper respiratory tract syndrome.

Diagnosis

Isolation of B. bronchiseptica from an animal with respiratory tract disease provides a reasonable assumption that the organism is playing at least some role in disease. More confidence can be had when the specimen is obtained from lower respiratory tract samples compared with nasal or oropharyngeal swabs, and from animals at lower risk of being colonized.

Management

Antimicrobial therapy appears to be unnecessary in uncomplicated cases in dogs and likely in other animal species. Antimicrobials may reduce the duration of disease, and amoxicillin/clavulanic acid and trimethoprim–sulfa are thought to be most effective.[148] Complete and rapid response is not necessarily expected because viral coinfections are common. More aggressive care may be required in serious cases.

Humans

Clinical presentation

Upper and lower respiratory tract infections can occur. These can range from mild sinusitis or bronchitis to pneumonia and rarely severe infections including necrotizing pneumonia.[139,143–145,150] Pertussis-like illness may be present. Extraintestinal infections such as surgical site infections and bloodstream infections are rare.[139]

Diagnosis

Definitive diagnosis is obtained by isolation of *B. bronchiseptica* from a patient with respiratory tract disease as this organism is not commonly found in healthy individuals. Cross-reactivity may lead to false-positive *B. pertussis* results with immunofluorescence testing.[145]

Management

Antimicrobial therapy should be based on the antibiogram. Published data are inadequate to determine optimal treatment regimens. Unlike *B. pertussis*, *B. bronchiseptica* rarely responds to macrolide antimicrobials, common first-line treatments for pertussis.[145] Poor response to macrolide therapy for pertussis should result in consideration of the possibility of *B. bronchiseptica* infection if immunofluorescence testing was the sole means of diagnosis. Doxycycline has been used to treat

vaccine-associated disease.[140] Other aspects of therapy depend on the severity of disease.

Prevention

Preventive efforts are directed largely at immunocompromised pet owners. Situations posing a high-risk for *B. bronchiseptica* exposure should be limited. New pets should not be obtained directly from animal shelters, pet stores, or similarly crowded facilities, and animals with respiratory tract disease should not be obtained. Boarding in kennels should be avoided if at all possible. If boarding is required, facility owners should be queried about the presence of animals with respiratory tract disease.

While a modified live vaccine is available for dogs, and vaccination has been shown to reduce *B. bronchiseptica* shedding after experimental challenge,[151] vaccination is not necessarily a useful measure to reduce the risk of zoonotic transmission. Modified live vaccination of immunocompromised humans is contraindicated,[140] and the potential for exposure of people to modified live *B. bronchiseptica*, combined with reports of vaccine-associated infections, indicates that pets of immunocompromised persons should not be vaccinated with this vaccine, if possible. In situations where vaccination is required (i.e., in advance of boarding at a kennel), a note from the physician and/or veterinarian explaining the reason that vaccination is not recommended should be provided. If vaccination is ultimately required, the use of parenteral killed *B. bronchiseptica* vaccine should be considered. While less efficacious for the prevention of infection, there is no risk to the owner. If the intranasal modified live vaccination is chosen, immunocompromised owners should be made aware of the potential, albeit quite low, of zoonotic infection. Veterinary personnel, not pet owners, should restrain the animal during administration of the vaccine. Immunocompromised individuals should never restrain an animal that is being vaccinated with modified live vaccine because of the potential for inadvertent exposure if the animal struggles or sneezes. Young children, elderly individuals, and immunocompromised individuals should be 2–3 m away during vaccine administration, or ideally in a different room. Care should be taken to avoid gross contamination of the animal with vaccine; however, some contamination of the animal's hair coat is likely inevitable, and hand hygiene should be emphasized for high-risk people handling animals after vaccination.

It is unclear whether pertussis vaccination of humans confers cross-protection against *B. bronchiseptica* and whether inadequately vaccinated individuals are at higher risk of infection.[145]

High-risk individuals should avoid contact with animals with potentially infectious respiratory disease. Screening of healthy pets for *B. bronchiseptica* colonization is not recommended. The prevalence of colonization is relatively low for most household pets, and inadequate information is available about the sensitivity of testing or optimal protocols. Similarly, testing of new pets is not indicated, even those from high-risk sources. Treatment of animals shedding *B. bronchiseptica* is not indicated as there is no information about whether decolonization therapy could be efficacious or whether it can reduce the risk of transmission. Good general hygiene practices should greatly reduce any risk of *B. bronchiseptica* transmission.

Brucella canis

Introduction

Brucellae are non-spore-forming gram-negative coccobacilli and important zoonotic pathogens. Virtually all human *Brucella* infections occur from direct or indirect exposure to animals.[152] The most clinically relevant Brucellae are *Brucella abortus* (primarily from cattle), *Brucella melitensis* (primarily from goats and sheep), and *Brucella suis* (swine). *B. canis* is associated with dogs and is a zoonotic pathogen, but is the least common cause of human brucellosis.[152] The zoonotic risk is highly variable and depends largely on an individual's contact with breeding dogs. It is of minimal consequence to people in contact with nonbreeding pet dogs.

Geographic distribution/epidemiology

The international distribution of *B. canis* has not been reported; however, it has been detected in numerous countries and is probably widely dis-

seminated. The prevalence may be higher in certain regions, such as the southeastern United States.[153] New Zealand and Australia appear to be *B. canis* free. Widespread transportation of dogs from and between kennels can facilitate the spread of this pathogen.[154]

Most seroprevalence studies have reported antibodies against *B. canis* in approximately 3.7–9.4% of stray and shelter dogs and 0–1% of pet dogs.[155–158] Occasional studies have reported higher rates, including a study that reported up to 43% prevalence in regions in China.[159] In general, the seroprevalence is probably low, particularly among household pets. Seropositivity was only identified among free-roaming dogs in one study, with *B. canis* antibodies present in 9% of stray and 0% of household dogs.[158] Close contact can result in the transmission of *B. canis* between dogs, though months of cohabitation are typically required for transmission.[160]

After exposure, bacteremia usually develops in approximately 3 weeks, at which time the bacterium localizes to genital tissues and can seed continuous or recurrent bacteremia for months or years.[153] Infected dogs can shed *B. canis* in urine, vaginal discharge, tissue from aborted fetuses, semen, and, to a lesser extent, other secretions such as saliva, nasal discharge, and milk.[161] Dog–dog transmission can occur via various routes, with ingestion and inhalation being most commonly reported by some studies[161] and the venereal route by others.[153] Vertical transmission may also occur.[161]

Human infections

The risk of infection is low in people that do not have contact with breeding dogs, but is relatively high in people who handle breeding dogs and who are exposed to reproductive tissues and fluids from infected dogs.[162] The incidence of human infection is unclear, and *B. canis* infection may be underdiagnosed because of a general lack of access to specific serological testing, failure to attempt diagnosis, and lack of cross-reactivity of *B. canis* with other pathogenic *Brucella*.[163,164] There are few reports of human infections, with only approximately 30 cases reported since *B. canis* was first described, but it is unclear whether that is because the disease is truly rare or underdiagnosed. Though an outbreak involving six people has been reported, most cases have been sporadic, single infections.[162]

People are relatively resistant to *B. canis* infection, particularly compared with other *Brucella* species, and severe disease is rare. Human cases of *B. canis* infection are almost invariably in people that report contact with dogs, most often contact with aborting bitches; however, reported contact with infected or breeding animals is not universal. Clear evidence of routes of transmission is currently lacking, but it is likely that most people become infected by inadvertent ingestion of *B. canis* from reproductive tissues or fluids or through contamination of mucous membranes or abraded skin. Urine may also be a source of infection, particularly from intact male dogs.[162]

Animals

Clinical presentation

Subclinical infections are common, but *B. canis* infection can cause a wide range of disease. *B. canis* is a leading cause of spontaneous abortion in dogs.[153,161] Late-term abortion is common, but decreased fertility with early embryonic death, stillbirths, and birth of weak puppies can also occur. Lymphadenopathy may be present as the sole sign of disease or in combination with reproductive disease. *B. canis* should always be considered in animals examined for reproductive failure.[153] Male dogs can develop orchitis and epididymitis with testicular enlargement in acute infection and atrophy with chronic disease. *B. canis* is also an important cause of diskospondylitis in dogs.[165] Less common manifestations include pyogranulomatous dermatitis, osteomyelitis, and endophthalmitis.[153,166,167] Mortality is low but morbidity can be high.[161]

Diagnosis

Isolation of *B. canis* is the gold standard for diagnosis. Blood culture is most often successful in the first 8 weeks after infection; however, a single negative result does not rule out *B. canis* infection.[161] *B. canis*-specific serological tests can be used, and a positive result in conjunction with consistent clinical signs can provide a presumptive diagnosis.

Serological tests may be negative during the first 3–8 weeks of infection,[161] so retesting of suspected cases with initial negative serological results is indicated. A rapid slide agglutination test (RSAT) can be used as a screening test. It has a high negative predictive value, but its specificity and corresponding positive predictive value are limited based on cross-reaction with other bacteria such as *Bordetella* and *Pseudomonas*.[155] A modified RSAT (ME-RSAT) increases the specificity by inactivating some cross-reacting IgM antibodies; however, it is still a screening test.[153] Positive RSAT results should be further investigated using tube agglutination test, agar gel immunodiffusion (AGID), and/or culture. The tube agglutination test is usually positive 2 weeks after exposure or bacteremia.[153] An AGID positive result is considered diagnostic, though animals are not usually positive until 12 weeks postinfection.[161] Other serological tests are available, including indirect fluorescent antibody (IFA) test and ELISA, with variable sensitivity and specificity.[161] Urine culture can be performed; however, the sensitivity may be low.[168]

Management

Treatment of *B. canis* with antimicrobials is often unrewarding, and long-term cure is not expected.[161] If antimicrobial therapy is elected, monotherapy should be avoided. Combinations of a tetracycline and streptomycin have been used with some success, but long-term treatment is required and resolution of infection is difficult, likely because of the difficulty in eliminating intracellular bacteria.[153] Enrofloxacin has also been used with some anecdotal success.[169] Neutering removes the main reservoir sites and may be a useful measure in combination with antimicrobial therapy.

Humans

Clinical presentation

Clinical presentation of *B. canis* infection can be identical to that of brucellosis from other *Brucella* spp., particularly as fever of unknown origin.[170–172] It usually starts as an acute febrile illness, often with headache, malaise, weakness, myalgia, and back pain. Prolonged fever may be present and is suggestive of brucellosis. Other clinical presentations include granulomatous hepatitis, gastroenteritis, hepatosplenomegaly, endocarditis, and oral lesions.[162,163,170,173] Clinical signs, particularly those early in disease, are usually nonspecific and may be present for weeks before other signs are evident.

Diagnosis

A history of contact with dogs is important to obtain as they are the only known reservoir. A history of contact with dogs from breeding kennels, particularly kennels with abortions or other reproductive problems should further increase suspicion.

Serology and blood culture are most commonly used for diagnosis.[163] B. canis will not be detected by standard serological tests targeting the smooth surface antigens of B. abortus.[163] Therefore, B. canis should be considered in patients with clinical signs consistent with brucellosis but a negative B. abortus antigen test, and culture should be performed, especially in patients with a history of dog contact. B. canis-specific serological tests, including agglutination tests and indirect ELISA, should be used wherever available. Culture is often required for diagnosis because of the lack of cross-reactivity with other Brucella serological tests and uncommon availability of species-specific serological assays.[163]

Management

Tetracyclines are most commonly used to treat human infections; however, monotherapy is associated with high relapse rates so combination therapy with rifampin or streptomycin is recommended.[152] Combination of trimethoprim–sulfamethoxazole and rifampin, a quinolone, or an aminoglycoside may be used in children less than 8 years of age and in pregnant women, where tetracyclines are contraindicated.[152,162] Ceftriaxone has also been used with anecdotal success.[163] Mortality rates are low, even in untreated individuals. Deaths are usually from endocarditis or meningitis.

Prevention

The lack of information regarding risk factors or routes of transmission limits objective recommen-

dations for prevention of zoonotic transmission. While objective information regarding relative susceptibility to B. canis infection is not available, brucellosis has a greater impact on young, immunocompromised, and pregnant individuals, and it should be assumed that this includes B. canis. These individuals should likely avoid contact with dogs from breeding kennels, particularly those that have had, or are encountering, problems with abortion or decreased fertility. Aborting bitches are a high-risk source of infection since large numbers of organisms can be present in aborted placental tissues and fluids[153] and should be avoided as much as possible. There should be an emphasis on routine hygiene practices, particularly hand hygiene, with added precautions taken around aborting bitches. This includes the use of gloves and protective outerwear when handling the dog or potential infected fluids, or having contact with a contaminated environment.[153] B. canis should be considered and investigated in breeding kennels that have encountered reproductive problems including stillbirths, birth of weak puppies, or poor fertility rates.

Urine from clinically normal dogs is typically considered a low-risk fluid for disease transmission; however, the potential for healthy male dogs to shed B. canis should be considered. Good general hygiene practices to avoid contact of urine with mucous membranes or abraded skin, or inadvertent ingestion, are reasonable in all situations but are particularly important in intact male dogs that may have been exposed to B. canis. This would include dogs that have been exposed to infected animals and dogs in breeding kennels with undiagnosed reproductive problems.

The risk posed by dogs with nonreproductive tract disease such as diskospondylitis is unclear. Information regarding B. canis shedding by infected animals is currently lacking, and it is unclear whether there is a realistic, or high, risk of exposure. In the absence of specific data, good general hygiene practices should be used. Contact with urine from intact male dogs should be avoided. The risks of zoonotic infection are probably quite low.

Preventing unrestricted outdoor access may reduce the risk of exposure since B. canis is much more common in stray dogs versus household pets. Neutering may also be useful through decreasing the likelihood of high-risk contact with other dogs.

Measures to decrease the prevalence of *B. canis* are desirable but control of *B. canis* in kennels can be difficult. Positive dogs should not be bred and should be neutered. Testing should be performed to identify all infected animals. While treatment can be attempted, the optimal measure is removal of infected animals from the facility.[153] If treatment is undertaken, periodic testing using culture and serological assays should be performed.[162] Infected dogs should not have any direct or indirect contact with uninfected dogs. To declare a kennel free of *B. canis*, three consecutive negative samples, collected monthly from all animals, must be obtained.[174] Subsequently, serological testing and quarantine (1 month) of all new dogs should be performed to reduce the risk of reinfection. Annual testing of breeding facilities has been recommended.[153] *B. canis* is susceptible to most disinfectants, including 70% ethanol, peroxygens, accelerated hydrogen peroxide, and bleach. There is no vaccine.

Campylobacter spp.

Introduction

Campylobacteriosis, infection with *Campylobacter* species, is a common disease in humans and many domestic animal species. Diarrheic disease is most common, but systemic manifestations can occur. Most human cases of campylobacteriosis are foodborne, but companion animals are a potential source of infection and the true role of pets in human campylobacteriosis may be underestimated. The wide range of different *Campylobacter* strains that can be found and the common presence of some *Campylobacter* species or subspecies in healthy individuals complicate diagnosis and assessment of the role of pets in human illness.

Etiology

Campylobacter is a genus of gram-negative microaerophilic curved bacteria (Figure 2.3) that contains at least 37 species and subspecies. Most

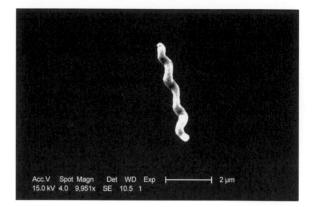

Figure 2.3   Scanning electron microscope image of *Campylobacter jejuni* (public domain, Centers for Disease Control and Prevention, Dr. Patricia Fields and Dr. Collette Fitzgerald).

Campylobacter species and subspecies are not generally pathogenic to humans or animals, but some may cause disease in a range of individuals. *Campylobacter* can be grouped in various ways, including thermophilic/nonthermophilic and based on catalase status. In general, most pathogenic *Campylobacter* spp. are thermophilic and catalase positive, and most diagnostic testing and research studies focus on thermophilic species. The introduction of PCR testing, with its ability to detect and differentiate species with diverse growth requirements, has led to increased information about the prevalence and diversity of *Campylobacter* in healthy animals.

Epidemiology

Campylobacter species can be found in humans and animals worldwide. They are gastrointestinal commensals of wildlife, food animal, and companion animal species and are commonly present in the feces of healthy dogs and cats. *Campylobacter jejuni* is the main human pathogen and is found in many animals. *Campylobacter coli* and *Campylobacter hyointestinalis* are predominantly found in pigs, while the main hosts of *Campylobacter upsaliensis* are dogs and cats. However, despite these general tendencies, there can be a range of *Campylobacter* species found within animal species. The variable growth of different species under dif-

ferent culture conditions and with different selective media can have a significant impact on reported prevalences and species distributions. Recent culture-independent studies have shown that the prevalence and diversity of *Campylobacter* colonization may be underestimated.[175]

Dogs

C. upsaliensis is the most common species found in dogs in most reports,[176–179] with *C. jejuni* being the most common catalase-positive species (Table 2.1).[176,177,180] *C. coli*, *Campylobacter lari*, and *Campylobacter helveticus*, among other species, are uncommonly identified.[175,181–183] Some studies have produced variable results, particularly when using molecular diagnostic methods. For example, *Campylobacter gracilis*, a human pathogen, was reported to be most common in rural dogs in a recent study.[175] Multiple species can be found in some dogs.[182,184]

Dogs housed in crowded conditions such as kennels or shelters are more likely to shed *Campylobacter*, irrespective of disease status.[181,185]

Table 2.1 *Campylobacter* colonization in dogs.

Group	Prevalence (%)	Reference
Healthy	47	177
Diarrheic	60	177
Dogs in animal shelter	51	186
Pet dogs	22	214
Stray dogs	51	214
Healthy dogs	56	182
5- to 12-month-old dogs	76	182
Healthy dogs	21	195
Young pet dogs	76	178
Puppies	29	183
Healthy	38	179
Healthy	1.7 (*C. jejuni* only)	215
Healthy	1.2 (*C. jejuni* only)	179

Table 2.2 *Campylobacter* colonization in cats.

Group	Any species (%)	Reference
Healthy	44	177
In animal shelter	75	186
Healthy cats in quarantine facility	58	216
Healthy	16 (*C. jejuni* only)	217
Healthy	1.6 (*C. jejuni* only)	218
Healthy	42	6
Less than 1 year of age	0.8	219

Young dogs (<6 months) also have higher shedding rates.[177,178,185–187] There may be seasonality to *Campylobacter*, though results are variable with some studies indicating higher rates in spring, summer, or fall.[185,188] Long-term carriage is suspected to occur, at least for some *Campylobacter* species in some individuals, as demonstrated by the detection of the same strain of *C. upsaliensis* over 21 months or longer in some dogs.[178]

Cats

Colonization of healthy cats is common (Table 2.2). *C. upsaliensis*, *C. helveticus*, and *C. jejuni* have all been reported as the predominant species in different studies.[6,177,181] Intensive housing, young age, winter sampling, and outdoor access are reported risk factors.[177,186,189] Duration of shedding has not been well investigated, but one study of cats reported a median duration of 44 days.[190]

Other species

There is limited information about *Campylobacter* in other companion animal species. Campylobacteriosis has been diagnosed in ferrets,[191] and *Campylobacter* colonization has been reported in diverse species such as hamsters and a pet turtle.[187,192,193] Concern has been raised about pet hamsters as potential reservoirs of human campylobacteriosis,[187] but clear evidence is lacking.

Role of *Campylobacter* in disease in dogs and cats

Studies comparing the prevalence of *Campylobacter* isolation from diarrheic and nondiarrheic animals have reported conflicting results. Some studies have reported similar rates in both groups,[6,186–188,194] while one study reported an association between the presence of *C. jejuni* and *C. upsaliensis* and diarrhea, but only in animals less than 1 year of age.[195] Coinfections with other enteropathogens may occur.

The true role of *Campylobacter* in diarrhea in dogs and cats is difficult to determine, largely because of the high prevalence in healthy animals. Experimental infection with *Campylobacter* has yielded variable results, with mild disease reproduced in puppies but no illness in kittens.[196–198] It is likely that some *Campylobacter* species, particularly *C. jejuni*, are potentially pathogenic in dogs and cats but that colonization occurs much more commonly. *C. coli* is also likely a potential pathogen, albeit rare. The role of *C. helveticus* and *C. upsaliensis* is even less clear.

Humans

The epidemiology of *Campylobacter* in humans is quite different from that in companion animals. *Campylobacter* is clearly an important pathogen in humans and is one of the most commonly diagnosed causes of enteric disease worldwide. The infectious dose can be low, with, at times, ingestion of as few as 500 organisms able to cause disease, though higher doses (>10⁴) are typically required to more consistently cause disease.[199] *C. jejuni* and *C. coli* are regarded as the main pathogenic *Campylobacter* species; however, there is increasing evidence that the role of other species may be underestimated. *Campylobacter fetus* is the most important cause of extraintestinal campylobacteriosis.[200] As with other animal species, *Campylobacter* species can be found in asymptomatic humans, albeit at lower rates than in animals (Table 2.3). *Campylobacter concisus* seems to predominate. Colonization with the main pathogenic species appears to be rare.

Transmission to humans

Infection is fecal–oral. Most infections are foodborne, but waterborne infections may also occur.

Table 2.3 *Campylobacter* colonization in humans.

Group	Prevalence (%)	Reference
Healthy children	*C. concisus*: 33	220
Healthy, nonfarm residents	0	221
Healthy, farm residents	5	221
Healthy individuals	3 (all *C. concisus*)	222
Healthy children	6.4 (thermotolerant only)	223
Healthy infants	6.4	224

Various studies have implicated pets as sources of infection. Having a pet with diarrhea has been identified as a risk factor for campylobacteriosis in three case-control studies, including one involving infants.[201–203] Pet puppy ownership was identified as a risk factor for campylobacteriosis is children less than 3 years of age.[204] Recent acquisition of a new pet dog has also been identified as a risk factor for campylobacteriosis.[205] In other studies, 16% of sporadic *C. jejuni* infections were linked to exposure to diarrheic kittens, and 30% of cases in a study of university students were associated with pet cats.[206] Indistinguishable isolates of *C. jejuni* were recovered from a girl with diarrhea and her pet dog,[207] yet as with any study of concurrent isolation of a pathogen, the source of infection and direction of transmission cannot be ascertained.

Overall, the epidemiological and case-report data strongly suggest a role of pets in some cases of human campylobacteriosis, although dwarfed by foodborne infection. Less information is available regarding risks posed by individual *Campylobacter* species, something that is of particular relevance with respect to species more commonly associated with companion animals. There is increasing evidence that *C. upsaliensis*, while perhaps not pathogenic in dogs, is a potential cause of disease in humans. The variable ability of diagnostic laboratories to isolate this species may lead to underdiagnosis.[208] *C. upsaliensis* was the second most common species in a study of quinolone-resistant *Campylobacter* in California, but only accounted for 4% of isolates.[208] A report of isolation of indistinguishable isolates of *C. upsaliensis* from a person with bloody diarrhea and her pet dog supports concerns about dogs as a source of human infection.[209] Concurrent isolation of *C. upsaliensis* from a person with diarrhea and her cat has also been reported.[210] Highly related *C. upsaliensis* isolates were also recovered from both a pet cat and fetoplacental material of a pregnant woman following spontaneous abortion.[210] Issues regarding the pathogenicity of *C. upsaliensis* are critical because of the high prevalence of this species in healthy dogs and cats. In humans, it appears that *C. upsaliensis* infection is usually subclinical; however, self-limited diarrhea to severe illness with spontaneous abortion or hemolytic–uremic syndrome can develop.[210,211] There is also some evidence of species specificity among *C. upsaliensis*, with canine and human strains clustering differently by amplified fragment length polymorphism (AFLP) typing.[212]

Emergence and dissemination of antimicrobial-resistant *Campylobacter* spp. is an important public health concern. This is assumed to be most related to antimicrobial use in food animals, but antimicrobial-resistant *Campylobacter* spp. have been isolated from pets.[213] Strains of antimicrobial-resistant *C. jejuni* from people and pets containing the same resistance mechanisms have been identified.[213] Presumably, pets acquired resistant species from food animal or food sources. Once a pet is shedding antimicrobial-resistant *Campylobacter*, there is the potential for transmission to humans, so the role of pets in disseminating these strains should not be dismissed.

Animals

Clinical presentation

Most infected animals have no signs of disease. Clinical disease is most common in young animals, particularly those less than 6 months of age. Diarrhea is the predominant clinical sign, ranging from mild to severe and bloody. Anorexia, vomiting, and abdominal pain may also occur. Extraintestinal infections such as bacteremia and cholecystitis are rare but have been reported. Neither clinical signs nor character of diarrhea are indicative of campylobacteriosis over other diarrheal diseases.

Diagnosis

Diagnosis of campylobacteriosis is challenging, largely because of the high prevalence of colonization in healthy animals. Fecal cytology is used by some to detect curved, "*Campylobacter*-like" organisms, yet this is of marginal utility because of the presence of similarly appearing organisms such as *Helicobacter*, *Arcobacter*, and *Anaerobiospirillum*. At best, detection of *Campylobacter*-like organisms is mildly suggestive of disease.

Fecal culture is currently the standard for diagnosis, although interpretation can be difficult because of the presence of *Campylobacter* in a large percentage of healthy animals. False-negative results are also a concern since *Campylobacter* require specific culture conditions, and labs without experience with the organism may have poor recovery rates. Different species grow better under different conditions,[176] and individual culture methods are not optimal for all species. The use of multiple methods can increase culture yield,[176] but may be impractical in diagnostic laboratories. Typically, diagnostic laboratories use methods optimized for *C. jejuni* and *C. coli*, the most clinically important species. Determination of the *Campylobacter* species is important. At a minimum, determination of catalase positive (*C. jejuni*, *C. coli*) versus catalase negative is important, since catalase-positive species are more likely to be clinically relevant. Molecular methods are preferred for speciation. PCR can be used to detect *Campylobacter* from feces, but the clinical utility is currently unclear. PCR has the potential to be more sensitive and rapid, and able to detect a broader range of species, but it is unclear whether increased sensitivity will truly help diagnose this disease. At this point, detection of *C. jejuni* or *C. coli* in a diarrheic animal should be taken as a presumptive diagnosis, with the understanding that it could still just represent colonization. The relevance of detection of other species is unclear. Concurrent diagnostic testing is required to detect coinfection with other pathogens.

Management

Antimicrobial treatment of animals with diarrhea is reasonable, despite it being unclear whether treatment actually has any effect on outcome. Treatment is perhaps best reserved for moderate to severe cases because of the often self-limited nature of mild disease. Optimal treatment regimens are not known. Erythromycin, fluoroquinolones, and second-generation cephalosporins are often recommended,[206] but the relative efficacy is unclear. Treatment appears to be more successful at controlling clinical signs than elimination of the bacterium.

Treatment of healthy carriers is not typically recommended because of a lack of evidence of efficacy or need. Treatment may not be effective at eliminating *Campylobacter* in colonized animals, especially those in high-risk environments such as pet stores or kennels, and could simply increase antimicrobial resistance.

Humans

Clinical presentation

Diarrhea is the main clinical manifestation, ranging from mild and self-limited to severe and prolonged. Acute enteritis, indistinguishable from various other types of enteritis, is common. Fever, headache, malaise, and myalgia may precede fever by 12–24 hours.[200] Diarrhea may range from loose to watery stools, which may be bloody. Defecation frequency may be high. Abdominal pain and cramping may accompany diarrhea and be relieved by defecation. Spontaneous resolution after a few days is common, but prolonged diarrhea (>1 week) may occur. Relapse may also occur following apparent clinical resolution.

In more serious cases, acute colitis may occur and is characterized by fever, abdominal cramps, and bloody diarrhea of 1 week or greater duration.[200] Some patients may develop severe disease, and toxic megacolon is a very rare complication.[225]

Acute abdominal pain in the absence of diarrhea is a rare presentation. Pain may be concentrated in the lower right quadrant and mimic appendicitis, as with *Yersinia pseudotuberculosis*.[200] In such cases, diagnosis is often made postoperatively on fecal cultures submitted following unremarkable exploratory surgery.

Bacteremia is uncommon with *C. jejuni* and *C. coli*, as are extraintestinal infections such as meningitis and endocarditis. Spontaneous abortion caused by *C. upsaliensis* has been reported.[210]

Extraintestinal infections are typically caused by *C. fetus* subsp. *fetus*. This species has a predilection for vascular sites, and infection is often manifested as endocarditis or pericarditis.[200] Abscessation of various body sites may occur, as can meningoencephalitis. Diarrhea or other signs of enteric disease are uncommonly present.

Guillain–Barre syndrome is a rare but important complication of *C. jejuni* infection. This acute, progressive inflammatory demyelinating polyneuropathy is believed to occur in approximately 1/2000 infections, typically 2–3 weeks after diarrheic illness.[226] This syndrome can also be caused by other infectious agents, but *C. jejuni* is believed to be the cause of 20–50% of cases.[226–228] A more common postinfectious condition associated with *C. jejuni* is a reactive arthritis, which is estimated to occur in 9% of infected individuals.[229] *C. jejuni* has also been linked to alpha-chain disease in humans, an immunoproliferative small bowel disorder.

Diagnosis

Diagnosis of campylobacteriosis in humans is easier compared with companion animals because of the lower prevalence of colonization. Therefore, detection of *Campylobacter* can be associated with disease with greater confidence. However, some healthy individuals may carry *Campylobacter* at any given time, so false positives can certainly occur.

Fecal cytology is sometimes used for a rapid, presumptive diagnosis. This is particularly useful early in disease and with freshly passed (<2 hours) samples. Evaluation of feces with darkfield or phase-contrast microscopy is most useful to assess both morphology and the characteristic darting motility of *Campylobacter*.[230,231] Identification of *Campylobacter*-like organisms on Gram stain can be used but only has a sensitivity of 50–75%.[232] In contrast with animals, the specificity is believed to be high.[200]

Culture is most commonly used. Proper sample handling and rapid submission are critical to reduce false-negative cultures. The culture methods used will have an impact on the recovery of the organism, and consideration must be given to the laboratory methods when evaluating results. Methods that are able to detect both thermophilic and nonthermophilic species are important. Testing for only thermophilic species will be adequate for *C. jejuni* and *C. coli*, but not necessarily *C. fetus, C. upsaliensis*, and many other species, which are non-thermophilic or have variable ability to grow at 42°C. Additionally, the type of culture media used can have a significant effect, particularly for *C. upsaliensis* as it is often susceptible to antimicrobials used in selective media.[211] The use of combinations of media is optimal but not always performed. Because of the fastidious nature of *Campylobacter*, a single negative culture does not rule out campylobacteriosis.

Management

Campylobacterioisis is often self-limited, with spontaneous resolution after a few days. Specific aspects of management vary with severity of disease. Supportive therapy is an important aspect of treatment of diarrheic patients. Oral rehydration with glucose or electrolyte-containing solutions may be required, with intravenous fluid therapy needed in some patients.[200]

Antimicrobial treatment is most commonly recommended in patients with high fever, bloody diarrhea, patients passing stools more than eight times per day, patients whose symptoms have not lessened or are worsening by the time diagnosis is made, or patients whose symptoms have persisted for more than 1 week.[200] If antimicrobials are to be used, early treatment is ideal as positive effects of antimicrobial therapy have been reported in children treated early in disease[233] but not in those where treatment was initiated a few days after culture results.[234] A macrolide is often recommended as first-line therapy.[200] *Campylobacter* spp. are usually susceptible to macrolides, as well as tetracyclines, aminoglycosides, quinolones, and chloramphenicol. The emergence and dissemination of antimicrobial-resistant strains is a concern. Ciprofloxacin is often used for the treatment of macrolide-resistant strains, but quinolone resistance is increasing. Tetracyclines may be effective but should not be used in children <8 years of age.

Treatment of extraintestinal infections varies depending on the organ system affected. Antimicrobials are indicated in all situations, and erythromycin should be avoided because of the

prevalence of resistance in *C. fetus*, the main cause of extraintestinal infection.[235,236] Choice of antimicrobial should be based on the *Campylobacter* species and *in vitro* susceptibility testing results.

Prevention

Certain animal populations can be assumed to be much higher risks for zoonotic transmission. These would include young puppies and kittens and animals recently obtained from pet stores, shelters, or kennels. Young animals are more likely to be shedding *Campylobacter* spp., have fecal accidents, and have very close contact with people. Particular care should be taken around these individuals, particularly with respect to handling feces and fecal contamination. Due to the high risk of shedding among young animals, they should be avoided by high-risk humans (very young, elderly, immunocompromised). If a high-risk individual wishes to obtain a new pet, an older animal from a household should be considered to reduce the risk of *Campylobacter* exposure.

Diarrheic animals are similarly high risk, both because of the potential for shedding zoonotic *Campylobacter* species and the potential for environmental contamination by diarrhea. Care should be taken when handling diarrhea because of many potential zoonotic pathogens, including *Campylobacter*. Diarrhea accidents in the house should be cleaned up with care. However, since many healthy animals carry *Campylobacter*, efforts focused solely on the management of diarrheic animals are insufficient. Care must be taken with routine fecal handling and hygiene practices to reduce the risk of exposure.

Because of the susceptibility of *Campylobacter* to acidic conditions, it has been suggested that ingestion with substances such as fatty foods, milk, and water, which facilitate rapid passage through the stomach, could facilitate infection with lower doses.[200] It is thus possible that low-dose exposure from pets during normal activities might be associated with lower risk than corresponding low-dose exposure in food. However, this is rather hypothetical, and there is clear evidence of an association of pets with human infection. It may be reasonable to consider the role of food ingestion in pet-associated campylobacteriosis, as one might surmise that *Campylobacter* exposure from pets could be of higher consequence when the organism is ingested along with foods. Good hygiene and food handling practices should minimize this risk.

Screening of healthy pets for *Campylobacter* colonization is not indicated. There are enough concerns about methodology that results could not necessarily be interpreted with confidence. More importantly, there is little information to guide actions in response to either positive or negative results. Considering the high prevalence of colonization in healthy animals, the ability to reduce the risk of fecal–oral infection with routine hygiene practices, and the lack of an indication to treat colonized animals, positive results would have little impact on animal management. Similarly, negative results only indicate a single point-in-time status, might represent a false-negative result, and would provide no assurance that the animal will not shed *Campylobacter* on a subsequent day. Therefore, recommendations for handling the animal would be essentially the same with either result, with an emphasis on routine precautions. Even in households containing high-risk humans, there is no indication to test given the reasons listed above and the need for high-risk personnel to take care around pets at all times because of a variety of potential pathogens.

Transmission of *Campylobacter* in veterinary clinics, either animal-to-animal or zoonotic, has not been reported but is certainly possible. As with households, all diarrheic animals should be handled with extra care in veterinary clinics because of the potential for various infectious agents. Diarrheic animals should be housed in isolation if possible and handled with contact precautions. Careful attention should be paid to routine hygiene and infection control practices.

Capnocytophaga spp.

Introduction

Capnocytophaga canimorsus and *Capnocytophaga cynodegmi* are uncommon but important causes of infection, particularly in certain high-risk groups. While the incidence of disease is low, it is often severe and can be rapidly fatal. The severity of

disease combined with the relatively ubiquitous nature of these two organisms in dogs highlights the risks associated with dog bites to high-risk individuals. Clinical infections in animals are rare (or at least rarely diagnosed).

Etiology

The genus *Capnocytophaga* consists of seven species: *C. canimorsus*, *C. cynodegmi*, *C. gingivalis*, *C. granulosa*, *C. haemolytica*, *C. ochracea*, and *C. sputigena*. These are fastidious gram-negative capnophilic anaerobes that inhabit the oral cavity. *C. canimorsus* and *C. cynodegmi* are associated with zoonotic transmission.

The fastidious nature of *Capnocytophaga* initially created difficulties with isolation and identification. It was first isolated in 1976 from a person following a dog bite but was initially classified as CDC group dysgonic fermenter 2 (DF-2). Seventeen human infections were reported the following year,[237] but details about the organism were slow to emerge because of its fastidious nature. It was given its current name in 1989[238] and knowledge about the genus has increased, though understanding of many aspects is still quite superficial.

Geographic distribution/epidemiology

C. canimorsus is a common inhabitant of the canine and, to a lesser degree, feline oral cavity. Colonization rates of 26–74% in dogs and 18–57% in cats have been reported.[239–242] Clinical infections of animals are rare. Less is known about *C. cynodegmi*. Recent evidence indicates that it might also be very common in healthy dogs and cats, as a study reported detection of *C. cynodegmi* by PCR from 86% of dogs and 84% of cats.[240] There are reports of *C. cynodegmi* bronchitis and pneumonia in a dog[243] and pneumonia in a cat with pulmonary carcinoma.[244]

Human *C. canimorsus* infections have been reported in the United States, Canada, Europe, Australia, and South Africa,[245] and likely occur throughout the world. Infections are more common in men and people >50 years of age.[246–248] Asplenic and other immunocompromised individuals are at highest risk.[248,249] Human infections are rare, with one study estimating the incidence rate at 0.67 infections per million population.[248] Despite the rarity of infection, *Capnocytophaga* is of concern because of the potential for severe disease and the much higher infection rate for the immunocompromised. Less is known about *C. cynodegmi*, although it can certainly cause disease.[250,251]

Capnocytophaga infections occur following bites, scratches, or other close contacts. While both *C. canimorsus* and *C. cynodegmi* can cause zoonotic infections, *C. canimorsus* infections are much more common and more severe.[248] Most reported infections are associated with exposure to dogs, with infections from cats, and rarely rabbits, having also been identified.[246,247,252–254] Bites are the most common source of infection, but other reported routes of infection include scratches, pets licking ulcers, and cats biting peritoneal dialysis tubing, as well as situations where no obvious route of exposure was reported in people that had close contact with animals.[246,255–259] There are also two separate reports of veterinarians becoming infected after being struck by fractured dog or cat teeth during dental procedures.[260,261]

Animals

Clinical presentation

Disease appears to be very rare in animals, despite the high incidence of bites. There are two reports of clinical infections in animals following dog bites: one in a rabbit and the other a dog.[262,263] There are also reports of *Capnocytophaga* sp. sinusitis and rhinitis in a cat,[264] *C. cynodegmi* lower respiratory tract infection in a cat with pulmonary carcinoma,[244] and *C. cynodegmi* pneumonia in a dog.[243] It is unclear whether this is a truly rare disease in animals or whether infections are not detected because of lack of routine culture and difficulty isolating the organism.

Diagnosis

Diagnosis of *Capnocytophaga* infection in animals relies on culture, as described below. Because of the fastidious nature of *Capnocytophaga* species and difficulties with definitive identification, PCR may be a better diagnostic tool.

Management

The small number of cases in animals provides little objective guidance. Based on *in vitro* susceptibility patterns, amoxicillin or ampicillin are reasonable first-line options. Clindamycin and fluoroquinolones are also likely to be effective based on *in vitro* susceptibility.[245]

Humans

Clinical presentation

The clinical presentation can be highly variable. The typical incubation period from a bite until the first clinical signs is approximately 5 days, with 7 days from bite to hospitalization.[265] Initial signs may be restricted to local inflammation that could be due to infection or trauma. As infection progresses, cellulitis, purulent discharge, lymphangitis, and regional lymphadenopathy may develop.[266] Systemic signs may be noted concurrently, including fever (78–85%), chills (46%), myalgia (31%), vomiting (31%), diarrhea or abdominal pain (21–26%), malaise (26%) dyspnea (23%), confusion (23%), and headache (18%).[245,247,266] Rapid onset of fulminant disease may also occur, and disseminated intravascular coagulation (DIC) is not uncommon.[247] This occurs mainly in asplenic or granulocytopenic individuals but has been reported in people without known risk factors.[267] Rapid progression can occur, with overwhelming infection resulting in multiple organ failure and DIC within 24 hours of onset of the first signs of disease. Other manifestations such as lymphocytic meningitis, endocarditis, pneumonitis, or cerebral abscess may occur, with or without apparent cellulitis.[253,268–271] Recently, a series of infections in preterm infants was published, with the suggestion that *Capnocytophaga* might be a cause of some occult cases of chorioamnionitis and preterm birth.[272]

Diagnosis

Definitive diagnosis currently involves culture, usually blood culture.[245,248] Culture of other specimens such as CSF and the infected wound may also be diagnostic. However, isolation and identification of *Capnocytophaga* spp. can be difficult. Some automated blood culture systems that are used in diagnostic laboratories may not be optimal for isolation of *Capnocytophaga* because they contain polyanethole-sulfonate, which inhibits *Capnocytophaga* growth.[245] Successful isolation of *Capnocytophaga* spp. is facilitated by specialized culture because of very slow growth on routine screening media as well as requirements for high levels of iron in the culture media and a CO_2-rich environment. The small, slow-growing colonies can be easy to overlook, particularly if mixed infection or contaminants are present. Gram-negative rods can be seen on blood smears of some patients with overwhelming infection.[273] While not specific for *Capnocytophaga*, this finding in a high-risk individual who has had a bite or other potential exposure should indicate a high potential for infection. In less severe infections, cytological examination of the buffy coat may be useful. Similarly, gram-negative rods may be seen in aspirates or swabs taken from the infection site or CSF. Methods to provide an earlier suspicion of *Capnocytophaga* infection are useful because of the slow growth of this organism and corresponding delays in culture results. *Capnocytophaga* should be suspected when laboratory reports of fastidious gram-negative rods are received. The use of molecular methods is appealing because of the potential for much more sensitive and faster diagnosis.[274] While currently there is limited clinical availability, molecular methods may become the main diagnostic options in the future.

Management

Prompt treatment is critical. *Capnocytophaga* infection should be considered in all infections that occur following a dog bite or other close contact, particularly in asplenic or otherwise immunocompromised individuals. Because of the slow-growing nature of *Capnocytophaga* and the difficulty in isolating it, empirical antimicrobial therapy should be started whenever there is a reasonable suspicion of *Capnocytophaga* infection. Penicillins tend to be effective *in vitro*. Amoxicillin/clavulanic acid may be preferable to amoxicillin alone because beta-lactamase-producing strains have been identified.[246,256] Erythromycin, clindamycin, doxycycline, rifampin, quinolones, carbapenems, vancomycin, and third-generation cephalosporins are also typically effective *in vitro*.[275]

Reported mortality rates can be high (13–33%)[247–249,257] and the prognosis is very poor in people with DIC and/or septicemia.[247] It is possible that many milder infections are not diagnosed and are successfully treated with empirical antimicrobial therapy. Progression may be more rapid and severe in asplenic individuals, immunocompromised, alcoholics, and persons on corticosteroids,[246] but reported mortality rates in otherwise healthy individuals can be similarly high.[266]

Prevention

Capnocytophaga spp., particularly *C. canimorsus*, are commensal microorganisms and potentially ubiquitous in dogs and cats. Therefore, there will be a constant risk of exposure. Testing of pets for colonization is not useful because of the high prevalence of colonization, difficulties in accurately detecting the organism and the lack of information indicating what to do with a positive animal. There is no indication to treat pets to attempt to eliminate *Capnocytophaga* colonization, even in households with high-risk individuals. No evidence exists indicating whether eradication is possible or that it would be an effective control measure. Given the high prevalence and typical difficulty in eradicating commensal microorganisms from their natural niche, it is unlikely that eradication therapy would be successful.

Prevention of *Capnocytophaga* infection involves bite avoidance and proper care of bite wounds. Bite avoidance is a critical aspect in households with high-risk individuals. Avoidance and proper management of scratches is also important. People should prevent contact of pets with wounds, especially contact with a dog's mouth. Pets should not be allowed to have contact with (particularly lick) open wounds or ulcers. While there are only two reports of dental procedure-associated infections in veterinarians, proper eye and face protection should be used whenever veterinary dental procedures are performed because of the high likelihood of exposure to *Capnocytophaga*. Veterinary personnel who are asplenic may be at a particularly high risk of infection and should take particular care to avoid bites, scratches, or direct contact with saliva from dogs and cats.

High-risk individuals such as people without a functional spleen must be aware of the risks associated with *Capnocytophaga* infection. Education regarding this rare but devastating infection should be mandatory for all such patients, and measures that must be taken in response to a bite or scratch must be clearly presented and understood. Antimicrobial prophylaxis is indicated in any high-risk individual that has been bitten by a dog or cat or where there has been contact of an ulcer or wound with dog or cat saliva.[245] Whether this should also apply to people that have been scratched is unknown.

The presence of a high-risk person in the household does not preclude pet ownership. Given the low incidence of disease, measures that can be taken to reduce exposure, and prophylactic treatment options after exposure, the emphasis should be on patient (and physician) education.

Chlamydophila felis

C. felis (*Chlamydophila psittaci* var. *felis*) is an obligate intracellular bacterium of the Chlamydiaceae family. It is a cause of ocular and upper respiratory tract disease in cats, characterized by conjunctivitis, sneezing, fever, transient inappetence, and mild nasal discharge.[276] It is also suspected to be a cause of keratitis, abortion, neonatal mortality, and infertility.[276] Transmission is presumably through direct contact with infected animals and fomites, and potentially through aerosols.[276] Some infected animals may be long-term or even persistent shedders following infection. Conjunctival, gastrointestinal, and reproductive shedding can occur. *C. felis* shedding has been reported in 0.3% of clinically normal cats[277–279] and up to 20% of cats with conjunctivitis.[276,280]

There are reports of zoonotic *C. felis* infection from cats,[281–287] but these are small in number and generally weak. Reports have consisted of keratoconjunctivitis and upper and lower respiratory tract infections, primarily in immunocompromised individuals. Most predated the availability of testing to definitively distinguish *C. felis* from related organisms. In some cases, cats were implicated based on having the same clinical signs as the owner without isolation of *C. felis* from the cat,

with isolation of *C. felis* from cats but no specific diagnosis of *C. felis* infection in owners, or based on serology that is nonspecific. Evidence supporting zoonotic transmission in many cases was circumstantial and relatively weak, and it is unclear whether *C. felis* truly poses a risk. A review of published cases of zoonotic infections concluded that there is evidence that *C. felis* may occasionally cause keratoconjunctivitis in people, but there is little evidence supporting its role as a cause of pneumonia or serious systemic disease.[288] In only one case of keratoconjunctivitis in an immunocompromised patient was there definitive evidence of zoonotic transmission.[281] Considering the small number and unconvincing nature of most reports and the low prevalence of *C. felis* shedding by healthy cats, the risk is likely minimal.

C. felis is presumably spread primarily through direct contact, especially by the hands. Good hand hygiene practices are likely the most important protective factor. While the risk is presumably low, immunocompromised individuals should exercise added caution and restrict contact with cats displaying signs of disease consistent with *C. felis* infection.

Chlamydophila psittaci

Introduction

Chlamydophila psittaci, formerly *Chlamydia psittaci*, is the cause of psittacosis (ornithosis) in humans and avian chlamydiosis in birds. Both "psittacosis" and the colloquial term "parrot fever" are testaments to the role of psittacine birds (e.g., parrots, cockatoos, parakeets, lories, lovebirds, budgerigars) in transmission of this pathogen to humans. However, it is clear that *C. psittaci* is not limited to psittacines and can be found in various avian species.

Etiology

C. psittaci is a gram-negative intracellular bacterium that was first thought to be a virus, then a *Rickettsia*. It was eventually identified as a *Chlamydia* sp. and subsequently changed to *Chlamydophila*, although the term "chlamydiosis" is still commonly used. It is an obligate intracellular bacterium with a biphasic development cycle involving the infectious form (elementary body) and metabolically active form (reticulate body).[289] There are six avian serovars that are relatively host specific in terms of avian hosts, but all are considered to be readily transmitted to humans.[289]

Geographic distribution/epidemiology

C. psittaci is widely disseminated in birds internationally. Most reports of human infections have come from North America and Europe,[290] but this is likely because of underreporting of psittacosis in many other regions. Initial reports of human infections involved large outbreaks associated with psittacines, particularly parrots. Human infections have subsequently been associated with contact with numerous bird species, including pigeons,[291,292] poultry,[293,294] ducks,[295] and canaries.[296] Successful isolation of *C. psittaci* has been reported from approximately 465 bird species among 30 different orders.[289]

Avian colonization with *C. psittaci* is most common in psittacines and variable between species and facilities.[289,297,298] In some facilities, the majority of birds are infected;[289] however, this is probably not the norm. Transmission between birds primarily occurs through feces and nasal discharges of commingled birds or those housed in close proximity. Fecal shedding is intermittent and more common with overcrowding, stress, nutritional deficiency, chilling, breeding, laying, or handling. The duration of shedding is variable but can last for several months. Large numbers of *C. psittaci* can be found in feces and respiratory secretions of shedding birds. These factors explain why colonization rates may be very high in large breeding operations. While less commonly considered as pets, *C. psittaci* may be common in racing pigeons, with seroprevalence rates of up to 60%.[289] Both infected and colonized birds can be sources of human infection, and colonization of apparently healthy pet birds is a concern because of the close contact of some pet birds with their owners. In contrast to earlier reports of large avian outbreaks, often with high mortality, most contemporary

reports involve sporadic cases, smaller outbreaks, and low mortality.[289]

Psittacosis is uncommonly diagnosed, with 935 human cases reported to the CDC from 1988 to 2003[299] and 91 reported between 2002 and 2007.[300] The incidence of psittacosis is likely underestimated because of the lack of diagnostic testing and the nonspecific nature of disease.[290] People with exposure to pet birds and poultry are at higher risk of infection, with most human cases associated with exposure to psittacines.[301] Sporadic cases and outbreaks have been reported in pet store workers, bird park staff, bird park visitors, and pet bird owners.[298,302–304] High seroprevalence rates have also been reported in zoo workers.[305] While the incidence of disease may be high in such groups, it has been suggested that regular infection of those individuals might confer protection against severe disease.[298]

Subclinical or mild infections may be more common than currently understood. A study in Belgium reported detection of *C. psittaci* by PCR in pharyngeal swabs of 12.7% of participants, ranging from 22% of people with daily contact with birds to 0.8% in people with no contact with birds.[290] Similarly, *C. psittaci* was detected in 31% of pet bird breeders in another study, all of which had infected birds in their colonies.[298] Sixty-seven percent of positive individuals (including all that were positive both on PCR and culture) reported recent mild respiratory illness but none had sought medical attention, providing further support that mild disease may be markedly underdiagnosed.

Mixing of large numbers of birds and widespread dissemination of groups of birds to pet stores can result in exposure of many individuals and create the potential for outbreaks. *C. psittaci* was identified in a shipment of over 700 pet birds from a Florida distributor, which resulted in respiratory disease in 10.7% of people in households exposed to birds from the affected shipment.[303]

While there is currently no objective evidence indicating that certain groups (e.g., the very young, elderly, immunocompromised) are at higher risk of disease or severe disease, it is reasonable to consider that they might be predisposed.

Zoonotic transmission mainly occurs through inhalation of contaminated material.[290] *C. psittaci* can be dispersed in the air in respiratory droplets or through aerosolization of dried respiratory secretions or feces.[301] While the organism is not particularly hardy when exposed to environmental effects, it can persist for over a month if protected by organic debris such as feces and litter.[301] Mouth-to-beak contact, bites, inadvertent ingestion of contaminated material, and handling infected birds are other possible routes of transmission.[290] Transient exposure can be enough to result in zoonotic infection.[301] An outbreak of psittacosis involving 12 people who visited a bird park in Japan is an example of the transitory degree of contact that can lead to infection.[302]

Little information is available about zoonotic transmission of C. psittaci from non-avian companion animals, yet there are reports of zoonotic infections from dogs.[306] Clear evidence of dog–human transmission is lacking however, as the C. psittaci-infected dogs were sharing a household with canaries and a parrot.

Animals

Clinical presentation

Disease in birds can be variable and depends on factors such as the C. psittaci strain, host species and individual susceptibility. Disease is typically nonspecific and difficult to differentiate clinically from various other illnesses. Common signs include lethargy, anorexia, and ruffled feathers.[301,307] Mucopurulent nasal and ocular discharge, diarrhea, and excretion of green to yellow-green urates are frequently observed. Chronic conjunctivitis, enteritis, air sacculitis, pneumonitis, and hepatosplenomegaly are common, particularly in psittacines.[289,307] Other manifestations include pericarditis, nasal adenitis, peritonitis, and sudden death.

There have been few reports of C. psittaci infection in other companion animals. These include pleuritis, recurrent keratoconjunctivitis, and severe respiratory disease in dogs.[306,308]

Diagnosis

Avian chlamydiosis should be considered in psittacines with nonspecific disease, but diagnosis may be difficult. A combination of methods may be required for optimal sensitivity. Culture is the gold standard. In live birds, conjunctival, choanal, and cloacal swabs should be tested. Intermittent shedding limits the sensitivity of this approach and collection of samples over 3–5 consecutive days has been recommended.[301] Samples can be pooled to reduce costs. Culture of liver biopsy specimens is also useful.[301] Specialized culture facilities with biosafety level 3 containment are required and not widely available, so clinicians should ensure that they have access to an appropriate laboratory before collecting specimens.

Serological testing can also be used. Single positive samples indicate either previous exposure or current infection, and are of limited use. False-negative samples can also be obtained with single samples collected early in disease or when antimicrobial treatment was initiated early in the disease process. A fourfold increase in the titer is required to confirm avian chlamydiosis. Elementary body agglutination (EBA), IFA test, and complement fixation (CF) can be used.[301] CF testing is more sensitive than the other methods.

Antigen testing is a useful alternative, and a combination of positive antigen test with consistent clinical signs provides a relatively sound diagnosis. False-positive reactions can occur from cross-reaction with other antigens and false negatives can occur with low antigen levels or intermittent shedding. ELISA and fluorescent antibody (FA) test are available. Direct PCR testing is available from numerous diagnostic laboratories; however, there are no standard methods.[301] PCR has the potential to provide a highly sensitive and specific result if methods are properly developed, and the test is performed using appropriate quality control.

Management

Treatment can be difficult and should be performed under the guidance of an experienced avian veterinarian. Doxycycline is the drug of choice. Initially, antimicrobials should be administered directly, not in food or water, because sick birds may not eat or drink adequate volumes to obtain a therapeutic dose.[301] Forty-five days of treatment is recommended, except for budgerigars, where 30 days is adequate.[301]

Treated birds are susceptible to reinfection so the cage and other environmental sources must be properly disinfected near the end of the treatment period but before treatment ends. Posttreatment testing is recommended no sooner than 2 weeks after completion of treatment.[301]

Prophylactic treatment of birds is not recommended because of the potential for adverse effects of therapy and emergence of antimicrobial resistance in *C. psittaci* and other bacteria.[301]

Humans

Clinical presentation

Psittacosis typically develops 5–15 days after exposure; however, longer incubation periods have been reported.[301,309] Illness can range from mild flu-like disease to severe systemic illness with pneumonia and encephalitis.[290] Early signs include an acute onset of headache, chills, fever, malaise, and myalgia. Respiratory disease may not be apparent initially, but a nonproductive cough usually develops.[301] Splenomegaly and nonspecific rash may also be noted. Severe respiratory disease can develop, and *C. psittaci* is an important cause of atypical pneumonia. Uncommon manifestations include endocarditis, myocarditis, hepatitis, arthritis, keratoconjunctivitis, and ocular adnexa lymphoma.[296,301,309] In contrast to the earlier literature, which reported relatively high (15–20%) mortality rates, fatal infections are now rare (~1%).[298,301,310] Fatalities still occur, however, particularly if there is no prompt diagnosis and treatment.[311] Older reports documented a very high mortality rate in pregnant women (80% vs. 20% overall).[310] It is unclear whether there is currently an increased risk of severe outcome in pregnant women, but it is not unreasonable considering the effects of pregnancy on immune function.

Diagnosis

Diagnosis can be difficult. It is often not attempted early in disease because of the nonspecific signs and influenza-like presentation. Identification of bird contact, even transient and indirect, is an important risk factor. Testing for psittacosis should be strongly considered in patients with a history of contact with birds (especially sick psittacines) and the presence of influenza-like illness.

The case definition for psittacosis is clinical signs compatible with the disease plus laboratory confir-

mation by (1) isolation of *C. psittaci* from respiratory secretions; (2) detection of a fourfold or greater increase in serum antibody against *C. psittaci* by CF, or microimmunofluorescence (MIF) to a reciprocal titer of >32 between paired acute and convalescent samples; or (3) detection of IgM against *C. psittaci* by MIF to a reciprocal titer of >16. Probable cases are those with compatible clinical signs and an epidemiological link with a confirmed human or avian case or suggestive serology such as a single high antibody titer (>32 by CF or MIF).[301] Most often, diagnosis is based on clinical signs and paired antibody titer using MIF testing. In cases that are promptly treated, antimicrobial therapy can diminish the antibody response and evaluation of a third serum sample collected 4–6 weeks after the first sample may be useful.[301] While MIF testing is more sensitive than CF testing, there can be some cross-reaction with other Chlamydiae.[290,301] The organism can be successfully isolated from sputum, pleural fluid, or blood during acute illness; however, culture is uncommonly performed because biosafety level 3 containment is required. PCR can provide a sensitive and specific diagnosis, and, though increasingly available, it is not yet routinely used as a diagnostic tool.

Management

Doxycycline or tetracycline is the drug of choice. Mild to moderate cases can be treated orally for at least 10 days.[301,309] Patients with severe disease should be treated with intravenous doxycycline hyclate, with treatment continued for 10–14 days after resolution of fever.[301] If tetracyclines are contraindicated (children <8 years of age, pregnant women), macrolides may be used, although *in vivo* efficacy has not been reported.

Person-to-person transmission has been suggested but not confirmed,[301] and if it occurs, it is presumably rare. Accordingly, enhanced infection control practices such as droplet or contact precautions are not indicated for patients with psittacosis.[301]

Prevention

Good general husbandry practices are important both to reduce the risk of human exposure and to reduce susceptibility of birds to infection. Good routine hygiene practices should be used, including hand hygiene after contact with birds or their environment. Mouth-to-beak contact should be avoided.

In multi-bird environments, cages should be positioned such that transfer of fecal material between cages is prevented. Direct contact between different birds, or groups of birds, should be limited. Cage litter should be a material that does not produce dust (e.g., newspaper). Cages, food, and water bowls should be cleaned daily with soiled bowls emptied, scrubbed with soap and water, disinfected, and rinsed.

Cage cleaning is likely a high-risk activity because of the potential for aerosolization of infectious particles from contaminated feces and other secretions. When cleaning cages or handling potentially infected birds, gloves, cap, eye protection, and a respirator (N95 or greater) should be worn.[301] It is unreasonable to assume that all bird owners will take such precautions during routine cleaning and handling, and unbarriered contact with clinically healthy birds in household situations is presumably relatively low risk. Nevertheless, any close contact with psittacines should be considered a risk of infection, and people choosing not to use routine protective measures should know that they are assuming an increased risk. Whenever cages are cleaned, the litter should be sprayed with water before removal to reduce the risk of aerosolization.

In veterinary clinics and diagnostic laboratories, cap, eye protection, gloves, and an N95 or better respirator should be used when handling infected (or potentially infected) birds or tissues and when performing necropsy.[301] Necropsy should be performed in a biosafety cabinet after wetting the carcass to reduce the risk of aerosolization.[301] Protective equipment should also be worn whenever entering a room housing an infected bird, as simply being in a room with infected birds was identified as a risk factor in an outbreak among bird park personnel.[302]

In multi-bird environments, affected birds should be isolated. Ideally, they should be in a separate room because of the potential for aerosol transmission. Optimal ventilation should be provided to reduce the risk of transmission to people entering the room. Transmission between rooms with properly maintained ventilation systems is unlikely.[301] Contact with the bird and its environment should be restricted. Potentially contaminated bedding should be double bagged prior to disposal. The floor should be sprayed lightly with water before cleaning to reduce aerosolization of *C. psittaci*. Vacuuming and pressure washing should be avoided because of the potential for aerosolization. If vacuums are used, they should be equipped with properly functioning HEPA filters. All potentially contaminated surfaces should be disinfected after the removal of organic debris. Most disinfectants are effective against *C. psittaci*,[289] provided they are used properly. Immunocompromised people should not have contact with infected birds or enter a room where an infected bird is present.

The risks associated with psittacines living in nursing homes, long-term care facilities, childcare facilities, and other locations where high-risk individuals are present are not well studied. A combination of the potential for subclinical shedding, aerosolization, and likely exposure of high-risk individuals is of concern. It is unclear whether pet birds, especially psittacines, are appropriate for such facilities. At a minimum, people operating and living in these facilities should be aware of the potential risks, and a plan should be in place to reduce the risk of exposure. Pet birds should be housed in an area that is easy to observe and contain. They should not be in areas where there is frequent passage of people. Cages should only be cleaned by staff using a standard protocol that reduces the risk of aerosolization of infectious materials. Direct contact between birds and residents should be prevented. There must be a commitment to provide veterinary care for sick birds and ensure that proper diagnostic testing is performed, if indicated.

All people that work with birds, particularly in aviaries, breeding operations, and pet stores, should be informed about the risks associated with psittacosis. They should ensure that their physician is aware of this increased risk, and they should be more proactive in seeking medical attention if they develop respiratory or flu-like disease.[301]

People that have had contact with a confirmed or probable case of avian chlamydiosis should seek prompt medical attention if they develop a respiratory or flu-like disease so that treatment can be initiated.[301] Broader investigation of human exposure may be initiated since psittacosis and avian chlamydiosis are reportable diseases in many jurisdictions.

People wishing to purchase a pet bird should ensure that it comes from a flock that is free of apparent disease; however, this certainly does not preclude subclinical *C. psittaci* carriage. People should not purchase birds that have signs of disease consistent with *C. psittaci* infection or birds that have been in contact with sick birds. Mixing of birds from different sources should be avoided if possible.

The role of screening in infection prevention is unclear. Screening has been recommended for birds in certain situations, such as those in public bird encounter exhibits, schools, and long-term care facilities.[301] However, the value of screening is limited by test sensitivity and specificity, as well as the potential for infection after screening. Screening is probably most justifiable in a closed environment where there is no further introduction of birds. Culture or a combination of culture and PCR is probably most useful for screening. Multiple samples may be required to increase the confidence of negative results. Treatment of infected birds in high-risk environments is reasonable, with subsequent testing to determine whether *C. psittaci* has been eliminated. Screening might also be a reasonable consideration in households with immunocompromised individuals. Serological screening is not particularly useful because it provides little information about the current status of the animal, since IgG can persist in the absence of active infection.[301]

Clostridium difficile

Introduction

C. difficile is an important human pathogen and the leading cause of antimicrobial- and hospital-associated diarrhea in people. It is also a cause of enteric disease in various animal species and can be isolated from the feces of healthy animals, including dogs and cats. Its role as a zoonotic pathogen is currently unclear. There is, however, some evidence suggesting that transmission of *C. difficile* between humans and companion animals can occur.

Etiology

C. difficile is a gram-positive spore-forming anaerobic bacterium. Its primary reservoir is the intestinal tracts of various species. It can be found in the environment in human and veterinary hospitals, farms, and households. Despite the frequency with which it is found, the role of the environment in the transmission of infection is unclear. There is also concern that food might be a source of infection, but this has yet to be proven.

Geographic distribution/epidemiology

Despite a lack of information from some regions, it is likely that *C. difficile* is present in human and animal populations worldwide. A small percentage of healthy humans carry *C. difficile* in their intestinal tract. The prevalence of colonization has not been adequately investigated but is likely less than 2%, with higher rates in certain groups such as those in hospitals or long-term care facilities, people being treated with antimicrobials or chemotherapeutic agents, and infants. The main risk factors for *C. difficile* infection (CDI) in humans are hospitalization, chemotherapy, and antimicrobial therapy. Various other factors may also increase risk.

As with humans, *C. difficile* can be isolated from the feces of a small percentage of companion animals. Studies have reported 0–10% colonization rates in healthy dogs and cats in households, with higher rates in shelters, breeding operations, and veterinary hospitals.[312–316] Risk factors for CDI and colonization have not been as extensively studied in companion animals. In animals, CDI appears to be more commonly a community-associated disease rather than hospital-associated, and a history of antimicrobial therapy is less often present either with CDI or *C. difficile* colonization.

Evidence of zoonotic transmission of CDI is currently circumstantial at best, but is of concern. Studies comparing human and animal isolates have reported that the same strains can be found in both groups. This does not necessarily indicate interspecies transmission and cannot provide information about the direction of transmission. Very high rates of *C. difficile* colonization have been reported in dogs that visit human hospitals,[317] although it is unclear whether the source was people or the hospital environment. Contact with human hospitals and contact with children were risk factors for *C. difficile* colonization in one study of therapy dogs.[318] Being treated with antimicrobials was, not surprisingly, also associated with *C. difficile* acquisition.[318] Additionally, antimicrobial treatment of a human in the household was a risk factor for colonization in the dog, presumably from increased risk of *C. difficile* colonization in the person with subsequent direct or indirect transmission to the pet. A recent study reported that living with an immunocompromised owner was a significant risk factor for *C. difficile* colonization in dogs,[319] further supporting interspecies transmission. These reports, while far from definitive, provide reasonable suspicion of the potential for transmission of *C. difficile* between humans and animals, in both directions, and it is prudent to consider *C. difficile* zoonotic until proven otherwise.

Pathophysiology

CDI is associated with proliferation of toxigenic strains of *C. difficile* in the intestinal tract and production of bacterial toxins. Toxin A, an enterotoxin, and toxin B, a cytotoxin, are the best-studied virulence factors. An additional toxin, CDT (binary toxin), may be present in some isolates, although the role of this toxin in disease is not clear. These toxins exert effects locally and produce enteric disease of varying severity.

Animals

Clinical presentation

Animals with CDI may have disease ranging from mild self-limited diarrhea to severe hemorrhagic gastroenteritis that can be fatal. Most cases are mild and not associated with antimicrobial therapy or hospitalization.

Diagnosis

There are two main approaches that can be used to attempt to diagnose CDI: detection of the organism or detection of its main toxins (toxin A and toxin B).

Detection of *C. difficile* as the sole diagnostic tool is questionable. The main problem with this approach is the presence of both toxigenic and nontoxigenic *C. difficile* in some healthy dogs and cats. While highly sensitive, antigen ELISA testing cannot differentiate toxigenic and nontoxigenic strains, nor can it determine whether toxins are actually being produced. Culture has the same limitations and requires days and an experienced laboratory. "Toxigenic culture," which combines culture with detection of toxin genes, eliminates problems with detection of nontoxigenic strains but cannot determine whether *C. difficile* toxins are actually causing disease or whether the animal is simply colonized. The same applies to real-time PCR targeting toxin genes.

Detection of toxins in feces is a preferred approach but has some limitations. The gold standard is the cell cytotoxicity assay; however, it is not generally available because it is time-consuming, technically demanding, and costly. While commercial ELISAs have been shown to perform well in humans and some other animal species, one study reported moderate to poor sensitivity and specificity of commercial ELISAs in dogs,[320] resulting in limitations in both positive and negative predictive values.

At this point, the use of a combination of toxin testing and antigen detection is recommended for the diagnosis of CDI, but this is based on expert advice, not objective data. Concurrent detection of toxin by ELISA and detection of *C. difficile* by culture or antigen ELISA provides a strong index of suspicion of CDI. Detection of toxins with failure to identify *C. difficile* should be interpreted with caution. If *C. difficile* was not detected by culture at an appropriate laboratory, a highly sensitive antigen ELISA or a validated PCR assay, it is quite possible that the toxin ELISA result is falsely positive. Such cases should be considered as a *possible* CDI. Antigen or culture positive but toxin negative results are difficult to interpret because of the marginal sensitivity of available toxin tests. They should be considered as a *possible* diagnosis of CDI in an animal with diarrhea and no other identifiable cause of diarrhea, as such test results cannot be considered definitive.

Management

Supportive therapy is the mainstay of treatment. This may consist of intravenous fluids, oncotic support, nutritional support, and anti-inflammatories. Metronidazole is commonly used. Toxin binders such as di-tri-octahedral smectite are sometimes used, but clinical efficacy is unclear.

Humans

Clinical presentation

The clinical presentation of CDI can range from inapparent disease or mild diarrhea to severe (and sometimes fatal) fulminant pseudomembranous colitis and toxic megacolon.[321–324] In mild cases, diarrhea may be the predominant or only clinical sign. Varying degrees of fever, abdominal discomfort, and cramping may be present.[322–325] Melena and hematochezia are rare. Leukocytosis is variably present.[326]

Patients with severe CDI may be dehydrated, with electrolyte disturbances, hypoalbuminemia, hypotension, renal failure, systemic inflammatory response syndrome (SIRS), or sepsis. Pseudomembranous colitis, toxic megacolon, and intestinal perforation are uncommon but potentially fatal complications.[326,327]

Diagnosis

Detection of C. difficile toxins in feces is the clinical standard for diagnosis,[328] but testing is only moderately specific and false-negative results are not uncommon.[326] While the cell cytotoxicity assay is the gold standard for toxin detection, it is not, in itself, highly sensitive, nor is it readily available. Various commercial ELISAs are available, and they generally have good correlation with the cell cytotoxicity assay, albeit often with reduced sensitivity. It has recently been stated that the sensitivity of ELISAs makes them a suboptimal approach to testing,[326] but a better alternative is not currently available. Use of a two-step procedure, whereby a highly sensitive antigen ELISA is performed, with positive results subsequently tested by toxin ELISA, has been recommended.[326] Negative antigen ELISA results have an excellent negative predictive value, and combined positive antigen and toxin

ELISAs have an excellent positive predictive value. Interpretation of antigen positive but toxin negative samples is more problematic as they could be a result of low sensitivity of the toxin ELISA or indicate colonization, not infection. Real-time PCR to detect toxin B genes is increasingly being used as a sensitive and rapid screening test[329] in hospitalized patients.

Identification of pseudomembranous colitis by colonoscopy is strongly suggestive, despite colonoscopy actually being relatively insensitive for diagnosis of CDI.[321]

Management

If the patient is receiving antimicrobials, these should be discontinued if possible.[326] Metronidazole is the drug of choice in mild to moderate CDI, with oral vancomycin recommended in patients with severe CDI.[326] Antiperistaltic agents should be avoided. Supportive care may be required. Colectomy may be indicated in severe cases.

Prevention

Objective recommendations for prevention of zoonotic transmission are difficult to make because of the paucity of information regarding if, and how, this occurs. Reducing recognized risk factors such as antimicrobial use is an obvious recommendation but may not be possible. Similarly, attention should be paid to prudent use of antimicrobials in animals to decrease the likelihood of C. difficile shedding.

The potential for C. difficile shedding by healthy animals complicates control measures. However, if one assumes that diarrheic animals pose the highest risk because of a greater likelihood of environmental contamination and shedding of larger numbers of C. difficile, general recommendations can be made. All diarrheic animals should be considered infectious because of the number of different pathogens they could be shedding. They should be isolated as much as possible. Care should be taken when handling stool. Any stool passed in a house should be cleaned promptly, ideally while wearing gloves. C. difficile spores are resistant to most disinfectants. Household bleach (1 : 10–1 : 100 dilution) should be used on smooth surfaces that will not be damaged by bleach, provided the surface has been cleaned. Thirty minutes contact time should be provided. Hands should be washed with soap and water after glove removal and after any contact with the animal or its feces. Hand washing is preferred over use of alcohol-based hand sanitizers because *C. difficile* spores are resistant to alcohol and physical removal of spores by hand washing is required. Diarrheic animals should not be allowed to sleep on beds. Feces that have been passed outside should be promptly removed because *C. difficile* spores can persist for years. Care should be taken to avoid contact with feces-contaminated hair coats, something that is a particular concern in long-haired cats. Litter boxes should be carefully cleaned and disinfected, as is discussed elsewhere.

Clostridium perfringens

C. perfringens is a gram-positive anaerobic spore-forming bacterium that is a common commensal of virtually all animal species and is also found widely in the environment. *C. perfringens* can cause a variety of diseases in humans and animals. The most common is enteric disease, which involves two main pathophysiologies. One is food poisoning, where disease is caused by ingestion of preformed enterotoxin that is produced by growth of enterotoxigenic strains of *C. perfringens* in improperly handled food. The other involves growth of *C. perfringens* in the intestinal tract with corresponding intraluminal production of various bacterial toxins. This can cause disease ranging from mild diarrhea to necrotic or hemorrhagic enterocolitis in many species. Clostridial myonecrosis (gas gangrene) is an uncommon but potentially devastating infection caused by growth of *C. perfringens* in compromised muscle. Infections of other systems and bacteremia can occur but are uncommon.

C. perfringens is a common canine and feline commensal and can be found in the intestinal tract of the vast majority of healthy and diarrheic animals. There has been minimal investigation of the potential for transmission of *C. perfringens* between companion animals and humans. Pets are probably rarely associated with infections in

humans. The incidence of nonfoodborne *C. perfringens*-associated disease in people in the community appears to be low, and considering the high prevalence of *C. perfringens* colonization in healthy companion animals and the apparently low incidence of human disease, zoonotic transmission seems unlikely. If it occurs, transmission would be via the fecal–oral route, so basic hygiene practices should greatly reduce any risk. Contact with feces should be avoided. Stool should be removed from yards and public places, taking care to avoid contamination of the hands in the process of stool removal. Hands should be washed thoroughly after removing feces or having any contact with areas contaminated with feces. Hand washing should be used instead of hand sanitizers because *C. perfringens* spores are alcohol resistant. Particular care should be taken with diarrheic animals because they may shed very high numbers of *C. perfringens* and are more likely to contaminate the environment. All diarrheic animals should be considered infectious because of the potential for various zoonotic pathogens, such as *Salmonella*.

C. perfringens food poisoning is associated with growth of enterotoxin-producing strains of *C. perfringens* in improperly stored foods. The source of contamination is usually the actual food item. However, *C. perfringens* can be inoculated into food products by food handlers. It is plausible that *C. perfringens* from companion animals could contaminate food via the hands of food handlers or the food preparation environment. Proper hand washing before handing food and keeping pets off kitchen counters or similar food preparation or storage surfaces should greatly reduce any risk.

Wounds potentially contaminated with *C. perfringens* should be washed immediately with soap and water.

Corynebacterium ulcerans

C. ulcerans is pleomorphic gram-positive rod-shaped bacterium that is a member of the *Corynebacterium diphtheriae* group. It is primarily an animal pathogen and has received the most attention as an infrequent cause of mastitis in dairy cattle. There are emerging concerns about the role of this bacterium in human disease and companion animals as a potential source of infection. *C. ulcerans* is related to *C. diphtheriae*, the cause of diphtheria in humans. Some *C. ulcerans* strains are able to produce diphtheria toxin,[330] the production of which is associated with classical diphtheria and cutaneous diphtheria, as well as other manifestations of infection. Strains of *C. ulcerans* that lack the ability to produce diphtheria toxin may still be able to cause disease.[331] Diphtheria has largely been eliminated from many regions because of successful vaccination programs, and *C. ulcerans* may represent an emerging problem and may be the most common cause of classical diphtheria in some areas.

The epidemiology of human *C. ulcerans* infection is not well understood. Increases in the incidence of *C. ulcerans* infection have been reported in different regions, with *C. ulcerans* typically surpassing *C. diphtheria* in disease incidence.[330,332] For example, no cases of human diphtheria were diagnosed in France between 1990 and 2001, yet 19 cases were diagnosed between 2002 and 2008, with 12 of those caused by *C. ulcerans*.[332] Among those were four cases of pseudomembranous pharyngitis, skin ulcers, otorrhea, bacteremia, and neurological symptoms. Underlying factors were present in a majority of patients, including immunosuppressive disorders, diabetes, and chronic renal disease.

C. ulcerans can also be carried in the pharynx of healthy animals. The role of colonized individuals in disease transmission is unknown as person-to-person transmission has never been reported.[333] Cattle have been considered the main reservoir of *C. ulcerans*, and consumption of raw milk products is a recognized risk factor for human infection. The association between cattle (or milk products) and human infection is far from absolute, and in fact, cattle may not even be the main source of infection. Pigs were recently implicated as a potential source,[334] but more attention has been focused on household pets. Various studies have implicated pets in human infections, including fatal infections, with varying strengths of evidence. Isolates recovered from dogs and cats can be among the predominant human ribotypes,[330,333,335] although typing comparisons are limited in their ability to infer a true risk of interspecies transmission. Human *C. ulcerans* infections have been associated with dogs,[332,336] though clear evidence of involvement of pets is variable. In one study, 10 of 12

patients with *C. ulcerans* infection reported contact with domestic animals, with none reporting contact with dairy animals or a recent travel history.[332] Colonization of family members with *C. ulcerans* was not identified in any of the four investigated households. More convincing evidence of pet involvement is provided from two households where indistinguishable strains of *C. ulcerans* were isolated from patients and their dogs.[332] Similarly, indistinguishable strains were found in two healthy dogs and a woman with fatal *C. ulcerans* infection.[337] The dogs lived on a farm where the woman had stayed shortly before becoming ill, and *C. ulcerans* was not identified from any cattle, cats, guinea pigs, or bulk tank milk on the farm. In another study, the same strain was found in an immunocompromised woman and her dog.[333] These reports provide strong evidence of interspecies transmission and suggest that pets were the source, though definite confirmation of the direction of transmission is impossible.

There has been limited investigation of the epidemiology of *C. ulcerans* in companion animals. *C. ulcerans* was isolated from the nares of 1/60 healthy dogs in a Brazilian animal shelter[331] and 1/65 dogs in a Japanese shelter.[335] Studies of broader populations or other companion animal species are currently lacking. With the existing data, it is reasonable to assume that *C. ulcerans* can be found in healthy pets, but that this is likely an uncommon event.

The appropriate response to diagnosis of *C. ulcerans* in pets, in terms of investigation and management, is unclear. Testing the pets of people who have been diagnosed with *C. ulcerans* is a reasonable consideration, but the lack of good data regarding the prevalence of *C. ulcerans* in the normal pet population hampers making a logical and reasonable interpretation of results. Negative results would not completely exclude the pet as a source of infection because of the retrospective nature of testing. What to do with positive pets is a tougher question, particularly since the prevalence is unclear. The approach to management of a colonized pet would vary greatly depending on how common colonization is in the general pet population, whether certain pets are more likely to transmit the organism to people, whether pets actually transmit *C. ulcerans* to humans or whether transmission is usually in the opposite direction, whether colonized pets pose a realistic risk to all people or just high-risk individuals, whether infection control measures can be used to reduce the risk of transmission, and whether there is the ability to successfully decolonize pets. In two reports, colonized dogs were treated with amoxicillin but were still positive on subsequent sampling and were euthanized.[332,333] In another report, one healthy dog that carried *C. ulcerans* in its nares continued to shed the organism for 3 months but successful eradication was apparently achieved through administration of ciprofloxacin.[331] In another report, two colonized dogs were treated with enrofloxacin, but *C. ulcerans* was isolated from one of the dogs plus a previously positive cat after the treatment course. All dogs and cats were then treated with spiramycin and metrondaizole, with apparent resolution.[337] Given the potential severity of disease, it is understandable that significant concern would be present about a colonized dog; however, euthanasia of the animal is a rather draconian measure, and there is currently no evidence indicating whether this is an appropriate response. If there are significant public health concerns about the presence of a colonized animal in the household, decolonization therapy, ideally based on *in vitro* susceptibility testing, could be considered, along with concurrent infection control measures aimed at reducing droplet/contact-based transmission.

Coxiella burnetii

Introduction

C. burnetii is an obligate intracellular gram-negative bacterium and the cause of Q fever, an acute febrile illness. This organism can infect a wide range of animals, but small ruminants (sheep, goats) and cattle are the main reservoirs and the most commonly implicated sources of infection. Zoonotic infections from companion animals can occur, and the role of pets in Q fever may be overlooked.

Geographic distribution/epidemiology

Q fever is present worldwide, with the exception of some geographically isolated countries, but rates are variable. High endemic rates are present in some regions. Many reports of cat-associated Q fever have come from Atlantic Canada and Japan; however, it is unclear whether this represents a true geographic predisposition or reporting bias.

C. burnetii can be identified in healthy cats. Prevalence data are variable and likely depend on region, study population, and laboratory technique. Reports of seroprevalence in cats range from 2% to 42%,[338–342] with higher rates in stray cats.[339] A PCR-based study of uterine biopsies identified *C. burnetii* DNA in 8.5% of cats in Colorado, USA,[343] while a study of cat serum in Korea and Japan detected *C. burnetii* DNA in 1.4% of samples.[339] *C. burnetii* was isolated from vaginal swabs from 31% of cats in another Japanese study.[344] There are fewer studies in dogs. Most have reported seroprevalence rates of 0–12%, with one study reporting antibodies against *C. burnetii* in 48% of hospitalized dogs and 66% of stray dogs.[345] High seroprevalence rates were present in wildlife in the region, which could represent the source of exposure and explain the uncommonly high rate reported in that study. Dogs that have contact with sheep may have a higher seroprevalence.[346]

C. burnetii is highly infectious with a few organisms able to cause clinical infection in healthy individuals. Infected animals can shed *C. burnetii* in feces, urine, and milk, but placenta and uterine secretions are most commonly implicated in transmission. Most infections are from inhalation of infectious aerosols, though contact transmission and ingestion can also transmit infection.[347] Direct contact with an infected animal is not always reported and simply being in an endemic area can result in disease.[347,348] Most infections are associated with periparturient animals because of the large numbers of *Coxiella* shed at that time; placentas of infected sheep can contain up to 10^9 organisms per gram.[348] *C. burnetii* can also be found in ticks,[349,350] and while ticks are potentially important for facilitating a sylvatic cycle in reservoir species, the role of ticks in the transmission of disease to humans is unclear and likely minimal.

Companion animals have been implicated in Q fever[351,352] and cats may be the most important reservoir in urban areas.[342] As with ruminants, most infections are associated with contact with periparturient pets,[351–356] and a study in Atlantic Canada identified contact with stillborn kittens and exposure to parturient cats as risk factors for Q fever.[353] In contrast, a study from Austria reported no influence of dog or cat ownership on seroprevalence.[357] Regardless, numerous outbreaks of Q fever have been reported from contact with periparturient cats.[351,352,354,356] One outbreak associated with an infected cat that had delivered stillborn kittens involved 33 people, 2.8% of the population of the town, with 42% of infected individuals living in four neighboring buildings.[354] Close contact with periparturient cats is not required for transmission, and simply being in the same house or room may be adequate.

Dog-associated Q fever is uncommonly reported and is likely very rare, but can occur. Three members of one family developed Q fever after contact with an infected parturient dog.[358] Close contact with the dog during parturition and cleaning up uterine fluid contaminated areas was reported in that case. Another report implicated a periparturient dog as a source of Q fever in one or more household members,[359] although this report is less convincing. The dog had ingested raw deer liver, which was thought to be the source of exposure, although infection of the dog or deer was not confirmed. A case of Q fever in a person was linked to a dog obtained from a sheep research facility with an ongoing Q fever outbreak.[360] Whether this represented direct transmission from the dog or indirect transmission from sheep-associated contamination of the dog's hair coat is unclear. The latter is possible, based on a report of Q fever that occurred after washing a sheepdog whose coat was soiled with sheep placenta.[361]

Q fever has also been reported as an occupational risk in companion animal veterinary practice, with reports of zoonotic infections[362] and higher seroprevalence rates compared with the general population.[363]

Animals

Clinical presentation

Humans are the only species known to regularly develop illness following C. burnetii exposure,[348] and infections in companion animals are typically subclinical. Fever, anorexia, and lethargy can develop in cats after experimental infection. Sple-

nomegaly in the absence of other abnormalities has been reported in dogs.[364] Abortion, stillbirth, and birth of weak puppies and kittens can occur.[358]

Diagnosis

Identification of seroversion is the main method, as is discussed below for humans. PCR-based testing of tissues can also be performed but is less available. Culture is uncommonly performed.

Management

Little is known about treatment since few companion animals develop overt clinical infections. Successful elimination of C. burnetii from cats using minocycline (5 mg/kg PO for 4 weeks) has been reported.[365] It is unclear whether treatment of subclinically infected animals is indicated, particularly nonpregnant animals.

Humans

Clinical presentation

Some individuals may simply seroconvert with no evidence of disease; this may account for 50–60% of infected individuals.[347] Severity of disease is often related to intensity of exposure, and with intense contact, there may be a shorter incubation period. Acute disease can be highly variable and typically develops 14–30 days after exposure.[358] The classical presentation is flu-like illness with fever, headache, sweats, cough, myalgia, and arthralgia.[347,348] Rash is rare. Concurrent pneumonia or hepatitis is common. Usually, pneumonia is mild, but severe pneumonia, including acute respiratory distress syndrome, can develop.[347] Hepatosplenomegaly may be present. The triad of fever, hepatitis, and atypical pneumonia is strongly suggestive of Q fever.[347] One problematic aspect is the wide range of clinical presentations that can occur with Q fever, and virtually any body system can be affected. This can complicate diagnosis, which is of concern as prompt diagnosis and treatment are required to reduce the risk of chronic disease. Infection in pregnant women can result in spontaneous abortion, premature birth, and low birth weight.

Chronic Q fever is estimated to develop in 0.76% of acute cases.[366] This occurs more commonly in pregnant women, immunosuppressed individuals, and people with heart valve or vascular abnormalities.[347] Endocarditis is the most common form of chronic disease, occurring in 60–70% of chronic cases.[366] Chronic Q fever is estimated to account for 3–5% of all endocarditis cases.[366] Uncommon manifestations of chronic disease include osteomyelitis, granulomatous hepatitis, and chronic pulmonary infections.[347] Chronic Q fever has also been implicated as a cause of chronic fatigue syndrome.[367]

Diagnosis

Perhaps the main limitation for diagnosis is lack of consideration of Q fever. This is particularly true in people that do not report contact with periparturient ruminants, since physicians may overlook pet contact and the potential association with Q fever. Q fever should not be considered solely an occupational disease of farmers, veterinarians, or slaughterhouse workers.[347] Rather, it should be considered an endemic environmental disease in areas where it is known to occur, and Q fever should be considered in all patients with the appropriate clinical presentation.

Identification of seroconversion is the main diagnostic method. Immunofluoresence is most commonly used and is highly sensitive and specific.[347] The most widely used tests detect phase I and II antibodies. Phase II antibodies tend to be present in acute disease, while phase I antibodies may remain elevated with chronic disease.[347] A titer of 200 or greater for IgG and 50 or greater for IgM against phase II antibodies indicates recent infection, while an IgG titer of 800 or greater against phase I antibodies suggests chronic infection.[368] Specific cutoffs, however, may vary between laboratories. Phase II antibodies tend to be detectable within 2 weeks of infection in most patients, and within 3 weeks in 90% of patients, and a lack of detectable antibody response at 4 weeks suggests that Q fever is not present.[347] Echocardiography should be performed in infected individuals to detect valvular lesions and direct therapy aimed at reducing the risk of infectious endocarditis.[347]

Isolation of C. burnetii is rarely attempted because it requires biosafety level 3 containment due to the high infectivity and potential use as a bioterrorism agent. PCR may be useful for rapid identification of C. burnetii but is currently of limited availability.

Management

Treatment is indicated for all infections, even those that are subclinical.[347] Early treatment is important to reduce the risk of chronic disease. The main treatment for acute disease is doxycycline, except in patients that are allergic to the drug, pregnant women, and children younger than 8.[347] Erythromycin has been shown to be unreliable,[369] but other macrolides such as clarithromycin may be efficacious, although convincing data are currently lacking. Fluoroquinolones are effective in vitro, but in vivo data are limited.[370] They may be preferred in the management of meningoencephalitis because of better CNS penetration.[347] Treatment of pregnant women is complicated because the main drug used is contraindicated during pregnancy. Treatment with trimethoprim–sulfamethoxazole during pregnancy can reduce the incidence of spontaneous abortion, intrauterine growth retardation, fetal death, premature delivery, and oligohydramnios; however, it is often not curative and postpartum therapy for chronic disease is commonly required.[371]

Monotherapy with doxycycline is not recommended for chronic cases. The combination of doxycycline and hydroxychloroquine has been shown to require shorter treatment duration and result in fewer relapses than a tetracycline and a fluoroquinolone.[372] Current recommendations are to treat with this combination for at least 18 months, with longer therapy required in some cases.[347] Doxycycline plus a fluoroquinolone for a minimum of 3–4 years has been proposed for people unable to tolerate hydroxychloroquine.[373] Monitoring antibody titers is commonly performed every 3–4 months during treatment and every 3 months after cessation of treatment.[347] Surgery is an important component of treatment of many patients with valvular disease.

Prevention

The greatest risk of pet-associated Q fever comes from periparturient animals, particularly cats, so efforts should be focused on that group.

Immunocompromised individuals and pregnant women should avoid contact with periparturient and newborn animals. People with cardiac valvular disease should also take extra precautions, not because of increased susceptibility to infection but because of increased likelihood of serious consequences should they become infected. Because of the potential for aerosol transmission, high-risk individuals should avoid areas where animals are giving birth, or where they have done so recently. With small ruminants, *C. burnetii* can be isolated from air for up to 2 weeks after parturition.[374] Persistence of airborne contamination following parturition in cats and dogs is not known, but prudence dictates that high-risk people should avoid birthing areas for at least a few days after birth.

Good infection control practices should be used during contact with periparturient cats and dogs, particularly during delivery. All periparturient animals should be considered potentially infected, although the risk is likely highest with cats. Particular care should be taken when handling periparturient stray cats because of higher seroprevalence rates. Pregnant cats or dogs should deliver in a well-ventilated area. This should be away from human living and food preparation areas. Contact with placenta and uterine secretions should be avoided. Gloves should be worn during the birthing process, handling newborn animals, handling the mother after delivery, and when cleaning up contaminated areas. Care should be taken to prevent cross-contamination, and hands must be washed after glove removal. Potentially contaminated bedding should be removed using gloves and disinfected or discarded. *C. burnetii* is quite hardy and can persist in the environment. It is highly resistant to disinfectants, dessication, and ultraviolet light. It can survive for months on wool[348] and likely weeks or months on typical indoor surfaces.

Care should be taken with animals in contact with common reservoir species, especially those in contact with periparturient sheep. Good hygiene practices should be used when handling dogs that may have had contact with placenta or uterine fluids. Household pets should not have direct contact with periparturient ruminants and should not be allowed to have contact with, or ingest, placenta or uterine secretions. Because the ingestion of *C. burnetii* can result in infection, dogs and cats

should not be fed raw meat from potential reservoir hosts.

Duration of infection of pets is unknown. As such, breeding of infected animals should be avoided to reduce high-risk exposure at the time of parturition, as well as the potential for abortion, fetal abnormalities, and birth of weak offspring.

Routine testing of pets for *C. burnetii* is not indicated. Testing should be restricted to diagnosis of clinical infection in pets and as part of human infection investigation.

Edwardsiella tarda

This gram-negative bacterium of the Enterobacteriaceae family is present widely in aquatic environments, most often associated with freshwater and freshwater fish, reptiles, and amphibians.[375] Gastroenteritis, sometimes severe, is the most common clinical infection in humans, but infections of virtually any body system can occur.[375-377] Immunocompromised individuals, children, and the elderly are predominantly affected.[376] Human exposure is typically through contact with contaminated freshwater or animals. Pet-associated infections appear to be rare. A pet turtle was implicated as a source of *E. tarda* gastroenteritis in a person.[378] Protracted diarrhea was also reported in an infant, with the *E. tarda* isolated both from the child and from an aquarium in the home.[379] The overall incidence and risk of disease is presumably very low. Basic hygiene practices, such as hand hygiene after contact with aquatic pets or aquarium water, and restriction of contact of high-risk individuals with aquaria and their contents should suffice.

Ehrlichia canis

E. canis is the cause of canine monocytotropic ehrlichiosis, a tick-borne disease. Dogs and wild canids are the reservoirs. It is present in tropical and temperate regions worldwide.[380] It has been suggested that a variant or subspecies of *E. canis* is the cause of Venezuelan human ehrlichiosis (VHE).[381] *E. canis* is closely related to *Ehrlichia chaffeensis*, and VHE is very similar to the disease caused by *E. chaffeensis*, human monocytic ehrlichiosis (HME).

While dogs may be the reservoir for human *E. canis* infections, particularly VHE, direct transmission of *E. canis* from dogs to humans is not possible, and tick control is the most important preventive measure.

Ehrlichia chaffeensis

E. chaffeensis is the cause of the tick-borne disease human monocytic ehrlichiosis (HME). Like other *Ehrlichia*, *E. chaffeensis* is an obligate intracellular gram-negative bacterium. The natural cycle likely involves deer or rodents as reservoir hosts, with occasional transmission to other species such as humans and dogs. Transmission involves ticks, predominantly *A. americanum*, *Dermacentor variabilis*, and *I. pacificus*.[7] Based on the geographic distribution of competent tick vectors, *E. chaffeensis* is almost exclusively reported in the United States, particularly the south-central, southeastern, and mid-Atlantic regions, as well as California.[382] Disease is most commonly identified from May to August.[383]

In immunocompetent humans, HME typically produces an influenza-like disease with fever, headache, and malaise. Severe multisystem disease may sometimes develop, particularly in immunocompromised individuals.[383] In the immunocompromised, infection tends to follow a more rapid course than typically encountered in immunocompetent individuals, with serious sequelae such as adult respiratory distress syndrome, renal failure, meningoencephalitis, coagulopathy, and gastrointestinal hemorrhage occurring more frequently.[7]

The role of *E. chaffeensis* as a cause of disease in dogs is unclear. Dogs can be experimentally infected, with resulting signs including fever, anterior uveitis, vomiting, epistaxis, erythema multiforme, lymphadenopathy, and thrombocytopenia, and natural infections with similar signs have been reported.[120,384,385]

Experimentally infected dogs can carry *E. chaffeensis* for months, raising the possibility that dogs could be a natural reservoir. However, direct transmission between mammalian species does not occur, so infected dogs are not a direct risk to humans.

As with some other tick-borne diseases, it is possible that dogs could be mechanical vectors by bringing infected ticks into contact with humans; however, if this occurs, it is probably uncommon. Tick avoidance and control measures are the most important aspects of infection prevention.

Ehrlichia ewingii

E. ewingii is the cause of canine granulocytotropic ehrlichiosis and human ewingii ehrlichiosis.[383,386] It has been reported over a limited range of the southern and southeastern United States.[7] Human ewingii ehrlichiosis appears to occur mainly in immunocompromised individuals, with similar signs as HME (*E. chaffeensis* infection) but less severe.[387] In dogs, it can cause polyarthritis as well as a nonspecific illness with fever, depression, and lethargy.[386] Less commonly, neurological manifestations, vomiting, or diarrhea may be present.

As with many other *Ehrlichia*, *E. ewingii* is a tick-borne pathogen, primarily transmitted by *A. americanum* (lone star tick). Direct transmission between mammals does not occur, and infected dogs are not a direct risk to humans. Dogs could act as mechanical vectors by bringing infectious ticks into the household. Tick control measures for both dogs and humans are required to reduce the risk from *E. ewingii*.

Eikenella corrodens

E. corrodens is a fastidious gram-negative rod-shaped bacterium that is part of the commensal oral microflora in humans and some animal species. It is most commonly associated with human and animal bite wounds,[388–390] often as a coinfection with other bacteria.[129] The most common clinical presentation is that of an indolent ulcer that develops gradually, with a week or more passing between the time of injury and signs of infection.[129] *E. corrodens* can be found commonly in the oral cavity of healthy dogs, with 62% of supragingival plaque samples positive in one study.[391] There are only a limited number of reports of dog bite-associated infections; however, the scope of the problem may be underestimated because of the fastidious nature of the organism and difficulty isolating and identifying it using normal laboratory procedures.[391,392]

Prevention of zoonotic *E. corrodens* infections involves reducing the incidence of dog bites and proper postbite management. The bacterium is typically susceptible to penicillins, second- and third-generation cephalosporins, fluoroquinolones, and tetracyclines.[129] Beta-lactamase production is uncommon but, when present, can usually be inhibited by clavulanic acid or sulbactam.[129]

Enterococcus spp.

Enterococci are gram-positive cocci that can be found widely in the intestinal tract of most species. The two most important species are *Enterococcus faecium* and *Enterococcus faecalis*. They are opportunistic pathogens and are uncommon causes of infection in otherwise healthy individuals in the community. They are most important as hospital-associated pathogens in human and veterinary medicine. Enterococci are inherently resistant to various antimicrobials (e.g., cephalosporins, clindamycin, some penicillins, trimethoprim) and have an impressive ability to develop further resistance. MDR enterococci, particularly vancomycin-resistant enterococci (VRE),[393] are an important problem in human medicine and an emerging issue in companion animals. While colonization with VRE is rare in companion animals,[394–396] there have been sporadic reports of infection or colonization in household pets.[397,398] Most reports have been from Europe and some have reported high VRE rates, such as a study reporting 48% vancomycin resistance among canine enterococci in The Netherlands.[399] A link between VRE carriage in dogs and avoparcin use in food animals in Europe has been suggested as an explanation for the high rates in some European studies. While the link to avoparcin has not been proven, a subsequent Dutch study, performed 5 years after avoparcin use was banned, reported no VRE in 100 dogs.[400] Currently, VRE infections are very rare in companion animals, but one concern is that should VRE rates in people in the community increase, this could be reflected in companion animals.

While the focus on VRE is reasonable, MDR but vancomycin-susceptible enterococci are currently more common in animals and should not be overlooked. Studies of healthy dogs in Denmark and dogs with antimicrobial exposure in Finland reported low prevalences of resistance to various antimicrobials,[394,401] whereas a study of healthy dogs in the community in Portugal reported higher rates of resistance to most antimicrobials[402] and a study of dogs presenting to a veterinary hospital in Italy reported frequent resistance to fluoroquinolones, tetracyclines, macrolides, rifampin, and tetracycline.[395] High rates of tetracycline and macrolide resistance in *E. faecalis* were also reported in dogs from private homes and kennels in Belgium.[403] Therefore, even in the absence of VRE in companion animals, pets might constitute a potential reservoir of MDR enterococci in households.

Currently, there is little information regarding zoonotic transmission of enterococci. Few studies have compared commensal animal and human strains, investigated intrahousehold transmission between humans and animals, or evaluated animal contact as a risk factor for human enterococcal infection. One study identified clonal complex 17 *E. faecium*, an important human epidemic clone, in a dog,[394] providing support to the hypothesis that interspecies, intrahousehold transmission can occur. Indeed, the risk may be highest for pets, with humans transmitting VRE to their pets. However, the potential establishment of a pet reservoir of MDR opportunistic bacteria, as is evident with MRSA, should not be dismissed, despite this likely being of limited importance at this point in time.

Screening of pets for enterococcal colonization, including VRE, is not indicated, even in the presence of human infection. Enterococci are commensals and MDR enterococci will commonly be found. Investigation of pets as part of a comprehensive outbreak evaluation, including testing of household human contacts, is reasonable but would be a rare scenario. There are no objective guidelines regarding management of pets colonized with MDR enterococci. Treatment is not indicated as elimination of a commensal gastrointestinal organism is very unlikely and treatment could lead to further resistance. Good household hygiene measures, particularly hand hygiene and avoiding contact with feces, are likely the most important. Animals with clinical MDR enterococcal infections should be handled in households and veterinary clinics using contact precautions and with close attention to personal hygiene.

Escherichia coli

E. coli is a gram-negative member of the Enterobacteriaceae family that is relatively ubiquitous among humans, animals, and the environment. This highly diverse species includes both harmless commensals and highly pathogenic strains.

Verotoxigenic *E. coli*

The main zoonotic disease concern involves verotoxigenic *E. coli* (VTEC), particularly *E. coli* O157:H7. These strains produce verotoxins (also known as Shiga toxins) and can cause disease ranging from mild self-limited diarrhea to bloody diarrhea, hemorrhagic colitis and hemolytic uremic syndrome. The organism can be commonly found in the intestinal tracts of healthy cattle, sheep, and goats,[404] and the main source of human infections is contaminated food. Higher rates of vertoxigenic *E. coli* (VTEC) shedding have been reported in dogs with acute and chronic diarrhea compared with healthy dogs;[405] however, it is unclear whether there was a causal association. Experimental infection with O157 and non-O157 VTEC strains has reproduced disease in dogs.[406] VTEC-associated gastroenteritis has also been reported in a cat,[407] but a case-control study could not identify an association between VTEC shedding and diarrhea in cats.[408]

Colonization of healthy dogs and cats is rare, with reported rates of 0–5.9% of healthy pets,[405,409,410] and pets are rarely (if ever) a source of human infection. Case-control studies have not identified pet ownership or contact as a risk factor for *E. coli* O157 infection and contact with dogs was identified as a protective factor in one study[411] but zoonotic transmission from dogs has been described.[412,413] One instance involved isolation of indistinguishable isolates of *E. coli* O157 from a child, pony, and dog.[413] A more suggestive report involved an outbreak in a family, which was attributed to contact by a child with two farm dogs that were colonized with *E. coli* O157.[412] Cattle on the farm were also colonized with this strain yet there was no contact between the child and cattle. While environmental infection or indirect transmission from cattle could not be excluded, transmission from the dogs was considered likely because they were shown to be shedding the same strain and

because close contact had occurred. The dogs were most probably infected from cattle feces, and the likelihood of *E. coli* O157 shedding in dogs and cats not exposed to farm animals or farm environments is presumably very low.

Risk reduction involves decreasing the likelihood of colonization of pets (and potentially contamination of the hair coat) and reducing exposure to feces. Contact between cattle and household pets should be restricted. Dogs and cats should not be allowed to have access to cattle manure. Proper handling of feces from pets is important, as is routine hand hygiene. VTEC shedding is higher in dogs with chronic or acute diarrhea than healthy dogs,[405] so particular care should be taken with diarrheic pets. The overall risk of *E. coli* O157 from pets is quite low.

Other types

Other potential concerns regarding *E. coli* in pets are opportunistic infections such as wound infections contaminated with *E. coli* from animals. This has not been specifically investigated, but it is likely that breaks of normal barriers, such as wounds, would allow for the development of infections should the site become contaminated with *E. coli* of animal origin. Standard hygiene practices involving animal contact, handling of feces, and care of broken skin should greatly reduce any risks.

There is evidence that generic *E. coli* can be transmitted between people and pets in households. A study evaluating *E. coli* from dogs and their owners reported within-household sharing of *E. coli* (the presence of indistinguishable strains) in 9.8% of households.[414] No factors associated with intra-household sharing of *E. coli* have been reported. Similarly, there has been concern about the potential for dogs to act as reservoirs of uropathogenic *E. coli*. One study reported the presence of *E. coli* containing urovirulence genes in 26% of dogs, with one or more of the same genes found in both dogs and owners in 2% of households.[415] There was also an association between a history of urinary tract infection in a female owner and the presence of urovirulence factors in *E. coli* from their dogs. The potential role of dogs in human urinary tract infections must still be resolved. For both household sharing of generic *E. coli* and dogs carrying uro-pathogenic *E. coli*, a critical aspect that needs to be determined is the direction of transmission. Current studies that have found the same *E. coli* in people and pets have not been able to determine whether dogs were the source of infection, whether dogs were infected by their owners, or whether both humans and dogs might have been infected from the same source.

Francisella tularensis

Introduction

Tularemia is an uncommon human infection caused by *F. tularensis*. It is of concern because of the potential severity of disease and classification as a potential bioterrorism agent. It is highly infectious, with as few as 25 organisms being able to cause infection in humans.[416] Human infections are most commonly from contact with infected wildlife (especially rabbits) or insect vectors. Transmission from pets is uncommon but can occur, with cats posing the greatest risk.

Etiology

F. tularensis is a gram-negative coccobacillus belonging to the alphaproteobacteria group. There are two main types: type A (*F. tularensis* subsp. *tularensis*) and type B (*F. tularensis* subsp. *holarctica*). Type A strains are found almost exclusively in North America, are highly virulent for rabbits, and are associated with a tick–rabbit cycle of infection.[417,418] Type B strains have a more complex cycle involving multiple animals (e.g., rodents, muskrats, beavers), insects (e.g., ticks, mosquitoes), and water. Type B strains are found throughout the Northern Hemisphere. Both can cause infections in humans, although type A strains tend to cause more severe illness.[418]

Geographic distribution/epidemiology

F. tularensis is endemic in most regions of the Northern Hemisphere between 30 and 71 degrees N. However, there is much variability in the incidence and endemicity of disease within this region. For example, in the United States, most cases occur in the central regions of the country.

Tularemia is a predominantly wildlife-associated infection, so it is more common in rural and semirural regions. This bacterium can infect a vast range of species, including more than 100 species of mammals; several species of birds, fish, and amphibians; and at least 50 species of insects.[419] In general, only a small number of animal species are important in any geographic region.[417] Most human cases are associated with contact with wildlife reservoirs, their insect vectors, or contaminated environment. Insects are considered the true biological vectors of disease, being both reservoir hosts and vectors.[418] In North America, the most important sources of infection are the cottontail rabbit, wild hares, and rodents, as well as ticks that feed on those species.[418] The wood tick (*Dermacentor andersonii*), American dog tick (*D. variabilis*), Pacific Coast tick (*D. occidentalis*), and lone star tick (*A. americanum*) are the most important tick vectors. In Europe, cricetine rodents (e.g., meadow voles, lemmings, muskrats) and hares are the main animal reservoirs, with mosquitoes being another important source of transmission.

Seroprevalence rates of 3.7–22% in cats and 0–14.2% in dogs have been reported.[420–422] Dogs are relatively resistant to tularemia and infections are rare despite frequent exposure. Cats appear to be more susceptible to infection. Infections are often linked to contact with wild animals such as through hunting or exposure to carcasses of dead rabbits, or contact with small rodents.[423,424] Direct transmission from infected animals can occur through bites or scratches, or perhaps through aerosols over short distances. Ingestion of contaminated food (especially carcasses) and water can also be involved, as can numerous blood-feeding insect vectors.

Humans are most commonly infected either from handling infected wildlife during hunting and trapping or from insect bites.[425] Companion animals are not true reservoirs of *F. tularensis* but can be sources of infection following exposure to a reservoir animal or insect vector. Human infections have been associated with cats, dogs, prairie dogs, and a hamster. Most cat-associated infections occur as a result of bites and scratches,[419,426–430] with ulceroglandular disease being the most common. Cat ownership was associated with disease in a case-control study of a Swedish outbreak, though it is unclear whether this was a true causal relationship.[425] The limited numbers of reports of dog–human infections have implicated other types of contact, with less than convincing evidence. One outbreak was attributed to inhalation of contaminated aerosols generated by a seropositive dog shaking itself,[431] although the link was somewhat tenuous. Licking by a puppy who had contact with rabbits was suspected as the source of infection of a young girl,[418] a conclusion that is rather presumptive. A single case of hamster-associated tularemia has been reported—a bite infection in a young child.[432] An outbreak of tularemia occurred from contact with wild-caught prairie dogs.[433]

Tularemia is an occupational risk in veterinary practice. While the incidence of disease is low, close contact with numerous animals and the potential for bites and scratches indicate an increased risk in endemic areas. Infections of veterinarians in the absence of obvious exposure (e.g., bite, scratch) have been reported, including tularemia septicemia.[419] One small study identified elevated *F. tularensis* titers in 14% of veterinarians in Fairbanks, Alaska,[419] a prevalence that is presumably much greater than in the general public. This risk is probably quite variable between regions. Seventy-five percent of veterinarians in the Alaska study had treated infected cats or dogs, a rate that is much higher than would be expected in most regions. Tularemia was also associated with laceration of a veterinarian's hand while spaying a cat.[434]

Animals

Clinical presentation

A range of clinical signs can be present in infected cats, although a comprehensive description of the clinical presentation is lacking. Various combinations of fever, depression, lymphadenopathy, splenomegaly, hepatomegaly, oral and lingual ulceration, draining abscesses, icterus, and panleukopenia may be present.[424,435,436]

If clinical illness develops in dogs, it is typically mild with brief fever, anorexia, lethargy, lymphadenopathy, and anorexia.[423,437] Uveitis and conjunctivitis have also been reported.[418]

Little information is available regarding other companion animal species. High death rates were identified in hamsters during an investigation of a hamster bite-associated case. Unfortunately, none of the hamster carcasses were available for testing for definite confirmation of tularemia.[432] High mortality among infected prairie dogs has been reported.[433]

Diagnosis

Clinical and hematologic data are rather nonspecific. Detection of microscopic agglutinating (MA) antibody is most commonly used to diagnose tularemia. While laboratory criteria may vary, titers from 1:140 to 1:160 are typically found in infected dogs. Titers above 1:20 are usually considered diagnostic in cats.[418] False-negative serological testing is not uncommon in cats,[435] as they tend to produce a lesser antibody response. IFA testing has also been used, with a fourfold difference between acute and convalescent titers indicating infection. A single IFA titer of >1:160 also suggests active infection. ELISAs used in humans are of unknown usefulness in animals and are not currently recommended.[418] FA testing or PCR can be performed on infected tissues.[435] Definitive diagnosis is based on isolation of *F. tularensis*; however, this is not commonly performed because biosafety level 3 containment is required.

Management

There is currently little information guiding treatment choices in companion animals. Disease may be self-limited in dogs,[437] but treatment is probably indicated because of the potential for zoonotic transmission. Based on extrapolation from humans, gentamicin may be the drug of choice. Doxycycline, chloramphenicol, and enrofloxacin are other options.[418] Initial treatment should be for 7–14 days. Surgical excision of localized draining masses is indicated, in conjunction with antimicrobial therapy.

Humans

Clinical presentation

The clinical manifestation depends on the virulence of the *F. tularensis* strain, route of entry, and immune status of the host.[417] There are six classic forms: ulceroglandular, glandular, oculoglandular, pharyngeal, typhoidal, and pneumonic, although these are general categorizations that can overlap.[417] Ulceroglandular tularemia is the most common, accounting for 21–87% of cases.[425] Regardless of the form, clinical signs usually start abruptly, with the average incubation period being 3–5 days (range <1–21 days).[417] Fever, chills, malaise, anorexia, and fatigue are typical initial signs. After several days, the fever usually abates but then recurs accompanied by other clinical signs.

The ulceroglandular form is characterized by pronounced inflammation at the site of inoculation along with localized lymphadenopathy. A red, painful papule is evident initially, followed by progression to ulceration with a raised border. Lymphangitis is rare unless there is a secondary infection.

Glandular tularemia, the second most common form, is present when patients have local or regional lymphadenopathy in the absence of an evident skin lesion. Lymphadenopathy may persist for prolonged periods, well after the febrile stage of illness so the history of febrile disease may not be reported, thereby complicating diagnosis. Suppuration of lymph nodes can occur with ulceroglandular or glandular forms.

Oculoglandular tularemia is uncommon, accounting for <5% of cases.[417] It develops from infection of the conjunctiva from aerosols, splashes, or contaminated fingers. Disease is usually unilateral. Lid edema, conjunctivitis, chemosis, and small conjunctival ulcers or papules may be present.[417] There may be associated periauricular, submandibular, or cervical lymphadenopathy.

Pharyngeal tularemia is rare and occurs after the ingestion of contaminated food, water, or droplets. Fever and exudative pharyngitis or tonsillitis, with or without ulceration, are typical. A membrane similar to a diphtheritic one may be identified. Local lymphadenopathy may be present.

Pneumonic tularemia occurs after the inhalation of infectious aerosols or hematogenous dissemination. It can be found in 7–20% of cases.[438]

Typhoidal tularemia is a default diagnosis for cases with fever but no prominent lymphadenopathy or characteristics of other forms. It can account for 5–30% of cases[439] and can be very severe.

Any form of tularemia can result in chronic, debilitating disease with chronic lymph node suppuration or persistent fatigue.[417]

Diagnosis

Clinical suspicion is a key component because routine laboratory tests are nonspecific. As with many zoonotic diseases, failure to consider tularemia is a problem. While this disease may be more readily considered in endemic regions, the focus is often on hunters and other people with wildlife exposure. These are certainly high-risk groups but it is important that tularemia be considered in people without those classical risk factors, including pet owners.

F. tularensis is rarely identified on smears or biopsies. It does not grow readily on routine culture media, and the use of specific culture methods is restricted to a limited number of laboratories because of the need for biosafety level 3 containment. Serological testing is most commonly used for diagnosis but is suboptimal because of the inherent time delay from infection to seroconversion. Antibodies against *F. tularensis* may be detected by tube agglutination, microagglutination, hemagglutination, and ELISA.[417] Microagglutination assay is sensitive and is often used. A tube agglutination titer of 1:160 or greater, or a microagglutination titer of 1:238 or greater provides a presumptive diagnosis. However, both IgG and IgM titers may persist for years, thereby limiting the interpretation of single test results, especially if there have been previous opportunities for infection. Therefore, identification of seroconversion, with a fourfold or greater rise in antibody titer between acute and convalescent samples, is required for a more convincing diagnosis.

More efforts have been made recently to develop rapid diagnostic tests because of concerns about bioterrorist use of *F. tularensis*. Direct FA testing of smear and biopsies, antigen detection in urine, and PCR are some of the tests being evaluated, but only PCR is currently widely used.[417]

Management

Streptomycin is the drug of choice for all forms, except in very rare cases where meningitis is present.[417] Gentamicin is an acceptable alternate.[440] Doxycycline has been used but has a higher relapse rate, perhaps because it is bacteriostatic. Similar results have been obtained for chloramphenicol. Surgical incision and drainage of abscessed lymph nodes may be required.

The prognosis for ulceroglandular disease is favorable. Morbidity and mortality are greater with typhoidal tularemia, but with prompt diagnosis and appropriate treatment, mortality rates for both forms are less than 4%.[417,440] Poor prognostic indicators include the presence of serious comorbidities, delayed diagnosis, and/or symptoms lasting a month or more prior to treatment, significant pulmonary involvement, typhoidal disease, renal failure, and inappropriate antimicrobial therapy.[441]

Prevention

Cats should be kept indoors, particularly in rural areas where tularemia is endemic in wildlife. Similarly, dogs should be supervised when outside and contact with rabbits and other wildlife should be restricted. Tick avoidance practices, for both people and pets, are indicated. Animals that venture outside, particularly into wooded areas, should be checked for ticks after returning to the house, with any identified ticks promptly and properly removed. In tularemia endemic areas, pet rabbits should ideally be housed indoors to reduce the risk of infection from wildlife or insect vectors. Because many pet–human infections are associated with bites or scratches, routine measures to reduce these should be implemented. While the risk from pet hamsters and similar rodents is presumably very low, good handling practices should be used to reduce the risk of bites. Contact between pet rodents and wild rodents should be prevented since wild rodents were suspected to be the source of tularemia in a hamster.[432]

Wild-caught animals should not be kept as pets, particularly those from tularemia-endemic regions. Dead animals brought home by pets in endemic areas should be removed carefully. The use of gloves, mask, and eye protection has been recommended.[417]

Infected animals and any items potentially contaminated with infectious secretions should be handled with gloves, gown, full-face protection or eye protection, and an N95 respirator. It is unknown how long infected animals shed *F. tularensis*, but using these precautions throughout the entire treatment period is prudent. Similar measures should be used in animals that are treated at home;

however, isolation and treatment in a veterinary hospital are preferred to outpatient therapy because of the ability for better containment. Owners wishing to manage infected animals as outpatients must be clearly informed of the potential risks and required infection control precautions. Necropsy of animals suspected of having tularemia should only be performed by experienced personnel, in facilities with appropriate biocontainment. *F. tularensis* is susceptible to most disinfectants, if used properly.

Screening of healthy pets is not indicated, nor is prophylactic therapy for pets that are exposed to wildlife. People that have had contact with a potentially infected animal do not require prophylactic treatment but should promptly report to a physician if any early signs of disease occur, such as fever, chills, and myalgia.

Helicobacter spp.

Helicobacter spp. are gram-negative, microaerophilic curved to spiral-shaped bacteria that resemble *Campylobacter* spp. They are uniquely adapted to survival in the acidic environment of the stomach, and gastric colonization with *Helicobacter* spp. is common in many species.

The most important species is *Helicobacter pylori*, a significant human pathogen that can be found in humans worldwide. It is the leading cause of gastritis and peptic ulceration, as well as a major risk factor for development of gastric carcinoma and gastric B-cell lymphoma. Gastric colonization with *H. pylori* is very common, occurring in 70–90% of people in developing countries and 25–50% of people in developed countries.[442] It is believed that humans are the major, if not sole, reservoir of *H. pylori*.[443] Transmission is presumably mainly through the fecal–oral route, and higher rates of colonization can be found in people living under suboptimal sanitary conditions.[443] It can also be found in saliva and dental plaque, which suggests that oral–oral transmission could also occur. Many other *Helicobacter* species have been isolated from humans, although they are much less common than *H. pylori*.[444] The role of different "non-*H. pylori* helicobacters" (NHPHs) in human disease is not well understood, but they have been associated to gastritis and gastric carcinoma.[445]

Initially, NHPHs were termed *"Helicobacter heilmannii,"*[446] but it is clear that NHPH does not constitute a single species and earlier reports of *H. heilmannii* could involve many different species. More recently, *H. heilmannii* was divided into two types: type 1 and type 2. Type 1 is now thought to represent one species, found most commonly in pigs and designated *Helicobacter suis.*[447] In contrast, type 2 is now known to consist of multiple different species, including *Helicobacter felis, Helicobacter bizzozeronii, Helicobacter salomonis, Helicobacter cynogastricus, Helicobacter baculiformis,* and *"Candidatus H. heilmannii."*[444]

The diversity of NHPH that can be found and the increasing recognition of NHPH in animals has led to the investigation of the potential role of animals in human infection. The understanding of *Helicobacter* spp. in companion animals is relatively superficial, and frequent changes in nomenclature have complicated matters further. Studies have identified *Helicobacter* spp. in the gastric mucosa or oral cavity of a large percentage (56–100%) of healthy dogs and cats.[444,448–450] *Helicobacter* spp. infection in dogs and cats is usually subclinical; however, gastritis can occur. Limited information is available regarding *Helicobacter* species in dogs and cats, but *H. bizzozeronii* appears to predominate in dogs.[451,452] Various other species have been identified in dogs and cats, including *H. cynogastricus, H. felis, H. baculiformis,* and *H. salomonis.*[445,447,453–455] *H. heilmannii* has been identified in rabbits,[452] while *Helicobacter mustelae* and *Helicobacter muridarum* have been found in ferrets and mice, respectively, and a wide range of other *Helicobacter* spp. have been identified in various other mammalian species. *H. pylori* has not been identified in dogs and has only been reported in colony-raised cats.[456,457] The clinical relevance of *Helicobacter* infection in dogs and cats is unclear, but chronic vomiting and weight loss have been attributed to *Helicobacter.*[458] Since diagnosis in these cases is made on finding *Helicobacter* in gastric biopsies, which can also be found in biopsies from healthy animals, proof of causation is currently lacking.

The relevance of exposure of humans to *Helicobacter* spp. from dogs and cats is unclear. Interpretation of studies describing a high prevalence of *Helicobacter* spp. can be difficult because speciation of *Helicobacter* is not always performed. *H. felis* was isolated from both a patient with gastric ulcers and her dog, and it was suggested that infection was acquired from the dog.[445] Another report described the detection of *"H. heilmannii"* from a child with chronic gastritis and two pet dogs.[459] Transmission of *"H. heilmannii"* from a pet cat to its owner was also suspected in another report, which provided stronger evidence because *"H. heilmannii"* isolates from the human and pet were indistinguishable.[460] In these reports, the direction of transmission is impossible to determine and common-source exposure cannot be excluded. Nonetheless, finding animal-associated *Helicobacter* species in humans with disease and in their pets is suggestive of zoonotic transmission. Few studies have specifically compared *Helicobacter* isolates from humans and animals. One such study reported that *"H. heilmannii"* isolates from dogs and cats were type 2, which is rare in humans.[451]

Less information is available regarding the potential for transmission of *H. pylori*, the main human pathogen. This species has been isolated from commercially reared cats, but not household pets.[448] Since this species obviously can colonize or infect cats, there is some concern about pets as a reservoir, but this has not been proven. Given the high prevalence of *H. pylori* in humans and the potential for exposure of dogs and cats, it is reasonable to assume that the canine and feline stomach are somewhat inhospitable environments for this species and that *H. pylori* colonization is rare, if it exists. Studies of *H. pylori* infection in people have not identified pet contact as a risk factor.[461] The exception is a study of shepherds in Sardinia that identified a very high prevalence of *H. pylori* antibodies among shepherds compared with family members and blood donors,[462] yet the study relied on serology and relatively superficial analysis was performed, so it is unclear whether this could truly represent a causal association or whether the serology was adequately specific to differentiate *H. pylori* antibodies from NHPH.

The route of zoonotic transmission, if it does occur, is presumably fecal–oral, though the presence of some *Helicobacter* spp. in feline and canine saliva suggests that contact with saliva could also be a route of exposure. It is unlikely that *Helicobacter* is a major zoonotic concern. Circumstantial evidence suggests that interspecies transmission may occur, but animals probably play a minor role, if any, in human disease. Basic household hygiene measures like hand washing and avoiding contact with feces should be adequate. The potential for saliva-associated transmission could be more concerning because of the potential for greater face-to-face or hand-to-face contact between people and their pets.

Leptospira spp.

Introduction

Leptospirosis is one of the most widespread zoonotic diseases in the world, although infections from companion animals are uncommon. Disease can occur in both humans and many animal species, and range from mild to fatal. Among animals commonly kept as pets, disease is most common in dogs, particularly those that spend time in forests or swampy areas. Other companion animal species, including cats and rodents, may also be infected and potentially act as sources of human infection. Zoonotic transmission from pets is thought to be rare but possible. The risk may be greatest among veterinary personnel, but infections have been reported in pet owners, including transmission from clinically healthy pets.

Etiology

Leptospirosis is caused by members of the *Leptospira* spp., a complex group of long, thin, spiral-shaped gram-negative bacteria (Figure 2.4).[463] Nomenclature and classification of *Leptospira* can be confusing. *Leptospira interrogans* includes more than 200 serovars, but about 10 are responsible for most of the disease seen in dogs and cats (Table 2.4). Related serovars are also classified into serogroups, many of which have the same name as one of the serovars within them (which adds to the confusion). Serogroups are capitalized while serovars are not, and neither should be italicized.[464] Each serovar has one or more reservoir or maintenance host species, in which infection is typically subclinical but where infected individuals shed bacteria in their urine and can therefore infect incidental hosts (Table 2.4). Infection is usually much more severe in incidental hosts, but they do not

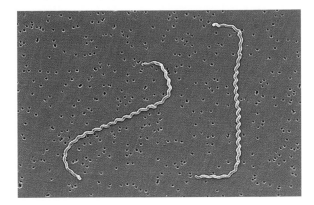

Figure 2.4 Scanning electron microscope image of *Leptospira interrogans* (public domain, photo credit: Janice Haney Carr).

Table 2.4 Common serovars of *L. interrogans* sensu lato in dogs and humans (adapted from Moore et al.[474] and Greene et al.[494]).

Serovar	Primary reservoir host	Other incidental domestic animal hosts
Bratislava	Rat, pig, horse	Cow, horse
Autumnalis	Mouse	Cow
Icterohemorrhagiae	Rat	Cow, horse, pig, cat, guinea pig
Pomona	Cow, pig, skunk, opossum	Horse, sheep, goat, rabbit, cat, guinea pig
Canicola	Dog	Cow, horse, pig, cat, raccoon
Bataviae	Dog, rat, mouse	Cow, cat
Hardjo	Cow	Pig, horse, sheep
Gryppotyphosa	Vole, raccoon, skunk, opossum	Cow, pig, sheep, goat, rabbit, gerbil, guinea pig

shed the organism for as long as reservoir hosts.[465] The potential for long-term shedding by dogs infected with the dog-adapted serovar canicola is a particular concern, as is shedding of icterohemorrhagiae by rats.

Geographic distribution/epidemiology

Leptospira can be found throughout the world, although there is variation among geographic areas in both the prevalence and predominant serovars. *Leptospira* can survive for prolonged periods of time in warm, wet environments, particularly in a neutral to alkaline pH, but it does not multiply outside a host.[465] Accordingly, leptospirosis has a seasonal trend in temperate climates, being more frequently diagnosed at the end of the summer and in early fall.[466,467] The incidence of leptospirosis in tropical climates is relatively constant year-round.[465]

Transmission of leptospires can be direct or indirect. Direct transmission involves skin or mucous membrane contact with infected urine, venereal discharge, or tissues from an infected animal. Transmission is more likely to occur through broken skin, but even intact skin can be penetrated if it is soft or mascerated from moisture.[463,464] The bacteria can occasionally be transmitted by bites,[464] although leptospires are generally not shed in saliva. Indirect transmission may be more common and occurs through contact with soil, water, food, or bedding that has been contaminated with leptospires, mainly from infected urine.

Once leptospires penetrate the skin or mucous membranes of a host, they enter the bloodstream and begin to multiply rapidly. The bacteria then invade other tissues including the kidneys, liver, spleen, CNS, eyes, and genital tract, and continue to multiply. Following the development of a humoral immune response, the organisms are cleared from most tissues, but frequently, a nidus of infection will persist in the proximal renal tubules. Leptospires can survive and replicate in this location for weeks or months, resulting in leptospiruria and damage to renal tubules, potentially leading to renal insufficiency or failure.

Leptospirosis in companion animals

Seroprevalence data are variable and, in addition to geographic location, can be impacted by the test used, vaccination status of tested animals, and interpretation criteria. Seroprevalence rates of 3–25% in pet dogs, 4.9–84% in stray dogs, and 14–49% in kenneled dogs have been reported.[468–472]

Table 2.5 Serovar distribution in dogs with leptospirosis.

Region	Serovars (%)
Trinidad and Tobago[507]	Mankarso: 48 Icterohemorrhagiae: 33 Autumnalis: 41 Copenhageni: 16
Ontario, Canada[473]	Autumnalis: 31 Bratislava: 16 Grippotyphosa: 12 Icterohemorrhagiae: 7.9 Canicola: 6.0
Southern Germany[508]	Grippotyphosa: 31 Saxkoebing: 24 Icterohemorrhagiae: 17 Canicola: 12
Japan[468]	Icterohemorrhagiae: 62 Autumnalis: 15 Canicola: 9.8 Hebdomadis: 6.2 Australis: 3.3
Chiapas, Mexico[469]	Pyrogenes: 73 Tarassovi: 27
United States[474]	Grippotyphosa: 29 Autumnalis: 21 Pomona: 18 Canicola: 13 Bratislava: 10 Icterohemorrhagiae: 7.0
Michigan, United States[476]	Grippotyphosa: 54 Bratislava: 21 Canicola: 9.2 Icterohemorrhagiae: 2.8

Predominant serovars in different regions are listed in Table 2.5. Determination of prominent serovars can help infer important sources of infection, as long as the limitations of testing methods are understood. For example, grippotyphosa and pomona are usually acquired from urban wildlife (raccoons, skunks), while canicola is acquired from dogs and icterohemorrhagiae from rats.[466] The potential for cross-reaction between different serovars must be considered. For example, serovar autumnalis is commonly reported in some regions, yet autumnalis titers may rise quickly following infection with other serovars and autumnalis titers may be more of a general indicator of leptospirosis than specific identification of the serovar that is involved.

Both seroprevalence and incidence of disease are increasing in some regions, and leptospirosis has been described as a reemerging disease in North America.[473,474] This reemergence may have occurred for many reasons, including a change in the predominant serovars, increased numbers of raccoons and other urban wildlife, increased infection of urban wildlife and perhaps climate changes that favor the survival of the organism in the environment.[466,473,475]

Reported risk factors for seropositivity or disease in dogs include livestock exposure; wildlife exposure; exercise outside of fenced yards; being a working, herding, or hound dog; living in periurban regions; and living in urban versus rural regions.[473,476–478] Conflicting data about urban versus rural or working dogs may reflect the prevalence of leptospirosis in urban wildlife in different regions. Overall, these risk factors relate to the potential for exposure through direct or indirect contact with wildlife and livestock.

While more attention is focused on dogs, leptospirosis can occur (and may be underdiagnosed) in cats.[479] A study of feral cats in Spain reported seropositivity in 14% of cats with a higher rate (20%) of detection of leptospires in organs.[471] Serovars icterohemorrhagiae, ballum, and sejroe were identified. A study from Greece reported seropositivity in 31% of healthy domestic cats, with autumnalis, bratislava, and bataviae as the most common,[480] while a Scottish study found antibodies against *Leptospira* hardjo, autumnalis, and icterohemorrhagiae in 9.2% of cats.[481]

Leptospirosis can also occur in a variety of other companion animals, and given reports of zoonotic infections, less common pets such as rats may actually pose a much higher relative risk compared with dogs and cats.[482–484] In particular, species such as rats that are recognized as subclinical carriers of *Leptospira* are a concern.

Human infection

While it has been called one of the most common zoonotic diseases, the incidence of human infection in most regions is low, such as the 0.06/100,000

persons incidence rate that has been reported in Germany.[485] There are numerous potential sources of exposure, and occupational and recreational risk factors have been clearly identified. Occupationally, veterinarians, farmers, slaughterhouse workers, animal caretakers, and sewer system workers are at increased risk.[465] Recreational exposure can occur through various outdoor activities such as freshwater swimming, boating, hiking, hunting, and adventure races.[24,464,465,486] Immunocompromised individuals, infants, and young children are at greater risk of complications, and children in general are at increased risk of exposure because of the nature of contact with animals and the environment, and the associated (low) level of hygiene.

Zoonotic infections from pets

Information regarding zoonotic transmission from companion animals to humans is limited and is dominated by anecdotal or poorly documented reports. However, it is clear that transmission can occur and that pet owners and veterinary personnel may be at risk. There are reports of zoonotic leptospirosis in veterinary personnel with infections acquired from rats. In one situation, a small animal veterinarian developed leptospirosis after having contact with urine from an apparently healthy rat that was being examined.[482] Gloves were not worn, and some skin abrasions were present on the person's hands. The limited number of published reports is overshadowed by larger numbers of anecdotal reports of infections in veterinarians and veterinary technicians. These anecdotal reports seem to be increasing in some areas, coinciding with the apparent reemergence of leptospirosis in pet animal species. Whether this represents a true increased risk, better diagnosis, or simply more widespread discussion of cases is unclear. Accordingly, the incidence and risk factors for occupational infection in veterinary personnel are poorly understood.

Studies of veterinarians have identified seropositivity rates of 1–2.9%,[487–490] although without a control group, it is difficult to determine whether these rates are higher than a comparable nonveterinary population. Interestingly, in one study, having treated an animal with "influenza-like illness," a description that could include animals with mild leptospirosis was associated with seropositivity.

There are multiple reports of zoonotic leptospirosis in pet owners from contact with apparently healthy rats, based on the diagnosis of leptospirosis in the person and subsequent identification of the same serovar in the pet rat.[483,484] Poorly described cases of infections from dogs have also been reported. In one situation, a dog owner developed leptospirosis after having contact with urine from his infected dog.[491] In another report, a person developed leptospirosis 7–10 days after his dog had "urinary incontinence."[492] Both the person and dog were seropositive. The person took the dog swimming in a nearby river almost daily, so it is difficult to determine whether the person was infected by the dog or whether they were both infected by the same environmental source.

While there is little information regarding infections from cats, cat ownership was identified as a risk factor for seropositivity in people in one American study.[493]

Animals

Clinical presentation

The clinical manifestations of leptospirosis in an animal vary depending on the age and immunity of the host, virulence of the serovar, and the environment in which the organism is found.[465] Subclinical infections appear to be the most common form.[472] Clinical disease is rarely reported in cats, even when leptospiremia and histological renal and hepatic damage are present.[494] The incubation period is approximately 5–14 days, but this can range from a few days to as many as 30 days.

Leptospirosis may result in fever, vomiting, abdominal pain, diarrhea, inappetence, severe weakness, depression, stiffness, or myalgia. Signs may be peracute, acute, subacute, or chronic in nature. Peracute infection results in massive leptospiremia followed rapidly by death, with few other clinical signs.[494] In acute infections, early signs may include pyrexia, shivering, muscle tenderness, subsequent vomiting, dehydration, signs of coagulopathy, and vascular collapse, often leading to death before renal or hepatic signs can develop. Subacute infection is more common, with fever,

anorexia, vomiting, dehydration, and polyuric renal failure, potentially leading to oliguric or anuric renal failure. Petechial and ecchymotic hemorrhages may be noted on mucous membranes and elsewhere on the body.[465] Serovars grippotyphosa, canicola, and bratislava tend to cause primarily renal damage. Hepatic damage is more commonly associated with serovars icterohemorrhagiae and pomona, signs of which tend to be more common in dogs less than 6 months of age. However, signs may vary by outbreak, geographic region, and host, even within the same serovar.[494] Respiratory signs may also be seen in 3–20% of cases, due to vascular damage to the lungs or as a direct effect of leptospiral toxins.[465,494] Signs of CNS involvement in dogs are usually limited to stiffness, disorientation, and posterior paresis.[495,496] Severe gastrointestinal inflammation, sometimes resulting in the development of intestinal intussuceptions, has also been reported.[494]

Diagnosis

Laboratory abnormalities include leukocytosis, thrombocytopenia, elevated hepatic enzymes and bilirubin, azotemia, and hyperglycemia.[465] Glucosuria, proteinuria, pyuria, hematuria, and granular casts may be identified.[494] The majority of dogs with leptospirosis (83–100%) are already in renal failure at the time of veterinary examination.[465,494]

The standard serological test used for the diagnosis of leptospirosis in dogs is the microscopic agglutination test (MAT), a test that is "somewhat serovar specific,"[465] meaning that the highest titer tends to be against the infecting serovar but crossreactivity with other serovars is not uncommon. Diagnosis is typically based on a fourfold rise in antibody titer over 3 weeks or a single high titer, if the dog was not vaccinated in the last 3 months.[494] A single titer of 1:800 is usually used as the cutoff, but some have recommended the use of 1:3200 or higher.[465,479] Titers may be negative during the first 7–10 days of infection, and early antimicrobial therapy may decrease the magnitude of the rise in titer. Vaccination can cause an increase in titer; however, this rarely exceeds 1:800, and high titers are typically short lasting.[497] Additionally, because serovar canicola is host adapted to dogs, dogs may shed this serovar in their urine without developing a titer over 1 : 100.[465] ELISAs for IgG and IgM have also been developed, which can help detect infection earlier in the clinical phase than the MAT and differentiate vaccine- versus disease-induced titers. However, these tests are not currently widely available. Regardless, while commonly used, serological tests have been reported to be poor predictors of urine shedding.[498]

A macroscopic slide agglutination test (MSAT) and an indirect hemagglutination assay (IHA), which were developed for use in humans, have also been used to detect recent infection in dogs and can be used in other species without modification.[494] The IHA has good specificity and sensitivity compared with MAT and ELISA, and is very simple to perform.[499] Detection of leptospires in urine using darkfield microscopy is uncommonly performed and can be associated with false-negative results, so it is only useful as an adjunctive test.[465] A low dose of a diuretic such as furosemide can be given to well-hydrated animals prior to sample collection to help increase the recovery of leptospires.[494] Because of the fastidious nature of the organism, culture is rarely performed, though it can be performed on blood, urine, or tissues (i.e., liver, kidney).[465] FA testing can be used with body fluids and tissues, and is useful for the diagnosis of leptospirosis, but it cannot differentiate different serovars.[465] Various PCR-based tests have been used in dogs and are available from some commercial labs, but require further study to determine their diagnostic sensitivity and reliability.[494]

Management

Treatment depends on the animal's condition and body systems that are involved, as well as the severity of disease and may include intravenous fluids, plasma, or whole blood transfusion; gastroprotectants; diuretics; or other supportive or specific treatments.[494] Early antimicrobial therapy is very important to reduce leptospiremia and further organ damage. Penicillins (e.g., ampicillin) are the empiric antimicrobials of choice.[494] Following treatment of acute infection, an alternate antimicrobial therapy to clear the carrier state is required. Options include doxycycline, tetracycline, and possibly macrolides (e.g., erythromycin), although the latter have not been well studied. Doxycycline can also

be used for initial therapy in dogs and may be advantageous in animals with marked renal dysfunction but minimal hepatic dysfunction. The survival rate for dogs with leptospirosis, if properly treated, ranges from 78% to 88%.[465]

All animals with leptospiruria should be treated with antimicrobials due to the associated public health risk, regardless of the severity of disease. Once an animal begins treatment, shedding of viable organisms should cease within 24–48 hours. Objective data regarding time to cessation of shedding are not available, and shedding may recur if antimicrobial therapy is withdrawn before renal colonization is completely eliminated.[494]

Humans

Clinical presentation

Infection in humans may range from subclinical, to a self-limited flu-like illness, to fulminant, rapidly fatal disease.[24,463,464] The incubation period is 5–14 days but can be as long as 30 days.[500] A large percentage (~90%) of infected individuals have subclinical or mild infections.[24] Nonspecific signs and symptoms such as fever, headache, chills, muscle aches, vomiting, jaundice, anemia, conjunctival suffusion without purulent discharge, myalgia of the calf and lumbar regions, and transient rash are present initially.[24,500] This occurs during the bacteremic/septicemia phase, which lasts for approximately 1 week.[24] It may be followed by an immune-mediated phase, which is characterized by return of fever along with complications such as jaundice and hepatic dysfunction (Weil's disease), uveitis, lymphadenopathy, aseptic meningitis, renal disease, myositis, and purpuric rash.[24,500] Aseptic meningitis is more common in children less than 14 years of age.[464] These severe complications occur in approximately 10% of individuals.[500]

Diagnosis

Isolation of leptospires from blood and CSF can be successful, particularly early in disease, with isolation from urine possible after 7–10 days of illness.[24] Culture requires special media and specific conditions, can take from a few days to as long as 16 weeks, and is of low sensitivity. Therefore, it is not a particularly useful tool for clinical diagnosis. Darkfield microscopy can be used to evaluate smears, but this is also of low diagnostic yield. *Leptospira* can also be seen with light microscopy on silver stain and immunostain preparations. Shedding of organisms in the urine can be intermittent; therefore, multiple samples need to be collected, and the overall sensitivity of visualization techniques is limited.

Because of the limitations of culture and direct visualization, serological testing is the standard for diagnosis; however, seroconversion can be delayed, transient, or absent in some individuals.[24] MAT is performed at reference laboratories and involves comparison of acute and convalescent samples. Other simpler, more rapid tests are available, including the MSAT, IHA, IgM immunoassays, and latex agglutination tests. The sensitivity of these tests is usually low during the first week of clinical disease, but increases after that.[501] PCR has also been used to detect leptospiral DNA in clinical samples.[501] This technique is more reliable than serology or culture for early diagnosis and will likely become more widely used as the availability of molecular testing increases.

Management

Penicillins have traditionally been used as the first-line treatment, but ceftriaxone has been shown to be an effective alternative. Doxycycline and cefotaxime are also reasonable alternative treatments based on one open-label clinical trial.[502] Jarisch–Herxheimer reactions may occur in people treated with penicillin.[24,464]

The case fatality rate in people with leptospirosis is generally 1–5%, but has been reported to be as high as 18% in patients presenting to an emergency department and >20% depending on location.[503,504] The mortality rate for anicteric leptospirosis tends to be very low.[464] An increased risk of mortality has also been associated with dyspnea, oliguria, leukocytosis >12,900/mm^3, repolarization abnormalities on ECG, and alveolar infiltrates on thoracic radiographs.[503] Prophylactic antimicrobial therapy should be considered in pregnant women that have been exposed because of the potential for spontaneous abortion.[500]

Prevention

Reducing exposure of animals

Identification and avoidance of high-risk environmental sites is an important consideration, although it is potentially difficult and hard to implement. Wet areas with drainage from potentially infected cattle, deer, or wildlife are of higher risk, particularly with slow-moving, warm, and alkaline water.[465] Obviously, avoidance is not possible in some situations, and high-risk sites may be difficult to determine without good information about the local prevalence of leptospirosis in different animal populations.

Since rodents can be a source of exposure, rodent infestation should be eliminated whenever present.[465] Pet rodents should be restricted from having any contact with wild rodents. Preventing roaming of pets will help reduce contact with infected wildlife.

Vaccination of animals

Vaccination of dogs is a potential control measure[465] but has some limitations. Vaccines only include selected serovars, and cross-protection is limited. The potential efficacy of vaccination is thus dependent, in part, on the serovar distribution in the region compared with the serovars present in the vaccine. In some regions, there is good correlation between vaccine and disease strains, but this is not universal.

Initial vaccines against canicola and icterohemorrhagiae likely played an important role in the marked decline of this serovar in dogs and humans.[466] With the increase in leptospirosis that was identified in some areas in the 1990s and the shift in the most common serovars away from canicola and icterohemorrhagiae to grippotyphosa, pomona, bratislava, and autumnalis, different vaccines were needed. Currently, there are bacterin vaccines available for serovars canicola and icterohemorrhagiae, serovars grippotyphosa, and pomona, or all four. A subunit vaccine protecting against these four serovars is also available. These vaccines provide some cross-protection with other serogroups, but this is incomplete,[494] and the potential emergence of autumnalis as an important serovar in some areas may limit the impact of vaccination as current vaccines do not include this serovar.

The impact of vaccination on urine shedding must be considered, as reduction of shedding, not just prevention of disease, is important from a zoonotic disease standpoint. Vaccines that prevent disease but result in infected animals becoming healthy shedders could be counterproductive, or at least unhelpful for the protection of human health. Data on this matter are conflicting, as are opinions. For example, a vaccine against canicola and icterohemorrhagiae was able to reduce morbidity and mortality in experimentally challenged dogs; however, 13% of vaccinated adult dogs became renal carriers.[505] This is of concern because infected animals, while clinically healthy, would be a potential source of infection for other animals and humans. An earlier study reported no urine shedding among vaccinated dogs; however, only six animals were studied.[506] More study is needed on this subject to make proper conclusions.

Vaccination has a role in the protection of dogs and humans, but it must be remembered that vaccination does not provide complete protection against urine shedding, and it should not be used as the sole preventive measure. Vaccination should be considered in dogs that, by nature of their location or management, are at reasonable risk of exposure and when vaccine strains are consistent with strains present in dogs in the region. Vaccination should also be considered in households with high-risk individuals to reduce the risk of infection and severe disease.

Leptospire shedding by pets

In general, an animal infected by a non-host-adapted serovar will shed for a relatively short period of time, while an animal infected with a host-adapted serovar may shed for prolonged periods, if not lifelong. For example, a dog infected with serovar grippotyphosa will shed the bacterium in urine for up to 6 weeks, while a dog infected with canicola can shed for life.[466] Fortunately, canicola is uncommon in most regions, and most infected dogs will only shed for a short period of time. This decreases the population of apparently healthy shedders. Proper antimicrobial treatment is highly effective at eliminating shedding, and animals usually cease shedding shortly

(24–48 hours) after antimicrobials are started. Therefore, early and appropriate diagnosis and treatment are critical. Some individuals have expressed concern that canicola shedding could persist in some dogs following treatment, yet there is currently no evidence to support that suspicion.

While urine shedding receives the most attention, leptospires can also be shed in other fluids and tissues, and contact with saliva is a potential route of infection that should not be ignored.[500] This emphasizes the need for contact precautions and good general hygiene when handling infected (or potentially infected) animals.

Handling infected animals

In veterinary clinics, infected animals (or animals with a reasonable likelihood of having leptospirosis) should be isolated and handled with contact precautions. Direct or indirect contact with urine must be avoided. Barrier clothing such as a dedicated lab coat, isolation gown, or coveralls should be used for any contact with the animal or its environment. Gloves should be worn and hands should be washed thoroughly after glove removal. Urine should be handled carefully and assumed to be infectious. Blood and other potentially infected fluids or tissues (e.g., saliva, CSF) should be handled with similar caution.[465] The entire animal should be considered infectious because of the potential for urine contamination of the hair coat. Face protection or eye protection and a mask should be used for any procedure that might create infectious aerosols or splashes, such as restraining a fractious, urine-contaminated animal. The animal's environment should also be considered infectious. Cages and runs should be cleaned and disinfected regularly. Leptospires are susceptible to many disinfectants, including bleach and iodophors, as well as drying.[465] Power washing should not be performed because of the potential for aerosolization of leptospires. Cleaning areas with a hose should also be avoided, at least until proper disinfection has been performed, because of the risk of exposure through splashing. Infected animals should not be walked and allowed to urinate in areas used by other animals. Confining animals to the clinic and having them urinate in the cage or in a dedicated run that can be properly disinfected is the ideal approach. If this is not possible, then the animal should be walked in an area that is not used by other animals or people, does not drain into a water source, and ideally is in an area and on a surface that allows for good exposure to sunlight.

It is important to remember that leptospires can occasionally be shed in the urine of even healthy, vaccinated dogs. While intensive infection control measures are not practical when handling all routine (non-leptospirosis) cases, consideration should be given to practical measures that could reduce the risk of infection from an apparently healthy host. For example, routine glove use is a good practice whenever skin lesions are present, since contact of urine from an apparently healthy rat with skin abrasions has been implicated in human infection.[482]

Prophylactic treatment of exposed persons

Prophylactic treatment with doxycycline can be considered for people at high risk through exposure to potentially contaminated fresh water, such as hikers or other outdoor enthusiasts in high-risk regions.[464,500] Similar prophylactic treatment could be considered for individuals exposed to urine from infected pets; however, adequate incidence data are not available to determine whether this is truly indicated.

Listeria monocytogenes

Listeriosis is an important foodborne disease caused by the saprophytic gram-positive bacterium *L. monocytogenes*. In healthy people, listeriosis is usually manifested as an acute, self-limited febrile gastroenteritis.[509] More serious, including fatal, infections can occur, particularly in the elderly, neonates, pregnant women, transplant recipients, and persons with hematologic malignancy, chronic liver disease, renal failure, or impaired cell-mediated immunity.[510,511] Fetal death can occur with infection during pregnancy.[511]

L. monocytogenes can be found widely in the environment and on food products. Listeriosis is rarely identified in companion animals. In dogs and cats, nonspecific signs including vomiting, diarrhea, and fever are most commonly reported. Rare cases

of neurological disease have been diagnosed in dogs and cats,[512–514] as well as dermatologic disease,[515] and one case of suspected miscarriage in a dog.[516] A study from Japan reported *L. monocytogenes* shedding in feces by 0.9% of healthy dogs.[517]

Transmission of *L. monocytogenes* from a person to puppies was reported via feeding newborn puppies human breast milk.[518] There is minimal concern about the transmission of *L. monocytogenes* from companion animals to people. Human exposure to *L. monocytogenes* is almost exclusively from food and environmental sources. Since listeriosis in companion animals is very rare, the risks to humans are probably negligible. Localized cutaneous listeriosis in farmers and veterinarians after contact with aborted calves and infected poultry has been reported,[509] so there is a theoretical possibility of cutaneous infection after handling infected companion animals or animal feces; however, the risks must be exceedingly low. General hygiene practices such as avoiding contact with feces and vomit from animals, careful attention to hand hygiene, restricting contact with infected skin sites, proper sharps management, good wound care following injury associated with animals, and hand washing after contact with bodily fluids from animals should virtually negate any risks.

Mycobacterium avium complex (MAC)

Introduction

MAC includes subspecies of *M. avium* and the related organism *Mycobacterium intracellulare*. Infections in humans and companion animals are uncommon. There is currently no evidence that MAC can be transmitted directly between humans and companion animals, in either direction, but the limited study and the potential severity of disease in some immunocompromised individuals indicates that consideration should be given to the potential for MAC as a zoonotic pathogen.

Etiology

Mycobacteria are a diverse group of acid-fast bacteria, and nomenclature and speciation have only been recently improved through the use of sequence-based methods. MAC species and sub-species are the most common nontubercular myco-bacteria involved in human and animal infection. While often discussed as a singular entity, MAC actually involves a diverse and often poorly under-stood group of organisms.

There is no consensus about what truly consti-tutes a MAC organism, with some classifying MAC as only involving true subspecies of *M. avium* and others including closely related (but distinct) species like *M. intracellulare*. It is likely that new information will become available regard-ing appropriate identification and taxonomy with further advancement of genomic techniques.

Often, four main groups are discussed in rela-tion to MAC. *M. avium* subsp. *avium* is the cause of avian tuberculosis (TB) and also a cause of disease in other animal species, including humans. It is also referred to as the avian tubercle bacillus, *Mycobacterium tuberculosis avium* or simply *M. avium*.[519] While typically discussed as a single entity, it is evident that there are various environ-mental and host-associated types.[519]

Recent study has indicated genotypic differences between isolates from birds and those from humans, pigs, and the environment, and this has led to a recommendation that *M. avium* subsp. *hom-inissuis* be recognized.[520] Infections with this sub-species have been identified in both humans and household pets, including birds.[521–523] It has been suggested that this subspecies is the main cause of MAC infection in children and that, therefore, the environment rather than birds or other MAC animal hosts may be the most important source of infection.[521] *M. avium* subsp. *silvaticum* is primarily associated with TB-like disease in pigeons and is also known as the wood pigeon bacillus, *M. avium* subsp. *columbae*, or *Mycobacterium silvaticum*.

M. avium subsp. *paratuberculosis* is the cause of Johne's disease in cattle and is also referred to as Johne's bacillus, *Mycobacterium johnei*, or *Mycobacterium paratuberculosis*. A link between this organism and Crohn's disease has been suggested, but this is controversial and far from definitive.

M. intracellulare was first isolated from a child that died of disseminated infection and has subse-quently been isolated from various animals and the environment.[524,525] It was previously known as *Nocardia intracellularis* or *Mycobacterium battey*.[519]

The most important MAC organism in compan-ion animals and humans has typically been assumed to be *M. avium* subsp. *avium*. It is the cause of virtually all disseminated infections in immunocompromised humans, while *M. intra-cellulare* is the main cause of pulmonary MAC infections in immunocompetent individuals.[519] However, recent studies have identified the pre-dominance of *M. genavense*, not *M. avium* in pet birds.[526,527] *M. genavense* is not a MAC organism but is another nontuberculous *Mycobacterium*, and it has also been reported as a cause of pneumonia in a rabbit,[528] disseminated infection in a cat,[529] lymph-adenitis in a dog,[530] and conjunctivitis in ferrets.[531] Human infections have been reported, predomi-nantly in HIV/AIDS patients.[532] It is clear that our knowledge of mycobacteria is still limited and that changes in our understanding of this diverse genus are likely.

Geographic distribution/epidemiology

MAC and *M. avium* in particular are presumably found worldwide. As a broad group, they are ubiq-uitous and commonly found in soil and water, par-ticularly in acidic conditions with high organic matter.[533] Understanding of the natural ecology of MAC organisms is limited. Some are thought to be primarily environmental bacteria, while others appear to be human and animal pathogens with limited ability to survive in the environment.[519] Many have excellent environmental survival prop-erties and can persist for years. They can be found in biofilms and even in treated water supplies. Thus, exposure to MAC may be a very common event, with rare clinical consequences since MAC are relatively avirulent in normal human or animal hosts.

Identification of sources of infection, risk factors for transmission, and related issues is complicated by the potentially long time from exposure to man-ifestation of infection. Months, or even years, may pass from the time of exposure to development of disease.[534] The main routes of infection of humans or animals are thought to be inhalation and inges-tion. Water sources such as swimming pools and hot tubs have been implicated in clusters of infec-tions.[535] Ingestion of MAC in pasteurized milk has been proposed as a source of infection, particularly in young children.[536] Companion animals are thought to be exposed mainly from the environment, either with true environmental mycobacteria or through contact with feces from infected birds.[533] Person-to-person transmission has not been reported, nor has direct animal-to-human transmission.

Human MAC infections are reported most often in developed countries, but that may simply reflect the availability of specific diagnostic testing. The incidence of infections may be increasing, though the apparent increases in disease rates may simply be due to better diagnostic testing.

The incidence of MAC infection in companion animals appears to be very low. This may be partly from variable diagnostic testing, but it is probably true given the minimally pathogenic nature of MAC, particularly in otherwise healthy animals.

The risk of zoonotic infection is unclear. Infection of both animals and humans with the same MAC species or subspecies can certainly occur; however, it is not known whether infected humans or animals pose a risk to other individuals. There are no reports of direct interspecies transmission of MAC, and it could be that human and animal infections are all from other (i.e., environmental) sources. Yet, the absence of proof of transmission does not indicate an absence of risk. The risks to immunocompetent individuals are probably negligible, but prudence is appropriate when dealing with high-risk individuals, particularly HIV/AIDS patients.

Animals

Clinical presentation

Disseminated disease is the most common manifestation in dogs, with extensive granulomatous lesions in the liver, spleen, mesenteric lymph nodes, and intestinal tract.[537-539] Vague signs such as weight loss, lethargy, fever, lymphadenopathy, diarrhea, and hematochezia may be present, but these may be variable and intermittent in nature.[522,540,541]

Cats typically develop lymphadenopathy and subcutaneous swelling, particularly around the head and face, with weight loss, anorexia, and fever.[533,542] Disseminated disease can also occur and

has been reported in both immunocompromised and immunocompetent cats.[543-545] Cutaneous infections may also occur.[546]

While *M. avium* is associated with birds, clinical infections in pet birds are uncommon. Classical tuberculous disease can occur, involving the respiratory tract or other body systems,[523,547] as can hepatic or multifocal disease that may be characterized by various vague and nonspecific signs like weight loss, inappetence, ascites, and melena.[523,548] Infections have been reported in various other species, including ferrets.[549]

Diagnosis

Detection of acid-fast organisms on cytological samples is suggestive of MAC infection but not diagnostic.[533] Isolation of MAC is the standard for diagnosis and allows for definitive identification of the *Mycobacterium* species. PCR can be performed on tissues or fluid samples.[541,550,551] This is most useful when there are large numbers of organism present and is currently of limited availability.

Management

In dogs, treatment is often unrewarding because of the advanced nature of disease at the time of diagnosis. There is limited objective information regarding options. Clarithromycin, clofazimine, tetracyclines, rifabutin, ethambutol, and rifampin can be considered, typically in combination therapy, but the relative efficacy is unknown.

Treatment may be more rewarding in cats because of the lower incidence of disseminated disease. Surgical removal of infected tissues should be considered, when possible. Doxycycline, clofazimine, and clarithromycin have been used as sole or in combined medical therapy.

Humans

Clinical presentation

Three main syndromes are encountered: pulmonary disease, disseminated infection, and cervical lymphadenitis. Infections can occur at other body sites but are uncommon.

Pulmonary MAC infection typically occurs in immunocompetent individuals with an estimated incidence of 0.9–1.3 cases/100,000 persons.[552,553] Underlying chronic lung disease is the most significant risk factor for the development of symptomatic MAC pulmonary infection.[554] Older, slim women are disproportionately represented.[554,555] It is a chronic and often nonspecific disease that may be difficult to differentiate clinically from other chronic pulmonary diseases.

Disseminated disease mainly occurs in people with advanced HIV/AIDS and was extremely rare prior to 1980. The disease incidence likely peaked in the 1990s, with a substantial decline since then because of more effective antiretroviral and prophylactic antimicrobial regimens.[534] The greatest risk is to patients with severely depressed CD4+ cell counts, and disease is rarely identified in individuals with >100 CD4+ cells/mm^3. Disseminated disease can occur in other immunocompromised populations such as children with primary immunodeficiencies and patients with hairy cell leukemia.[556,557]

Cervical lymphadenitis is quite rare with approximately 300 reported cases annually in the United States;[552] however, more cases presumably go undiagnosed. This is typically a disease of children, especially those less than 3 years of age. Cervical, mediastinal, or intra-abdominal lymph node enlargement may be present.[534]

Diagnosis

Isolation of MAC is the standard for diagnosis, but false-positive results can occur because of carriage of MAC at certain body sites in the absence of infection. This is a particular problem with respiratory disease as MAC can commonly be found in the sputum of healthy individuals.[558] Diagnosis of pulmonary disease requires the presence of consistent clinical signs and one or more of (1) detection of acid-fast bacilli and granulomas or isolation of MAC from histological specimens, (2) three positive sputum cultures without positive smears, (3) two positive sputum cultures with one positive smear, or (4) isolation of moderate to heavy (2+ or greater) growth of MAC or detection of moderate to large numbers of MAC on a smear from bronchial wash samples.[558] Diagnosis of disseminated disease involves isolation of MAC from infected sterile sites such as blood, bone marrow, liver, or spleen.[534] Similarly, diagnosis of MAC lymphadeni-

tis involves the isolation of MAC from the affected lymph node. Histological evidence of granulomatous inflammation with the presence of acid-fast organisms is suggestive but not diagnostic.

Management

Treatment can be difficult and requires long-term therapy with a combination of two or more active drugs, such as clarithromycin or azithromycin, ethambutol, rifabutin, rifampin, amikacin, and streptomycin.[534] Duration of treatment is long and may not be effective. The general consensus is that treatment of pulmonary MAC infection should be continued for 12 months after sputum cultures have become negative, commonly leading to 18–24 months of treatment.[534]

Prevention

The risk of interspecies transmission of MAC, or at least clinically relevant interspecies transmission, is minimal. Presumably, the greatest risk involves pets with clinical infections (and therefore the potential for shedding of large numbers of MAC) and immunocompromised household contacts. In households with infected pets, contact with the infected site should be avoided as much as possible. External infections should be covered with an impermeable dressing if possible. High-risk individuals should limit contact with the pet, particularly the infected site, and should not participate in bandage changing or similar activities that would result in close contact with the infected site or contaminated materials. Hand hygiene should be performed after contact with the infected site or contaminated materials, and routinely after contact with the pet. While it has been recommended that households with immunocompromised members should not keep MAC-infected pets,[533] this is hard to justify if basic control measures can be implemented.

In households with infected humans, general hygiene practices involving pets are warranted to decrease the risk of contamination or infection of the pet, but the likelihood of this causing a problem is minimal. Good attention to hand hygiene and restricting contact of the pet with the infected site are practical measures that may be more important for other pathogens.

There is no indication to screen healthy pets for MAC carriage, even in situations where a human is infected or when a high-risk individual is present in the household. MAC can be found in various locations, including the environment, and isolation of MAC from a pet would provide little indication of risk. Difficulties in isolation, speciation, and typing further weaken screening.

Despite the traditional association of birds and *M. avium*, there is inadequate information indicating a risk is posed by pet birds in households, even in households containing high-risk individuals. The risks are probably greater for other pathogens such as *C. psittaci* in such households.

Mycobacterium bovis

Introduction

M. bovis is the agent of bovine TB but has one of the broadest host ranges of all known pathogens.[559] Along with *M. tuberculosis*, it is a cause of "tubercular" disease in humans and various animal species. It has exhibited a resurgence in some regions where it was once controlled or eradicated as a result of the presence of wildlife reservoirs that are difficult or impossible to completely control. It is subject to rigorous surveillance and control programs in most developed countries through testing of food animals and pasteurization of milk products. Animal infections are uncommon, but given the broad host range and potential public health implications, this disease continues to attract attention.

Etiology

M. bovis is an intracellular "tubercle-producing" *Mycobacterium* sp. that is closely related to *M. tuberculosis*. It is believed that *M. bovis* is evolutionarily a subtype of *M. tuberculosis*.[533]

Geographic distribution/epidemiology

The relative importance of *M. bovis* varies geographically. Domestic cattle are the natural host and main reservoir of this pathogen and have been the focus of most investigations and control efforts, but all terrestrial mammals are believed to be susceptible to infection.[560] The establishment of *M. bovis* in wildlife reservoirs has complicated control measures. Various wildlife species are important reservoirs in some regions. For example, the European badger and deer are the main wildlife reservoirs in the United Kingdom and Ireland,[561,562] while opossums are important wildlife reservoirs in New Zealand.[563] Human–human transmission is the main route of transmission in areas where *M. bovis* has been controlled in cattle and through pasteurization of milk.[561]

M. bovis accounts for approximately 1–2% of human TB cases in the United States,[24] with *M. tuberculosis* being of much greater concern. The relative impact of *M. bovis* compared with *M. tuberculosis* presumably varies among different geographic regions, with *M. bovis* accounting for a minority of human infections in virtually all regions. Most human *M. bovis* infections are from the ingestion of unpasteurized dairy products,[564] with children at highest risk.[559] In areas where pasteurization is mandatory, infection rates are very low and are most often associated with occupational inhalation of *M. bovis*, particularly in slaughterhouse workers.[565]

M. bovis infection has been reported in both dogs and cats,[560,566–569] but the incidence is low. Cats may have increased susceptibility.[533] The most likely routes of exposure of companion animals probably vary with the type of reservoir. In areas where cattle or wild ruminants are the reservoir, most infected animals are probably exposed through ingestion of infected carcasses, unpasteurized dairy products, and offal.[570,571] Ingestion of infected small mammals like badgers and opossums is also possible; however, direct respiratory exposure cannot be excluded since infections have been reported in dogs that have been bitten by badgers or squirrels.[569] The number of organisms excreted by badgers in feces is low,[559] and the risk of exposure through contact with badger feces (or other infected animals) is unclear but likely low. Contrary to earlier reports, it appears that *M. bovis* only survives for days to weeks in the environment, with shorter survival in sunlight and during summer months.[559] The role of the environment in infection is unclear.

The incidence and risk factors for transmission to or between companion animals have not been adequately evaluated. A study of 20 cats exposed to an infected cat did not detect any transmission.[571] In contrast, an earlier study during major outbreaks identified *M. bovis* in 4/9 dogs and 24/52 cats on infected farms.[572] Whether this represented transmission by dogs and cats or widespread common-source infection is impossible to determine. The discharging sinus of an infected cat was suspected as the source of infection in one cluster of feline cases.[570] Respiratory transmission is also a possible concern, since it is known to occur between badgers.[559] Vertical transmission may be possible, as demonstrated by seropositivity of kittens from an infected cat.[571,572]

The risk and incidence of transmission of *M. bovis* from companion animals to humans is also unclear. Concurrent infection of people and pets in the same household has been identified.[573] Cross-sectional studies identifying concurrent colonization indicate the possibility of interspecies transmission; however, the direction of transmission cannot be determined nor can common-source infection be excluded. Direct transmission of *M. bovis* resulting in cutaneous disease was reported in a veterinarian that had contact with an alpaca with pulmonary *M. bovis* TB.[574] The route of infection was not clear; however, the veterinarian had direct contact with the sick alpaca during examination and euthanasia, and her hands were contaminated with blood during venipuncture. These reports provide adequate evidence to support a risk of transmission of *M. bovis* from infected companion animals to humans. The overall risk of transmission from companion animals to humans appears to be low, largely based on the rarity of disease in companion animals. If *M. bovis* infection is, or becomes, more common in a region, then the risks would increase. Immunocompromised individuals, particularly those with HIV/AIDS, are at increased risk of primary infection and reactivation of latent infection.[575]

Animals

Clinical presentation

The type of infection relates to the route of exposure. Nonspecific signs such as lethargy, anorexia, weight loss, and fever may be the sole initial abnormalities.[560] Even with advanced disease, clinical signs may be vague and nonspecific.[560,572] While signs of classical tuberculous respiratory tract disease (fever, weight loss, cough, inappetence) may be present,[566] granulomatous disease of other systems may be present concurrently or as the sole problem.[560]

Inhalation exposure will predominantly result in respiratory tract disease, with or without the involvement of other systems. Oral exposure is more likely to result in abdominal tract or disseminated disease.[560] Liver, mesenteric, and deep lymph node involvement is common following gastrointestinal exposure. Severe disseminated disease can occur as a consequence of exposure through any route.[571] Discharging abscesses or bite wounds accounted for 6/12 infections in one report in cats,[567] highlighting the nonspecific nature of illness. Conjunctivitis, abdominal mass, and mesenteric lymph node enlargement have also been reported.[567,568] Skin lesions may be common in cats and may appear similar to cat leprosy, which is predominantly caused by the nontuberculous *Mycobacterium lepraemurium*.[576]

Diagnosis

Diagnosis can be difficult due to the nature of disease and nonspecific presentation. Often, diagnosis is made late in disease or at necropsy. Identification of acid-fast bacilli, particularly in the presence of granulomatous inflammation, is strongly suggestive of mycobacterial disease but cannot differentiate *M. bovis* from other mycobacteria. Misdiagnosis as neoplasia is possible, particularly if acid-fast stains are not evaluated.[560] Isolation of *M. bovis* from infected tissue is the current main method for obtaining a definitive diagnosis.[567] *M. bovis*-specific PCR testing of tissues may become another option but is not yet widely available.

Intradermal tuberculin testing with purified protein derivative (PPD) of *M. tuberculosis* is inconsistent and unreliable in dogs and cats.[533,577] While infected animals might respond, so do animals infected with *M. tuberculosis* and other mycobacteria. Intradermal skin testing with bacilli Calmette–Guerin, an attenuated *M. bovis* strain, may be more reliable for both *M. bovis* and *M. tuberculosis* but can induce future false-positive PPD testing results and cannot differentiate between *M. bovis* and *M. tuberculosis*.[533] An alternate form of tuberculin testing in dogs involves evaluation of body temperature increase in response to subcutaneous injection of PPD, with a 1.1°C rise in body temperature over 2–12 hours interpreted as a positive response.[533] This test does not appear to work well with cats, and diagnosis is that species is best based on biopsy, culture, histology, and/or necropsy.

Management

There is little information available regarding treatment of infected pets. Prolonged therapy (months) is required. Possible treatment options include combinations of rifampin, clarithromycin, fluoroquinolones, ethambutol, and isoniazid.[533] Surgical excision of infected areas is ideal, if possible. However, it has been recommended that infected pets should not be treated but rather should be euthanized because of the potential risk for transmission to humans.[560,571] It is difficult to determine whether this is a reasonable recommendation given the lack of objective evidence. Certainly, pet to human transmission of *M. bovis* appears to be rare, and some infections (perhaps especially in cats) may be relatively mild and respond to treatment.[567,568] Therefore, a case-by-case approach considering animal and human factors is warranted. However, given the potential severity of disease in people and the lack of information regarding appropriate treatments, along with the typically advanced state of illness in the pet by the time of diagnosis, serious consideration should be given to whether attempting treatment is appropriate. Treatment should probably not be attempted if there is no clear understanding of the duration and cost of treatment and commitment from the owners to follow treatment recommendations and implement good infection control practices.

Humans

Clinical presentation

M. bovis infection is indistinguishable clinically and radiographically from *M. tuberculosis* infec-

tion, which is discussed in more detail below.[559] Extrapulmonary infections can occur, particularly in children, where cervical lymphadenitis, intestinal tuberculosis, and meningitis are more commonly found.[24] Disseminated infections are rare and of greatest concern in people with HIV/AIDS.[578]

Latent infection can occur, as with *M. tuberculosis*, and people with latent infection can develop disease in the future and pose a risk for transmission to others.[24]

Diagnosis

Isolation of *M. bovis* is the standard for diagnosis, but specialized laboratories are required for the isolation and differentiation from *M. tuberculosis*. Acid-fast stains of tissue or body fluids can lead to a suspicion of mycobacterial infection, but cannot differentiate *M. bovis* from other acid-fast organisms. Tuberculin skin test is typically positive; however, this does not differentiate *M. bovis* from *M. tuberculosis*.

Management

Objective information regarding treatment is lacking, and most recommendations are based on information regarding the treatment of *M. tuberculosis*.[24] Combinations of three or more drugs such as isoniazid, rifampin, ethambutol, or streptomycin should be used.[24,574] Pyrazinamide resistance is common, but multidrug resistance is rare.[24] Nine to twelve months of treatment should be provided.[24]

Prevention

The risk to humans from infected companion animals is difficult to quantify. Diagnosis of *M. bovis* in a pet should result in investigation as to whether human contacts may have been infected from the pet or exposed to the same source of infection. It is unclear whether pets that reside on farms with endemic *M. bovis* infection pose a greater public health risk. There have been conflicting data, but it is certainly reasonable to consider that this might be the case. In the absence of specific

Table 2.6 General recommendations for management of companion animals on farms with endemic *Mycobacterium bovis* in cattle and in regions where *M. bovis* is endemic in wildlife.

On farms with endemic *M. bovis* in cattle	Protection from wildlife
Do not feed dogs and cats raw milk	Keep cats in the house
Keep house cats in the house and barn cats out of the house	Do not allow dogs or cats to roam freely
Keep barn cats away from peoples' faces	Do not allow dogs and cats to have access to carcasses of dead animals
Do not allow dogs to roam freely	
Use good preventive measures to keep pets healthy and reduce their susceptibility to infection	

data, general recommendations have been made (Table 2.6).[577]

Control (or ideally eradication) of *M. bovis* in cattle and wildlife is an important factor, since decreasing the natural reservoirs will reduce the risk of exposure of companion animals.

As discussed above, it has been recommended that infected pets not be treated and be promptly euthanized, although the necessity for such a definitive measure in all cases is questionable. If infected pets are not euthanized, careful application of infection control practices in the veterinary clinic and household are required. All individuals that have (or might have) contact with the infected animal must be informed of the risks, understand them, and take appropriate actions. There is no objective information about the relative efficacy or need for various infection control precautions. In veterinary clinics, infected animals should be isolated because of the potential for zoonotic and nosocomial infection, the latter of which was suspected in a cluster of infections in cats.[576] Contact and respiratory precautions should be used. The hospital environment is of minimal concern as a source of infection, but thorough cleaning and disinfection with a product with a claim of efficacy against mycobacteria are still useful routine practices. Mycobacteria are more resistant to disinfection than most vegetative bacteria but can be killed with proper cleaning and disinfection practices. Particular care must be taken with items that have contact with high risk and/or sterile sites like bronchoscopes and surgical equipment as there is a realistic potential for transmission if these items are contaminated.

In households, contact with infected animals should be restricted. Close contact, particularly face-to-face contact, must be avoided. External lesions should be covered with an impermeable barrier if possible. Barrier precautions and mask should be used when close contact is required. Hand hygiene and related routine hygiene measures should be judiciously implemented.

It has also been recommended that cats exposed to *M. bovis*-infected animals be euthanized.[571] It is difficult to determine whether this is a reasonable response, and balancing the apparent low incidence of infection of animals and the low reported incidence of pet-to-human transmission with public health risks is complicated. A case-by-case approach, considering risk of infection, risk of transmission, susceptibility of the human population, potential for other sources of exposure of the human population, along with other factors, is probably more justifiable.

Testing with tuberculin skin test or interferon gamma release assay is recommended for people that have had contact with an infected person.[24] It is reasonable to apply the same criteria for people that have had contact with infected pets, although close and prolonged contact is presumably required for transmission.

Mycobacterium lepraemurium

This nontuberculosis mycobacterium species is the, or more likely a, leading cause of murine and feline leprosy. This disease is rare in cats and is most commonly reported in New Zealand, The Netherlands, Australia, and Canada (British Columbia)[579,580] and causes single or multiple granulomas in the skin and subcutaneous tissues. This difficult-to-culture organism is closely related to MAC.[519] There is no relation to human leprosy, caused by *Mycobacterium leprae*, and there is no evidence of zoonotic transmission of this organism.[581] Cats most likely become infected after being bitten by infected rodents.

Mycobacterium marinum, Mycobacterium fortuitum, and *Mycobacterium chelonae*

M. marinum, M. fortuitum, and *M. chelonae* are nontuberculous mycobacteria that may be transmitted from fish (or their environment) to humans.[582] *M. marinum* is classified as an immediately growing species, while *M. fortuitum* and *M. chelonae* are classified as rapidly growing species. *M. marinum* is the species most commonly associated with human disease. The main reservoirs for these mycobacteria are freshwater and marine fish, and they can be found in fish (and amphibians) worldwide. Human infection is uncommon and is frequently misdiagnosed,[583] but strongly associated with contact with fish or fish tanks. Clinically healthy individuals are most often affected, but disease has also been reported in high-risk groups such as transplant recipients.[584] Identification of fish and fish tank contact is a critical factor in suspecting this disease.

In fish, these mycobacteria can cause chronic progressive granulomatous disease,[585] but mycobacteria can also be found in clinically healthy fish or fish with other diseases. A study of predominantly freshwater fish reported isolation of *Mycobacterium* spp. from 36% of fish with no pathological evidence of mycobacterial infection.[586] In the same study, *Mycobacterium* spp. were isolated from 29% of batches of healthy fish. Studies of the prevalence of mycobacterial colonization in pet fish in households have not been reported. It is prudent to assume that all aquaria are contaminated.

These mycobacteria are also the cause of "fish tank granuloma" or "swimming pool granuloma" in humans. Logically, infection is predominantly caused by exposure to contaminated fish tanks or swimming pool water. Indirect infections can occur, as highlighted by a report of infection in a young child from contact with a bucket used to clean an aquarium.[587] Most infections occur within

2–3 weeks of exposure. While prolonged contact or the presence of other skin lesions presumably increases the risk, minimal contact, such as simply touching the water with a finger to check the temperature, was suspected as the cause of infection in a transplant recipient.[588]

Infection is characterized by small papules that often progress to shallow ulcerations with crusting. Ascending invasion can occur and resemble sporotrichosis. Progression to deeper infections, such as tenosynovitis, arthritis, and osteomyelitis, is possible but rare.[583] More aggressive disease may be present in transplant recipients,[584] and probably other immunocompromised individuals.

There are no standard guidelines for treatment of infected humans. Rifampin plus ethambutol, doxycycline, minocycline, clarithromycin, or trimethoprim–sulfamethoxazole are typically used for at least 3 months.[589] Longer treatment may be required in transplant recipients.[584]

Prevention of disease associated with pet fish largely involves reducing contact with contaminated water, proper hygiene, and careful handling of items in aquaria. Aquarium water should not be dumped into kitchen or bathroom sinks, or into bathtubs. Areas contaminated by water during aquarium maintenance should be promptly cleaned. Care should be taken when handling items in aquaria, particularly rocks and hard corals, as skin trauma could predispose to infection. Contact with aquarium water should be avoided by persons with compromised immune systems[584,590] or skin lesions. If contact with aquarium water is inevitable, those individuals should wear disposable gloves and carefully wash their hands immediately after glove removal. Proper hand hygiene is important for all people having contact with aquaria. Items used to clean aquaria, such as buckets, should be used only for aquarium cleaning. Particular care should be taken if fish have signs of granulomatous disease.

Mycobacterium tuberculosis

Introduction

M. tuberculosis is a pathogen of significant public health concern, both historically and in modern times. Like *M. bovis*, *M. tuberculosis* is a highly pathogenic tubercle-causing mycobacterium. Humans are the reservoir host of *M. tuberculosis*, and TB is predominantly a disease of humans; however, sporadic cases have been reported in various companion animal species. Dogs, cats, and pet birds are all susceptible to *M. tuberculosis* infection, and infections in companion animals are believed to be exclusively human in origin.[591–593] Infection of dogs seems to be much more common than cats.

Identification of the same strain of *M. tuberculosis* in a person and his or her pet has been reported[592,594] and strongly supports interspecies transmission, though the incidence and risk factors have not been quantified. The role of companion animals in human disease has been minimally investigated, yet it is clear that interspecies transmission can occur among close contacts.

A particular problem in human medicine in recent years has been the dissemination of antimicrobial resistant strains. MDR and extensively drug-resistant (XDR) TB are significant public health concerns. These have not yet been reported in animals, but there is no reason to suspect that this will not occur as a result of transmission from humans.

Etiology

M. tuberculosis is an aerobic, non-spore-forming, acid-fast bacillus. It is a slow-growing organism both *in vitro* and *in vivo*. It is closely related to *M. bovis*, the other organism capable of causing tubercular disease.

Geographic distribution/epidemiology

M. tuberculosis is present in humans worldwide. Approximately one-third of the world's population is infected, with approximately 8 million new cases and 2 million deaths occurring annually.[595] Human infection rates vary greatly between regions, with high rates of disease in sub-Saharan Africa and some parts of Eastern Europe. Infections tend to concentrate in crowded populations with poor hygiene and inadequate access to medical care. Large numbers of infected individuals have latent infections, with no clinical signs but the potential for developing symptomatic disease. The

distribution of *M. tuberculosis* in companion animals is unknown; however, it likely reflects a combination of the distribution in humans and degree of companion animal contact.

Transmission is predominantly via inhalation of contaminated aerosols and droplets, liberated during coughing, sneezing, or talking.[596] Close and prolonged contact is usually required for efficient transmission, and brief contact carries little risk.[596] Infection almost always occurs indoors. *M. tuberculosis* strains can vary in their infectivity, and brief casual contact resulted in disease transmission one outbreak,[597] but this is uncommon.

TB is rare in dogs but can occur,[593,598–600] usually (if not invariably) after close and prolonged contact with an infected person. The incidence of transmission from humans to companion animals is not well understood. Transmission of subclinical infection might be relatively common, as evidenced by a study that reported isolation of *M. tuberculosis* from 15% of healthy dogs and cats in regular contact with infected people.[598] In contrast, another study did not identify *M. tuberculosis* from any of the 29 exposed dogs.[601] More recent studies of dogs and TB are lacking, and this is a clear knowledge deficit considering increasing concerns regarding TB in the human population.

Transmission from infected people to pet birds has been reported.[602,603] Very close contacts such as feeding a bird food that was prechewed by the infected person or mouth-to-beak feeding have been features of some case reports.[602,603]

Animals

Clinical presentation

Infections are often subclinical.[593] When clinical disease does occur, granulomatous respiratory disease is most common.[591,600] Signs such as fever, weight loss, anorexia, and nonproductive cough are common. Gastrointestinal signs may be evident alone or concurrent with respiratory tract disease. In such cases, vomiting, weight loss, anorexia, anemia, and diarrhea are common.[533,593] It has been suggested that gastrointestinal TB is more common in cats.[533] Disseminated disease can be present and result in a wide range of clinical signs, depending on the systems that are involved.[600]

Diagnosis

Definitive antemortem diagnosis can be difficult. Physical examination and diagnostic imaging may indicate the presence of abscesses or tubercles. Regional lymphadenopathy and effusions may also be present. Cytological examination of smears or aspirates can indicate the presence of acid-fast organisms but is not specific as other mycobacteria and a few other bacterial types are also acid-fast positive. Isolation of M. tuberculosis is the gold standard, but it can be slow and difficult. Selective methods are required for successful isolation. Histological examination cannot distinguish between different Mycobacterium spp. Molecular testing of tissues and exudates can provide a rapid and specific diagnosis of M. tuberculosis. Tuberculin testing is inconsistent and unreliable in dogs and cats.[533]

Management

There is little information available about optimal treatment regimens. Disease is often quite advanced by the time TB is suspected or diagnosed.[600] Some individuals have advocated prompt euthanasia of infected animals because of the poor prognosis and human health risks.[591,593] A standard recommendation for euthanasia is probably inappropriate considering the apparent low likelihood of animal-to-human transmission; however, the potential for human infections cannot be dismissed when determining the treatment plan, and a clear understanding and acceptance by the owner of the public health risks and required control measures must be assured. Important aspects that need to be considered include whether the owner can afford to attempt treatment of the animal (with no clear evidence of effective therapy and long-term treatment being required), whether they are committed to administer medications over a prolonged period of time, whether the disease is potentially treatable, the status of other household members with respect to TB infection or exposure, and the presence of risk factors for serious disease in people in the household (e.g., HIV/AIDS). Prompt euthanasia may be reasonable in many cases because of the public health risk, severity of disease, and/or inability to implement adequate preventive measures. If treatment is attempted, there are no clear guidelines to follow. The use of monotherapy is

not recommended because of the potential for the presence or emergence of antimicrobial resistance. Isoniazid, rifampin, ethambutol, and pyrazinamide are possible options,[533] with a combination of isoniazid, rifampin, and ethambutol having been recommended for dogs.[593] Long-term therapy (6–12 months) may be required, and if there is no commitment and financial ability from owners to pursue a proper treatment course, euthanasia should be elected.

Humans

Clinical presentation

Early infection is asymptomatic, and the onset of clinical disease may be slow and insidious. Fever, weight loss, chills, cough, and night sweats are typical signs that develop with pulmonary TB.[24] Cough is usually productive, and hemoptysis may develop with advanced disease.[596] Extrapulmonary manifestations include meningitis, lymphadenitis, septic arthritis, and osteomyelitis.[24] Any organ can potentially be affected. No signs or symptoms are apparent with latent TB infection.

Diagnosis

Isolation of M. tuberculosis from sputum or other body fluids (e.g., bronchial fluids, gastric aspirates, pleural fluid, CSF, urine) is the most common method of diagnosis.[24,604] Sputum testing is relatively insensitive.[604] Typically, testing of two or three consecutive (daily) morning sputum samples is recommended.[24,596] Isolation of M. tuberculosis requires specialized laboratories and patience, since detection may take weeks.[24] Rapid testing methods are therefore desirable. PCR can be used for the detection of M. tuberculosis from respiratory tract samples, but available tests are not as accurate for other specimens. Acid-fast staining of samples can be a rapid test; however, it cannot differentiate TB from infection by other similar-appearing organisms. Enzyme-linked immunospot (ELISpot) testing of bronchoalveolar lavage (BAL) fluid has a good sensitivity and reasonable specificity (91% and 79%, respectively) for diagnosis of pulmonary TB.[605] Thoracic radiographs can be highly suggestive but not definitive.[596] Characteristic findings include a patchy or nodular infiltrate in the apical or subapical posterior areas of the upper lung lobes in the superior segment of a lower lung lobe.[596] Identification of cavities further strengthens suspicion of TB.

Tuberculin skin testing (TST) has been the most commonly used test to diagnose latent TB infection. Interferon gamma release assays (IGRAs) are now more widely available; however, consensus is lacking whether IGRAs should be primary tests or used to confirm positive TST results.[606,607] TST is not appropriate for the diagnosis of active disease as the test may be negative in approximately 20% of individuals with active TB.

Management

Prolonged antimicrobial therapy is required, with a minimum of 6 months' treatment of susceptible TB and 18 months for MDR TB.[604] Detailed treatment information is beyond the scope of this book, but combinations of isoniazid, rifampin, ethambutol, and pyrazinamide are commonly used.[24]

Prevention

The risk to humans from infected companion animals is unclear. Overall, the risks of zoonotic transmission are probably low, and risks to humans are probably much greater from the person who originally infected the pet than from the pet itself. While transmission from human-to-pet has been documented, subsequent pet-to-human transmission has not been reported. The potential for transmission certainly cannot be dismissed, and it is unclear whether lack of reports indicates minimal risk or minimal investigation. Accordingly, infected animals should be treated or euthanized. Maintaining a nontreated animal is highly questionable ethically because of the potential for ongoing exposure of people and other animals.

Since pets, particularly dogs, can release *M. tuberculosis* in respiratory secretions and droplets, care must be taken to reduce any possible risks, particularly when one considers the potential severity of human infection. Feces and vomitus can also be infectious. Therefore, infected animals should be handled with contact and respiratory precautions to reduce the risk of exposure. Close contact with infected animals, particularly coughing animals, should be prevented. Hand hygiene should be performed after every contact, and after contact with potentially contaminated items such as food and water bowls. Infected animals that are undergoing treatment should be isolated as much as possible from uninfected individuals. Contact with people or animals outside the household should be prevented. It is not known how long animals remain potentially infectious after the start of treatment.

Recommendations for management of exposed and subclinically infected animals are difficult to make. It is likely that the risk of transmission from a pet without a clinical infection is minimal;[593] however, there is inadequate information to state this with certainty. If *M. tuberculosis* infection is diagnosed (or suspected) in a pet, a prompt investigation of the status of household contacts is indicated because of the almost absolute association between infection in pets and the presence of an infected household individual.[599] Investigation of household (and other close) contacts for undiagnosed clinical infection as well as exposure is indicated. In humans, exposure is defined as contact in an enclosed environment for days or weeks, not minutes or hours, and this criterion is reasonable for contact with infected animals. Treatment is indicated for most persons found to be TST positive after contact with an infected human,[596] and it is reasonable to apply the same criteria to those in contact with an infected pet.

In households where humans have been diagnosed with TB, the pet should be evaluated to ensure that it is not concurrently actively infected. A pet with no signs of respiratory tract disease likely poses minimal risk; however, thoracic radiographs should be considered to provide an added degree of confidence. Tuberculin testing of exposed pets is not recommended because of the inconsistent nature of results. Sputum culture could be considered but is hard to justify in a clinically normal dog and would likely be of very low yield. General household infection control practices to reduce animal–human contact and to improve hygiene should be applied, as described above, to reduce the risk of human–animal infection. There is currently no indication that pets exposed to infected individuals should be treated prophylactically.

Veterinary personnel caring for, or performing necropsies on, infected animals must implement infection control practices to reduce the risk of infection. Contact and respiratory precautions are indicated. While the risk of transmission from veterinary patients is presumed to be much lower than that from human patients to human healthcare workers, the risk should not be assumed to be absent. A strong positive tuberculin reaction was identified in a person who necropsied an infected dog, suggesting that they were exposed during the procedure.[594] While it cannot be stated that there was no previous exposure, this finding supports the need for implementation of good routine infection control practices.

Pasteurella multocida

Introduction

P. multocida is a gram-negative coccobacillus that is commonly found in the oral cavity and intestinal tract of various animal species. It is an opportunistic pathogen that can cause disease in humans and animals. Most human infections are associated with exposure to dogs and cats. While bites are a common inciting factor, normal household interaction between people and their pets has also been associated with disease transmission. Other *Pasteurella* species such as *Pasteurella dagmatis* can also be involved,[608,609] but are less common.

Geographic distribution/epidemiology

P. multocida can be found in healthy animals worldwide. It has been isolated from dogs, cats, rabbits, and rats,[133,317,610] as well as noncompanion animals. Colonization rates are particularly high (up to 90%) in cats.[611]

Colonization of humans is uncommon, and most colonized individuals have underlying upper or lower respiratory tract disease and a history of contact with animals.[612]

Pathophysiology

Various types of contact with animals have been implicated in human infections. Bite infections are common, and *Pasteurella* spp. are the most commonly reported causes of cat-bite infections.[613] Infections can also occur secondary to other animal contact, such as scratches, licking open wounds and surgical incisions, or routine household contact.[614–616] Infection from a cat biting a person's dialysis tubing has been reported.[617] One review of the literature reported that 72% of *P. multocida* meningitis infections were associated with animal contact without bites,[618] while another reported that licking was the most common type of inciting contact in patients with meningitis.[619] However, it is unclear whether nonbite contacts are truly the most common source of infection because it is possible that bite-associated infections are not published since that route of infection is well known. Regardless, it is clear that contact with animals, be it bites, scratches, licks, or casual contact, can result in *P. multocida* transmission. A small percentage of infections have no known animal contact; however, it is possible that animal contact was unreported or animals were involved indirectly.

Infections appear to be most common in the very young, the elderly, immunocompromised people, and people undergoing dialysis.

Animals

Clinical infections are uncommon, and the vast majority of animals harboring *P. multocida* have no clinical abnormalities. Bite infections are the most common problems. The main exception is in rabbits where *P. multocida* is a leading cause of upper respiratory tract disease.[133]

Humans

Clinical presentation

Skin and soft tissue infections predominate, both from bites and other sources. These can range from mild, superficial infections to severe cellulitis, tenosynovitis, and abscessation. Cat bites may be more severe as their thin, pointed teeth can cause deep puncture wounds. Respiratory tract infections, including sinusitis, bronchitis, and pneumonia, can also develop.[620–622] Less commonly, septic arthritis, urinary tract infection, osteomyelitis, meningitis, necrotizing fasciitis, peritonitis, endocarditis, septicemia, and infections of other sites can be encountered.[608,614,615,623–625] Systemic infections are typically confined to very young or elderly individuals, immunocompromised individuals, or those with significant comorbidities.[608]

Diagnosis

Isolation of *P. multocida* from an infected site is relatively straightforward. Because this organism is not considered a normal inhabitant of humans, isolation is typically indicative of infection.

Management

Specific treatment will depend on the location of infection. Incision and drainage may be required for soft tissue abscesses. Antibiogram can guide antimicrobial selection, but penicillin or amoxicillin/clavulanic acid are typically highly effective.[617] Because bite infections are often polymicrobial, broad spectrum coverage with efficacy against staphylococci, streptococci, and anaerobes is indicated in the absence of culture results. The prognosis is excellent for skin and soft tissue infections, and other minor manifestations of disease. The prognosis is poorer for meningitis, septicemia, and endocarditis.

Prevention

Bite and scratch avoidance measures, as well as prompt and appropriate treatment following such incidents, are important. Antimicrobials expected to be effective against *P. multocida* should be used for postbite prophylaxis. There is no indication for screening of healthy animals for *P. multocida* colonization. Because it is a common commensal, it should be assumed that all companion animals are shedding the bacterium. Pets should not be allowed to have contact with wounds, surgical incisions, or skin lesions. Pets should not be allowed to lick peoples' faces and ears, especially young children[626] and individuals with a nonintact tympanic membrane.[627] Decolonization therapy is not indicated to attempt to eradicate *P. multocida*, either prophylactically or following infection of a human

contact. There is no evidence that decolonization therapy could be effective, and there is no indication that it is needed. Measures to reduce exposure, particularly to high-risk individuals, should be the focus of preventive measures. Direct or indirect contact of a pet's oral secretions with nonintact skin must be avoided, and good hygiene measures should be used for all pet–human contacts. Particular attention to good general hygiene measures should be taken by people in contact with infants because of reports of serious infection such as septicemia and meningitis in infants in the absence of bites, scratches, or licks,[616,628] suggesting indirect transmission through other people. Considering the disproportionately large number of reports of disease in dialysis patients,[614,617,629] extra care should also be taken by this population. Animals should not have contact with invasive devices and associated instruments such as dialysis tubing.[617]

There is no evidence that contact with an animal with a clinical *P. multocida* infection carries more risk for zoonotic transmission than contact with clinically healthy animal; however, it is prudent to use appropriate barriers and hygiene measures to reduce the risk of transmission from infected sites.

Plesiomonas shigelloides

This gram-negative bacterium is an infrequent cause of acute diarrhea in people. It typically causes mild self-limited diarrhea but can cause severe, bloody, mucoid diarrhea. Disease is most common in children less than 2 years of age.[630] Infections in adults are often associated with ingestion of raw shellfish.[631] Extraintestinal infections can occur, mainly in immunocompromised individuals.[632,633] This bacterium is predominantly associated with water and soil environments and is quite common in the intestinal tract of aquatic animals.[634,635] Infection is via the fecal–oral route, predominantly through ingestion of contaminated water or food.

Its role in enteric disease of animals is currently unclear. It has been implicated as a pathogen in cats,[636,637] but evidence is limited. Studies have reported isolation of *P. shigelloides* from 4% to 8% of healthy dogs and 10% of healthy cats.[630,634] There is presumably significant geographic variation in the prevalence of colonization of pets.

Concern has been raised about dogs and cats as a possible source of infection because similar strains have been found in humans and animals.[634,638] Reptiles may also be a source of infection, and infection of a zoo worker who handled a sick snake has been reported.[639] However, other evidence for zoonotic transmission from companion animals is currently minimal. Routine practices for handling feces and animals should be adequate to greatly reduce any risk. These include avoiding contact with animal feces, careful attention to hand hygiene after direct or indirect contact with feces, and hand hygiene after contact with animals (especially diarrheic animals).

Rat-bite fever

Introduction

Rat-bite fever is a syndrome associated with two different bacteria: *Streptobacillus moniliformis* and *Spirillum minus*. Infections are primarily associated with bites or scratches from rats and other rodents. Because there are similarities in clinical presentation and often no identification of the causative agent, they are considered together. Both organisms are difficult to identify, so rat-bite fever may be underdiagnosed.

Etiology

S. moniliformis (previously referred to as *Streptothrix muris ratti*, *Nocardia muris*, and *Actinomyces muris ratti*, among others) is the sole member of the *Streptobacillus* genus and the most common cause of rat-bite fever in North America and Europe.[640] It is a pleomorphic, microaerophilic, gram-negative bacillus that requires specialized culture methods for growth. The difficulty in isolating this organism may result in underestimation of its role in disease. This bacterium is also the cause of Haverhill fever, which occurs following ingestion.

S. minus is a spiral-shaped gram-negative to gram-variable bacterium that is the most common cause of rat-bite fever in Asia. It cannot be cultured using artificial media, greatly limiting our under-

standing of the organism and perhaps its role in disease.

Geographic distribution/epidemiology

S. moniliformis can be found worldwide but is most commonly identified in rat-bite fever in North America.[641] This bacterium is a commensal of rats and many other rodents, and can be found in the nasopharynx or inner ear of up to 100% of healthy wild and laboratory rats.[640,642] Wild mice are not generally considered to be natural hosts of *S. moniliformis*; however, there have been reports of rat-bite fever following mouse bites,[643,644] and *S. moniliformis* was isolated from wild mice on a farm in Australia.[645]

Transmission is predominantly via bites and scratches of rats and other rodents, though a history of a bite or scratch is not always present.[646,647] Infections have been reported following handling of rats[646] or through skin lesions.[648] Fatal infection developed following a minor superficial finger wound from a contaminated cage.[649] Rat-bite fever has also been reported following bites from a gerbil and ferret, as well as noncompanion animal species.[640,650] *S. moniliformis* DNA can be found in the mouths of dogs that have had contact with rats,[651] and dog bite-associated transmission has been suspected in a small number of cases.[252,644] Close contact with rats such as kissing and sharing food has also been implicated in disease transmission.[652,653]

The epidemiology of rat-bite fever from *S. minus* is similar, with most infections caused by rat bites. *S. minus* can be isolated from the oropharynx of 25–100% of wild rats, depending on the geographic region.[654] Little is known about other animal sources of *S. minus*. It is unclear whether that is because rats are the sole or main host, or because of the difficulty identifying *S. minus* and correspondingly little investigation. Infection from ingestion of the organism does not occur.

Children appear to be at greatest risk of rat-bite fever.[655,656] It is unclear whether this relates to inherently increased susceptibility or a greater likelihood of exposure. People that work with rodents, have rodents as pets, or live in areas with high wild rodent populations are also at increased risk.

Animals

Clinical presentation

S. moniliformis is a nonpathogenic commensal in rats. It has been associated with chronic joint abscess formation in wild mice on a single farm,[645] as well as sepsis, multifocal abscessation, polyarthritis, and nephritis in laboratory mice.[657,658] It can also cause disease in guinea pigs.[640]

Diagnosis

Identification of *S. moniliformis* in animals is difficult because of the fastidious nature of the organism and specialized culture conditions that are required. Given the high prevalence of colonization of rats, and potentially other rodents, and the difficulty in testing, there is little reason to attempt to isolate the organism apart from a situation where investigation of the source of human infection is being performed.

For both organisms, molecular methods may facilitate screening, but there are few situations when screening of rodents would be indicated.

Management

There is no indication to treat known or suspected carriers of *S. moniliformis* or *S. minus*.[659] No information is available regarding the efficacy or need for decolonization therapy. Considering the typical difficulties encountered in eradicating a commensal from its normal body site, decolonization therapy would likely be ineffective.

Humans

Clinical presentation

The clinical presentation varies between the two causative agents. For *S. moniliformis*, disease usually develops 2–3 days after exposure, although in some cases, the incubation period may be greater than 3 weeks.[640] An abrupt onset of a high fever (which may be relapsing), headache, chills, vomiting, severe migratory arthalgia, and myalgia are common initially.[641] A few days later, a nonpruritic maculopapular, morbilliform, petechial, vesicular, or pustular rash erupts, most commonly over the soles, palms, and extremities. Severe diarrhea may develop, particularly in children.[655] Polyarthritis develops in 50–70% of affected individuals. This most commonly involves the knees, followed by the ankles, elbows, wrists, shoulders, and hip. There is no ulceration at the site of inoculation and no regional lymphadenopathy. Fever usually resolves spontaneously within 3–5 days, and the remaining symptoms resolve within 2 weeks. Occasionally, relapsing fever and arthritis may be encountered. Uncommonly, complications such as endocarditis, myocarditis, pericarditis, meningitis, pneumonia, amnionitis, and anemia, as well as abscesses of virtually any body site, will develop. Haverhill fever, which occurs following ingestion, is more likely to present with severe vomiting and to have an associated pharyngitis.

Despite being considered together with *S. moniliformis*, rat-bite fever caused by *S. minus* is somewhat different clinically. The bite wound usually heals initially, but in contrast with *S. moniliformis*, 1–4 weeks later, the site becomes painful, swollen, and purple, and regional lymphadenopathy develops. The skin lesion often subsequently ulcerates.[641] Development of the skin lesion is accompanied by fever, chills, headache, and malaise, but rarely arthritis and myalgia. During the first week of fever, a rash erupts over the face, scalp, trunk, and extremities. The rash fades during afebrile periods. In untreated individuals, a relapsing fever for a duration of 3–4 days occurs with intervening afebrile periods of 3–9 days.[641] As with *S. moniliformis*, serious sequalae such as endocarditis, myocarditis, and other complications can develop but are rare.

Diagnosis

Collection of a thorough history is critical as initial signs may be dismissed as a benign viral infection, particularly with *S. moniliformis* infection. Presumptive diagnosis is often made based on clinical signs and a history of a rat bite. In patients with fever and a history of a rat bite, the two main differential diagnoses are rat-bite fever and leptospirosis.[641]

Direct identification of pleomorphic bacteria on smears from blood or infected sites is suggestive of *S. moniliformis* infection, particularly when no organisms are isolated using routine culture methods. Specific culture for *S. moniliformis* can be performed using enriched media and microaero-philic conditions; however, this may not be readily available. PCR is a more promising technique[660] but not widely available for routine diagnostic testing. Serological testing is available, but its role in clinical diagnosis is unclear.

Diagnosis of *S. minus* infection is difficult because of the inability to isolate the organism. Diagnosis involves the identification of spirochetes in blood or samples from infected sites, typically using Giemsa staining.[641] Serological testing is not available. PCR could be a useful tool but is not widely available.

Management

Penicillin is the drug of choice for both *S. monili-formis* and *S. minus*. Oral tetracycline is recommended for patients with penicillin allergy, although other drugs such as erythromycin, chloramphenicol, and ceftriaxone may be effective. Typically, response to therapy is good with resolution of most symptoms in 5–7 days. Endocarditis is a concern and is uniformly lethal without antimicrobial therapy.[641] The prognosis is reasonable with prompt institution of therapy; however, the optimal treatment for endocarditis is not known because of the rarity of disease and lack of objective study. Untreated *S. minus* infections usually resolve within 1–2 months, but relapsing fevers may continue for years.[661]

Overall, rat-bite fever has a mortality rate of 7–10% in untreated patients.[659]

Prevention

Bites from wild and pet rodents are the cause of the vast majority of infections, and the most important preventive measure is reducing bites. Wild rodent control should be used to reduce the risk of rodents living in or around houses and subsequent exposure of people or pet rodents. Control measures involving pet rodents largely involve proper socialization and handling to reduce the risk of bites. Particular attention should be paid to children because of the apparent overrepresentation of children in rat-bite fever cases. Any rodent bite should be thoroughly cleaned. Prophylactic therapy with oral penicillin might be useful;

however, the efficacy and need for this is unknown. Educating patients about signs of rat-bite fever and ensuring that prompt treatment is provided if signs consistent with the disease are identified may be as useful. It is also possible that infection could occur when cleaning rat cages if wounds are present on the hands,[640] so cages should be regularly inspected for sharp edges that could cause injuries and gloves should be worn over any skin lesions when cleaning cages or handling rats. Close contact with a rat's oral microflora, such as through kissing or sharing food, should be avoided. Hands should be washed after handling rats or having contact with their environment to reduce the risk of oral infection (Haverhill fever).

Screening of healthy rats is not indicated. Failure to identify either causative agent would not indicate a lack of risk because of limited information about optimal screening methods and the potential for false-negative results. Similarly, as a common commensal, it would not be surprising to find one of these bacteria in healthy rats. Certainly, removal of a positive rat from the household would not be indicated because of the high prevalence of colonization but low incidence of disease. Even in situations where rat-bite fever has been diagnosed in a person, screening of pet rats is unlikely to be rewarding, beyond testing to determine the source of infection if there were multiple different potential sites of exposure. There is no evidence indicating that decolonization therapy is needed or potentially effective, and treatment of colonized rats is not recommended.

Rickettsia felis

R. felis is an intracellular flea-borne pathogen that causes flea-borne spotted fever (cat flea rickettsiosis) in people. Microbiologically, it is classified in the spotted fever group, along species such as *Rickettsia rickettsii* (the cause of Rocky Mountain spotted fever [RMSF]) and *Rickettsia typhi* (murine typhus), but clinically, it can be indistinguishable with both spotted fever group and typhus group (*Rickettsia prowazekii*, *R. typhi*) infections.[662] *R. felis* is transmitted by the cat flea (*Cterocephalides felis*) and has been found in *C. felis* in countries in five continents, including the United States, Mexico, Brazil, Chile, Algeria, Portugal, Israel, Spain,

Australia, New Zealand, and South Korea.[662,663] It may be common in fleas in some regions, as evidenced by a study reporting detection of *R. felis* DNA in 36% of *C. felis* pools from California.[664] There are also occasional reports of detection of *R. felis* from other potential flea and tick vectors such as *Ctenocephalides canis*, *Xenopsylla cheopsis*, *R. sanguineus*, and *Ixodes ovatus*;[662] however, *C. felis* is the only recognized vector as it is the only species that has been shown to be able to maintain infected progeny through transovarial transmission.[665] Opossums are suspected as being a reservoir host in some regions,[662] but considering the wide international distribution of *R. felis*, other reservoir hosts are likely present. *R. felis* has been found on fleas from various animal species internationally, including cats, dogs, wild rodents, monkeys, hedgehogs, and a horse.[662] Studies of seroprevalence of cats in the United States have reported rates of 8–11%.[36,666] The prevalence in dogs is less clear because of minimal study and cross-reaction with other *Ricksettsia*, but a study from Spain reported that serum samples from 16% of dogs reacted only against *R. felis*, suggesting that exposure may be common, at least in some regions.[667] It is unclear if *R. felis* is a pathogen in domestic animals, and experimental infection of cats failed to produce any clinical abnormalities.[668]

Since it was first recognized in 1990,[669] human infections have been reported in the United States (Texas and California), Mexico, Brazil, France, Spain, Germany, Thailand, Laos, and Tunisia.[662,663,670–672] It is suspected that the disease is present worldwide wherever *C. felis* is present. The incidence of disease is unknown, and it is possible that some cases are misdiagnosed as murine typhus (*R. typhi*), RMSF (*R. rickettsii*), or typhus (*R. prowazekii*) in areas where both diseases may be present.[663,664]

Human infections can occur following a bite from an infected flea. Despite the name, *C. felis* is not cat specific and readily infests dogs and rodents, so lack of history of exposure to potential wildlife reservoirs or cats does not result in dismissing the possibility of *R. felis* infection. Infections are usually relatively mild and characterized by fever, myalgia, headache, and skin lesions.[663] A maculopapular rash is typical for ricksettsiosis and is usually present,[673] but skin lesions more similar to rickettsial pox (*Rickettsia akari* infection) have

also been reported.[674] Other signs such as abdominal pain, vomiting, neurological abnormalities (meningitis, photophobia, hearing loss), hepatitis, and pulmonary disease may also be present.[662,671,674] Severe infections requiring hospitalization are uncommon but have been reported.[663]

Diagnosis can be difficult. Culture is extremely difficult and unlikely to be successful outside of specialized laboratories. Serology can be performed, but cross-reaction among various *Rickettsia* is common. Serology can provide an indication that rickettsial disease is likely but not identify the specific agent. PCR can be more specific, although some assays may require subsequent enzyme restriction, sequencing, or hybridization to differentiate *R. felis* from related species like *R. typhi*.[664]

Short-term treatment of infected humans with doxycycline is the most common approach for rickettsial disease.[675] A single dose may be adequate.

The role of pets as a source of human disease is unclear. *R. felis* cannot be transmitted directly between animals and humans. It requires a bite from an infected flea. However, pets could be sources of infected fleas. Dogs and cats do not need to be infected with *R. felis* to play an indirect role in human disease, as they could be a host for fleas that had been infected (or whose ancestors had been infected) by feeding on an infected reservoir host. The ability of the organism to be maintained in cat fleas for up to 12 generations without feeding on another infected host supports concern for this delayed, indirect route. Inter-cat transmission via infected fleas has been reported,[668] giving further support to the potential for indirect cat–human transmission via infected fleas. However, there is no objective information regarding the potential for cats to act as sources of human infection. In the absence of definitive evidence, it is reasonable to consider cats infected with *C. felis* as a potential, albeit likely low, source of human infection. The risks are presumably higher in areas where *R. felis* has been diagnosed in humans. Cats that have outdoor access are at greater risk of flea exposure and a greater likelihood of encountering fleas infected by wildlife reservoirs.

Prevention of animal and human infections involves flea avoidance and flea control, as is discussed elsewhere.

Rickettsia rickettsii

R. rickettsii is the cause of RMSF, a regionally important and potentially life-threatening tick-borne disease. RMSF is a disease of the Americas that occurs throughout much of the United States, along with areas of western Canada, Mexico, Central America, Colombia, Argentina, and Brazil.[364] *R. rickettsii* is primarily transmitted by *D. andersoni* (wood tick) and *D. variabilis* (American dog tick).[364] *A. americanum* (lone star tick) and *R. sanguineus* (brown dog tick) may also be involved.[364] Ticks can become infected from feeding off infected reservoir hosts (rodents, small mammals, birds), as well as through horizontal or venereal transmission.[364] Ticks can infect incidental hosts such as humans and companion animals during feeding; however, they must be attached for a minimum of 5–20 hours for transmission to occur.[364,676]

Disease in humans and companion animals is typically vague, particularly early in the disease. Upper respiratory tract signs and symptoms are commonly present. A rash is a classical finding with RMSF; however, it does not develop in all infected individuals and is present in the first 3 days of illness in less than 50% of people.[364,676] Therefore, clinical suspicion of RMSF may be low early in disease, particularly in the absence of reported exposure to ticks in an endemic area. Neurological disease, along with hepatic and renal involvement, may develop, along with other severe manifestations such as meningoencephalitis, myocarditis, gangrene, and DIC.[364,676] Mortality rates in humans are 1.4–4%,[677,678] with higher rates in children. Untreated, mortality rates are much higher,[677] with rates among the highest for any tick-borne disease. Prompt treatment is important as a main prognostic factor is timeliness of appropriate treatment.[676]

There is no risk of transmission of *R. rickettsii* directly from infected animals to people, since ticks are required for natural transmission. Pets pose two main potential risks with respect to RMSF. One is as a source of infected ticks. Pets could carry infected ticks into the household, and ticks could subsequently leave the dog and attach to a human host. Another potential risk is human exposure to infectious hemolymph when removing infected ticks, since there is the potential for human exposure through contact of mucous membranes or nonintact skin if ticks are crushed during removal.[676,679] The greatest relevance of pets and RMSF may be as a sentinel of exposure, since pets and humans could encounter infected ticks in the same environment.[680] This was demonstrated by a situation where two dogs died of RMSF, and their owner developed a fatal RMSF infection 2 weeks after the death of the second dog.[680]

Prevention of RMSF involves tick avoidance, regular inspection for ticks, careful removal of ticks, and use of tick control medication. These are covered in more detail in Chapter 1. Careful examination of people and pets for ticks is important in endemic regions, particularly after walking in high-risk areas (e.g., wooded areas). Because ticks require 5–20 hours to transmit *R. rickettsii*, regular and careful examination for ticks, followed by proper removal of any identified ticks, should be a highly effective preventive measure. Care should be taken to avoid crushing the tick during examination and removal, and direct contact with the tick should be avoided. If skin lesions are present on the hands, gloves should be worn. Hands should be washed after removing ticks or after contact with ticks on animals.

Identification of RMSF in a pet should lead to consideration of the potential for human exposure. People developing early signs of disease that could be attributable to RMSF should ensure that they receive prompt medical attention and that their physician is informed about the potential exposure. Conversely, RMSF should be considered in pets whose owners have been diagnosed with RMSF.

Salmonella spp.

Introduction

Salmonella is a broad genus containing a range of serovars that can cause enteric and multisystem disease in humans and animals. Human salmonellosis is most commonly associated with foodborne infection, but transmission of *Salmonella* from pets can occur. The risk is greatest with reptiles, but zoonotic transmission involving various other animal species has been documented.

Etiology

Salmonellae are gram-negative enteric bacteria that are normally found in a wide range of mammals, reptiles, amphibians, birds, and insects. They are opportunistic pathogens that can be found in a variable percentage of healthy individuals, depending on the animal species and associated risk factors.

Salmonella enterica subspecies *enterica* comprises the majority of over 2400 serotypes that are currently known. Serotypes in this subspecies predominantly infect and colonize mammals and birds. Some *Salmonella* serotypes are host adapted, preferring or solely infecting an individual species. *Salmonella* Typhi, *Salmonella* Paratyphi, and *Salmonella* Sendai are host adapted for humans and do not infect other species, but most serotypes show little host adaptation and can infect a broad range of species. *Salmonella* can survive for long periods of time in the environment. Antimicrobial resistance has emerged as a serious problem, and MDR *Salmonella* can be isolated from companion animals.[681–685] While inherently no more virulent than susceptible *Salmonella*, antimicrobial-resistant strains are a concern because of the treatment difficulties that may be encountered in situations when antimicrobial therapy is indicated.

Geographic distribution/epidemiology

Salmonella spp. can be found in humans and animals worldwide. Typhoid fever, caused by *S.* Typhi and *S.* Paratyphi is a global health problem but is nonzoonotic and relates solely to direct or indirect human–human transmission. The incidence of nontyphoidal salmonellosis appears to be increasing in many countries, with an estimated doubling of cases in the United States over the past two decades.[686] Approximately 1.4 million cases are estimated to occur annually in the United States.[687] Transmission is by the fecal–oral route. Most cases of salmonellosis are foodborne, through ingestion of live salmonellae in contaminated food products.

Most recent studies indicate that *Salmonella* is uncommonly present in healthy dogs, being identified in only 0–2.9% of household pet or shelter dogs[215,317,688–691] and 6.3% of stray dogs.[691] Much higher rates can be identified in dogs fed raw meat,[692,693] and *Salmonella* shedding was 23 times as likely in pet therapy dogs fed raw meat compared with non-raw-meat-fed dogs.[694] Contamination of raw meat intended for pet feeding is common (5.9–80%),[692,695–697] and eating a single meal of *Salmonella*-contaminated meat can result in fecal shedding for up to 1 week in healthy dogs.[698]

Colonization rates are also low (0.4–1.7%) in healthy cats.[219,683,699] Outdoor cats may have higher colonization rates from ingestion of colonized or infected birds, particularly songbirds. There has been less investigation of the impact of raw meat feeding on cats, but presumably this practice is associated with more frequent colonization. Colonization of dogs and cats is transient, and natural elimination of *Salmonella* over a relatively short period of time (a few weeks) is expected. Long-term or persistent colonization should not occur, and repeated isolation of *Salmonella* from a dog or cat likely indicates repeated exposure as opposed to persistent infection.

Colonization rates are much higher in various reptile species, with up to 75% reported in a study of pet turtles.[700] Multiple *Salmonella* strains can be found in the same individual.[701] *Salmonella* can be isolated from reptile housing environments, including water.[702] Reptiles can shed the bacterium intermittently, a factor that complicates testing, and can be found at various body sites. *Salmonella* can be found in a small percentage (1.6–2.7%) of healthy pet birds.[703,704] Less is known about other domestic species, and some exotic species have been identified as commonly carrying *Salmonella*, such as the 28% rate reported in pygmy hedgehogs.[705] *Salmonella* can be isolated from a small percentage (0.4%) of fish aquaria.[704]

Zoonotic infections have been reported in association with various pet species. Reptiles are the greatest concern, and large numbers of zoonotic infections occur each year. One report estimated 74,000 reptile- or amphibian-associated salmonellosis cases in the United States per year.[706] Another study reported that 14% of all nontyphoidal salmonellosis cases were caused by reptiles.[707] Numerous outbreaks have been attributed to contact with small turtles,[708–710] typically involving young children. Overrepresentation of children less than 1 year of age has been reported for reptile-associated salmonellosis.[711] Infections have been associated with numerous other reptiles such as iguanas, snakes, and bearded dragons. Contact with reptiles was identified as a risk factor in a study of sporadic *Salmonella* infections in infants.[712] Infections have occurred in household members that reported no contact with reptiles or their environment, despite finding the same *Salmonella* strain in both the person and animal, suggesting that indirect transmission from other family members or contamination of the general household environment can also occur.[702] Life-threatening infections can be encountered.[713] Outbreaks have also occurred from handling contaminated frozen rodents sold as snake food.[714,715] Pet rodents, including rats, mice, and hamsters can also be sources of infection.[716,717]

Transmission of *Salmonella* from dogs and cats to people can occur in households, shelters, and veterinary clinics. One investigation of outbreaks in three veterinary clinics and one shelter identified 18 human infections.[685] Outbreaks of salmonellosis have been linked to people handling *Salmonella*-contaminated raw animal-based treats like pig ears.[718,719] Concerns are also present about exposure to *Salmonella* from raw pet food diets, although human infections have not been documented. Outbreaks of human and pet salmonellosis have been associated with contact with contaminated dry pet foods.[720–722]

Other species may also be involved, with human infections reported in association with uncommon pets such as pygmy hedgehogs and sugar gliders.[723–725] Pygmy hedgehogs should be considered high-risk animals based on the number of reports of human infection compared with the relative rarity of these animals in households.

Exposure is through the ingestion of *Salmonella*. The infectious dose is likely highly variable and depends on both bacterial and host factors. Approximately 10^6 bacteria was the median dose required to cause disease in a study of healthy human volunteers;[686] however, some outbreaks have been associated with ingestion of much lower numbers. Variation in infectious dose likely involves numerous factors such as gastric acidity, the endogenous microflora, and the immune response. In particular, persons with HIV/AIDS are at much greater (20- to 100-fold) risk of salmonellosis.[726] Reduction of the gastric acid barrier

may be an important risk factor, and proton pump inhibitor administration was implicated in one case of repeated turtle-associated salmonellosis in an immunocompetent adult.[727] Immunocompromise and old age are associated with increased risk of extraintestinal infections.[728,729] Immunocompromise or underlying chronic disease are associated with increased mortality.[730]

Animals

Clinical presentation

Most animals that have *Salmonella* in their intestinal tracts do not have any signs of disease. In dogs, salmonellosis can range from mild self-limited diarrhea to severe hemorrhagic gastroenteritis and septicemia. Young and old dogs are most commonly affected, and fever, vomiting, diarrhea, abdominal pain, and lethargy are common.[731] Diarrhea may be mucoid, watery, or hemorrhagic, and the character of diarrhea cannot indicate or rule out salmonellosis. In severe cases, dehydration, toxemia, hypovolemia shock, and septicemia may be present. Death is uncommon but can occur with severe cases. Disease is similar in cats. Hypersalivation may also be present in this species, associated with vomiting. Clinical signs are presumably similar in other companion animal species that develop salmonellosis, but many species (especially reptiles) rarely or never develop clinical infections. After resolution of clinical infection, dogs and cats tend to shed *Salmonella* for a short period of time, up to 8 weeks in some cases. Long-term or persistent colonization postinfection is not recognized.

Diagnosis

Isolation of *Salmonella* from feces is the standard for the diagnosis of salmonellosis. Isolation of the bacterium from blood or other sterile body sites is diagnostic for invasive infections. The sensitivity of single fecal samples is unknown and is likely variable. Isolation of *Salmonella* from feces requires the use of enrichment and selective media, and an appropriate laboratory is important. Fecal samples are believed to be superior to rectal swabs because of the larger amount of fecal material available for enrichment culture. The number of samples required is unknown. In horses, five serial negative samples are considered the standard for declaring a horse "*Salmonella* free." It is unknown whether this applies to other species. It is likely that single samples do not provide optimal sensitivity and that multiple samples would be more effective. The number of samples required and the true benefit of testing multiple samples are unclear. PCR testing is becoming more widely available and may offer improvements in sensitivity and turnaround time. However, validation of PCR for the detection of *Salmonella* is currently lacking, and the efficacy of such testing is unclear. Increased sensitivity may be useful but could be problematic if PCR is able to detect very low (and perhaps clinically irrelevant) levels of *Salmonella* in feces or DNA from dead salmonellae passing through the intestinal tract. There is potential for PCR to be a useful diagnostic tool; however, further test evaluation is needed.

Management

Treatment is restricted to management of clinical salmonellosis. There is no indication to treat healthy carriers. There is no evidence that antimicrobials are effective for eradication of *Salmonella* colonization, and there is evidence that colonization is transient. Antimicrobial treatment could also increase the risk of antimicrobial resistance and antimicrobial-associated diarrhea, and is not recommended. Attempts made by turtle breeders to produce "*Salmonella*-free" turtles through the use of antimicrobials have just resulted in production of turtles carrying antimicrobial-resistant *Salmonella*.

Management of salmonellosis depends on the nature and severity of disease. In mild cases, close observation for dehydration and other consequences of diarrhea and anorexia may be adequate. Fluid therapy may be indicated in more severe or prolonged cases, with possible need for adjunctive therapy such as nutritional support and colloids. Antimicrobial use in salmonellosis is controversial. There is no evidence that antimicrobials are effective against enteric salmonellae or that they decrease the severity or duration of diarrhea. Antimicrobials, if used, are directed against systemic manifestations of salmonellosis to prevent or treat bacteremia and secondary infections such as arthritis, meningitis, and pneumonia, which are rare, especially in immunocompetent adult animals. Antimicrobials are not typically recommended in dogs and cats with uncomplicated gastroenteritis but may be indicated in animals with severe disease, as well as young and old animals, immunosuppressed animals, or animals with significant comorbidities. Drug choice should be based on *in vitro* susceptibility testing.

Humans

Clinical presentation

Gastroenteritis is the most common clinical manifestation of salmonellosis. Severity of disease is variable and similar to disease caused by many other enteropathogens. Typically, nausea, vomiting, and diarrhea are present.[686] Diarrhea may be of variable character and volume, and sometimes includes blood. Fever, abdominal cramping, malaise, headache, and chills may be present concurrently.[686] Diarrhea is usually self-limited in otherwise healthy individuals, lasting 3–7 days.[686] Fever usually resolves within 48 hours. Bacteremia can occur and be intermittent or sustained. This can lead to extraintestinal infections of virtually any body site, particularly heart valves, CNS, bone, joints, and urinary tract.[686]

Diagnosis

Gastrointestinal salmonellosis is diagnosed by isolation of *Salmonella* spp. from feces.[24] Extraintestinal infections are diagnosed by isolation of *Salmonella* from blood, urine, or any other infected body site.[24] Determination of whether the patient has typhoidal (human source) or nontyphoidal (likely food or animal source) salmonellosis is important.

Management

Salmonellosis is usually self-limited, and treatment is directed at replacement of fluid and electrolyte losses, when needed.[686] The use of antimicrobials in uncomplicated disease in low-risk individuals has been controversial. A meta-analysis indicated that antimicrobial treatment did not have any positive effect on length of illness but was associated with increased risk of relapse, prolonged isolation of *Salmonella* from feces, and adverse drug reactions.[732] Accordingly, antimicrobials are not indicated for the treatment of uncomplicated *Salmonella* gastroenteritis.[24,686] Antimicrobials should be considered in people at increased risk of invasive infection, including neonates, people older than 50 years of age, immunosuppressed individuals, and people with cardiac valvular or endovascular abnormalities (including prosthetic vascular grafts).[686]

Treatment of extraintestinal infections depends on the site of infection. Prolonged antimicrobial therapy or surgical intervention may be required.

Prevention

Exposure to *Salmonella* is an inherent risk of contact with animals because any animal could be shedding *Salmonella* at any time. However, the prevalence of shedding is low for most animal species, and good general infection control practices, particularly routine hand hygiene, avoiding contact with feces, and preventing contact of pets with food and food preparation or storage areas should reduce the risks. Other specific preventive measures vary with the animal species.

Reptiles

All reptiles should be considered to be *Salmonella* carriers. There is no known way to declare a reptile *Salmonella* free, and screening of reptiles is not recommended. Antimicrobial treatment is not indicated to attempt to eradicate colonization. Children under 5 years of age and other high-risk individuals (elderly, pregnant, immunocompromised) should avoid all contact with reptiles. Reptiles should not be kept in households with these individuals, regardless of how the animals are housed or managed. One cannot confidently prevent direct or indirect contact, as evidenced by infections in people with no contact with reptiles or their enclosures.[702] Small turtles should be avoided in all households with children. Small turtles are easily handled by children and may be put into their mouths or kissed. The sale of turtles with a shell length of less than 4 in. was (still at the time of

writing) banned in the United States, but small turtles are still readily available in that country, as well as other countries without such a ban. Careful attention should be paid to hand hygiene. Contact with reptile enclosures should be restricted and associated with good hygiene practices. Children should never be allowed to play in, or have contact with, reptile enclosures, as there are anecdotal reports of salmonellosis in children from such exposure. Allowing reptiles to roam freely around the house likely increases the risk of environmental contamination and exposure, and is not recommended.

Because salmonellosis has been associated with contact with frozen rodents sold as snake food, care should be taken when handling them. Frozen rodents should be stored in a sealed container if they are stored in a freezer containing human food. They should be defrosted in a sealed container on the bottom shelf of a refrigerator or, ideally, in a small refrigerator used only for reptile food. Contact with kitchen surfaces should be avoided. Any areas that might have been contaminated should be promptly cleaned and disinfected. Hands should be washed immediately after contact with rodents.

Care should be taken around aquatic reptiles. Aquaria should have covered tops to prevent inadvertent contact with water. Pets such as cats should never be allowed to drink from aquaria. Aquarium water should not be dumped down kitchen or bathroom sinks or bathtubs. Any water spills should be promptly cleaned, and hands should be washed after cleaning aquaria or having any contact with water or other contents.

Dogs and cats

Because of the strong association between feeding raw meat and *Salmonella* shedding (and less clear risk of salmonellosis) in pets, this feeding practice should be discouraged. It is particularly important to discourage this when there are high-risk people or animals (young or elderly, immunocompromised, pregnant, significant comorbidities) in the household. If raw meat products are fed, careful attention must be paid to reduce the risk of inadvertent exposure. Raw meat for animal use should be kept in a sealed, leak-proof container on the bottom shelf of the refrigerator, or ideally in a separate refrigerator. It should be prepared and handled as per food intended for human consumption with care to prevent cross-contamination of surfaces and human foods. Contact with raw meat should be avoided and hands washed after handling meat or anything that has been in contact with meat. Uneaten food should not be left in food bowls because of the potential for *Salmonella* growth and exposure of household members. Food bowls should be cleaned and disinfected regularly to prevent accumulation of biofilm and persistence of *Salmonella*. However, complete disinfection of *Salmonella*-contaminated bowls is very difficult. Stainless steel bowls without any scratches or other defects are preferable to plastic bowls.

While presumably of much lower risk, *Salmonella* contamination of dry (kibble) pet foods has been associated with human infection. High-risk individuals should avoid direct contact with pet foods and food bowls. Pets should not be fed in the kitchen. Hands should be washed after contact with pet food.

Cats should be kept inside to reduce the risk of exposure to *Salmonella* from wildlife, particularly songbirds. If cats are allowed outdoors, outdoor access should be restricted any time there are reports or evidence of songbird deaths, because outbreaks of salmonellosis are common in these birds and can result in exposure of cats. Houses with outdoor cats should not have bird feeders, to decrease the risk of exposure to birds (and to protect the birds from the cats).

If an infected or colonized dog or cat has been identified, careful attention to general hygiene practices and avoiding contact with feces is important. Close contact with the pet should be avoided, particularly contact with the perineum and areas that may have been stained with feces. Hands should be washed after contact with the animal and cleaning up feces.

Birds

While *Salmonella* shedding rates tend to be low in pet birds, basic measures such as proper cage cleaning and hand hygiene should be undertaken to reduce the risk of exposure to feces. Pet birds should not be allowed to have free access to kitchens or other food preparation, storage, or consumption areas.

Other species

Salmonella shedding rates are quite variable among other exotic species and are not well understood for many species. High rates have been reported for some animals, such as pygmy hedgehogs. In the absence of data regarding *Salmonella* carriage, it should be assumed that all exotic animals are potentially infectious and managed in that manner. Households with children under 5 years of age or with other high-risk individuals (elderly, pregnant, immunocompromised) should avoid these species.

Screening

Testing of animals for *Salmonella* carriage is not recommended. Screening offers little information that can be used for prevention of disease or assessment of risk. A negative result simply indicates the status of the individual on that day, with the added potential of a false-negative result. A positive sample also only reflects a single point in time, and *Salmonella* shedding is transient. Logical infection control decisions cannot be made on such an assessment. All reptiles should be considered *Salmonella* carriers, even with negative results. All other individuals could be carriers at any given time, and management practices should reflect that possibility.

Veterinary clinics

Routine isolation of all animals with potentially infectious diarrhea is a standard recommendation, along with handling such individuals using contact precautions. Consideration should be given to where dogs are walked to reduce the risk of exposure of other hospitalized patients or dogs from the general public. Personal hygiene, especially hand hygiene, should be emphasized. Colonized individuals should likely be handled in a similar manner, although it is unlikely that the *Salmonella* status of healthy animals would be known. Because the prevalence of *Salmonella* colonization in the general dog and cat population is so low, concerns about colonized animals mainly involves animals fed raw meat. Some veterinary hospitals routinely impose enhanced infection control precautions on all raw-fed animals. This can include isolation of all individuals, normal housing but use of contact precautions, and/or using a dedicated area to walk raw-fed dogs. Many veterinary hospitals prohibit the feeding of raw meat to hospitalized patients to reduce the risks of exposure of staff and other patients. Raw-animal-based treats should not be fed to hospitalized animals.

All reptiles should be considered *Salmonella* positive and handled with appropriate contact precautions and attention to hygiene.

Staphylococcus aureus

Introduction

S. aureus is an important opportunistic pathogen that has the ability to colonize and infect a wide range of species, including humans, other mammals, birds, and reptiles (Table 2.7). While it can be part of the commensal microflora, it is an important cause of disease in some species, particularly humans.

Etiology

S. aureus is a gram-positive bacterium that is a commensal and opportunistic pathogen in many species. It is a coagulase-positive *Staphylococcus*

species, the most important pathogenic *Staphylococcus* species in humans, and well adapted for colonization of mucosal and skin surfaces of various animal species.

S. aureus can possess a wide array of potential virulence factors, and the role that many of these play in the actual development of disease is variable. Some virulence factors facilitate adhesion to and colonization of host tissues. Others encode secreted enzymes and toxins that are responsible for invasion as well as local and distant disease. Special attention has been paid to a select group of toxins, particularly the Panton–Valentine leukocidin (PVL), which may have a role in severe methicillin-resistant *S. aureus* (MRSA) skin and soft tissue infections, as well as necrotizing fasciitis and necrotizing pneumonia in humans,[733–736] and toxic shock syndrome toxin-1 (TSST-1), which causes toxic shock syndrome.[737] *S. aureus* has an impressive ability to acquire resistance to antimicrobials. While naturally susceptible to virtually every antibiotic class ever developed, many *S. aureus* strains have become resistant to a range of antimicrobials. Of greatest concern is MRSA, which is resistant to virtually all beta-lactam antimicrobials (penicillins, cephalosporins, carbapenems) and often to a number of different antimicrobial classes. This is conferred by the presence of the *mecA* gene, a gene that encodes an altered penicillin-binding

Table 2.7 Comparison of *Staphylococcus* species.

Species	Main hosts	Zoonotic	Comments
S. aureus	Humans, less commonly dogs, cats	Yes	Emerging concerns with MRSA; may be more human–pet transmission
S. pseudintermedius	Dogs, less commonly cats	Uncommonly	Increasing reports of human infections but still very uncommon; human exposure and colonization may be common
S. schleiferi coagulans	Dogs, less commonly cats	Rare	Little evidence of zoonotic transmission
Coagulase-negative staphylococci	Humans, dogs, cats, other animals	Rare to no	Most are minimally pathogenic and common, and not a relevant zoonotic disease concern

protein (PBP2a) with low affinity to beta-lactam antimicrobials.

Geographic distribution/epidemiology

Humans

S. aureus is a common commensal in humans that can be found in the nasal passages of approximately 30% of healthy humans worldwide. It can also be found on the skin, and in the respiratory and gastrointestinal tracts. Three main colonization patterns are recognized: persistent colonization, intermittent colonization, and noncarriers. Persistently colonized individuals harbor *S. aureus* for prolonged periods of time, potentially lifelong. Intermittently colonized individuals frequently harbor *S. aureus* but regularly eliminate colonization and then become recolonized following subsequent exposure. Noncarriers appear to be refractory to colonization, and *S. aureus* is unable to establish itself in their nasal passages or elsewhere. Transient contamination of body sites, especially skin surfaces, can occur in all groups but does not represent colonization.

As is typical for an opportunistic pathogen, clinical *S. aureus* infections typically occur following breaks to the body's normal defenses, such as skin lesions, insertion of invasive devices, surgical incisions, and factors affecting the immune system. However, *S. aureus* infections also occur in the absence of recognizable risk factors.

Staphylococcal food poisoning can occur secondary to the growth of enterotoxin-producing strains of *S. aureus* in improperly handled or prepared food. This is of limited relevance in terms of zoonotic transmission from companion animals, although it is possible that colonized animals could be sources of enterotoxigenic *S. aureus* that could indirectly contaminate food.

MRSA is a tremendous problem in humans and has been for years. It has been stated that hospital-associated MRSA reached pandemic status in the 1980s and that the pandemic continues unabated.[738] It is a leading cause of hospital-associated infections internationally and has been estimated to result close to 100,000 invasive infections and over 18,000 deaths in the United States annually.[739] It has also emerged as an important cause of community-associated disease in people with no contact with the healthcare system and few or no identifiable risk factors for multidrug resistant (MDR) infection. Community-associated MRSA has reached epidemic proportions in many areas with infections ranging from skin and soft tissue infection to necrotizing fasciitis and necrotizing pneumonia. MRSA is the leading cause of community-associated skin and soft tissue infections in some areas. Community-associated MRSA infections are of particular concern for certain groups, including athletes, First Nations communities, military recruits, institutionalized individuals, men that have sex with men, IV drug users, and certain animal-contact groups.[734,740–742]

As with methicillin-susceptible *S. aureus*, MRSA is an opportunistic pathogen that can be found in healthy individuals. A small but apparently increasing percentage of the general population (0.8–3.3%) carry MRSA at any given time, predominantly in their nasal passages.[743–745] Colonized individuals do not have signs of disease and typically never develop an MRSA infection. In general, colonized individuals are not at higher risk of developing an infection except in certain situations such as when undergoing surgery. However, should they get an infection, they are at higher risk of it being an MRSA infection and thus more difficult to treat.[746,747] Colonized individuals may also transmit MRSA to other susceptible individuals. This large pool of colonized individuals allows for continuous circulation of MRSA in the population and complicates control measures.

Animals

While *S. aureus* is considered to be predominantly a human pathogen, it can be found in many animal species, including 12–14% of dogs and 4.3–20% of cats.[748–750] Whether *S. aureus* should truly be considered a commensal in those species is unclear. It is possible that isolation of *S. aureus* represents transient colonization or contamination acquired from humans, particularly in dogs where *Staphylococcus pseudintermedius* is the predominant coagulase-positive species. A study of dogs and their owners reported that in 50% of households where *S. aureus* was isolated from both a dog and family member, the *S. aureus* strains were indistinguishable, strongly suggesting interspecies transmission.[749] The situation with cats is less clear. Given the higher apparent prevalence of *S. aureus* in cats in some studies and the lack of another predominant commensal coagulase-positive *Staphylococcus* sp., it is possible that *S. aureus* is a true feline commensal though this is far from certain. Regardless, *S. aureus* can be found in a small but still appreciable percentage of healthy dogs and cats (and likely other companion animal species). Risk factors for colonization have not been adequately investigated, and may relate to human contact.

Much of the recent attention regarding *S. aureus* in dogs and cats has been focused on MRSA, both in terms of animal health and zoonotic disease. The emergence of MRSA in dogs and cats appears to be a direct reflection of MRSA in the human population, with MRSA infections in pets being noted after MRSA emerged as an important cause of disease in the general population and with MRSA strains from animals usually reflecting predominant humans strains.[318,751–756] Currently, MRSA can be isolated from 0% to 3.3% of healthy dogs and from 0% to 4% of healthy cats.[749–751,757–759] As opposed to the situation in humans, most MRSA cases in companion animals are community associated, although hospital-associated transmission can certainly occur.[755,760,761] Being owned by a human healthcare worker and participation in hospital visitation programs have been identified as risk factors for MRSA colonization in dogs and are logical based on the increased likelihood of exposure to colonized people.[318,752] Contact with children has also been identified as a risk factor.[318] While these, and potentially other, risk factors should be considered, MRSA can be identified in any animal and the absence of known risk factors should not lead to excluding MRSA from consideration. As with methicillin-susceptible *S. aureus*, colonized animals typically have no signs of infection and may never develop a clinical infection. In humans and horses, MRSA colonization is known to be a risk factor for clinical MRSA infection in certain circumstances (e.g., after admission to hospital).[746,762] It is reasonable to assume that this also applies to dogs and cats, though this is not yet proven.

An interesting aspect of MRSA in companion animals involves the types that are found. MRSA strains found in companion animals are typically those most prevalent in humans in their area.[752,755,756,760,763,764] This provides further support

to the hypothesis that MRSA in pets is a close reflection of MRSA in humans and that changes in MRSA in humans can be subsequently noted in pets. Recently, livestock-associated MRSA caused by sequence type 398 (ST398) MRSA has emerged as an important problem in people in some countries, particularly northern Europe.[765,766] This strain has also been identified in a small number of dogs.[767,768] Whether the small number of recently reported infections in pets indicates an expansion of the range of this strain or rare, aberrant infections is as of yet unclear.

MRSA has also been isolated from other companion animal species, including rabbits, reptiles, and pet birds.[769–771] Prevalence data are lacking, but it is reasonable to assume that infection and colonization are rare in most species, and that infection is typically acquired from infected or colonized humans.

Interspecies transmission

Given the ecology of MRSA and the relatively small number of people and animals that household pets typically encounter, MRSA in pets is ultimately human in origin. Despite this, infected or colonized animals can pose a risk to human contacts. There are significant concerns about the role of pets in human MRSA infection, but detailed information about the frequency, risk factors, and direction of transmission is lacking.

Colonization of people in contact with infected or colonized dogs and cats has been widely reported.[752,756,772–776] Finding important human MRSA strains in pets combined with the close nature of contact between people and pets raises concerns about zoonotic transmission. Pets have been implicated as sources of infection for humans in households.[773,775] This has been based on circumstantial evidence, given that concurrent colonization of people and pets with the same MRSA strain supports interspecies transmission but cannot determine the direction of transmission. It is likely that human-to-animal transmission occurs as least as commonly, if not more often, than animal-to-human transmission. Regardless, while information from most studies should be considered preliminary and circumstantial, it is very likely that interspecies transmission can occur in households and in veterinary clinics and that MRSA,

Table 2.8 Reported MRSA colonization rates of veterinary personnel.

Study population	Country*	Prevalence (%)	Reference
Small animal veterinarians at internal medicine conference	United States	4.4	[777]
Veterinary technicians at internal medicine conference	United States	12	[777]
Veterinarians	Denmark	3.9	[779]
Small animal veterinary clinic staff	United Kingdom	18	[760]
Small animal veterinary surgeons	United States	17	[781]
Veterinarians attending to MRSA infected dogs and cats	United Kingdom	12.3	[764]
Veterinarians not knowingly attending to MRSA-infected dogs and cats	United Kingdom	4.8	[764]
Veterinary conference attendees	Czech Republic	0.7	[782]

* Country where sampling was performed. Some individuals may have been from other countries.

while human in origin, is a relevant zoonotic pathogen.

There may also be occupational health risks for veterinary personnel. Numerous studies of MRSA colonization in veterinary personnel have been performed, generally reporting high (up to 18%) colonization rates (Table 2.8).[760,777–780] It cannot be determined with certainty that these colonization rates reflect acquisition of MRSA from animals; however, the identification of higher rates than present in the general population (1.5–3%)[744,745] and the similarity between human and animal strains provide support of occupational origin.

Transmission is assumed to be primarily from direct contact between an infected or colonized individual and a susceptible individual. MRSA can be found in the environment in households and veterinary clinics,[783–785] and indirect transmission through environmental sources is certainly possible, but has not been well studied. Aerosol transmission is unlikely but theoretically possible over short distances in coughing or sneezing individuals, or through other circumstances when infectious aerosols or liquid splatters are created.

Animals

Clinical presentation

A wide range of opportunistic infections can occur. Pyoderma, otitis, and soft tissue infections are most common, but infection of virtually any body site can be encountered. There are no clinical signs that would indicate *S. aureus* infection over any other opportunistic infection. Severe manifestations such as sepsis or necrotizing infections are rare.

MRSA infections may also occur at virtually any body site and are not distinguishable clinically from methicillin-susceptible infections or infections caused by other pathogens. Pyoderma and otitis are most commonly reported.[748,755,756,770,772,786–789] It is possible that MRSA infections are more commonly associated with human contact (e.g., wounds or surgical site infections contaminated by hands of owners or veterinary personnel) are more likely to be caused by *S. aureus* (including MRSA), but objective data are lacking.

Diagnosis

Clinical signs are not diagnostic (or suggestive). Cytological examination of infected tissues can indicate that a staphylococcal infection is likely but cannot differentiate *S. aureus* from other staphylococci. Culture of *S. aureus* from an infected body site is the standard for diagnosis; however, interpretation of culture results from nonsterile body sites like skin is complicated by the fact that *S. aureus* can be found as a commensal. This is less of a concern than with coagulase-negative staphylococci, and typically, isolation of *S. aureus* is interpreted as at least a presumptive diagnosis, but consideration of the possibility of false-positive culture results is important.

Identification of MRSA involves further testing of *S. aureus* isolates to detect phenotypic resistance and the presence of PBP2a or *mecA*. The latter two are currently rarely performed in veterinary diagnostic laboratories, and phenotypic identification is used. Problems may be encountered with laboratories that do not perform proper, or any, testing for methicillin resistance. Oxacillin resistance used to be the main indicator of MRSA. Oxacillin was used because it is more stable than methicillin *in vitro*, and oxacillin-resistant *S. aureus* is MRSA. However, it was subsequently shown that oxacillin is a poor inducer of resistance *in vitro* in some strains, so the current recommendation is to use cefoxitin, a better inducer of resistance. Cefoxitin-resistant *S. aureus* should be considered MRSA. Issues regarding testing and reporting of MRSA are a significant concern, and veterinarians should ensure that the laboratory they use performs testing for methicillin resistance and follow standard (i.e., Clinical and Laboratory Standards Institute [CLSI]) guidelines. If MDR *S. aureus* that are not reported as MRSA are identified, testing should be repeated to confirm results because MDR methicillin-susceptible *S. aureus* are uncommon.

Screening for MRSA colonization is rarely indicated, as discussed below. If it is required, there is currently minimal information to guide sampling. Nasal and rectal swabs are the most common sites screened. It is not unusual to find discrepant nasal and rectal swab results, and it is evident that sampling of only one site will result in underdiagnosis.

Management

Management of staphylococcal infections is highly variable because of the diverse nature of disease. Treatment is based on the nature of the infection and the antibiogram. Sole use or combinations of systemic antimicrobials, local antimicrobials, topical biocides, and other medical and surgical approaches may be considered. If a discrete abscess is present, incision and drainage alone may be adequate. However, discrete abscessation, a common presentation in humans, is rare in animals. MRSA should be considered resistant to all beta-lactams. Inducible clindamycin resistance is common in MRSA,[790,791] and erythromycin-resistant/clindamycin-susceptible MRSA should be considered clindamycin resistant in the absence of specific testing for inducible resistance by D-test. Fluoroquinolones should be avoided, regardless of *in vitro* susceptibility.

Humans

Clinical presentation

As a well-adapted opportunistic pathogen, *S. aureus* can cause a wide range of disease, including local and invasive infections and toxin-mediated syndromes. Localized infections are most common, including abscesses, cellulitis, wound infections, impetigo, and various other manifestation of skin and soft tissue infection.[792–794] Invasive infections can involve virtually any body system, with bacteremia, endocarditis, osteomyelitis, fasciitis, septic arthritis, pneumonia, and meningitis being the most common or concerning examples.[733,795,796]

Three main toxin-mediated syndromes are recognized: staphylococcal toxic shock syndrome, scalded skin syndrome, and staphylococcal food poisoning. The presence of specific toxin genes (TSST-1, exfoliative toxins A and B, and various enterotoxins, respectively) is required for these syndromes to develop. There is no evidence of zoonotic involvement in these syndromes.

S. aureus, both methicillin resistant and methicillin susceptible, is a leading cause of hospital-associated infections such as surgical site infections, bacteremia, and prosthetic device infections. Clinically, MRSA and methicillin-susceptible *S. aureus* infections are indistinguishable, whether in the community or in hospitals.

The severity of infection can be highly variable, ranging from mild skin infection to rapidly fatal necrotizing fasciitis, necrotizing pneumonia, septicemia, or toxic shock syndrome.

Diagnosis

Diagnosis requires culture and susceptibility testing. Isolation of *S. aureus* from an otherwise sterile body site is diagnostic.[24] Diagnosis of infections of superficial sites is somewhat more complicated because of the potential for colonization or contamination of the site, and culture results from superficial sites must be interpreted in light of the site of infection, sample type, number of *S. aureus* present (heavy growth vs. light growth), and whether other organisms were also isolated. While methicillin resistance is more common in hospitals, it is certainly present widely in the community, and it is inappropriate to assume that *S. aureus* will be methicillin susceptible based on the origin of infection or lack of recognized risk factors for MRSA.[733,792,797] Proper antimicrobial susceptibility testing must be performed on all *S. aureus* isolates.

Management

Treatment of *S. aureus* infection is highly dependent on the type, location, and severity of infection, and approaches can be highly variable. Antimicrobial susceptibility testing results are critical for most infections because of the potential for multidrug resistance. Some *S. aureus* isolates, particularly from community-associated infections, are susceptible to most antimicrobials, but methicillin and multidrug resistance are common and increasing in most regions. Empirical therapy with beta-lactam antimicrobials is commonly used for non-life-threatening skin and soft tissue infections in the community, but treatment failure rates parallel increases in methicillin resistance.

An important aspect to consider is that systemic antimicrobials are not required for the treatment of all infections. Incision and drainage alone may be adequate for treatment of abscesses (including those caused by MRSA) in otherwise healthy, afebrile patients with a localized abscess and no or mild cellulitis.[24] Oral antimicrobials should be used alongside incision and drainage when the patient is febrile or when there is moderate cellulitis. Hospitalization with more aggressive antimicrobial therapy (including coverage against MRSA) is indicated in immunocompromised patients and patients with limb-threatening infection or who appear toxic.[24] Treatment of other manifestations of *S. aureus* infection is variable and may range from outpatient systemic or topical antimicrobial therapy to hospitalization in an intensive care unit (ICU) and the need for surgical intervention.

Prevention

Public health concerns regarding pets and *S. aureus* have almost exclusively involved MRSA. It is unlikely that MRSA is truly more able to transfer from animals to humans. Rather, it is probably easier to detect and receives more attention. The potential role of pets in human methicillin-susceptible *S. aureus* infection currently receives little attention.

The true risk to humans from exposure to infected or colonized companion animals is completely unclear at this point. Given the epidemic of community-associated MRSA infections in people and endemic MRSA in human healthcare facilities, pets certainly play a minor role in overall human infections. However, there is ample evidence indicating that MRSA can be transmitted between humans and animals and that veterinary personnel are at increased risk for MRSA exposure. Therefore, the potential role of pets in human MRSA infections should be considered, but in a balanced manner.

Management of colonized pets in households

While the prevalence of MRSA colonization of pets is low, the sheer number of pets in households indicates that large numbers of colonized pets are residing, unknowingly, in thousands of households. Based on current recommendations for screening, which are discussed below, it would be uncommon for colonized pets to be identified. Accordingly, the use of good general hygiene measures around all pets is probably the most important preventive measure. However, if colonization status is known, colonized animals should be approached in a manner that would likely reduce the risk of transmission. Care should be taken not to overreact to identification of a colonized pet. Since pets tend to be colonized for only a short period of time and because of the strong link between MRSA in pets and their owners, it is likely that most colonized pets acquired MRSA from their owner. Therefore, the pet may be only one of multiple potential sources of infection in the household or other household members may already be colonized. The risk of the animal transmitting infection to other people would vary with the number of nonhousehold individuals encountered and their risk status, and would be greatest with animals in hospital visitation programs. Regardless, basic measures should be implemented to reduce the risk of transmission and facilitate elimination of MRSA from the pet. Household members should be aware of the high-risk sites on the pet, the nose and perineum, and avoid direct or indirect contact with those sites. Contact of high-risk human sites (nose, perineum, skin lesions) with the colonized pet should be prevented. People at higher risk for the development of MRSA infection should take particular care and probably should avoid all contact with the pet. Hands should be washed or a hand sanitizer should be used regularly after contact with the pet. Care should be taken when handling feces, which may also be contaminated. Items that are more likely to be contaminated, such as food or water bowls, should be handled with care and regularly cleaned and disinfected. Reducing overall duration and intensity of contact with the pet is indicated. To prevent transmission of MRSA from the pet to other animals, colonized cats should not be allowed outdoors. Dogs should be restrained by a leash whenever outside and not permitted to have contact with other dogs. Decolonization therapy is not indicated, as discussed below.

Typically, these are short-term measures. While MRSA can colonize various species, it does not seem well adapted to colonize companion animals for long periods of time. Unlike humans, where long-term or persistent colonization can occur, short-term colonization appears to be the norm in pets, with most pets eliminating MRSA within a few weeks as long as reinfection is prevented.[318,761,798,799]

Management of infected pets in households

General principles of MRSA control for infected pets are the same as those for colonized pets, and focus on restriction of contact with the animal, particularly areas of active infection and sites more likely to be colonized or contaminated. Animals with clinical infections may pose added challenges because of the potential heavy contamination of external body sites and the risk of exposure through home care. Animals with generalized pyoderma or extensive soft tissue infections probably pose the greatest risk. Infected sites should be covered by an impermeable dressing, whenever possible. Contact with the infected site should be minimized. If home care is required (e.g., bandage changing, bathing), clear instructions should be provided regarding infection control measures that should be undertaken to reduce the risk of MRSA transmission. If substantial infections are present and require intensive contact, consideration should be given to having the animal hospitalized during the initial treatment period, regardless of the severity of illness, to reduce the risk of exposure in the household. Similarly, if high-risk individuals are present in the household, especially if they are handling the pet, hospitalization of the pet during the treatment period should be considered.

Decolonization of pets

Active elimination of MRSA colonization in humans is a contentious issue. Active decolonization, often using topical antimicrobials such as mupirocin or fusidic acid, sometimes with concurrent oral antimicrobial therapy and antiseptic baths, is used as a means of MRSA control in humans in some situations in some regions. Even though long-term MRSA colonization can occur, the need for decolonization therapy in otherwise healthy individuals in the community is controversial and not universally recommended because of variable efficacy, questionable need, and concerns about the development of further resistance. Decolonization is most commonly used in specific populations, such as healthcare workers, patients undergoing surgical procedures, patients in ICUs, or individuals in households with recurrent MRSA infections.

In some respects, active elimination of MRSA colonization in dogs and cats could be desirable to reduce the risk of development of clinical infection or transmission to other individuals, including people. However, there is currently no evidence that therapy to eliminate colonization is indicated or even potentially efficacious in dogs and cats. Adequate topical application of an antimicrobial to the entire nasal passages of a dog or cat is not realistic, and incomplete treatment could lead to further resistance. Equally important is the apparent transient nature of MRSA colonization in companion animals. Since MRSA colonization appears to be transient in most if not all dogs and cats,[318,756,761] and the use of good general hygiene measures to reduce reinfection almost invariably results in spontaneous decolonization, it is questionable whether active decolonization is even indicated. The authors do not recommend any form of active decolonization therapy for pets.

Management of infected and colonized pets in veterinary clinics

Because of the potential risk that infected or colonized pets pose to veterinary personnel and patients, an enhanced level of infection control is required in veterinary hospitals. Ideally, infected or colonized animals are housed and treated in isolation. As MRSA is transmitted by contact, placing an animal in isolation reduces the risk of inadvertent transmission or contamination. If isolation is not possible for logistical or case management issues, management in a general ward area is possible. In that situation, particular care must be taken because of the potential for indirect transmission via veterinary personnel or equipment.

Regardless of the location, infected or colonized animals should be handled with barrier precautions: gloves and gowns. There is no indication for routine use of face or eye protection; however, some individuals may be more confident using a mask to reduce the risk of inadvertent hand–nose contact that could result in transmission of MRSA. Hand hygiene is critical, both as a routine tool and following contact with an infected or colonized animal. Hand hygiene should be performed after glove removal. Infected sites should be covered with an impermeable barrier dressing, if possible. This may not be an option in many cases, particularly otitis and generalized pyoderma. In all aspects of case management, care should be taken to avoid contamination of commonly used items such as bandage materials and clippers.

Screening/testing

There are few indications for MRSA screening in pets. For any screening program, a plan is required for interpretation of, and response to, the results. There must be clear (and different) recommendations for MRSA positive and negative results.

Testing of pets for MRSA colonization is not indicated in situations where MRSA has been identified in a person in a household,[800] nor is it indicated when high-risk humans are present in the household. Identification of a colonized pet would typically not lead to any specific recommendations since active decolonization would not be recommended, removal of the pet would be inappropriate and the emphasis would be on routine hygiene measures. Similarly, if the pet was negative, it would not be guaranteed that the pet was truly negative (at the time of sampling or thereafter), and the focus would be on hygiene measures to reduce the risk of human–pet transmission or pet–human transmission should the pet become colonized. Since there would be essentially no difference in response to the results, there is little justification to test.

The main situation where screening is currently recommended is when there are recurrent MRSA infections in humans in the household, but only if the entire household (human and animal) is being concurrently evaluated and a plan is made regarding how to deal with colonized people and pets.[800] Screening of infected animals after resolution of clinical disease might be useful in some circumstances to determine if colonization is still present. It is not unusual for animals to shed MRSA in their nose or gastrointestinal tract for a short period of time (a few weeks) after clinical resolution. If enhanced infection control practices are being used, screening could be performed to determine when to discontinue those practices.

Screening of pets is rarely indicated as a routine infection control tool in veterinary clinics, although it has been used as part of a comprehensive MRSA control plan in an equine hospital.[762] The usefulness of routine screening would depend on the population prevalence, disease incidence, financial resources, and risk adversity of the facility. If MRSA rates in the entire or a definable subset of the population are high, then routine testing of all or selected patients might be useful. This could be particularly true for animals undergoing surgery to reduce the risk of surgical site infections. However, given the low incidence of infection in most hospitals, the typical short hospital stay of veterinary patients, the time required to receive culture results, and the costs of testing, routine screening is rarely required or practical.

Optimal screening regimens are not known. A combination of nasal and rectal swabs is used by some, but objective data are lacking. It is also unclear whether a single round of testing is adequate. Two negative nasal–rectal pairs taken on different occasions (e.g., 1 week apart) has been recommended based on anecdotal data.

Screening of veterinary personnel

Routine screening of veterinary personnel is not indicated. While colonized veterinary personnel can certainly transmit MRSA, the need and efficacy of veterinary personnel screening has not been demonstrated. MRSA colonization rates in veterinary personnel are high, and it is likely that one or more colonized personnel are present in most large (and many small) veterinary hospitals. Given these high rates and the perpetual risk of exposure, it makes more sense to assume that personnel are colonized and structure routine infection control practices accordingly. Furthermore, it is unclear what actions would be taken in response to identifying colonized personnel. Decolonization therapy is questionable in this population because the high rates of colonization indicate a high likelihood of reexposure. Screening of staff is also associated with a host of legal, ethical, privacy, and occupational health issues that are best avoided unless there is clear evidence of need. The main situation where personnel screening might be considered is when there is epidemiological evidence of personnel-borne transmission and transmission continues despite enhancement of infection control practices. With a good routine infection control program, particularly careful attention to hand hygiene, the implications of colonized personnel in a veterinary hospital should be minimal. If screening is performed, human healthcare personnel must direct it and results must be kept confidential.

Removing infected or colonized pets from households

There is little indication to recommend removal of pets from households. *Temporary removal* could be considered in exceptional circumstances when pets are colonized and thought to be a source of infection, when implementation of good household infection control measures has not had an effect and as part of a comprehensive plan to eradicate MRSA from all individuals (human and animal) in the household. This would mainly be when recurrent MRSA infections were present and all people in the household were undergoing decolonization therapy. If good infection control measures involving the pet could not be implemented, then temporary removal of the pet could be considered. People would undergo decolonization therapy and the pet would be given time to naturally decolonize, with the pet returned to the household once it was deemed MRSA negative.

Staphylococcus pseudintermedius/ Staphylococcus intermedius

Introduction

S. pseudintermedius is a commensal and common cause of opportunistic infections in dogs and cats. Previously, *S. intermedius* was considered the common and clinically important canine *Staphylococcus* species, but it is now known that previous reports of *S. intermedius* in dogs and cats almost certainly were actually the closely related *S. pseudintermedius*.[801,802] Methicillin-resistant *S. pseudintermedius* (MRSP) is an emerging problem in animals, especially dogs. Human infections with *S. pseudintermedius* are rarely reported, but there is some potential for zoonotic transmission.

Etiology

S. pseudintermedius is a coagulase-positive *Staphylococcus* species that is closely related to *S. intermedius*.

Geographic distribution/epidemiology

S. pseudintermedius is a true canine commensal, with reported colonization rates of 31–68% in healthy dogs.[748,749,803,804] Higher rates (up to 100%) have been reported in puppies.[805] It is possible that colonization rates in adult dogs could be higher if multiple sites and enrichment culture methods were used, and it is reasonable to assume that a high percentage of healthy dogs are carrying *S. pseudintermedius* at some body site at any given time. Various body sites can be colonized, particularly the nasal passages, oral cavity, skin, and perineal mucosa.[803,804] Most colonized dogs do not have, and do not develop, clinical infection, but opportunistic infections of various body sites may occur, particularly the skin and ears. Colonization is less common (6.8–22%) in healthy cats.[749,750,806,807] As with dogs, opportunistic infections can develop but the influence of long-term or transient colonization on risk of disease is unknown. MRSP has emerged and disseminated widely in dogs and cats in recent years. It is considered a serious emerging problem in small animal veterinary medicine and one that requires urgent action to control its spread.[808] MRSP can be found in or on 1.5–17% of dogs and 1.2% of healthy cats.[748,749,757,758,809] As with susceptible staphylococci, MRSP is an opportunistic pathogen and colonization does not necessarily lead to disease. Antimicrobial exposure and hospital exposure are associated with MRSP versus methicillin-susceptible *S. pseudintermedius* infection in dogs,[810] but primary community-onset cases in the absence of antimicrobial exposure or hospitalization can occur.

There are limited reports of *S. intermedius* or *S. pseudintermedius* infection or colonization in humans. Most infections relate to dog bites, with one study reporting *S. (pseud)intermedius* in 18% of 34 dog-bite wounds.[811] Bacteremia,[812] pneumonia,[813] ear infections,[814,815] varicose leg ulcers,[816] an infected suture line,[811] and a brain abscess[816] have also been reported. A link to animals is often suggested but rarely proven. In one case, *S. (pseud) intermedius* was cultured from the ear fluid of a patient with otitis externa and from her pet dog.[814] Colonization with *S. pseudintermedius* occurs more often than infection but is still uncommon, with reported rates of 1–4% in veterinary personnel and pet owners.[749,817] Contact with pets may be a risk factor for *S. pseudintermedius* colonization of people. One study reported the presence of indistinguishable pet and human isolates in 44% of households where both a person and dog were colonized, suggesting that pets were the source of human colonization.[749] This study also indicated that regular hand washing after contact with pets was associated with less risk of *S. pseudintermedius* coloniza-

tion. Higher rates of colonization have also been reported in owners of dogs with deep pyoderma compared with nonpet owners.[818] Reports of MRSP infection are also limited. MRSP infections have been reported in a person with bacteremia and one with pneumonia, but interestingly, there was no known contact with dogs.[813,819] Transmission of MRSP between dogs and people is likely based on reports of indistinguishable isolates from people and dogs in veterinary clinics.[802,820] None of the individuals in those studies were reported to have developed disease. Therefore, while there is relatively strong evidence that *S. pseudintermedius* can be transmitted from animals to people in veterinary clinics and households, the clinical implications of this appear to be very limited given the extremely low number of reported infections in people.

Animals

Clinical presentation

S. pseudintermedius accounts for the vast majority of cases of pyoderma in dogs, and a lesser percentage in cats. It also causes a range of other infections including wound infections, surgical site infections, septic arthritis, osteomyelitis, urinary tract infections, endocarditis, liver abscess, peritonitis, and ocular infections.[821–826] The severity of disease is highly variable. Serious, including fatal, invasive infections can occur but are uncommon. Fatal toxic shock and cellulitis associated with *S. pseudintermedius* has been reported.[827] Necrotizing fasciitis, a rare but devastating disease, is most commonly associated with *Streptococcus canis* but *S. pseudintermedius* has also been implicated.[828] The same spectrum of disease is caused by MRSP, with a predominance of skin, ear, and other soft tissue infections.[810,829] Postoperative infections appear to be increasingly common.[810]

Diagnosis

Isolation of *S. pseudintermedius* from an infected site is the standard for diagnosis. Because this organism is a common commensal, care must be taken to avoid contamination with the resident microflora. One complicating factor in the diagnosis of *S. pseudintermedius* is the availability of proper speciation. Some diagnostic laboratories only provide superficial identification of staphylococci and may simply report "coagulase positive" or "coagulase positive non-aureus." Speciation is important for assessing zoonotic disease risks and proper antimicrobial susceptibility testing since some breakpoints differ between *S. aureus* and *S. pseudintermedius*. This includes testing to determine methicillin resistance, and false-negative results can easily be obtained if proper guidelines are not used.[830,831]

Management

Treatment of *S. pseudintermedius* infections is highly variable and depends largely on the site and severity of infection. Antimicrobial therapy (local, systemic, or a combination thereof) is usually required. Management of some MRSP infections can be complicated because of the high level of antimicrobial resistance. In general, MRSP isolates from dogs and cats are resistant to more antimicrobials than MRSA isolates, and in some situations, there may be few viable treatment options.

Humans

Clinical presentation

There are limited reports of *S. pseudintermedius* infection, so a clear description of the expected clinical presentation is not possible. It is presumed that *S. pseudintermedius* infection in humans could encompass a range of opportunistic infections, as is the case with other staphylococci.

Diagnosis

Diagnosis of *S. pseudintermedius* is based on bacterial culture. One area of concern is the possibility that *S. pseudintermedius* isolates could be misidentified as *S. aureus*, considering the similarity of *S. aureus* and *S. pseudintermedius* and the predominance of *S. aureus* among coagulase-positive staphylococci from humans. Misdiagnosis of *S. aureus* has been reported,[832] but this is probably a rare occurrence.

Management

Treatment of *S. pseudintermedius* infections is identical to the treatment of *S. aureus* infections. Antimicrobials are typically required and should be chosen based on susceptibility testing.

Prevention

There is currently limited concern regarding zoonotic transmission of *S. pseudintermedius*; however, given the evidence of transmission of this organism between species and the high level of antimicrobial resistance that can be present, it is prudent to take reasonable precautions to decrease the risk of human exposure.

In households, contact with infected sites should be avoided. Infected sites should be covered with an impermeable barrier, if possible, but this is not likely to be practical in most situations. Contact with mucous membranes should be restricted. Given the frequency of skin infections and the presence of *S. pseudintermedius* as a common commensal, avoidance of exposure is difficult to achieve. Therefore, there should be an emphasis on personal hygiene. Hand washing has been shown to be associated with decreased *S. pseudintermedius* colonization in dog owners[749] and should be performed after animal contact.

In veterinary clinics, a greater level of infection control is recommended, more to reduce the risk of transmission of MRSP to other animals. There is less concern about zoonotic transmission, although transmission of MRSP between people and patients can occur in veterinary hospitals. Establishing a population of colonized staff is undesirable as they could be sources of hospital-associated infection of patients. Animals with MRSP infection should be isolated in veterinary clinics whenever possible and handled with contact precautions.

There is little information regarding infection control practices for animals colonized with MRSP. There is no evidence that more aggressive infection control practices are required in households with colonized animals. There is currently also no evidence that eradication of *S. pseudintermedius* colonization is feasible or required. Elimination of commensal organisms from its ecological niche can be difficult. Administration of topical antimicrobials to eliminate *S. pseudintermedius* is unlikely to be practical or even feasible in most animals and could lead to even more resistance. Given the lack of evidence that decolonization is an effective control tool, the lack of evidence of efficacy of any approach toward decolonization, the minimal role of *S. pseudintermedius* in human disease, and the potential for emergence of further resistance with inadequate antimicrobial therapy, active decolonization is not currently recommended. Instead, an emphasis should be placed on routine hygiene and infection control precautions in households and veterinary clinics.

Staphylococcus schleiferi

S. schleiferi is comprised of two subspecies that differ based on their ability to produce coagulase. *S. schleiferi schleiferi* is coagulase negative, while *S. schleiferi coagulans* is coagulase positive. *S. schleiferi schleiferi* can be found in healthy humans, dogs, and cats,[750,758,786,833] and it is unclear whether it has a true species tropism. In contrast, *S. schleiferi coagulans* was first identified in dogs[834] and dogs may be the natural host, although it has also been reported in cats.[750] Neither appears to be highly pathogenic in humans, with most *S. schleiferi schleiferi* infections (like those caused by other coagulase-negative staphylococci) occurring in compromised hosts.[835]

Both subspecies can be found in healthy and diseased dogs and, to a lesser degree, cats. Skin infections are the most common manifestation of disease.[748,786,836] As with other staphylococci, emergence of methicillin resistance is a concern. There are increasing reports of methicillin-resistant strains in dogs and cats, particularly animals with pyoderma,[748,750,786,837] but methicillin-resistant *S. schleiferi schleiferi* and *S. schleiferi coagulans* can be found in healthy pets.[748,758]

Infections with either subspecies are uncommon in humans and mainly involve *S. schleiferi schleiferi*.[838–840] Opportunistic infections such as postoperative, implant, and wound infections are most commonly reported.[833,835,838,841] *S. schleiferi coagulans* infections appear to be extremely rare.[842]

The zoonotic disease risk with *S. schleiferi scheiferi* is probably extremely low to nonexistent because it is a human commensal and rare cause of disease. Similarly, the risks with *S. schleiferi coagulans* are probably very low because of the small number of reported human infections. A dog with otitis was hypothesized to be the source of *S. schleiferi coagulans* endocarditis in an immunocompromised person;[842] however, there was no investigation to confirm this suspicion. It is reasonable to assume that there could be some risk of zoonotic transmission, but this is likely low and of greatest concern in immunocompromised individuals.

The risks should be no greater with methicillin-resistant strains; however, the potential difficulty treating methicillin-resistant staphylococcal infections indicates that even if the risk of transmission is very low, some consideration should be taken for the reduction of potential risks. Animals with methicillin-resistant *S. schleiferi* infections should be handled with care, avoiding contact with infected sites and with an emphasis on good personal hygiene. Isolation of infected animals or other more aggressive measures do not appear to be indicated. The same measures should be taken by people with methicillin-resistant *S. schleiferi* infections to reduce the risk of transmission to pets. Screening of pets for colonization is not recommended.

Streptococcus canis

Introduction

S. canis is a beta-hemolytic *Streptococcus* spp. that can be part of the commensal microflora in dogs. It is a rare human pathogen, accounting for only 1% of streptococcal isolates in one study[843] but can cause a range of infections, including invasive disease.

Etiology

S. canis is a Lancefield group G *Streptococcus* (GGS) spp. Other members of this group include *Streptococcus anginosus*, *Streptococcus dysgalactiae* subsp. *dysgalactiae*, and *S. dysgalactiae* subsp. *equisimilis*, the latter of which is most commonly implicated in human disease.

Geographic distribution/epidemiology

S. canis is likely disseminated in the dog population worldwide; however, only limited data are available. While mostly associated with dogs, which are considered the primary animal reservoir, *S. canis* has been identified in other species including cats and cattle.[844–848]

Limited information is available regarding the prevalence of *S. canis* colonization of healthy animals. One study reported isolation of *S. canis* from the external ears of 2.8% of healthy dogs, versus 30% of dogs with otitis externa.[849] Upper respiratory tract and urogenital colonization have been identified in humans,[843] although it is unclear whether those represented true colonization or transient contamination.

Most human cases are community in origin, as with other GGS infections. Human infection via dog bite has been reported.[850] In the absence of bites, transmission from dogs has been hypothesized[851] and is logical, but has not been proven. Transmission is presumably from direct contact with infected or colonized individuals.

Animals

Clinical presentation

While a commensal, *S. canis* is also an opportunistic pathogen in dogs and cats. Most attention has been paid to necrotizing fasciitis, and *S. canis* is considered the primary cause of necrotizing fasciitis in dogs.[852] An association has been made between fluoroquinolone administration and *S. canis* necrotizing fasciitis.[853] Endocarditis, pericarditis, toxic shock syndrome, and various other milder opportunistic infections such as otitis externa have also been reported in dogs.[849,854–857] Skin infections, meningitis, sepsis, sinusitis, myocarditis, necrotizing fasciitis, and arthritis have been reported in cats.[845–848]

Diagnosis

Culture and susceptibility testing of infected sites is used to diagnose *S. canis* infection. Routine screening of pets for *S. canis* colonization is not indicated. If screening of pets is performed as part of a disease investigation, the optimal screening sites are unclear. Pharyngeal swabs are probably ideal, with possible addition of other sites such as the perineum, vagina, or oral cavity.

Management

Treatment of animals with clinical infections depends on the site of infection and antimicrobial susceptibility of the recovered isolate. Most isolates are susceptible to various antimicrobials, including penicillin.[855,858] Resistance to tetracycline, clindamycin, gentamicin, and enrofloxacin has been reported.[855,858] Fluoroquinolones must be avoided.

Decolonization therapy is not indicated to prevent either disease in animals or zoonotic transmission. There is no evidence that decolonization therapy could be successful or that it is needed.

Humans

Clinical presentation

Information regarding human disease is limited because specific identification of GGS is not commonly reported and because older reports predate differentiation of *S. canis* as a novel species. It has been suggested that the role of *S. canis* in human disease may be underestimated.[843,859,860] Soft tissue infections, urinary tract infections, bloodstream infections, bone infections, meningitis, and pneumonia have been reported.[843,851,859–861] Fatal infections can occur.[843]

Diagnosis

Routine culture of infected sites is used for diagnosis. Identification of *S. canis* versus more broad diagnosis of GGS requires additional biochemical or genotypic testing. This is not necessary for clinical management of cases but could provide useful information for elucidation of the potential source of infection.

Management

Management of *S. canis* infections is no different than other streptococcal infections. Treatment is based on infection and patient factors, along with antimicrobial susceptibility data. Isolates are often susceptible to most antimicrobials, including penicillin.[843] Successful resolution without antimicrobials may occur in superficial skin infections.[843]

Prevention

As a rare opportunistic pathogen in humans, specific preventive measures have not been investigated. Because *S. canis* is part of the commensal microflora in dogs, there may be a continual risk of exposure to people that interact with dogs. Measures to reduce colonization in dogs are impractical because elimination of a commensal is difficult, and there is no indication that it would be useful. General hygiene measures such as hand hygiene are probably the most effective approach. Contact with animals with *S. canis* infection could be of higher risk because of the presumably larger infectious burden, particularly with skin and soft tissue infections. Routine practices for handling infectious animals should be used, including restricting contact, hand hygiene after contact, and the use of barrier dressings wherever possible. This applies both in veterinary clinics and in households. Because a high percentage of reported human cases involve people with comorbidities or advanced age,[843,851,861] those individuals should take extra care. Similarly, people with skin wounds should avoid direct contact of their compromised sites with dogs.[859] There is no indication for screening of dogs for *S. canis* colonization nor is there an indication for screening of in-contact individuals following exposure to an infected animal.

Group A *Streptococcus* (GAS)

GAS is an important human pathogen, causing a wide range of disease. Pharyngitis ("strep throat") and pyoderma are the most common clinical presentations and are frequently encountered in people in the community.

Streptococcal pharyngitis is a very common childhood disease, accounting for 0.14–0.5 cases per child-year, and recurrent disease is not uncommon.[862] GAS also accounts for 4–10% of cases of pharyngitis in human adults. Severe invasive infections (bacteremia, pneumonia, necrotizing fasciitis, streptococcal toxic shock syndrome, puerperal sepsis) can also occur, and an estimated 9100 cases and 1350 deaths from invasive GAS infection occur each year in the United States, many among previously healthy children.[863]

It has been suggested that pets could be reservoirs of infection in households,[864–866] though supporting data are weak. Earlier studies reported identification of GAS colonization in pets;[867,868] however, these studies have been questioned because the methods used could have misidentified other streptococci as GAS.[869] In particular, earlier methods may have incorrectly identified groups C and G streptococci as group A. Considering groups C and G streptococci are commensals in dogs and cats, these prevalence data may not be accurate. Subsequent studies have not identified GAS from pets,[870] including pets of children with GAS infection.[869] Furthermore, an epidemiological study reported no correlation between the presence of pets in the household and recurrent streptococcal infection in humans.[871] Thus, the role of pets in GAS transmission has probably been overestimated.

Of greater concern is the potential for pets to act as sources of infection in households encountering recurrent GAS infection. Again, there is little evidence of a role of pets in disease transmission. A Swedish study reported isolation of GAS from ocular secretions, but not pharyngeal swabs, of two pets from 114 households with human GAS infection.[872] There was no difference in recurrence rates in families with pets versus those without, and there was no indication of direction of transmission.

Currently, there is little evidence that pets are a significant (or even uncommon) source of human infection. Guidelines from the Infectious Disease Society of America only recommend testing and treatment of household human contacts in specific situations and state that there is no credible evidence of the involvement of pets in recurrent disease.[873] Screening of pets for colonization is not indicated in response to sporadic human infections in a household. In situations where all household members are being screened because of recurrent disease, concurrent testing of pets may be considered but is likely of low utility. Optimal testing methods are not known. It is important that the diagnostic laboratory be aware of the reason for testing to ensure that proper identification of GAS is attempted. There is no information regarding management of colonized pets, if they are identified. Because of the low prevalence of colonization, it is likely that colonization is short term and naturally eliminated. Antimicrobial therapy may not be required, and attention to hygiene practices in association with pet contact may be all that is required. Empirical treatment of pets in households with sporadic or recurrent GAS infections is not indicated.

Streptococcus equi subsp. equi

This bacterium, more commonly referred to as *S. equi*, is a group C *Streptococcus* species that is predominantly associated with "strangles" in horses. Horses are the natural host and *S. equi* is endemic in horses internationally.

An important aspect in the diagnosis of *S. equi* infection is differentiation of *S. equi equi* from *S. equi* subsp. *zoepidemicus* (*Streptococcus zooepidemicus*). *S. zooepidemicus* is more commonly, albeit still rarely, diagnosed as a cause of disease in dogs. Some diagnoses of *S. equi* infection in dogs have subsequently been determined to be *S. zooepidemicus*. True *S. equi* infections in dogs appear to be extremely rare. There is a single published report of lymphadenopathy in a dog that lived on a horse farm.[874]

In humans, *S. equi* is of minimal relevance. Human infections have not been well documented. Considering the rarity of confirmed *S. equi* infections in dogs and humans, as well as the miniscule apparent risk of transmission of *S. equi* from infected horses to their caretakers, the risks associated with pets are presumably negligible.

S. equi subsp. zooepidemicus

More commonly known simply as *S. zooepidemicus*, this group C *Streptococcus* is primarily an equine opportunistic pathogen and is endemic in the horse population. This organism is rarely found in dogs but is a sporadic cause of respiratory tract disease. Most reports in dogs are from kennels, shelters, and research colonies,[875–877] that may reflect increased risk of transmission in concen-

trated and stressful situations, and exposure to other respiratory pathogens. Isolation of *S. zooepidemicus* from household pets is rare.[878] Clinical infections may range from typical upper respiratory tract disease to fatal hemorrhagic pneumonia.[876–880]

S. zooepidemicus is a rare pathogen in humans, most often causing pneumonia and glomerulonephritis, but also other infections such as meningitis and arthritis.[881–883] Infected milk and cheese are typically implicated as the sources of human infection, although horse–human transmission has also been documented.[883–885] The overall zoonotic risks involving *S. zooepidemicus* and pets are minimal. There is only a single published report of pet–human transmission of *S. zooepidemicus*. This involved a dog with respiratory tract disease and an owner that subsequently developed *S. zooepidemicus* infection with fever, headache, malaise, and stiffness in the neck and chest.[886] A healthy pet dog was also colonized with *S. zooepidemicus*, and the source of human or canine infection was not clear. Horses were present on the property, yet *S. zooepidemicus* was not isolated from any horse. There is also an unpublished report of a shelter worker who developed invasive streptococcal infection after being splashed in the eye while conducting a necropsy on a dog that died of *S. zooepidemicus* pneumonia. Unfortunately, the human *Streptococcus* isolate was not speciated and zoonotic transmission remains speculative in that case. When one considers that this organism is endemic in horses and few human cases are reported, the overall risks associated with animal contact must be low.

The single published report of zoonotic infection from a dog recommended the use of safety glasses and face masks when dealing with animals presenting with respiratory tract disease.[886] It is hard to justify such an approach for all animals with respiratory tract disease given the commonness of disease and extreme rarity of zoonotic infections and the lack of similar recommendations for handling horses with *S. zooepidemicus* infection. Certainly, prudence is never a bad idea when dealing with ill animals; however, close attention to routine infection control practices, especially hand hygiene, is probably adequate in most situations. Care should be taken to reduce the risk of close contact with respiratory secretions and aerosols, and mask and eye protection are not unreasonable when performing procedures that require close proximity to the respiratory tract of an infected animal, or when there it a high likelihood of the affected animal coughing in close proximity to the face of a person. It is difficult to recommend mask and eye protection as a standard of care for respiratory tract disease. This is certainly going to be impractical in household situations, and close adherence to good general hygiene and restriction of close contact with the animal's face are probably reasonable recommendations.

Yersinia enterocolitica

Y. enterocolitica is a gram-negative bacterium and the most common cause of enteric yersiniosis, an important but sporadic disease in humans. Most human cases are from the ingestion of contaminated food, particularly pork, and yersiniosis is the third most commonly reported cause of foodborne disease in some regions.[887] All ages can be affected, but disease is most common in children and young adults. Fever, abdominal pain, and diarrhea (sometimes bloody) are common.

The clinical relevance of Y. enterocolitica in dogs and cats is unclear. It may be a commensal as it can be isolated from a small percentage (<1–5%) of healthy dogs and cats,[887–889] and attempts to reproduce disease in dogs experimentally have failed.[890] However, it has been isolated from diarrheic dogs and cats fed contaminated raw pork,[891] and its role as a pathogen cannot be dismissed. It may be of greater concern in young dogs, where disease characterized by diarrhea, increased frequency of defecation, blood and mucus in stool, and tenesmus has been described.[892]

Isolation of indistinguishable serotypes of Y. enterocolitica from dogs, cats, and humans has been reported[893,894] and could indicate the potential for zoonotic transmission. However, it could also reflect common-source infection with no transmission from dogs or cats.

Very little is known about the potential for transmission of Y. enterocolitica from companion animals to humans. Pets are probably rarely, if ever, the source of human infections, but the potential cannot be discounted. Since this bacterium is transmitted by the fecal–oral route and can be shed both by diarrheic as well as clinically normal dogs and cats, general hygiene practices regarding contact with animal feces are important. This involves avoiding contact with feces, careful attention to hand hygiene, and reducing environmental contamination by properly removing feces.

Yersinia pestis

Introduction

Few diseases have had a greater impact on the human population historically than Y. pestis, the cause of plague. Plague is one of the oldest recognized diseases and has played an important role in human disease and development throughout history. While much less common today, Y. pestis is still a concern and causes infections in humans and animals alike.

Etiology

Y. pestis is a gram-negative coccobacillus belonging to the Enterobacteriaceae family. There are three geographic variants (orientalis, antiqua, mediaevalis), but these produce identical disease.

Geographic distribution/epidemiology

Y. pestis is widely distributed internationally and is endemic in many regions. It is most common in the tropics and subtropics, from 55 degrees North to 40 degrees South; however, within these regions, there are areas of endemic disease and areas where plague does not occur. Focally affected regions tend to be those that are semiarid, cooler areas adjacent to deserts. Y. pestis is poorly tolerant to environmental conditions like sunlight, high temperatures, and dessication. Australia and Antarctica are the only continents where plague has not been identified.[895] Internationally, most cases of plague are reported in focal regions of Asia and Africa.[895,896] In North America, most cases occur in the southwestern United States, particularly New Mexico, Arizona, Colorado, and California.[897–899] The geographic range tends to be stable during endemic cycles but expand to adjacent areas during epizootics. Disease is usually seasonal. Most human cases in the Northern Hemisphere occur between March and October.

Y. pestis circulates in multiple animal reservoirs but primarily lives in wild rodents. Thirty to forty different rodent species can serve as permanent natural reservoirs.[900] The bacterium is spread between rodents by infected fleas. Some natural reservoirs tend to be relatively resistant to plague and can be chronically bacteremic.[901] Chronically infected animals are an important reservoir because of the number of fleas they can infect over time. Other natural reservoirs, such as prairie dogs (*Cynomys* spp.), rock squirrels (*Spermophilus variegates*), and ground squirrels (*Spermophilus richardsoni*), are highly susceptible and have upwards of 100% mortality rates.[900]

Human infections are usually the result of a bite from an infected flea. Most often, this occurs following the death of an infected rat, when the fleas on the rat leave their dead host to look for a new blood meal. Transmission between humans by infected human fleas (*Pulex irritans*) is uncommon but possible. Direct transmission from infected people or animals can also occur. Human-to-human transmission is of greatest concern in individuals with pneumonic plague, who can spread *Y. pestis* through aerosols, resulting in subsequent cases of pneumonic plague. Overall, person-to-person transmission is extremely rare.[897]

Predatory species may become infected through ingestion of infected animals, and ingestion of infected prey is the most common source of plague in dogs and cats.[900]

Plague is uncommon in domestic pets, and cats are most often involved. Outdoor access and hunting are likely the primary factors associated with exposure of cats. A study of 60 plague-infected cats reported that 75% had hunted.[902] After ingestion of an infected rodent, *Y. pestis* can be found in the oropharynx of 50% of dogs and in the bloodstream of 20%. Seroprevalence studies have identified plague exposure in 2% of dogs and 3% of cats in California.[903]

Transmission of *Y. pestis* from companion animals to humans is uncommon and usually involves cats.[898,904,905] Cases have involved cats diagnosed with (or suspected of having plague) as well as clinically normal individuals. From 1977 to 1998, 23 cases of human plague from inhalation of *Y. pestis*-infected aerosols from cats were identified.[904] Approximately 25% of infected individuals were veterinary personnel, while the remainder was the people who took care of sick cats. Twenty percent of infected individuals died. Infections have been reported following face-to-face contact, bites, scratches, or caring for a sick cat.[904–906] Infection via face-to-face contact is of particular concern because of the potential for pneumonic plague, which is often fatal.[904,905] However, it may not always be possible to differentiate zoonotic transmission involving a cat from concurrent infection from infected fleas from the same rodent source.

Cat and dog fleas (*Ctenocephalides felis* and *C. canis*, respectively) have traditionally been considered inefficient vectors of *Y. pestis*;[907] however, it has recently been established that *C. felis* is a competent vector, albeit with a lower efficiency than many other flea species.[896] Pets may also act as transient hosts of other flea species, including highly efficient vectors from rodents, so flea infestation of pets is a significant concern.

Dogs are also a potential source of infection, although of lesser concern than cats. In a case-control study of households containing a plague survivor versus controls, having a sick dog in the household and sleeping in the same bed with the dog were associated with plague households.[909] Furthermore, within households of affected individuals, sleeping in the same bed as the dog was a risk factor. These suggest that close and prolonged contact with dogs, particularly sick dogs, may increase the risk of plague infection. Failure to use flea control measures on dogs and cats was identified as a possible risk factor for human plague in an endemic region in the United States.[909]

Other household pets such as rabbits are not considered reservoir hosts but can become infected during epizootics.[900] The human health risks associated with pet rabbits are minimal.

Fomite transmission is unlikely because of the poor environmental persistence of *Y. pestis*.[900]

In humans, there are three clinical forms: bubonic plague, septicemic plague, and pneumonic plague. Bubonic plague occurs as a result of cutaneous or mucous membrane exposure to *Y. pestis*. After inoculation, *Y. pestis* is carried by lymphatics to regional lymph nodes, where an intense inflammatory reaction ensues. Bacteremia commonly develops and can lead to sepsis, pneumonia, and infections of various body systems. Septicemic plague can develop following cutaneous exposure, particularly in elderly individuals.[910] Pneumonic plague can be primary (inhalation) or secondary (hematogenous spread to lungs). In primary pneumonic plague, *Y. pestis* is inhaled from infective aerosols generated by other individuals with pneumonic plague. This is of greatest concern early in disease when forceful coughing can spread infective aerosols over a distance of up to 2 m.[911] Secondary pneumonic plague occurs following hematogenous spread of *Y. pestis* to the lungs.

Animals

Clinical presentation

Cats have a similar susceptibility to plague as humans and can develop bubonic, septicemic, or pneumonic plague. Bubonic plague is most common and associated with the lowest mortality rate.[902] High fever, lymphadenopathy, dehydration, and hyperesthesia are common. A pain response will be elicited by palpation of enlarged lymph nodes. The submandibular, retropharyngeal, and cervical lymph nodes may be more commonly involved in cats that are infected through ingestion of infected prey. However, absence of lymphadenopathy does not rule out plague. Septicemic plague is usually characterized by septic shock. Fever, weakness, anorexia, vomiting, diarrhea, tachycardia, and hypotension are common.[900] Cats with pneumonic plague start with a high fever and rapidly deteriorate with signs of severe respiratory and systemic disease. Various other presentations can be present with infections of other body sites, but are uncommon.

Dogs are relatively resistant to *Y. pestis* and typically only develop mild disease, if any, characterized by fever and lymphadenopathy.[912]

Diagnosis

Plague should be considered in any febrile cat in an endemic area, particularly cats that are allowed outdoors to hunt or those that are flea infested. Confirmation of the diagnosis is critical because of the potential for zoonotic transmission. Isolation of *Y. pestis* from blood or fine-needle aspirates of infected tissues is definitive. Identification of seroconversion is diagnostic. A single antibody titer is not diagnostic because animals in endemic areas may have high titers from previous exposure. FA testing of direct smears can also be performed. Veterinarians should never attempt to isolate *Y. pestis* using in-house culture, and they should ensure that the diagnostic laboratory they use is capable of (and willing to) attempt to isolate this pathogen. Submission of samples to a government laboratory may be required. Cytological examination can be suggestive, through identification of a monomorphic population of bipolar staining coccobacilli.

Management

Treatment should begin immediately is cases where plague is suspected. In general, *Y. pestis* is susceptible to a wide range of antimicrobials. *Y. pestis* may appear susceptible to beta-lactams *in vitro*, *in vivo* resistance is typical. Gentamicin, chloramphenicol, or enrofloxacin are commonly used. A minimum of 21 days of treatment is required, and treatment should continue well past clinical resolution. Oral medications should be avoided during the initial treatment period to reduce the risk of bites associated with medication administration.

The prognosis is guarded and best if prompt and appropriate treatment is provided. A study of 119 feline plague cases reported a survival rate of 33%, with most survivors being cats with bubonic plague.[902] Experimental studies involving feeding cats infected mice have reported 50% survival of affected cats, without antimicrobial therapy or supportive care.[913,914] Septicemic plague is usually fatal, with most cats dying 1–2 days after the initial bacteremic event. Pneumonic plague is almost always fatal.

Humans

Clinical presentation

Bubonic plague is the classical form of disease. An incubation period of 2–6 days is followed by a sudden onset of fever, chills, headache, malaise, and pain over regional lymph nodes. Lymph nodes subsequently, and usually rapidly, enlarge. Single or multiple enlarged lymph nodes (buboes) may be present and can be extremely painful.

Septicemic plague is characterized by typical signs of gram-negative sepsis as well as prominent gastrointestinal symptoms such as nausea, vomiting, diarrhea, and abdominal pain.[897] Lymphadenopathy is not usually apparent. Multiorgan failure, DIC, and acute respiratory distress syndrome may develop. Secondary pneumonia, meningitis, or infection of other body systems may also develop.

Pneumonic plague is a highly fatal form. After a 1- to 3-day incubation period, there is a sudden onset of fever, chills, headache, myalgia, weakness, and chest discomfort.[895] Disease progresses rapidly and varying degrees of cough, hemoptysis, chest pain, difficulty breathing, and hypoxia develop.[897] Coughing can spread Y. pestis to close contacts, resulting in primary pneumonic plague.

Less commonly, localized cutaneous disease can develop at skin or mucous membrane sites inoculated with Y. pestis. Various other local manifestations can occur but are rare.[895]

Diagnosis

Clinical signs are highly suggestive in endemic areas where a patient has a known exposure. Definitive diagnosis of plague involves isolation of Y. pestis or demonstration of seroconversion. Cytological evaluation and culture of sputum, blood, aspirates from enlarged lymph nodes, or pharyngeal washes are commonly performed. Additional sites may be sampled depending on the type of disease (e.g., tracheal wash of patients with suspected pneumonic plague, CSF samples from suspected cases of meningitis). Enlarged lymph nodes are typically firm, so aspiration is usually performed following injection of 1–2 mL of saline. Seroconversion is evaluated by identification of a fourfold (or higher) increase in Y. pestis F1 antigen by passive hemagglutination testing titers of acute serum samples with those taken 4–6 weeks later.[895] IgG and IgM ELISA may also be used.[895] Presumptive diagnosis can be made by detection of Y. pestis F1 antigen using FA testing or a single positive antibody titer in an individual that was not previously vaccinated. Testing of smears using direct FA testing can be performed.

Management

Treatment for plague should be initiated as soon as plague is suspected based on clinical and epidemiological evidence. Streptomcyin is considered the most effective antimicrobial against Y. pestis, particularly in pneumonic plague.[895] Gentamicin is another option that is sometimes used. Chloramphenicol may be an alternative for bubonic or septicemic plague and is recommended for infection of areas of the body where aminoglycosides are unable to adequately penetrate (e.g., CNS, pleural cavity, eye).[895] Tetracyclines are sometimes used in uncomplicated plague. While sulfonamides have been used extensively, use of this class may be associated with higher mortality, increased complications, and longer duration of fever compared with treatment with other drugs.[915,916] Fluoroquinolones have been used in animals and would presumably be useful in humans; however, data regarding their use in human plague are currently lacking.[895] A recent concerning development has been the emergence of MDR Y. pestis.

Plague suspects with signs of respiratory disease should be placed in isolation and managed using respiratory droplet precautions.[917] Other potentially infected individuals should be managed with contact precautions, using gloves and gown as well as face protection or protective eyewear and mask for activities that could result in sprays or splashes.[895]

Prognosis varies with the type of disease and timing of diagnosis and treatment. Two hundred forty-seven cases were reported in the United States between 1980 and 1997, with a 15% mortality rate.[895] The main factors associated with mortality were a delay in seeking medical care and failure of the primary physician to recognize the potential for plague. These are of greatest concern in nonendemic areas. Untreated, mortality rates may be 50–80% in bubonic plague, and essentially 100% in septicemic and pneumonic plague.[895,897] In uncomplicated bubonic plague, systemic signs improve rapidly after the onset of appropriate therapy, and may resolve within 3–5 days. Buboes may remain enlarged and painful for weeks. Incision and drainage of buboes may be required, and should be done with care, as viable *Y. pestis* may be present. Pneumonic plague is the most serious form, and death usually occurs within 18–24 hours of onset of clinical signs in the absence of aggressive therapy.

In some situations, prophylactic antimicrobial treatment of potentially exposed people is indicated. This would include close contact with a pneumonic plague patient, potential exposure to *Y. pestis*-infected fleas, or contact with body fluids or tissues of an infected individual, as well as high-risk animal contact situations that are described below. Tetracyclines, chloramphenicol, or sulfonamides are typically used.[895]

Live-attenuated and formalin-killed *Y. pestis* vaccines are available; however, these do not provide protection against pneumonic plague. Vaccination is not typically useful during an outbreak because of the delay from vaccination to onset of protective immunity. Vaccination is typically reserved for people that are at particularly high risk, such as people working with *Y. pestis* and/or *Y. pestis*-infected animals. There is currently no general recommendation to vaccinate people working with animals in endemic areas.

Prevention

Households

The greatest risk of companion animal-associated transmission to humans comes from cats. All free-roaming or flea-infested cats in endemic areas should be considered at risk for plague exposure. Routine flea control should be used in dogs and cats in endemic areas. Preventing dogs and cats from having contact with wildlife, especially hunting, may help reduce direct transmission of *Y. pestis* to pets. Furthermore, keeping cats indoors should reduce the risk of exposure to and acquisition of infected fleas, and should be considered in endemic areas, particularly during periods of increased disease activity. Dogs and cats should not be allowed to come into contact with wild rodent burrows or dead rodents or lagomorphs. Routine measures to reduce the risk of rodent infestations in the house or yard such as containing garbage are important. A vaccine is not currently available for dogs and cats.

When plague has been identified in a person in the household, investigation of pets is indicated. Serological testing of pets should be considered during investigation of human cases;[903] however, seropositivity does not indicate that the pet was the source of infection. There has been minimal investigation of the potential for human-to-animal transmission of plague. It is certainly plausible, particularly from people with pneumonic plague, as is concurrent infection from the same source. Therefore, dogs and cats that have been exposed to *Y. pestis* should be treated prophylactically, typically with tetracycline or doxycycline.

When plague has been identified in a pet in the household, prophylactic treatment of human contacts is reasonable. Particular attention should be paid to people that have been in contact with a cat with pneumonic plague, have been bitten or scratched by a plague suspect, or have skin lesions consistent with flea bites. Otherwise, there should be close attention for the onset of fever or other clinical signs attributable to plague. Humans that have been in contact with plague suspects should seek medical attention if they are bitten, scratched, had contact with potentially infectious fluids, or have an abrupt onset of fever. Other pets should also be treated prophylactically. It is reasonable to keep infected cats in isolation at a veterinary clinic for the first 2–4 days of treatment, after which point the risk of *Y. pestis* transmission is quite low.

Wild-caught animals such as prairie dogs, particularly those from plague-endemic areas, should never be taken as pets. Sick or injured wildlife should only be handled by trained personnel.

Veterinary clinics

All cats with fever of unknown origin or submandibular or retropharyngeal lymphadenopathy in endemic regions should be considered plague suspects. Coughing cats with no underlying cause for respiratory disease should also be considered high risk.

Animals with suspected plague that are hospitalized in veterinary clinics should be isolated and handled with barrier precautions consisting of gloves and gown, as well as full face protection or eye protection and a mask. An N95 respirator should be used when handling animals with pneumonic plague because of the potential for aerosol transmission. Because of the high prevalence of oropharyngeal colonization in all animals infected with *Y. pestis*, great care should be taken when handling plague suspects to reduce the risk of bites. Any bite from a plague suspect should be lavaged thoroughly, and medical attention should be promptly obtained. There should be limited contact with plague suspects. The first 48–72 hours is the period of greatest risk. After that time, surviving animals are considered to be of low risk for transmission of *Y. pestis* if proper antimicrobial therapy has been initiated. Plague suspects should be closely examined for the presence of fleas, and if any evidence of flea infestation is identified, they should be treated with an adulticide. If live fleas are identified, pyrethrin or carbamate treatment of clinic areas where the cat has been is prudent, as well as treatment of any animals that may have had direct or indirect contact with the plague suspect or its fleas. All organic material, particularly pus-contaminated items, should be treated as biohazardous and carefully managed as per local regulations. All items that have come into contact with the animal should be disinfected or discarded after use. Routine disinfectants are effective against *Y. pestis* if used properly.

Care should be taken when collecting and handling diagnostic specimens from infected animals. Proper needle handling practices are critical, considering the high incidence of needlestick injuries in veterinary practices.

As with owners of pets with plague, prophylactic treatment of veterinary personnel who have been in contact with infected animals should be considered or close attention should be paid to the development of symptoms potentially associated with plague. High-risk exposure such as unbarriered contact with infected animals, contact with a cat with pneumonic plague, a bite from an infected cat, or a needlestick injury from an infected animal indicates the need for prophylactic antimicrobial therapy.

Y. pestis is also an important potential bioterrorism agent. While the likelihood of intentional release of *Y. pestis* in a nonendemic area is very low, veterinarians need to be aware of the disease as companion animals could be among the first individuals exposed.

Yersinia pseudotuberculosis

Y. pseudotuberculosis is a gram-negative bacterium in the Enterobacteriaceae family and an uncommon cause of both sporadic disease and outbreaks in humans. It can be found worldwide in a wide range of domestic and wild animals, including rodents, rabbits, deer, livestock, hedgehogs, and birds.[918–921] A small percentage of healthy dogs and cats can shed *Y. pseudotuberculosis* in feces. A study from Japan reported *Y. pseudotuberculosis* shedding by 4.1% of cats and 6.3% of dogs,[922] while a study from New Zealand reported colonization of 28% of stray cats.[921] Despite being a relatively common commensal in healthy animals, *Y. pseudotuberculosis* can cause clinical infections in companion animals. It has been implicated as a cause of enteritis in dogs and cats, though its presence in normal animals complicates the assessment of its role in enteritis. More convincing are reports of extraintestinal *Y. pseudotuberculosis* infections in animals, which appear to be more common in cats. Clinical presentation can be variable, with nonspecific signs such as lethargy, malaise, anorexia, and vomiting with focal abscessation in areas such as the liver, lungs, and kidneys.[923,924]

In humans, the most common clinical manifestation is mesenteric adenitis. This is characterized by acute abdominal disease, which may mimic appendicitis, as patients typically have fever and right lower quadrant abdominal pain.[925] Infection is typically self-limited. Erythema nodosum and polyarthritis are less common clinical presentations. Bloodstream infections are rare but can occur, particularly in individuals with underlying chronic diseases.

Most affected individuals are 5–14 years of age, with males infected three times more often than females.[926] Infections are most commonly reported in Europe and during winter months. The source of infection is typically believed to be fecal–oral exposure to *Y. pseudotuberculosis* from infected or colonized animals, contaminated environment or food and water.[926] The relative importance of those different sources is unclear.

Because rodents and birds commonly carry *Y. pseudotuberculosis*, and the potential exposure of many cats to these species, it has been suggested that cats may play a role in the transmission of this pathogen from those species to humans.[927] However, the actual evidence of transmission from companion animals to humans is minimal. Some reports have implicated pets as a possible source but with weak evidence. One report of a fatal infection in a person who had worked in a garden that a diarrheic cat may have defecated in has been used to implicate cats as a source of infection.[928] Another study implicated cats by finding *Y. pseudotuberculosis* in two children and a stray cat, as well as soil and sand.[928] Conclusions about zoonotic transmission from the cat are tenuous because concurrent isolation cannot determine direction of transmission or rule out common-source infection. Since this organism can be found in the environment and many other animal species, such as rodents, that could have both contaminated the environment and infected the cat, care should be taken when interpreting these studies. Concurrent infection of four children and their dog has also been reported,[929] but that could also indicate common-source infection.

Given the low incidence of disease and presence of *Y. pseudotuberculosis* in a small percentage of healthy animals, the risk of zoonotic transmission from companion animals is presumably very low. There is no information available about measures to reduce the risk of transmission from companion animals to humans. Since *Y. pseudotuberculosis* is transmitted via the fecal–oral route, and it can be shed in feces of animals, general hygiene practices regarding contact with animal feces are probably the most important. This involves avoiding contact with feces, careful attention to hand hygiene, and reducing environmental contamination by removing feces.

References

1. Goddard WW, Bennett SA, Parkinson C. *Anaerobiospirillum succiniciproducens* septicaemia: important aspects of diagnosis and management. *J Infect* 1998;37:68–70.
2. Malnick H. *Anaerobiospirillum thomasii* sp. nov., an anaerobic spiral bacterium isolated from the feces of cats and dogs and from diarrheal feces of humans, and emendation of the genus *Anaerobiospirillum*. *Int J Syst Bacteriol* 1997;47:381–384.
3. Yuen KY, Yung WH, Seto WH. A case report of *Anaerobiospirillum* causing septicemia. *J Infect Dis* 1989;159:153–154.
4. Anonymous. *Anaerobiospirillum* infection. *Commun Dis Scot* 1985;85:vii.
5. Malnick H, Jones A, Vickers JC. *Anaerobiospirillum*: cause of a "new" zoonosis? *Lancet* 1989;1:1145–1146.
6. Rossi M, Hänninen ML, Revez J, et al. Occurrence and species level diagnostics of *Campylobacter* spp., enteric *Helicobacter* spp. and *Anaerobiospirillum* spp. in healthy and diarrheic dogs and cats. *Vet Microbiol* 2008;129:304–314.
7. Walker DH, Dumler JS. *Ehrlichia chaffeensis*, *Anaplasma phagocytophilum* and other Ehrlichieae. In: Mandell GL, Bennett JE, Dolin R, eds. *Principles and Practice of Infectious Diseases*. Philadelphia: Elsevier, 2005, pp. 2310–2318.
8. Fera MT, La Camera E, Carbone M, et al. Pet cats as carriers of *Arcobacter* spp. in Southern Italy. *J Appl Microbiol* 2009;106:1661–1666.
9. Vandamme P, Falsen E, Rossau R, et al. Revision of *Campylobacter*, *Helicobacter*, and *Wolinella* taxonomy: emendation of generic descriptions and proposal of *Arcobacter* gen. nov. *Int J Syst Bacteriol* 1991;41:88–103.
10. Vandamme P, Pugina P, Benzi G, et al. Outbreak of recurrent abdominal cramps associated with *Arcobacter butzleri* in an Italian school. *J Clin Microbiol* 1992;30:2335–2337.
11. Aydin F, Gümüşsoy KS, Atabay HI, et al. Prevalence and distribution of *Arcobacter* species in various sources in Turkey and molecular analysis of isolated strains by ERIC-PCR. *J Appl Microbiol* 2007;103:27–35.
12. Ho HT, Lipman LJ, Gaastra W. *Arcobacter*, what is known and unknown about a potential foodborne zoonotic agent! *Vet Microbiol* 2006;115:1–13.
13. Lerner J, Brumberger V, Preac-Mursic V. Severe diarrhea associated with *Arcobacter butzleri*. *Eur J Clin Microbiol Infect Dis* 1994;13:660–662.
14. Vandenberg O, Dediste A, Houf K, et al. *Arcobacter* species in humans. *Emerg Infect Dis* 2004;10:1863–1867.
15. Wybo I, Breynaert J, Lauwers S, et al. Isolation of *Arcobacter skirrowii* from a patient with chronic diarrhea. *J Clin Microbiol* 2004;42:1851–1852.
16. Snelling WJ, Matsuda M, Moore JE, et al. Under the microscope: *Arcobacter*. *Lett Appl Microbiol* 2006;42:7–14.
17. Petersen RF, Harrington CS, Kortegaard HE, et al. A PCR-DGGE method for detection and identification of *Campylobacter*, *Helicobacter*, *Arcobacter* and

related *Epsilobacteria* and its application to saliva samples from humans and domestic pets. *J Appl Microbiol* 2007;103:2601–2615.

18. Houf K, De Smet S, Baré J, et al. Dogs as carriers of the emerging pathogen *Arcobacter*. *Vet Microbiol* 2008;130:208–213.

19. Shadomy SV, Smith TL. Zoonosis update. Anthrax. *J Am Vet Med Assoc* 2008;233:63–72.

20. Moore GE, Greene CE. Anthrax. In: Greene CE, ed. *Infectious Diseases of the Dog and Cat*. Philadelphia: Saunders Elsevier, 2006, pp. 312–315.

21. Lucey D. *Bacillus anthracis* (anthrax). In: Mandell GL, Bennett JE, Dolin R, eds. *Principles and Practice of Infectious Diseases*. Philadelphia: Elsevier, 2005, pp. 2485–2491.

22. Metcalfe N. The history of woolsorters' disease: a Yorkshire beginning with an international future? *Occup Med (Lond)* 2004;54:489–493.

23. Langston C. Postexposure management and treatment of anthrax in dogs—executive councils of the American Academy of Veterinary Pharmacology and Therapeutics and the American College of Veterinary Clinical Pharmacology. *AAPS J* 2005;7:E272–E273.

24. American Academy of Pediatrics. *Red Book: 2009 Report of the Committee on Infectious Diseases*, 28th ed. Elk Grove Village, IL: American Academy of Pediatrics, 2009.

25. Jernigan JA, Stephens DS, Ashford DA, et al. Bioterrorism-related inhalational anthrax: the first 10 cases reported in the United States. *Emerg Infect Dis* 2001;7:933–944.

26. Inglesby TV, O'Toole T, Henderson DA, et al. Anthrax as a biological weapon, 2002: updated recommendations for management. *JAMA* 2002;287:2236–2252.

27. Centers for Disease Control and Prevention. *E-IND Protocol: One Time Emergency Use of Liquid 5% Anthrax Immune Globulin for Treatment of Severe Anthrax*. Altanta, GA: Centers for Disease Control and Prevention, 2006.

28. Breitschwerdt EB. Feline bartonellosis and cat scratch disease. *Vet Immunol Immunopathol* 2008;123:167–171.

29. Chomel BB, Kasten RW, Henn JB, et al. *Bartonella* infection in domestic cats and wild felids. *Ann N Y Acad Sci* 2006;1078:410–415.

30. Avidor B, Graidy M, Efrat G, et al. *Bartonella koehlerae*, a new cat-associated agent of culture-negative human endocarditis. *J Clin Microbiol* 2004;42:3462–3468.

31. Duncan AW, Marr HS, Birkenheuer AJ, et al. Bartonella DNA in the blood and lymph nodes of Golden Retrievers with lymphoma and in healthy controls. *J Vet Intern Med* 2008;22:89–95.

32. Mexas AM, Hancock SI, Breitschwerdt EB. *Bartonella henselae* and *Bartonella elizabethae* as potential canine pathogens. *J Clin Microbiol* 2002;40:4670–4674.

33. Daly JS, Worthington MG, Brenner DJ, et al. *Rochalimaea elizabethae* sp. nov. isolated from a patient with endocarditis. *J Clin Microbiol* 1993;31:872–881.

34. Arvand M, Feil EJ, Giladi M, et al. Multi-locus sequence typing of *Bartonella henselae* isolates from three continents reveals hypervirulent and feline-associated clones. *PLoS One* 2007;2:e1346.

35. Slater LN, Welch DF. *Bartonella*, including cat-scratch disease. In: Mandell GL, Bennett JE, Dolin R, eds. *Principles and Practice of Infectious Diseases*. Philadelphia: Elsevier, 2005, pp. 2733–2748.

36. Case JB, Chomel B, Nicholson W, et al. Serological survey of vector-borne zoonotic pathogens in pet cats and cats from animal shelters and feral colonies. *J Feline Med Surg* 2006;8:111–117.

37. Celebi B, Kilic S, Aydin N, et al. Investigation of *Bartonella henselae* in cats in Ankara, Turkey. *Zoonoses Public Health* 2009;56:169–175.

38. Inoue K, Maruyama S, Kabeya H, et al. Prevalence of *Bartonella* infection in cats and dogs in a metropolitan area, Thailand. *Epidemiol Infect* 2009;137:1–6.

39. Guptill L, Wu CC, HogenEsch H, et al. Prevalence, risk factors, and genetic diversity of *Bartonella henselae* infections in pet cats in four regions of the United States. *J Clin Microbiol* 2004;42:652–659.

40. Chomel BB, Boulouis HJ, Maruyama S, et al. *Bartonella* spp. in pets and effect on human health. *Emerg Infect Dis* 2006;12:389–394.

41. Chang CC, Lee CC, Maruyama S, et al. Cat-scratch disease in veterinary-associated populations and in its cat reservoir in Taiwan. *Vet Res* 2006;37:565–577.

42. Kamrani A, Parreira VR, Greenwood J, et al. The prevalence of *Bartonella*, hemoplasma, and *Rickettsia felis* infections in domestic cats and in cat fleas in Ontario. *Can J Vet Res* 2008;72:411–419.

43. Kim YS, Seo KW, Lee JH, et al. Prevalence of *Bartonella henselae* and *Bartonella clarridgeiae* in cats and dogs in Korea. *J Vet Sci* 2009;10:85–87.

44. Chomel BB, Boulouis HJ, Petersen H, et al. Prevalence of *Bartonella* infection in domestic cats in Denmark. *Vet Res* 2002;33:205–213.

45. Jackson LA, Spach DH, Kippen DA, et al. Seroprevalence to *Bartonella quintana* among patients at a community clinic in downtown Seattle. *J Infect Dis* 1996;173:1023–1026.

46. Chang CC, Kasten RW, Chomel BB, et al. Coyotes (*Canis latrans*) as the reservoir for a human pathogenic *Bartonella* sp.: molecular epidemiology of *Bartonella vinsonii* subsp. *berkhoffii* infection in

coyotes from central coastal California. *J Clin Microbiol* 2000;38:4193–4200.

47. Chomel BB, Abbott RC, Kasten RW, et al. *Bartonella henselae* prevalence in domestic cats in California: risk factors and association between bacteremia and antibody titers. *J Clin Microbiol* 1995;33:2445–2450.

48. Gurfield AN, Boulouis HJ, Chomel BB, et al. Epidemiology of *Bartonella* infection in domestic cats in France. *Vet Microbiol* 2001;80:185–198.

49. Al-Majali AM. Seroprevalence of and risk factors for *Bartonella henselae* and *Bartonella quintana* infections among pet cats in Jordan. *Prev Vet Med* 2004;64:63–71.

50. Guptill L, Slater L, Wu CC, et al. Experimental infection of young specific pathogen-free cats with *Bartonella henselae*. *J Infect Dis* 1997;176:206–216.

51. Yamamoto K, Chomel BB, Kasten RW, et al. Experimental infection of specific pathogen free (SPF) cats with two different strains of *Bartonella henselae* type I: a comparative study. *Vet Res* 2002;33:669–684.

52. Abbott RC, Chomel BB, Kasten RW, et al. Experimental and natural infection with *Bartonella henselae* in domestic cats. *Comp Immunol Microbiol Infect Dis* 1997;20:41–51.

53. Arvand M, Viezens J, Berghoff J. Prolonged *Bartonella henselae* bacteremia caused by reinfection in cats. *Emerg Infect Dis* 2008;14:152–154.

54. Foil L, Andress E, Freeland RL, et al. Experimental infection of domestic cats with *Bartonella henselae* by inoculation of *Ctenocephalides felis* (Siphonaptera: Pulicidae) feces. *J Med Entomol* 1998;35:625–628.

55. Guptill L, Slater LN, Wu CC, et al. Evidence of reproductive failure and lack of perinatal transmission of *Bartonella henselae* in experimentally infected cats. *Vet Immunol Immunopathol* 1998;65:177–189.

56. Di Francesco A, Sanguinetti V, Gallina L, et al. Prevalence of antibodies to *Bartonella henselae* in dogs in Italy. *Vet Rec* 2007;161:489–490.

57. Diniz PP, Wood M, Maggi RG, et al. Co-isolation of *Bartonella henselae* and *Bartonella vinsonii* subsp. *berkhoffii* from blood, joint and subcutaneous seroma fluids from two naturally infected dogs. *Vet Microbiol* 2009;138:117–123.

58. Gary AT, Webb JA, Hegarty BC, et al. The low seroprevalence of tick-transmitted agents of disease in dogs from southern Ontario and Quebec. *Can Vet J* 2006;47:1194–1200.

59. Henn JB, Liu CH, Kasten RW, et al. Seroprevalence of antibodies against *Bartonella* species and evaluation of risk factors and clinical signs associated with seropositivity in dogs. *Am J Vet Res* 2005;66:688–694.

60. Solano-Gallego L, Bradley J, Hegarty B, et al. *Bartonella henselae* IgG antibodies are prevalent in dogs from southeastern USA. *Vet Res* 2004;35:585–595.

61. Gundi VA, Bourry O, Davous B, et al. *Bartonella clarridgeiae* and *B. henselae* in dogs, Gabon. *Emerg Infect Dis* 2004;10:2261–2262.

62. Diniz PP, Maggi RG, Schwartz DS, et al. Canine bartonellosis: serological and molecular prevalence in Brazil and evidence of co-infection with *Bartonella henselae* and *Bartonella vinsonii* subsp. *berkhoffii*. *Vet Res* 2007;38:697–710.

63. Duncan AW, Maggi RG, Breitschwerdt EB. Bartonella DNA in dog saliva. *Emerg Infect Dis* 2007;13:1948–1950.

64. Chomel BB, Kasten RW, Sykes JE, et al. Clinical impact of persistent *Bartonella* bacteremia in humans and animals. *Ann N Y Acad Sci* 2003;990:267–278.

65. Holmberg M, McGill S, Ehrenborg C, et al. Evaluation of human seroreactivity to *Bartonella* species in Sweden. *J Clin Microbiol* 1999;37:1381–1384.

66. Al-Majali AM, Al-Qudah KM. Seroprevalence of *Bartonella henselae* and *Bartonella quintana* infections in children from Central and Northern Jordan. *Saudi Med J* 2004;25:1664–1669.

67. Noah DL, Kramer CM, Verbsky MP, et al. Survey of veterinary professionals and other veterinary conference attendees for antibodies to *Bartonella henselae* and *B quintana*. *J Am Vet Med Assoc* 1997;210:342–344.

68. Breitschwerdt EB, Maggi RG, Duncan AW, et al. *Bartonella* species in blood of immunocompetent persons with animal and arthropod contact. *Emerg Infect Dis* 2007;13:938–941.

69. Podsiadly E, Chmielewski T, Sochon E, et al. *Bartonella henselae* in *Ixodes ricinus* ticks removed from dogs. *Vector Borne Zoonotic Dis* 2007;7:189–192.

70. Cotté V, Bonnet S, Le Rhun D, et al. Transmission of *Bartonella henselae* by *Ixodes ricinus*. *Emerg Infect Dis* 2008;14:1074–1080.

71. Billeter SA, Diniz PP, Battisti JM, et al. Infection and replication of *Bartonella* species within a tick cell line. *Exp Appl Acarol* 2009;49:193–208.

72. Telford SR, Wormser GP. *Bartonella* spp. transmission by ticks not established. *Emerg Infect Dis* 2010;16:379–384.

73. Chen TC, Lin WR, Lu PL, et al. Cat scratch disease from a domestic dog. *J Formos Med Assoc* 2007;106:S65–S68.

74. Carithers HA. Cat-scratch disease. An overview based on a study of 1,200 patients. *Am J Dis Child* 1985;139:1124–1133.

75. Magalhães RF, Cintra ML, Barjas-Castro ML, et al. Blood donor infected with *Bartonella henselae*. *Transfus Med* 2010;20:280–282.

76. Velho PE. Blood transfusion as an alternative bartonellosis transmission in a pediatric liver transplant. *Transpl Infect Dis* 2009;11:474.

77. Jackson LA, Perkins BA, Wenger JD. Cat scratch disease in the United States: an analysis of three national databases. *Am J Public Health* 1993;83: 1707–1711.

78. Breitschwerdt EB, Maggi RG, Nicholson WL, et al. *Bartonella* sp. *bacteremia* in patients with neurological and neurocognitive dysfunction. *J Clin Microbiol* 2008;46:2856–2861.

79. Centers for Disease Control and Prevention (CDC). Cat-scratch disease in children—Texas, September 2000-August 2001. *MMWR Morb Mortal Wkly Rep* 2002;51:212–214.

80. Zangwill KM, Hamilton DH, Perkins BA, et al. Cat scratch disease in Connecticut. Epidemiology, risk factors, and evaluation of a new diagnostic test. *N Engl J Med* 1993;329:8–13.

81. Gasquet S, Maurin M, Brouqui P, et al. Bacillary angiomatosis in immunocompromised patients. *AIDS* 1998;12:1793–1803.

82. Chomel BB, Kasten RW, Williams CA, et al. *Bartonella* endocarditis: a pathology shared by animal reservoirs and patients. *Ann N Y Acad Sci* 2009;1166:120–126.

83. Perez C, Hummel JB, Keene BW, et al. Successful treatment of *Bartonella henselae* endocarditis in a cat. *J Feline Med Surg* 2010;12:483–486.

84. Duncan AW, Maggi RG, Breitschwerdt EB. A combined approach for the enhanced detection and isolation of *Bartonella* species in dog blood samples: pre-enrichment liquid culture followed by PCR and subculture onto agar plates. *J Microbiol Methods* 2007;69:273–281.

85. Breitschwerdt E. *Treatment of* Bartonella *Infection in Dogs and Cats*. Raleigh, NC: Vector Borne Disease Diagnostic Laboratory, North Carolina State University, 2009.

86. Maman E, Bickels J, Ephros M, et al. Musculoskeletal manifestations of cat scratch disease. *Clin Infect Dis* 2007;45:1535–1540.

87. Margileth AM, Wear DJ, English CK. Systemic cat scratch disease: report of 23 patients with prolonged or recurrent severe bacterial infection. *J Infect Dis* 1987;155:390–402.

88. Cherinet Y, Tomlinson R. Cat scratch disease presenting as acute encephalopathy. *Emerg Med J* 2008;25:703–704.

89. Fouch B, Coventry S. A case of fatal disseminated *Bartonella henselae* infection (cat-scratch disease) with encephalitis. *Arch Pathol Lab Med* 2007;131:1591–1594.

90. Nishio N, Kubuta T, Nakao Y, et al. Cat scratch disease with encephalopathy in a 9-year-old girl. *Pediatr Int* 2008;50:823–824.

91. Patel SJ, Petrarca R, Shah SM, et al. Atypical *Bartonella henselae* chorioretinitis in an immunocompromised patient. *Ocul Immunol Inflamm* 2008;16: 45–49.

92. Pipili C, Katsogridakis K, Cholongitas E. Myocarditis due to *Bartonella henselae*. *South Med J* 2008;101:1186.

93. Ridder-Schröter R, Marx A, Beer M, et al. Abscessforming lymphadenopathy and osteomyelitis in children with *Bartonella henselae* infection. *J Med Microbiol* 2008;57:519–524.

94. Smith RA, Scott B, Beverley DW, et al. Encephalopathy with retinitis due to cat-scratch disease. *Dev Med Child Neurol* 2007;49:931–934.

95. Bonatti H, Mendez J, Guerrero I, et al. Disseminated *Bartonella* infection following liver transplantation. *Transpl Int* 2006;19:683–687.

96. Lejko-Zupanc T, Slemenik-Pusnik C, Kozelj M, et al. Native valve endocarditis due to *Bartonella henselae* in an immunocompetent man. *Wien Klin Wochenschr* 2008;120:246–249.

97. Martín L, Vidal L, Campins A, et al. *Bartonella* as a cause of blood culture-negative endocarditis. Description of five cases. *Rev Esp Cardiol* 2009;62: 694–697.

98. Caniza MA, Granger DL, Wilson KH, et al. *Bartonella henselae*: etiology of pulmonary nodules in a patient with depressed cell-mediated immunity. *Clin Infect Dis* 1995;20:1505–1511.

99. Margileth AM. Antibiotic therapy for cat-scratch disease: clinical study of therapeutic outcome in 268 patients and a review of the literature. *Pediatr Infect Dis J* 1992;11:474–478.

100. Bass JW, Freitas BC, Freitas AD, et al. Prospective randomized double blind placebo-controlled evaluation of azithromycin for treatment of cat-scratch disease. *Pediatr Infect Dis J* 1998;17:447–452.

101. Mofenson LM, Brady MT, Danner SP, et al. Guidelines for the prevention and treatment of opportunistic infections among HIV-exposed and HIV-infected children: recommendations from CDC, the National Institutes of Health, the HIV Medicine Association of the Infectious Diseases Society of America, the Pediatric Infectious Diseases Society, and the American Academy of Pediatrics. *MMWR Recomm Rep* 2009;58:1–166.

102. Hemsworth S, Pizer B. Pet ownership in immunocompromised children—a review of the literature and survey of existing guidelines. *Eur J Oncol Nurs* 2006;10:117–127.

103. Wardrop K, Reine N, Birkenheuer A, et al. Canine and feline blood donor screening for infectious disease. *J Vet Intern Med* 2005;19:135–142.

104. Heller R, Artois M, Xemar V, et al. Prevalence of *Bartonella henselae* and *Bartonella clarridgeiae* in stray cats. *J Clin Microbiol* 1997;35:1327–1331.

105. Arvand M, Klose AJ, Schwartz-Porsche D, et al. Genetic variability and prevalence of *Bartonella henselae* in cats in Berlin, Germany, and analysis of its genetic relatedness to a strain from Berlin that is pathogenic for humans. *J Clin Microbiol* 2001; 39:743–746.

106. Chomel BB, Carlos ET, Kasten RW, et al. *Bartonella henselae* and *Bartonella clarridgeiae* infection in domestic cats from The Philippines. *Am J Trop Med Hyg* 1999;60:593–597.

107. Kelly PJ, Meads N, Theobald A, et al. *Rickettsia felis*, *Bartonella henselae*, and *B. clarridgeiae*, New Zealand. *Emerg Infect Dis* 2004;10:967–968.

108. Rolain JM, Locatelli C, Chabanne L, et al. Prevalence of *Bartonella clarridgeiae* and *Bartonella henselae* in domestic cats from France and detection of the organisms in erythrocytes by immunofluorescence. *Clin Diagn Lab Immunol* 2004;11:423–425.

109. MacDonald KA, Chomel BB, Kittleson MD, et al. A prospective study of canine infective endocarditis in northern California (1999–2001): emergence of *Bartonella* as a prevalent etiologic agent. *J Vet Intern Med* 2004;18:56–64.

110. Kordick DL, Hilyard EJ, Hadfield TL, et al. *Bartonella clarridgeiae*, a newly recognized zoonotic pathogen causing inoculation papules, fever, and lymphadenopathy (cat scratch disease). *J Clin Microbiol* 1997;35:1813–1818.

111. Margileth AM, Baehren DF. Chest-wall abscess due to cat-scratch disease (CSD) in an adult with antibodies to *Bartonella clarridgeiae*: case report and review of the thoracopulmonary manifestations of CSD. *Clin Infect Dis* 1998;27:353–357.

112. Breitschwerdt E, Chomel B. Canine bartonellosis. In: Greene CE, ed. *Infectious Diseases of the Dog and Cat*. Philadelphia: Saunders Elsevier, 2006, pp. 518–524.

113. Beldomenico PM, Chomel BB, Foley JE, et al. Environmental factors associated with *Bartonella vinsonii* subsp. *berkhoffii* seropositivity in free-ranging coyotes from northern California. *Vector Borne Zoonotic Dis* 2005;5:110–119.

114. Diniz PP, Billeter SA, Otranto D, et al. Molecular documentation of *Bartonella* infection in dogs in Greece and Italy. *J Clin Microbiol* 2009;47: 1565–1567.

115. Henn JB, Vanhorn BA, Kasten RW, et al. Antibodies to *Bartonella vinsonii* subsp. *berkhoffii* in Moroccan dogs. *Am J Trop Med Hyg* 2006;74:222–223.

116. Just FT, Gilles J, Pradel I, et al. Molecular evidence for *Bartonella* spp. in cat and dog fleas from Germany and France. *Zoonoses Public Health* 2008; 55:514–520.

117. Solano-Gallego L, Llull J, Osso M, et al. A serological study of exposure to arthropod-borne pathogens in dogs from northeastern Spain. *Vet Res* 2006;37: 231–244.

118. Celebi B, Carhan A, Kilic S, et al. Detection and genetic diversity of *Bartonella vinsonii* subsp. *berkhoffii* strains isolated from dogs in Ankara, Turkey. *J Vet Med Sci* 2010;72:969–973.

119. Pappalardo BL, Correa MT, York CC, et al. Epidemiologic evaluation of the risk factors associated with exposure and seroreactivity to *Bartonella vinsonii* in dogs. *Am J Vet Res* 1997;58:467–471.

120. Breitschwerdt EB, Hegarty BC, Hancock SI. Sequential evaluation of dogs naturally infected with *Ehrlichia canis*, *Ehrlichia chaffeensis*, *Ehrlichia equi*, *Ehrlichia ewingii*, or *Bartonella vinsonii*. *J Clin Microbiol* 1998;36:2645–2651.

121. Kordick SK, Breitschwerdt EB, Hegarty BC, et al. Coinfection with multiple tick-borne pathogens in a Walker Hound kennel in North Carolina. *J Clin Microbiol* 1999;37:2631–2638.

122. Cherry NA, Diniz PP, Maggi RG, et al. Isolation or molecular detection of *Bartonella henselae* and *Bartonella vinsonii* subsp. *berkhoffii* from dogs with idiopathic cavitary effusions. *J Vet Intern Med* 2009;23:186–189.

123. Cockwill KR, Taylor SM, Philibert HM, et al. *Bartonella vinsonii* subsp. *berkhoffii* endocarditis in a dog from Saskatchewan. *Can Vet J* 2007;48: 839–844.

124. Fenollar F, Sire S, Wilhelm N, et al. *Bartonella vinsonii* subsp. *arupensis* as an agent of blood culture-negative endocarditis in a human. *J Clin Microbiol* 2005;43:945–947.

125. Breitschwerdt EB, Maggi RG, Varanat M, et al. Isolation of *Bartonella vinsonii* subsp. *berkhoffii* genotype II from a boy with epithelioid hemangioendothelioma and a dog with hemangiopericytoma. *J Clin Microbiol* 2009;47:1957–1960.

126. Lin WR, Chen YS, Liu YC. Cellulitis and bacteremia caused by *Bergeyella zoohelcum*. *J Formos Med Assoc* 2007;106:573–576.

127. Montejo M, Aguirrebengoa K, Ugalde J, et al. *Bergeyella zoohelcum* bacteremia after a dog bite. *Clin Infect Dis* 2001;33:1608–1609.

128. Shukla SK, Paustian DL, Stockwell PJ, et al. Isolation of a fastidious *Bergeyella* species associated with cellulitis after a cat bite and a phylogenetic comparison with *Bergeyella zoohelcum* strains. *J Clin Microbiol* 2004;42:290–293.

129. Steinberg JP, Del Rio C. Other gram-negative and gram-variable bacilli. In: Mandell GL, Bennett JE, Dolin R, eds. *Principles and Practice of Infectious Diseases*. Philadelphia: Elsevier, 2005, pp. 2751–2768.

130. Bemis DA, Shek WR, Clifford CB. *Bordetella bronchiseptica* infection of rats and mice. *Comp Med* 2003;53:11–20.

131. Egberink H, Addie D, Belák S, et al. *Bordetella bronchiseptica* infection in cats ABCD guidelines on prevention and management. *J Feline Med Surg* 2009; 11:610–614.

132. Mochizuki M, Yachi A, Ohshima T, et al. Etiologic study of upper respiratory infections of household dogs. *J Vet Med Sci* 2008;70:563–569.

133. Rougier S, Galland D, Boucher S, et al. Epidemiology and susceptibility of pathogenic bacteria responsible for upper respiratory tract infections in pet rabbits. *Vet Microbiol* 2006;115:192–198.

134. Speakman AJ, Dawson S, Binns SH, et al. *Bordetella bronchiseptica* infection in the cat. *J Small Anim Pract* 1999;40:252–256.

135. Englund L, Jacobs AA, Klingeborn B, et al. Seroepidemiological survey of *Bordetella bronchiseptica* and canine parainfluenza-2 virus in dogs in Sweden. *Vet Rec* 2003;152:251–254.

136. Gaskell RM, Dawson S, Radford A. Feline respiratory disease. In: Greene CE, ed. *Infectious Diseases of the Dog and Cat*. Philadelphia: Saunders Elsevier, 2006, pp. 145–154.

137. Binns SH, Dawson S, Speakman AJ, et al. Prevalence and risk factors for feline *Bordetella bronchiseptica* infection. *Vet Rec* 1999;144:575–580.

138. Helps CR, Lait P, Damhuis A, et al. Factors associated with upper respiratory tract disease caused by feline herpesvirus, feline calicivirus, *Chlamydophila felis* and *Bordetella bronchiseptica* in cats: experience from 218 European catteries. *Vet Rec* 2005; 156:669–673.

139. Dworkin MS, Sullivan PS, Buskin SE, et al. *Bordetella bronchiseptica* infection in human immunodeficiency virus-infected patients. *Clin Infect Dis* 1999;28: 1095–1099.

140. Gisel JJ, Brumble L, Johnson M. *Bordetella bronchiseptica* pneumonia following exposure to recently vaccinated canine. *Chest* 2007;132:7105.

141. Gisel JJ, Brumble L, Johnson M. *Bordetella bronchiseptica* pneumonia in a kidney-pancreas transplant patient after exposure to recently vaccinated dogs. *Transpl Infect Dis* 2009;12:73–76.

142. Huebner ES, Christman B, Dummer S, et al. Hospital-acquired *Bordetella bronchiseptica* infection following hematopoietic stem cell transplantation. *J Clin Microbiol* 2006;44:2581–2583.

143. Ner Z, Ross LA, Horn MV, et al. *Bordetella bronchiseptica* infection in pediatric lung transplant recipients. *Pediatr Transplant* 2003;7:413–417.

144. Llombart M, Chiner E, Senent C. Necrotizing pneumonia due to *Bordetella bronchiseptica* in an immunocompetent woman. *Arch Bronconeumol* 2006; 42:255–256.

145. Rath BA, Register KB, Wall J, et al. Persistent *Bordetella bronchiseptica* pneumonia in an immunocompetent infant and genetic comparison of clinical isolates with kennel cough vaccine strains. *Clin Infect Dis* 2008;46:905–908.

146. Stefanelli P, Mastrantonio P, Hausman SZ, et al. Molecular characterization of two *Bordetella bronchiseptica* strains isolated from children with coughs. *J Clin Microbiol* 1997;35:1550–1555.

147. Tamion F, Girault C, Chevron V, et al. *Bordetella bronchoseptica* pneumonia with shock in an immunocompetent patient. *Scand J Infect Dis* 1996; 28:197–198.

148. Ford RB. Canine infectious tracheobronchitis. In: Greene CE, ed. *Infectious Diseases of the Dog and Cat*. Philadelphia: Saunders Elsevier, 2006, pp. 54–61.

149. Berkelman RL. Human illness associated with use of veterinary vaccines. *Clin Infect Dis* 2003;37: 407–414.

150. Reina J, Bassa A, Llompart I, et al. Pneumonia caused by *Bordetella bronchiseptica* in a patient with a thoracic trauma. *Infection* 1991;19:46–48.

151. Jacobs AA, Theelen RP, Jaspers R, et al. Protection of dogs for 13 months against *Bordetella bronchiseptica* and canine parainfluenza virus with a modified live vaccine. *Vet Rec* 2005;157:19–23.

152. Young EJ. *Brucella* species. In: Mandell GL, Bennett JE, Dolin R, eds. *Principles and Practice of Infectious Diseases*. Philadelphia: Elsevier, 2005, pp. 2669–2674.

153. Hollett RB. Canine brucellosis: outbreaks and compliance. *Theriogenology* 2006;66:575–587.

154. Brower A, Okwumabua O, Massengill C, et al. Investigation of the spread of *Brucella canis* via the U.S. interstate dog trade. *Int J Infect Dis* 2007;11: 454–458.

155. Brown J, Blue JL, Wooley RE, et al. *Brucella canis* infectivity rates in stray and pet dog populations. *Am J Public Health* 1976;66:889–891.

156. Dahlbom M, Johnsson M, Myllys V, et al. Seroprevalence of canine herpesvirus-1 and *Brucella canis* in Finnish breeding kennels with and without reproductive problems. *Reprod Domest Anim* 2009;44:128–131.

157. Ebani VV, Cerri D, Fratini F, et al. Serological diagnosis of brucellosis caused by *Brucella canis*. *New Microbiol* 2003;26:65–73.

158. Lovejoy GS, Carver HD, Moseley IK, et al. Serosurvey of dogs for *Brucella canis* infection in Memphis, Tennessee. *Am J Public Health* 1976;66: 175–176.

159. Shang DQ. Investigation of *B. canis* infection in China. *Zhonghua Liu Xing Bing Xue Za Zhi* 1989; 10:24–29.

160. Carmichael LE, Joubert JC. Transmission of *Brucella canis* by contact exposure. *Cornell Vet* 1988;78: 63–73.

161. Pretzer SD. Bacterial and protozoal causes of pregnancy loss in the bitch and queen. *Theriogenology* 2008;70:320–326.

162. Lucero NE, Corazza R, Almuzara MN, et al. Human *Brucella canis* outbreak linked to infection in dogs. *Epidemiol Infect* 2010;138:280–285.

163. Lucero NE, Escobar GI, Ayala SM, et al. Diagnosis of human brucellosis caused by *Brucella canis*. *J Med Microbiol* 2005;54:457–461.

164. Lucero NE, Jacob NO, Ayala SM, et al. Unusual clinical presentation of brucellosis caused by *Brucella canis*. *J Med Microbiol* 2005;54:505–508.

165. Kerwin SC, Lewis DD, Hribernik TN, et al. Diskospondylitis associated with *Brucella canis* infection in dogs: 14 cases (1980–1991). *J Am Vet Med Assoc* 1992;201:1253–1257.

166. Ledbetter EC, Landry MP, Stokol T, et al. *Brucella canis* endophthalmitis in 3 dogs: clinical features, diagnosis, and treatment. *Vet Ophthalmol* 2009; 12:183–191.

167. Smeak DD, Olmstead ML, Hohn RB. *Brucella canis* osteomyelitis in two dogs with total hip replacements. *J Am Vet Med Assoc* 1987;191:986–990.

168. Serikawa T, Muraguchi T, Nakao N, et al. Significance of urine culture for detecting infection with *Brucella canis* in dogs. *Nippon Juigaku Zasshi* 1978;40:353–355.

169. Wanke MM, Delpino MV, Baldi PC. Use of enrofloxacin in the treatment of canine brucellosis in a dog kennel (clinical trial). *Theriogenology* 2006;66: 1573–1578.

170. Rousseau P. *Brucella canis* infection in a woman with fever of unknown origin. *Postgrad Med* 1985;78:249, 253–244, 257.

171. Rumley RL, Chapman SW. *Brucella canis*: an infectious cause of prolonged fever of undetermined origin. *South Med J* 1986;79:626–628.

172. Soloaga R, Salinas A, Poterallo M, et al. Bacteremia by *Brucella canis*. Isolation with the Bact-Alert system. *Rev Argent Microbiol* 2004;36:81–84.

173. Schoenemann J, Lütticken R, Scheibner E. *Brucella canis* infection in man. *Dtsch Med Wochenschr* 1986;111:20–22.

174. Johnson CA, Walker RD. Clinical signs and diagnosis of *Brucella canis* infection. *Compend Cont Educ Pract Vet* 1992;14:763–772.

175. Chaban B, Musil K, Himsworth CG, et al. Development of cpn60-based real-time quantitative PCR assays for the detection of 14 *Campylobacter* species and application to screening of canine fecal samples. *Appl Environ Microbiol* 2009;75:3055–3061.

176. Acke E, McGill K, Golden O, et al. A comparison of different culture methods for the recovery of *Campylobacter* species from pets. *Zoonoses Public Health* 2009;56:490–495.

177. Acke E, McGill K, Golden O, et al. Prevalence of thermophilic *Campylobacter* species in household cats and dogs in Ireland. *Vet Rec* 2009;164:44–47.

178. Hald B, Pedersen K, Wainø M, et al. Longitudinal study of the excretion patterns of thermophilic *Campylobacter* spp. in young pet dogs in Denmark. *J Clin Microbiol* 2004;42:2003–2012.

179. Parsons BN, Porter CJ, Ryvar R, et al. Prevalence of *Campylobacter* spp. in a cross-sectional study of dogs attending veterinary practices in the UK and risk indicators associated with shedding. *Vet J* 2009; 184:66–70.

180. Moreno GS, Griffiths PL, Connerton IF, et al. Occurrence of campylobacters in small domestic and laboratory animals. *J Appl Bacteriol* 1993;75:49–54.

181. Baker J, Barton MD, Lanser J. *Campylobacter* species in cats and dogs in South Australia. *Aust Vet J* 1999;77:662–666.

182. Engvall EO, Brändstrom B, Andersson L, et al. Isolation and identification of thermophilic *Campylobacter* species in faecal samples from Swedish dogs. *Scand J Infect Dis* 2003;35:713–718.

183. Hald B, Madsen M. Healthy puppies and kittens as carriers of *Campylobacter* spp., with special reference to *Campylobacter upsaliensis*. *J Clin Microbiol* 1997;35:3351–3352.

184. Koene MG, Houwers DJ, Dijkstra JR, et al. Strain variation within *Campylobacter* species in fecal samples from dogs and cats. *Vet Microbiol* 2008; 133:199–205.

185. Torre E, Tello M. Factors influencing fecal shedding of *Campylobacter jejuni* in dogs without diarrhea. *Am J Vet Res* 1993;54:260–262.

186. Acke E, Whyte P, Jones BR, et al. Prevalence of thermophilic *Campylobacter* species in cats and dogs in two animal shelters in Ireland. *Vet Rec* 2006; 158:51–54.

187. Fox JG, Hering AM, Ackerman JI, et al. The pet hamster as a potential reservoir of human campylobacteriosis. *J Infect Dis* 1983;147:784.

188. Sandberg M, Bergsjø B, Hofshagen M, et al. Risk factors for *Campylobacter* infection in Norwegian cats and dogs. *Prev Vet Med* 2002;55:241–253.

189. Wieland B, Regula G, Danuser J, et al. *Campylobacter* spp. in dogs and cats in Switzerland: risk factor analysis and molecular characterization with AFLP. *J Vet Med B Infect Dis Vet Public Health* 2005; 52:183–189.

190. Bender J, Shulman S, Averbeck G, et al. Epidemiologic features of *Campylobacter* infection among cats in the upper midwestern United States. *J Am Vet Med Assoc* 2005;226:544–547.

191. Fox JG, Curry C, Leathers CW. Proliferative colitis in a pet ferret. *J Am Vet Med Assoc* 1986;189: 1475–1476.

192. Fox JG, Zanotti S, Jordan HV, et al. Colonization of Syrian hamsters with streptomycin resistant *Campylobacter jejuni*. *Lab Anim Sci* 1986;36:28–31.

193. Harvey S, Greenwood JR. Isolation of *Campylobacter fetus* from a pet turtle. *J Clin Microbiol* 1985;21: 260–261.

194. Marks S, Kather E, Kass P, et al. Genotypic and phenotypic characterization of *Clostridium perfringens* and *Clostridium difficile* in diarrheic and healthy dogs. *J Vet Intern Med* 2002;16:533–540.

195. Burnens AP, Angéloz-Wick B, Nicolet J. Comparison of *Campylobacter* carriage rates in diarrheic and healthy pet animals. *Zentralbl Veterinarmed B* 1992; 39:175–180.

196. Prescott JF, Barker IK, Manninen KI, et al. *Campylobacter jejuni* colitis in gnotobiotic dogs. *Can J Comp Med* 1981;45:377–383.

197. Prescott JF, Karmali MA. Attempts to transmit *Campylobacter* enteritis to dogs and cats. *CMAJ* 1978;119:1001–1002.

198. Macartney L, Al-Mashat RR, Taylor DJ, et al. Experimental infection of dogs with *Campylobacter jejuni*. *Vet Rec* 1988;122:245–249.

199. Black RE, Levine MM, Clements ML, et al. Experimental *Campylobacter jejuni* infection in humans. *J Infect Dis* 1988;157:472–479.

200. Blaser MJ, Allos BM. *Campylobacter jejuni* and related species. In: Mandell GL, Bennett JE, Dolin R, eds. *Principles and Practice of Infectious Diseases*, 6th ed. Philadelphia: Elsevier, 2005, pp. 2548–2557.

201. Adak GK, Cowden JM, Nicholas S, et al. The Public Health Laboratory Service national case-control study of primary indigenous sporadic cases of *Campylobacter* infection. *Epidemiol Infect* 1995; 115:15–22.

202. Fullerton KE, Ingram LA, Jones TF, et al. Sporadic *Campylobacter* infection in infants: a population-based surveillance case-control study. *Pediatr Infect Dis J* 2007;26:19–24.

203. Gillespie IA, O'Brien SJ, Adak GK, et al. Point source outbreaks of *Campylobacter jejuni* infection—are they more common than we think and what might cause them? *Epidemiol Infect* 2003;130:367–375.

204. Tenkate TD, Stafford RJ. Risk factors for *Campylobacter* infection in infants and young children: a matched case-control study. *Epidemiol Infect* 2001;127:399–404.

205. Tam CC, Higgins CD, Neal KR, et al. Chicken consumption and use of acid-suppressing medications as risk factors for *Campylobacter* enteritis, England. *Emerg Infect Dis* 2009;15:1402–1408.

206. Fox JG. *Campylobacter* infections. In: Greene CE, ed. *Infectious Diseases of the Dog and Cat*, 3rd ed. Philadelphia: Elsevier, 2006, pp. 339–343.

207. Damborg P, Olsen KE, Møller Nielsen E, et al. Occurrence of *Campylobacter jejuni* in pets living with human patients infected with *C. jejuni*. *J Clin Microbiol* 2004;42:1363–1364.

208. Labarca JA, Sturgeon J, Borenstein L, et al. *Campylobacter upsaliensis*: another pathogen for consideration in the United States. *Clin Infect Dis* 2002;34:E59–E60.

209. Goossens H, Vlaes L, Butzler JP, et al. *Campylobacter upsaliensis* enteritis associated with canine infections. *Lancet* 1991;337:1486–1487.

210. Gurgan T, Diker KS. Abortion associated with *Campylobacter upsaliensis*. *J Clin Microbiol* 1994; 32:3093–3094.

211. Bourke B, Chan VL, Sherman P. *Campylobacter upsaliensis*: waiting in the wings. *Clin Microbiol Rev* 1998;11:440–449.

212. Damborg P, Guardabassi L, Pedersen K, et al. Comparative analysis of human and canine *Campylobacter upsaliensis* isolates by amplified fragment length polymorphism. *J Clin Microbiol* 2008; 46:1504–1506.

213. Acke E, McGill K, Quinn T, et al. Antimicrobial resistance profiles and mechanisms of resistance in *Campylobacter jejuni* isolates from pets. *Foodborne Pathog Dis* 2009;6:705–710.

214. Fernández H, Martin R. *Campylobacter* intestinal carriage among stray and pet dogs. *Rev Saude Publica* 1991;25:473–475.

215. Hackett T, Lappin MR. Prevalence of enteric pathogens in dogs of north-central Colorado. *J Am Anim Hosp Assoc* 2003;39:52–56.

216. Fox JG, Maxwell KO, Taylor NS, et al. "*Campylobacter upsaliensis*" isolated from cats as identified by DNA relatedness and biochemical features. *J Clin Microbiol* 1989;27:2376–2378.

217. López CM, Giacoboni G, Agostini A, et al. Thermotolerant campylobacters in domestic animals in a defined population in Buenos Aires, Argentina. *Prev Vet Med* 2002;55:193–200.

218. Hill SL, Cheney JM, Taton-Allen GF, et al. Prevalence of enteric zoonotic organisms in cats. *J Am Vet Med Assoc* 2000;216:687–692.

219. Spain CV, Scarlett JM, Wade SE, et al. Prevalence of enteric zoonotic agents in cats less than 1 year old in central New York State. *J Vet Intern Med* 2001; 15:33–38.

220. Man SM, Zhang L, Day AS, et al. *Campylobacter concisus* and other *Campylobacter* species in children with newly diagnosed Crohn's disease. *Inflamm Bowel Dis* 2009;210:1008–1016.

221. Padungtod P, Kaneene JB. *Campylobacter* in food animals and humans in northern Thailand. *J Food Prot* 2005;68:2519–2526.

222. Engberg J, On SL, Harrington CS, et al. Prevalence of *Campylobacter*, *Arcobacter*, *Helicobacter*, and *Sutterella* spp. in human fecal samples as estimated by a reevaluation of isolation methods for campylobacters. *J Clin Microbiol* 2000;38:286–291.

223. Fernández H, Kahler K, Salazar R, et al. Prevalence of thermotolerant species of *Campylobacter* and their biotypes in children and domestic birds and dogs in southern Chile. *Rev Inst Med Trop Sao Paulo* 1994;36:433–436.

224. Pazzaglia G, Bourgeois AL, Araby I, et al. *Campylobacter*-associated diarrhoea in Egyptian infants: epidemiology and clinical manifestations of disease and high frequency of concomitant infections. *J Diarrhoeal Dis Res* 1993;11:6–13.

225. McKinley MJ, Taylor M, Sangree MH. Toxic megacolon with *Campylobacter* colitis. *Conn Med* 1980; 44:496–497.

226. Mishu B, Blaser MJ. Role of infection due to *Campylobacter jejuni* in the initiation of Guillain-Barré syndrome. *Clin Infect Dis* 1993;17:104–108.

227. Kaldor J, Speed BR. Guillain-Barré syndrome and *Campylobacter jejuni*: a serological study. *Br Med J (Clin Res Ed)* 1984;288:1867–1870.

228. Rees JH, Soudain SE, Gregson NA, et al. *Campylobacter jejuni* infection and Guillain-Barré syndrome. *N Engl J Med* 1995;333:1374–1379.

229. Hannu T, Mattila L, Rautelin H, et al. *Campylobacter*-triggered reactive arthritis: a population-based study. *Rheumatology* 2002;41:312–318.

230. Karmali MA, Fleming PC. *Campylobacter* enteritis in children. *J Pediatr* 1979;94:527–533.

231. Paisley JW, Mirrett S, Lauer BA, et al. Dark-field microscopy of human feces for presumptive diagnosis of *Campylobacter fetus* subsp. *jejuni* enteritis. *J Clin Microbiol* 1982;15:61–63.

232. Sazie ES, Titus AE. Rapid diagnosis of *Campylobacter* enteritis. *Ann Intern Med* 1982;96:62–63.

233. Salazar-Lindo E, Sack RB, Chea-Woo E, et al. Early treatment with erythromycin of *Campylobacter jejuni*-associated dysentery in children. *J Pediatr* 1986;109:355–360.

234. Anders BJ, Lauer BA, Paisley JW, et al. Double-blind placebo controlled trial of erythromycin for treatment of *Campylobacter* enteritis. *Lancet* 1982; 1:131–132.

235. Francioli P, Herzstein J, Grob JP, et al. *Campylobacter fetus* subspecies *fetus* bacteremia. *Arch Intern Med* 1985;145:289–292.

236. Tremblay C, Gaudreau C, Lorange M. Epidemiology and antimicrobial susceptibilities of 111 *Campylobacter fetus* subsp. *fetus* strains isolated in Québec, Canada, from 1983 to 2000. *J Clin Microbiol* 2003; 41:463–466.

237. Butler T, Weaver RE, Ramani TK, et al. Unidentified gram-negative rod infection. A new disease of man. *Ann Intern Med* 1977;86:1–5.

238. Brenner D, Hollis D, Fanning G, et al. *Capnocytophaga canimorsus* sp. nov. (formerly CDC group DF-2), a cause of septicemia following dog bite, and *C. cynodegmi* sp. nov., a cause of localized wound infection following dog bite. *J Clin Microbiol* 1989;27: 231–235.

239. Mally M, Paroz C, Shin H, et al. Prevalence of *Capnocytophaga canimorsus* in dogs and occurrence of potential virulence factors. *Microbes Infect* 2009;11:509–514.

240. Suzuki M, Kimura M, Imaoka K, et al. Prevalence of *Capnocytophaga canimorsus* and *Capnocytophaga cynodegmi* in dogs and cats determined by using a newly established species-specific PCR. *Vet Microbiol* 2010;144:172–176.

241. Blanche P, Bloch E, Sicard D. *Capnocytophaga canimorsus* in the oral flora of dogs and cats. *J Infect* 1998;36:134.

242. Bailie WE, Stowe EC, Schmitt AM. Aerobic bacterial flora of oral and nasal fluids of canines with reference to bacteria associated with bites. *J Clin Microbiol* 1978;7.223–231.

243. Workman HC, Bailiff NL, Jang SS, et al. *Capnocytophaga cynodegmi* in a rottweiler dog with severe bronchitis and foreign-body pneumonia. *J Clin Microbiol* 2008;46:4099–4103.

244. Forman MA, Johnson LR, Jang S, et al. Lower respiratory tract infection due to *Capnocytophaga cynodegmi* in a cat with pulmonary carcinoma. *J Feline Med Surg* 2005;7:227–231.

245. Gaastra W, Lipman LJ. Capnocytophaga canimorsus. *Vet Microbiol* 2009;140:339–346.

246. Gill JV. Capnocytophaga. In: Mandell GL, Bennett JE, Dolin R, eds. *Principles and Practice of Infectious Diseases*. Philadelphia: Elsevier, 2005, pp. 2730–2732.

247. Janda JM, Graves MH, Lindquist D, et al. Diagnosing *Capnocytophaga canimorsus* infections. *Emerg Infect Dis* 2006;12:340–342.

248. van Dam AP, Jansz A. *Capnocytophaga canimorsus* infections in the Netherlands: a nationwide survey. *Clin Microbiol Infect* 2010. Epub ahead of print.

249. Kullberg BJ, Westendorp RG, van't Wout JW, et al. Purpura fulminans and symmetrical peripheral gangrene caused by *Capnocytophaga canimorsus* (formerly DF-2) septicemia—a complication of dog bite. *Medicine (Baltimore)* 1991;70:287–292.

250. Gerster JC, Dudler J. Cellulitis caused by *Capnocytophaga cynodegmi* associated with etanercept treatment in a patient with rheumatoid arthritis. *Clin Rheumatol* 2004;23:570–571.

251. Khawari AA, Myers JW, Ferguson DA, et al. Sepsis and meningitis due to *Capnocytophaga cynodegmi* after splenectomy. *Clin Infect Dis* 2005;40: 1709–1710.

252. Peel MM. Dog-associated bacterial infections in humans: isolates submitted to an Australian reference laboratory, 1981–1992. *Pathology* 1993;25: 379–384.

253. Sarma PS, Mohanty S. *Capnocytophaga cynodegmi* cellulitis, bacteremia, and pneumonitis in a diabetic man. *J Clin Microbiol* 2001;39:2028–2029.

254. Valtonen M, Lauhio A, Carlson P, et al. *Capnocytophaga canimorsus* septicemia: fifth report of a cat-associated infection and five other cases. *Eur J Clin Microbiol Infect Dis* 1995;14:520–523.

255. Chadha V, Warady BA. *Capnocytophaga canimorsus* peritonitis in a pediatric peritoneal dialysis patient. *Pediatr Nephrol* 1999;13:646–648.

256. Jolivet-Gougeon A, Sixou JL, Tamanai-Shacoori Z, et al. Antimicrobial treatment of *Capnocytophaga* infections. *Int J Antimicrob Agents* 2007;29:367–373.

257. Lion C, Escande F, Burdin JC. *Capnocytophaga canimorsus* infections in human: review of the literature and cases report. *Eur J Epidemiol* 1996;12:521–533.

258. Pers C, Tvedegaard E, Christensen JJ, et al. *Capnocytophaga cynodegmi* peritonitis in a peritoneal dialysis patient. *J Clin Microbiol* 2007;45:3844–3846.

259. Tierney D, Strauss L, Sanchez J. *Capnocytophaga canimorsus* mycotic abdominal aortic aneurysm: why the mailman is afraid of dogs. *J Clin Microbiol* 2006;44:649–651.

260. Chodosh J. Cat's tooth keratitis: human corneal infection with *Capnocytophaga canimorsus*. *Cornea* 2001;20:661–663.

261. de Smet MD, Chan CC, Nussenblatt RB, et al. *Capnocytophaga canimorsus* as the cause of a chronic corneal infection. *Am J Ophthalmol* 1990;109: 240–242.

262. van Duijkeren E, van Mourik C, Broekhuizen M, et al. First documented *Capnocytophaga canimorsus* infection in a species other than humans. *Vet Microbiol* 2006;118:148–150.

263. Meyers B, Schoeman JP, Goddard A, et al. The bacteriology and antimicrobial susceptibility of infected and non-infected dog bite wounds: fifty cases. *Vet Microbiol* 2008;127:360–368.

264. Frey E, Pressler B, Guy J, et al. *Capnocytophaga* sp. isolated from a cat with chronic sinusitis and rhinitis. *J Clin Microbiol* 2003;41:5321–5324.

265. Le Moal G, Landron C, Grollier G, et al. Meningitis due to *Capnocytophaga canimorsus* after receipt of a dog bite: case report and review of the literature. *Clin Infect Dis* 2003;36:e42–e46.

266. Pers C, Gahrn-Hansen B, Frederiksen W. *Capnocytophaga canimorsus* septicemia in Denmark, 1982–1995: review of 39 cases. *Clin Infect Dis* 1996; 23:71–75.

267. Hantson P, Gautier PE, Vekemans MC, et al. Fatal *Capnocytophaga canimorsus* septicemia in a previously healthy woman. *Ann Emerg Med* 1991;20: 93–94.

268. Gasch O, Fernández N, Armisen A, et al. Community-acquired *Capnocytophaga canimorsus* meningitis in adults: report of one case with a subacute course and deafness, and literature review. *Enferm Infecc Microbiol Clin* 2009;27:33–36.

269. Guay DR. Pet-assisted therapy in the nursing home setting: potential for zoonosis. *Am J Infect Control* 2001;29:178–186.

270. Ricciardi B, Galgani I, Trezzi M, et al. Cerebral abscess caused by *Capnocytophaga* spp in an immunocompetent subject: case report. *Infez Med* 2008;16: 162–163.

271. Sandoe JA. *Capnocytophaga canimorsus* endocarditis. *J Med Microbiol* 2004;53:245–248.

272. Lopez E, Raymond J, Patkai J, et al. *Capnocytophaga* species and preterm birth case series and review of the literature. *Clin Microbiol Infect* 2009. Epub ahead of print.

273. Ndon JA. *Capnocytophaga canimorsus* septicemia caused by a dog bite in a hairy cell leukemia patient. *J Clin Microbiol* 1992;30:211–213.

274. Gottwein J, Zbinden R, Maibach R, et al. Etiologic diagnosis of *Capnocytophaga canimorsus* meningitis by broad-range PCR. *Eur J Clin Microbiol Infect Dis* 2006;25:132–134.

275. Bremmelgaard A, Pers C, Kristiansen JE, et al. Susceptibility testing of Danish isolates of *Capnocytophaga* and CDC group DF-2 bacteria. *APMIS* 1989;97:43–48.

276. Sykes JE. Feline chlamydiosis. *Clin Tech Small Anim Pract* 2005;20:129–134.

277. Di Francesco A, Piva S, Baldelli R. Prevalence of *Chlamydophila felis* by PCR among healthy pet cats in Italy. *New Microbiol* 2004;27:199–201.

278. Kang BT, Park HM. Prevalence of feline herpesvirus 1, feline calicivirus and *Chlamydophila felis* in clinically normal cats at a Korean animal shelter. *J Vet Sci* 2008;9:207–209.

279. Low HC, Powell CC, Veir JK, et al. Prevalence of feline herpesvirus 1, *Chlamydophila felis*, and *Mycoplasma* spp DNA in conjunctival cells collected from cats with and without conjunctivitis. *Am J Vet Res* 2007;68:643–648.

280. Rampazzo A, Appino S, Pregel P, et al. Prevalence of *Chlamydophila felis* and feline herpesvirus 1 in cats with conjunctivitis in northern Italy. *J Vet Intern Med* 2003;17:799–807.

281. Hartley JC, Stevenson S, Robinson AJ, et al. Conjunctivitis due to *Chlamydophila felis* (*Chlamydia psittaci*

feline pneumonitis agent) acquired from a cat: case report with molecular characterization of isolates from the patient and cat. *J Infect* 2001;43:7–11.

282. Cotton MM, Partridge MR. Infection with feline *Chlamydia psittaci*. *Thorax* 1998;53:75–76.

283. Schmeer N, Jahn GJ, Bialasiewicz AA, et al. The cat as a possible infection source for *Chlamydia psittaci* keratoconjunctivitis in humans. *Tierarztl Prax* 1987; 15:201–204.

284. Regan RJ, Dathan JR, Treharne JD. Infective endocarditis with glomerulonephritis associated with cat chlamydia (*C. psittaci*) infection. *Br Heart J* 1979; 42:349–352.

285. Griffiths PD, Lechler RI, Treharne JD. Unusual chlamydial infection in a human renal allograft recipient. *Br Med J* 1978;2:1264–1265.

286. Grayston JT, Kuo CC, Wang SP, et al. A new *Chlamydia psittaci* strain, TWAR, isolated in acute respiratory tract infections. *N Engl J Med* 1986; 315:161–168.

287. Marrie TJ, Peeling RW, Reid T, et al. *Chlamydia* species as a cause of community-acquired pneumonia in Canada. *Eur Respir J* 2003;21:779–784.

288. Browning GF. Is *Chlamydophila felis* a significant zoonotic pathogen? *Aust Vet J* 2004;82.695–696.

289. Harkinezhad T, Geens T, Vanrompay D. *Chlamydophila psittaci* infections in birds: a review with emphasis on zoonotic consequences. *Vet Microbiol* 2009;135:68–77.

290. Harkinezhad T, Verminnen K, De Buyzere M, et al. Prevalence of *Chlamydophila psittaci* infections in a human population in contact with domestic and companion birds. *J Med Microbiol* 2009;58:1207–1212.

291. Magnino S, Haag-Wackernagel D, Geigenfeind I, et al. Chlamydial infections in feral pigeons in Europe: review of data and focus on public health implications. *Vet Microbiol* 2009;135:54–67.

292. Tanaka C, Miyazawa T, Watarai M, et al. Bacteriological survey of feces from feral pigeons in Japan. *J Vet Med Sci* 2005;67:951–953.

293. Gaede W, Reckling KF, Dresenkamp B, et al. *Chlamydophila psittaci* infections in humans during an outbreak of psittacosis from poultry in Germany. *Zoonoses Public Health* 2008;55:184–188.

294. van Droogenbroeck C, Beeckman DS, Verminnen K, et al. Simultaneous zoonotic transmission of *Chlamydophila psittaci* genotypes D, F and E/B to a veterinary scientist. *Vet Microbiol* 2009;135: 78–81.

295. Laroucau K, Vorimore F, Bertin C, et al. Genotyping of *Chlamydophila abortus* strains by multilocus VNTR analysis. *Vet Microbiol* 2009;137:335–344.

296. Ferreri AJ, Dolcetti R, Magnino S, et al. A woman and her canary: a tale of chlamydiae and lymphomas. *J Natl Cancer Inst* 2007;99:1418–1419.

297. Raso Tde F, Júnior AB, Pinto AA. Evidence of *Chlamydophila psittaci* infection in captive Amazon parrots in Brazil. *J Zoo Wildl Med* 2002;33:118–121.

298. Vanrompay D, Harkinezhad T, van de Walle M, et al. *Chlamydophila psittaci* transmission from pet birds to humans. *Emerg Infect Dis* 2007;13: 1108–1110.

299. Smith K, Bradley K, Stobierski M, et al. Compendium of measures to control *Chlamydophila psittaci* (formerly *Chlamydia psittaci*) infection among humans (psittacosis) and pet birds, 2005. *J Am Vet Med Assoc* 2005;226:532–539.

300. Centers for Disease Control and Prevention. Final 2007 reports of nationally notifiable diseases. *MMWR Morb Mortal Wkly Rep* 2008;57:903–913.

301. Smith KA, Stobierski MG, Tengelsen LA, et al. Compendium of measures to control *Chlamydophila psittaci* infection among humans (psittacosis) and pet birds (avian chlamydiosis), 2009, National Association of State Public Health Veterinarians, 2009.

302. Matsui T, Nakashima K, Ohyama T, et al. An outbreak of psittacosis in a bird park in Japan. *Epidemiol Infect* 2008;136:492–495.

303. Moroney JF, Guevara R, Iverson C, et al. Detection of chlamydiosis in a shipment of pet birds, leading to recognition of an outbreak of clinically mild psittacosis in humans. *Clin Infect Dis* 1998;26:1425–1429.

304. Ward C, Ward AM. Acquired valvular heart-disease in patients who keep pet birds. *Lancet* 1974;2: 734–736.

305. Raso TF, Carrasco AO, Silva JC, et al. Seroprevalence of antibodies to *Chlamydophila psittaci* in zoo workers in Brazil. *Zoonoses Public Health* 2009. Epub ahead of print.

306. Sprague LD, Schubert E, Hotzel H, et al. The detection of *Chlamydophila psittaci* genotype C infection in dogs. *Vet J* 2009;181:274–279.

307. Mohan R. Epidemiologic and laboratory observations of *Chlamydia psittaci* infection in pet birds. *J Am Vet Med Assoc* 1984;184:1372–1374.

308. Arizmendi F, Grimes JE, Relford RL. Isolation of *Chlamydia psittaci* from pleural effusion in a dog. *J Vet Diagn Invest* 1992;4:460–463.

309. Beeckman DS, Vanrompay DC. Zoonotic *Chlamydophila psittaci* infections from a clinical perspective. *Clin Microbiol Infect* 2009;15:11–17.

310. Rasmussen-Ejde R. Ueber eine durch Sturmvogel ubertragbare Lungenerkrankung auf den Faroern. *Zentralbl Bakteriol Naturwiss* 1938;143:89–93.

311. Petrovay F, Balla E. Two fatal cases of psittacosis caused by *Chlamydophila psittaci*. *J Med Microbiol* 2008;57:1296–1298.

312. al Saif N, Brazier JS. The distribution of *Clostridium difficile* in the environment of South Wales. *J Med Microbiol* 1996;45:133–137.

313. Borriello S, Honour P, Turner T, et al. Household pets as a potential reservoir for *Clostridium difficile* infection. *J Clin Pathol* 1983;36:84–87.

314. Clooten J, Kruth S, Arroyo L, et al. Prevalence and risk factors for *Clostridium difficile* colonization in dogs and cats hospitalized in an intensive care unit. *Vet Microbiol* 2008;129:209–214.

315. Madewell BR, Bea JK, Kraegel SA, et al. *Clostridium difficile*: a survey of fecal carriage in cats in a veterinary medical teaching hospital. *J Vet Diagn Invest* 1999;11:50–54.

316. Riley TV, Adams JE, O'Neill GL, et al. Gastrointestinal carriage of *Clostridium difficile* in cats and dogs attending veterinary clinics. *Epidemiol Infect* 1991; 107:659–665.

317. Lefebvre S, Waltner-Toews D, Peregrine A, et al. Prevalence of zoonotic agents in dogs visiting hospitalized people in Ontario: implications for infection control. *J Hosp Infect* 2006;62:458–466.

318. Lefebvre SL, Reid-Smith RJ, Waltner-Toews D, et al. Incidence of acquisition of methicillin-resistant *Staphylococcus aureus*, *Clostridium difficile*, and other health-care-associated pathogens by dogs that participate in animal-assisted interventions. *J Am Vet Med Assoc* 2009;234:1404–1417.

319. Weese JS, Finley R, Reid-Smith R, et al. *Clostridium difficile* in dogs and the home environment. European Conference of Clinical Microbiology and Infectious Diseases. Helsinki, Finland, 2009.

320. Chouicha N, Marks SL. Evaluation of five enzyme immunoassays compared with the cytotoxicity assay for diagnosis of *Clostridium difficile*-associated diarrhea in dogs. *J Vet Diagn Invest* 2006;18: 182–188.

321. Bartlett JG, Gerding DN. Clinical recognition and diagnosis of *Clostridium difficile* infection. *Clin Infect Dis* 2008;46(Suppl. 1):S12–S18.

322. Kyne L, Merry C, O'Connell B, et al. Factors associated with prolonged symptoms and severe disease due to *Clostridium difficile*. *Age Ageing* 1999;28: 107–113.

323. Bartlett JG. Clinical practice. Antibiotic-associated diarrhea. *N Engl J Med* 2002;346:334–339.

324. Kelly CP, Pothoulakis C, LaMont JT. *Clostridium difficile* colitis. *N Engl J Med* 1994;330:257–262.

325. Triadafilopoulos G, Hallstone AE. Acute abdomen as the first presentation of pseudomembranous colitis. *Gastroenterology* 1991;101:685–691.

326. Cohen SH, Gerding DN, Johnson S, et al. Clinical practice guidelines for *Clostridium difficile* infection in adults: 2010 Update by the Society for Healthcare Epidemiology of America (SHEA) and the Infectious Diseases Society of America (IDSA). *Infect Control Hosp Epidemiol* 2010;31:431–455.

327. Morgan OW, Rodrigues B, Elston T, et al. Clinical severity of *Clostridium difficile* PCR ribotype 027: a case-case study. *PLoS One* 2008;3:e1812.

328. Lyerly DM, Neville LM, Evans DT, et al. Multicenter evaluation of the *Clostridium difficile* TOX A/B TEST. *J Clin Microbiol* 1998;36:184–190.

329. Peterson LR, Manson RU, Paule SM, et al. Detection of toxigenic *Clostridium difficile* in stool samples by real-time polymerase chain reaction for the diagnosis of *C. difficile*-associated diarrhea. *Clin Infect Dis* 2007;45:1152–1160.

330. De Zoysa A, Hawkey PM, Engler K, et al. Characterization of toxigenic *Corynebacterium ulcerans* strains isolated from humans and domestic cats in the United Kingdom. *J Clin Microbiol* 2005;43: 4377–4381.

331. Dias AA, Silva FC, Pereira GA, et al. *Corynebacterium ulcerans* isolated from an asymptomatic dog kept in an animal shelter in the metropolitan area of Rio de Janeiro, Brazil. *Vector Borne Zoonotic Dis* 2010. Epub ahead of print

332. Bonmarin I, Guiso N, Le Flèche-Matéos A, et al. Diphtheria: a zoonotic disease in France? *Vaccine* 2009;27:4196–4200.

333. Lartigue MF, Monnet X, Le Flèche A, et al. *Corynebacterium ulcerans* in an immunocompromised patient with diphtheria and her dog. *J Clin Microbiol* 2005;43:999–1001.

334. Schuhegger R, Schoerner C, Dlugaiczyk J, et al. Pigs as source for toxigenic *Corynebacterium ulcerans*. *Emerg Infect Dis* 2009;15:1314–1315.

335. Katsukawa C, Kawahara R, Inoue K, et al. Toxigenic *Corynebacterium ulcerans* isolated from the domestic dog for the first time in Japan. *Jpn J Infect Dis* 2009;62:171–172.

336. Aaron L, Heurtebise F, Bachelier MN, et al. Pseudomembranous diphtheria caused by *Corynebacterium ulcerans*. *Rev Med Interne* 2006;27: 333–335.

337. Hogg RA, Wessels J, Hart J, et al. Possible zoonotic transmission of toxigenic *Corynebacterium ulcerans* from companion animals in a human case of fatal diphtheria. *Vet Rec* 2009;165:691–692.

338. Higgins D, Marrie TJ. Seroepidemiology of Q fever among cats in New Brunswick and Prince Edward Island. *Ann N Y Acad Sci* 1990;590:271–274.

339. Komiya T, Sadamasu K, Kang MI, et al. Seroprevalence of *Coxiella burnetii* infections among cats in different living environments. *J Vet Med Sci* 2003;65:1047–1048.

340. Marrie TJ, Van Buren J, Fraser J, et al. Seroepidemiology of Q fever among domestic animals in Nova Scotia. *Am J Public Health* 1985;75: 763–766.

341. Matthewman L, Kelly P, Hayter D, et al. Exposure of cats in southern Africa to *Coxiella burnetii*, the agent of Q fever. *Eur J Epidemiol* 1997;13:477–479.

342. Morita C, Katsuyama J, Yanase T, et al. Seroepidemiological survey of *Coxiella burnetii* in domestic cats in Japan. *Microbiol Immunol* 1994;38: 1001–1003.

343. Cairns K, Brewer M, Lappin MR. Prevalence of *Coxiella burnetii* DNA in vaginal and uterine samples from healthy cats of north-central Colorado. *J Feline Med Surg* 2007;9:196–201.

344. Nagaoka H, Sugieda M, Akiyama M, et al. Isolation of *Coxiella burnetii* from the vagina of feline clients at veterinary clinics. *J Vet Med Sci* 1998;60: 251–252.

345. Willeberg P, Ruppanner R, Behymer DE, et al. Environmental exposure to *Coxiella burnetii*: a seroepidemiologic survey among domestic animals. *Am J Epidemiol* 1980;111:437–443.

346. Boni M, Davoust B, Tissot-Dupont H, et al. Survey of seroprevalence of Q fever in dogs in the southeast of France, French Guyana, Martinique, Senegal and the Ivory Coast. *Vet Microbiol* 1998;64:1–5.

347. Hartzell JD, Wood-Morris RN, Martinez LJ, et al. Q fever: epidemiology, diagnosis, and treatment. *Mayo Clin Proc* 2008;83:574–579.

348. Marrie TJ, Raoult D. *Coxiella burnetii* (Q fever). In: Mandell GL, Bennett JE, Dolin R, eds. *Principles and Practice of Infectious Diseases*. Philadelphia: Elsevier, 2005, pp. 2296–2303.

349. Loftis AD, Reeves WK, Szumlas DE, et al. Rickettsial agents in Egyptian ticks collected from domestic animals. *Exp Appl Acarol* 2006;40:67–81.

350. Mantovani A, Benazzi P. The isolation of *Coxiella burnetii* from *Rhipicephalus sanguineus* on naturally infected dogs. *J Am Vet Med Assoc* 1953;122: 117–118.

351. Embil J, Williams JC, Marrie TJ. The immune response in a cat-related outbreak of Q fever as measured by the indirect immunofluorescence test and the enzyme-linked immunosorbent assay. *Can J Microbiol* 1990;36:292–296.

352. Kosatsky T. Household outbreak of Q-fever pneumonia related to a parturient cat. *Lancet* 1984;2: 1447–1449.

353. Marrie TJ, Durant H, Williams JC, et al. Exposure to parturient cats: a risk factor for acquisition of Q fever in Maritime Canada. *J Infect Dis* 1988;158: 101–108.

354. Marrie TJ, MacDonald A, Durant H, et al. An outbreak of Q fever probably due to contact with a parturient cat. *Chest* 1988;93:98–103.

355. Nausheen S, Cunha BA. Q fever community-acquired pneumonia in a patient with Crohn's disease on immunosuppressive therapy. *Heart Lung* 2007;36:300–303.

356. Pinsky RL, Fishbein DB, Greene CR, et al. An outbreak of cat-associated Q fever in the United States. *J Infect Dis* 1991;164:202–204.

357. Skerget M, Wenisch C, Daxboeck F, et al. Cat or dog ownership and seroprevalence of ehrlichiosis, Q fever, and cat-scratch disease. *Emerg Infect Dis* 2003;9:1337–1340.

358. Buhariwalla F, Cann B, Marrie TJ. A dog-related outbreak of Q fever. *Clin Infect Dis* 1996;23:753–755.

359. Laughlin T, Waag D, Williams J, et al. Q fever: from deer to dog to man. *Lancet* 1991;337:676–677.

360. Rauch AM, Tanner M, Pacer RE, et al. Sheep-associated outbreak of Q fever, Idaho. *Arch Intern Med* 1987;147:341–344.

361. Connolly JH. Q fever in Northern Ireland. *Br Med J* 1968;1:547–552.

362. Asano K, Suzuki K, Nakamura Y, et al. Risk of acquiring zoonoses by the staff of companion-animal hospitals. *Kansenshōgaku Zasshi* 2003;77: 944–947.

363. Abe T, Yamaki K, Hayakawa T, et al. A seroepidemiological study of the risks of Q fever infection in Japanese veterinarians. *Eur J Epidemiol* 2001;17: 1029–1032.

364. Greene CE, Breitschwerdt E. Rocky mountain spotted fever, murine typhuslike disease, rickettsialpox, typhus and Q fever. In: Greene CE, ed. *Infectious Diseases of the Dog and Cat*. Philadelphia: Saunders Elsevier, 2006, pp. 232–245.

365. Komiya T, Sadamasu K, Toriniwa H, et al. Epidemiological survey on the route of *Coxiella burnetii* infection in an animal hospital. *J Infect Chemother* 2003;9:151–155.

366. Fenollar F, Fournier PE, Carrieri MP, et al. Risks factors and prevention of Q fever endocarditis. *Clin Infect Dis* 2001;33:312–316.

367. Hickie I, Davenport T, Wakefield D, et al. Post-infective and chronic fatigue syndromes precipitated by viral and non-viral pathogens: prospective cohort study. *BMJ* 2006;333:575.

368. Fournier PE, Marrie TJ, Raoult D. Diagnosis of Q fever. *J Clin Microbiol* 1998;36:1823–1834.

369. Parker NR, Barralet JH, Bell AM. Q fever. *Lancet* 2006;367:679–688.

370. Yeaman MR, Mitscher LA, Baca OG. In vitro susceptibility of *Coxiella burnetii* to antibiotics, including several quinolones. *Antimicrob Agents Chemother* 1987;31:1079–1084.

371. Carcopino X, Raoult D, Bretelle F, et al. Managing Q fever during pregnancy: the benefits of long-term cotrimoxazole therapy. *Clin Infect Dis* 2007;45: 548–555.

372. Raoult D, Houpikian P, Tissot Dupont H, et al. Treatment of Q fever endocarditis: comparison of 2 regimens containing doxycycline and ofloxacin or hydroxychloroquine. *Arch Intern Med* 1999;159: 167–173.

373. Gami AS, Antonios VS, Thompson RL, et al. Q fever endocarditis in the United States. *Mayo Clin Proc* 2004;79:253–257.

374. Lennette EH, Welsh HH. Q fever in California. X. Recovery of *Coxiella burneti* from the air of premises harboring infected goats. *Am J Hyg* 1951;54: 44–49.

375. Janda JM, Abbott SL. Infections associated with the genus *Edwardsiella*: the role of *Edwardsiella tarda* in human disease. *Clin Infect Dis* 1993;17:742–748.

376. Mikamo H, Ninomiya M, Sawamura H, et al. Puerperal intrauterine infection caused by *Edwardsiella tarda*. *J Infect Chemother* 2003;9:341–343.

377. Pien FD, Jackson MT. Tuboovarian abscess caused by *Edwardsiella tarda*. *Am J Obstet Gynecol* 1995; 173:964–965.

378. Nagel P, Serritella A, Layden TJ. *Edwardsiella tarda* gastroenteritis associated with a pet turtle. *Gastroenterology* 1982;82:1436–1437.

379. Vandepitte J, Lemmens P, de Swert L. Human Edwardsiellosis traced to ornamental fish. *J Clin Microbiol* 1983;17:165–167.

380. Neer TM, Harrus S. Canine monocytotropic ehrlichiosis and neorickettsiosis. In: Greene CE, ed. *Infectious Diseases of the Dog and Cat*. Philadelphia: Saunders Elsevier, 2006, pp. 203–216.

381. Perez M, Bodor M, Zhang C, et al. Human infection with *Ehrlichia canis* accompanied by clinical signs in Venezuela. *Ann N Y Acad Sci* 2006;1078: 110–117.

382. Neer TM, Harrus S. Canine monocytotropic ehrlichiosis and neorickettsiosis. In: Greene CE, ed. *Infectious Diseases of the Dog and Cat*. Philadelphia: Saunders Elsevier, 2005, pp. 203–216.

383. Dumler JS, Madigan JE, Pusterla N, et al. Ehrlichioses in humans: epidemiology, clinical presentation, diagnosis, and treatment. *Clin Infect Dis* 2007;45 (Suppl. 1):S45–S51.

384. Yu DH, Li YH, Yoon JS, et al. *Ehrlichia chaffeensis* infection in dogs in South Korea. *Vector Borne Zoonotic Dis* 2008;8:355–358.

385. Zhang XF, Zhang JZ, Long SW, et al. Experimental *Ehrlichia chaffeensis* infection in beagles. *J Med Microbiol* 2003;52:1021–1026.

386. Greig B, Breitschwerdt E, Armstrong PJ. Canine granulocytic ehrlichiosis. In: Greene CE, ed. *Infectious Diseases of the Dog and Cat*. Philadelphia: Saunders, Elsevier, 2005, pp. 217–219.

387. Paddock CD, Folk SM, Shore GM, et al. Infections with *Ehrlichia chaffeensis* and *Ehrlichia ewingii* in persons coinfected with human immunodeficiency virus. *Clin Infect Dis* 2001;33:1586–1594.

388. Brook I. Management of human and animal bite wound infection: an overview. *Curr Infect Dis Rep* 2009;11:389–395.

389. Goldstein EJ. Bite wounds and infection. *Clin Infect Dis* 1992;14:633–638.

390. Griego RD, Rosen T, Orengo IF, et al. Dog, cat, and human bites: a review. *J Am Acad Dermatol* 1995;33:1019–1029.

391. Allaker RP, Langlois T, Hardie JM. Prevalence of *Eikenella corrodens* and *Actinobacillus actinomycetemcomitans* in the dental plaque of dogs. *Vet Rec* 1994;134:519–520.

392. Allaker RP, Young KA, Langlois T, et al. Dental plaque flora of the dog with reference to fastidious and anaerobic bacteria associated with bites. *J Vet Dent* 1997;14:127–130.

393. Reik R, Tenover FC, Klein E, et al. The burden of vancomycin-resistant enterococcal infections in US hospitals, 2003 to 2004. *Diagn Microbiol Infect Dis* 2008;62:81–85.

394. Damborg P, Sørensen AH, Guardabassi L. Monitoring of antimicrobial resistance in healthy dogs: first report of canine ampicillin-resistant *Enterococcus faecium* clonal complex 17. *Vet Microbiol* 2008;132:190–196.

395. Ossiprandi M, Bottarelli E, Cattabiani F, et al. Susceptibility to vancomycin and other antibiotics of 165 *Enterococcus* strains isolated from dogs in Italy. *Comp Immunol Microbiol Infect Dis* 2007; 31:1–9.

396. Rice EW, Boczek LA, Johnson CH, et al. Detection of intrinsic vancomycin resistant enterococci in animal and human feces. *Diagn Microbiol Infect Dis* 2003;46:155–158.

397. de Niederhäusern S, Sabia C, Messi P, et al. VanA-type vancomycin-resistant enterococci in equine and swine rectal swabs and in human clinical samples. *Curr Microbiol* 2007;55:240–246.

398. Devriese L, Ieven M, Goossens H, et al. Presence of vancomycin-resistant enterococci in farm and pet animals. *Antimicrob Agents Chemother* 1996;40: 2285–2287.

399. van Belkun A, van den Braak N, Thomassen R, et al. Vancomycin-resistant enterococci in cats and dogs. *Lancet* 1996;348:1038–1039.

400. Wagenvoort JH, Burgers DM, Wagenvoort TH, et al. Absence of vancomycin-resistant enterococci (VRE) in companion dogs in the conurbation of Parkstad Limburg, The Netherlands. *J Antimicrob Chemother* 2003;52:532.

401. Rantala M, Lahti E, Kuhalampil J, et al. Antimicrobial resistance in *Staphylococcus* spp., *Escherichia coli* and *Enterococcus* spp. in dogs given antibiotics for

chronic dermatological disorders, compared with non-treated control dogs. *Acta Vet Scand* 2004; 45:37–45.

402. Poeta P, Costa D, Rodrigues J, et al. Antimicrobial resistance and the mechanisms implicated in faecal enterococci from healthy humans, poultry and pets in Portugal. *Int J Antimicrob Agents* 2006;27: 131–137.

403. De Graef EM, Decostere A, Devriese LA, et al. Antibiotic resistance among fecal indicator bacteria from healthy individually owned and kennel dogs. *Microb Drug Resist* 2004;10:65–69.

404. Beutin L, Geier D, Steinrück H, et al. Prevalence and some properties of verotoxin (Shiga-like toxin)-producing *Escherichia coli* in seven different species of healthy domestic animals. *J Clin Microbiol* 1993; 31:2483–2488.

405. Sancak A, Rutgers H, Hart C, et al. Prevalence of enteropathic *Escherichia coli* in dogs with acute and chronic diarrhoea. *Vet Rec* 2004;154:101–106.

406. Wang J, Wang S, Yin P. Haemolytic-uraemic syndrome caused by a non-O157:H7 *Escherichia coli* strain in experimentally inoculated dogs. *J Med Microbiol* 2006;55:23–29.

407. Tanaka H, Kondo R, Nishiuchi C, et al. Isolation of verocytotoxin-producing *Escherichia coli* from cattle and pets. *Kansenshōgaku Zasshi* 1992;66:448–455.

408. Smith K, Kruth S, Hammermueller J, et al. A case-control study of verocytotoxigenic *Escherichia coli* infection in cats with diarrhea. *Can J Vet Res* 1998;62:87–92.

409. Roopnarine RR, Ammons D, Rampersad J, et al. Occurrence and characterization of verocytotoxigenic *Escherichia coli* (VTEC) strains from dairy farms in Trinidad. *Zoonoses Public Health* 2007;54: 78–85.

410. Worth AJ, Marshall N, Thompson KG. Necrotising fasciitis associated with *Escherichia coli* in a dog. *N Z Vet J* 2005;53:257–260.

411. Hancock DD, Besser TE, Rice DH, et al. Multiple sources of *Escherichia coli* O157 in feedlots and dairy farms in the northwestern USA. *Prev Vet Med* 1998; 35:11–19.

412. Hogg RA, Holmes JP, Ghebrehewet S, et al. Probable zoonotic transmission of verocytotoxigenic *Escherichia coli* O 157 by dogs. *Vet Rec* 2009;164: 304–305.

413. Trevena WB, Hooper RS, Wray C, et al. Vero cytotoxin-producing *Escherichia coli* O157 associated with companion animals. *Vet Rec* 1996;138:400.

414. Stenske KA, Bemis DA, Gillespie BE, et al. Comparison of clonal relatedness and antimicrobial susceptibility of fecal *Escherichia coli* from healthy dogs and their owners. *Am J Vet Res* 2009;70: 1108–1116.

415. Stenske KA, Bemis DA, Gillespie BE, et al. Prevalence of urovirulence genes *cnf*, *hlyD*, *sfa/foc*, and *papGIII* in fecal *Escherichia coli* from healthy dogs and their owners. *Am J Vet Res* 2009;70:1401–1406.

416. Oyston PC, Sjostedt A, Titball RW. Tularaemia: bio-terrorism defence renews interest in *Francisella tularensis*. *Nat Rev Microbiol* 2004;2:967–978.

417. Penn RL. *Francisella tularensis* (tularemia). In: Mandell GL, Bennett JE, Dolin R, eds. *Principles and Practice of Infectious Diseases*. Philadelphia: Elsevier, 2005, pp. 2674–2685.

418. Greene CE, DeBey BM. Tularemia. In: Greene CE, ed. *Infectious Diseases of the Dog and Cat*. Philadelphia: Saunders Elsevier, 2006, pp. 446–451.

419. Liles W, Burger RJ. Tularemia from domestic cats. *West J Med* 1993;158:619–622.

420. Berrada ZL, Goethert HK, Telford SR. Raccoons and skunks as sentinels for enzootic tularemia. *Emerg Infect Dis* 2006;12:1019–1021.

421. Leighton FA, Artsob HA, Chu MC, et al. A serological survey of rural dogs and cats on the southwestern Canadian prairie for zoonotic pathogens. *Can J Public Health* 2001;92:67–71.

422. Magnarelli L, Levy S, Koski R. Detection of antibodies to *Francisella tularensis* in cats. *Res Vet Sci* 2007;82:22–26.

423. Meinkoth KR, Morton RJ, Meinkoth JH. Naturally occurring tularemia in a dog. *J Am Vet Med Assoc* 2004;225:545–547, 538.

424. Woods JP, Crystal MA, Morton RJ, et al. Tularemia in two cats. *J Am Vet Med Assoc* 1998;212:81–83.

425. Eliasson H, Lindbäck J, Nuorti JP, et al. The 2000 tularemia outbreak: a case-control study of risk factors in disease-endemic and emergent areas, Sweden. *Emerg Infect Dis* 2002;8:956–960.

426. Quenzer RW, Mostow SR, Emerson JK. Cat-bite tularemia. *JAMA* 1977;238:1845.

427. Arav-Boger R. Cat-bite tularemia in a seventeen-year-old girl treated with ciprofloxacin. *Pediatr Infect Dis J* 2000;19:583–584.

428. Capellan J, Fong IW. Tularemia from a cat bite: case report and review of feline-associated tularemia. *Clin Infect Dis* 1993;16:472–475.

429. Cooper WR, Ewell NM. Cat scratch induced tularemia. *Va Med Mon* 1973;100:640–642.

430. Miller LD, Montgomery EL. Human tularemia transmitted by bite of cat. *J Am Vet Med Assoc* 1957;130:314.

431. Siret V, Barataud D, Prat M, et al. An outbreak of airborne tularaemia in France, August 2004. *Euro Surveill* 2006;11:58–60.

432. Centers for Disease Control and Prevention (CDC). Tularemia associated with a hamster bite—Colorado, 2004. *MMWR Morb Mortal Wkly Rep* 2005;53:1202–1203.

433. Avashia SB, Petersen JM, Lindley CM, et al. First reported prairie dog-to-human tularemia transmission, Texas, 2002. *Emerg Infect Dis* 2004;10:483–486.

434. Scheel O, Reiersen R, Hoel T. Treatment of tularemia with ciprofloxacin. *Eur J Clin Microbiol Infect Dis* 1992;11:447–448.

435. Baldwin CJ, Panciera RJ, Morton RJ, et al. Acute tularemia in three domestic cats. *J Am Vet Med Assoc* 1991;199:1602–1605.

436. Rhyan JC, Gahagan T, Fales WH. Tularemia in a cat. *J Vet Diagn Invest* 1990;2:239–241.

437. Gustafson BW, DeBowes LJ. Tularemia in a dog. *J Am Anim Hosp Assoc* 1996;32:339–341.

438. Jacobs RF, Condrey YM, Yamauchi T. Tularemia in adults and children: a changing presentation. *Pediatrics* 1985;76:818–822.

439. Ohara Y, Sato T, Fujita H, et al. Clinical manifestations of tularemia in Japan—analysis of 1,355 cases observed between 1924 and 1987. *Infection* 1991;19:14–17.

440. Evans ME, Gregory DW, Schaffner W, et al. Tularemia: a 30-year experience with 88 cases. *Medicine (Baltimore)* 1985;64:251–269.

441. Penn RL, Kinasewitz GT. Factors associated with a poor outcome in tularemia. *Arch Intern Med* 1987;147:265–268.

442. Kusters JG, van Vliet AH, Kuipers EJ. Pathogenesis of *Helicobacter pylori* infection. *Clin Microbiol Rev* 2006;19:449–490.

443. Blaser MJ. *Helicobacter pylori* and other *Helicobacter* species. In: Mandell GL, Bennett JE, Dolin R, eds. *Principles and Practice of Infectious Diseases*. Philadelphia: Elsevier, 2005, pp. 2557–2567.

444. Baele M, Pasmans F, Flahou B, et al. Non-*Helicobacter pylori* helicobacters detected in the stomach of humans comprise several naturally occurring *Helicobacter* species in animals. *FEMS Immunol Med Microbiol* 2009;55:306–313.

445. De Bock M, Van den Bulck K, Hellemans A, et al. Peptic ulcer disease associated with *Helicobacter felis* in a dog owner. *Eur J Gastroenterol Hepatol* 2007;19:79–82.

446. Heilmann KL, Borchard F. Gastritis due to spiral shaped bacteria other than *Helicobacter pylori*: clinical, histological, and ultrastructural findings. *Gut* 1991;32:137–140.

447. Baele M, Decostere A, Vandamme P, et al. *Helicobacter baculiformis* sp. nov., isolated from feline stomach mucosa. *Int J Syst Evol Microbiol* 2008;58:357–364.

448. Ghil HM, Yoo JH, Jung WS, et al. Survey of *Helicobacter* infection in domestic and feral cats in Korea. *J Vet Sci* 2009;10:67–72.

449. Happonen I, Linden J, Saari S, et al. Detection and effects of helicobacters in healthy dogs and dogs with signs of gastritis. *J Am Vet Med Assoc* 1998;213:1767–1774.

450. Recordati C, Gualdi V, Tosi S, et al. Detection of *Helicobacter* spp. DNA in the oral cavity of dogs. *Vet Microbiol* 2007;119:346–351.

451. Priestnall SL, Wiinberg B, Spohr A, et al. Evaluation of "*Helicobacter heilmannii*" subtypes in the gastric mucosas of cats and dogs. *J Clin Microbiol* 2004; 42:2144–2151.

452. Van den Bulck K, Baele M, Hermans K, et al. First report on the occurrence of '*Helicobacter heilmannii*' in the stomach of rabbits. *Vet Res Commun* 2005; 29:271–279.

453. Cattoli G, van Vugt R, Zanoni RG, et al. Occurrence and characterization of gastric *Helicobacter* spp. in naturally infected dogs. *Vet Microbiol* 1999;70:239–250.

454. Hänninen ML, Hirvi U. Genetic diversity of canine gastric helicobacters, *Helicobacter bizzozeronii* and *H. salomonis* studied by pulsed-field gel electrophoresis. *J Med Microbiol* 1999;48:341–347.

455. Van den Bulck K, Decostere A, Baele M, et al. *Helicobacter cynogastricus* sp. nov., isolated from the canine gastric mucosa. *Int J Syst Evol Microbiol* 2006;56:1559–1564.

456. Fox JG, Perkins S, Yan L, et al. Local immune response in *Helicobacter pylori*-infected cats and identification of *H. pylori* in saliva, gastric fluid and faeces. *Immunology* 1996;88:400–406.

457. Handt LK, Fox JG, Dewhirst FE, et al. *Helicobacter pylori* isolated from the domestic cat: public health implications. *Infect Immun* 1994;62:2367–2374.

458. Hermanns W, Kregel K, Breuer W, et al. *Helicobacter*-like organisms: histopathological examination of gastric biopsies from dogs and cats. *J Comp Pathol* 1995;112:307–318.

459. Fox JG. Gastric *Helicobacter* infections. In: Greene CE, ed. *Infectious Diseases of the Dog and Cat*. Philadelphia: Saunders Elsevier, 2006, pp. 343–351.

460. Dieterich C, Wiesel P, Neiger R, et al. Presence of multiple "*Helicobacter heilmannii*" strains in an individual suffering from ulcers and in his two cats. *J Clin Microbiol* 1998;36:1366–1370.

461. McIsaac WJ, Leung GM. Peptic ulcer disease and exposure to domestic pets. *Am J Public Health* 1999;89:81–84.

462. Dore MP, Bilotta M, Vaira D, et al. High prevalence of *Helicobacter pylori* infection in shepherds. *Dig Dis Sci* 1999;44:1161–1164.

463. Levett PN. Leptospira. In: Murray PR, Baron EJ, Jorgensen JH, et al., eds. *Manual of Clinical Microbiology*, 9th ed. Washington, DC: ASM Press, 2007, pp. 963–970.

464. Levett PN. Leptospirosis. *Clin Microbiol Rev* 2001;14:296–326.

465. Langston CE, Heuter KJ. Leptospirosis. A re-emerging zoonotic disease. *Vet Clin North Am Small Anim Pract* 2003;33:791–807.

466. Prescott J. Canine leptospirosis in Canada: a veterinarian's perspective. *CMAJ* 2008;178:397–398.

467. Weese JS, Peregrine AS, Armstrong J. Occupational health and safety in small animal veterinary practice: Part I—nonparasitic zoonotic diseases. *Can Vet J* 2002;43:631–636.

468. Iwamoto E, Wada Y, Fujisaki Y, et al. Nationwide survey of *Leptospira* antibodies in dogs in Japan: results from microscopic agglutination test and enzyme-linked immunosorbent assay. *J Vet Med Sci* 2009;71:1191–1199.

469. Jimenez-Coello M, Ortega-Pacheco A, Guzman-Marin E, et al. Stray dogs as reservoirs of the zoonotic agents *Leptospira interrogans*, *Trypanosoma cruzi*, and *Aspergillus* spp. in an urban area of Chiapas in Southern Mexico. *Vector Borne Zoonotic Dis* 2009;10:135–141.

470. Jittapalapong S, Sittisan P, Sakpuaram T, et al. Coinfection of *Leptospira* spp and *Toxoplasma gondii* among stray dogs in Bangkok, Thailand. *Southeast Asian J Trop Med Public Health* 2009;40: 247–252.

471. Millán J, Candela MG, López-Bao JV, et al. Leptospirosis in wild and domestic carnivores in natural areas in Andalusia, Spain. *Vector Borne Zoonotic Dis* 2009;9:549–554.

472. Scanziani E, Origgi F, Giusti AM, et al. Serological survey of leptospiral infection in kennelled dogs in Italy. *J Small Anim Pract* 2002;43:154–157.

473. Alton GD, Berke O, Reid-Smith R, et al. Increase in seroprevalence of canine leptospirosis and its risk factors, Ontario 1998–2006. *Can J Vet Res* 2009; 73:167–175.

474. Moore GE, Guptill LF, Glickman NW, et al. Canine leptospirosis, United States, 2002–2004. *Emerg Infect Dis* 2006;12:501–503.

475. Glickman L, Moore G, Glickman N, et al. Purdue University-Banfield National Companion Animal Surveillance Program for emerging and zoonotic diseases. *Vector Borne Zoonotic Dis* 2006;6:14–23.

476. Stokes JE, Kaneene JB, Schall WD, et al. Prevalence of serum antibodies against six *Leptospira serovars* in healthy dogs. *J Am Vet Med Assoc* 2007;230: 1657–1664.

477. Ward MP, Glickman LT, Guptill LE. Prevalence of and risk factors for leptospirosis among dogs in the United States and Canada: 677 cases (1970–1998). *J Am Vet Med Assoc* 2002;220:53–58.

478. Ward MP, Guptill LF, Wu CC. Evaluation of environmental risk factors for leptospirosis in dogs: 36 cases (1997–2002). *J Am Vet Med Assoc* 2004;225: 72–77.

479. Bolin CA. Diagnosis of leptospirosis: a reemerging disease of companion animals. *Semin Vet Med Surg (Small Anim)* 1996;11:166–171.

480. Mylonakis ME, Bourtzi-Hatzopoulou E, Koutinas AF, et al. Leptospiral seroepidemiology in a feline hospital population in Greece. *Vet Rec* 2005; 156:615–616.

481. Agunloye CA, Nash AS. Investigation of possible leptospiral infection in cats in Scotland. *J Small Anim Pract* 1996;37:126–129.

482. Baer R, Turnberg W, Yu D, et al. Leptospirosis in a small animal veterinarian: reminder to follow standardized infection control procedures. *Zoonoses Public Health* 2009;57:281–284.

483. Gaudie CM, Featherstone CA, Phillips WS, et al. Human *Leptospira interrogans* serogroup icterohaemorrhagiae infection (Weil's disease) acquired from pet rats. *Vet Rec* 2008;163:599–601.

484. Guerra B, Schneider T, Luge E, et al. Detection and characterization of *Leptospira interrogans* isolates from pet rats belonging to a human immunodeficiency virus-positive patient with leptospirosis. *J Med Microbiol* 2008;57:133–135.

485. Jansen A, Schöneberg I, Frank C, et al. Leptospirosis in Germany, 1962–2003. *Emerg Infect Dis* 2005;11: 1048–1054.

486. Monahan AM, Miller IS, Nally JE. Leptospirosis: risks during recreational activities. *J Appl Microbiol* 2009;107:707–716.

487. Whitney EA, Ailes E, Myers LM, et al. Prevalence of and risk factors for serum antibodies against *Leptospira* serovars in US veterinarians. *J Am Vet Med Assoc* 2009;234:938–944.

488. Schnurrenberger PR, Hanson LE, Martin RJ. Infections with *Erysipelothrix*, *Leptospira*, and *Chlamydia* in Illinois veterinarians. *Int J Zoonoses* 1978;5:55–61.

489. Robinson RA, Metcalfe RV. Zoonotic infections in veterinarians. *N Z Vet J* 1976;24:201–210.

490. Nowotny N, Deutz A, Fuchs K, et al. Prevalence of swine influenza and other viral, bacterial, and parasitic zoonoses in veterinarians. *J Infect Dis* 1997;176:1414–1415.

491. Vincent C, Munger C, Labrecque O. La leptospirose: cas de transmission d'un chien a un humain. Quebec City, QC: Reseau d'Alerte et d'Information Zoosanitaire (RAIZO) Bulletin Zoosanitaire [no. 51], 2007.

492. Allard R, Bedard L. Explanatory notes on statistics for reportable disease and other infectious diseases under surveillance, period 3, year 2006 (weeks 9–12 [26 February 2006 to 25 March 2006]). Montreal, Quebec: Montreal Public Health Department, 2006.

493. Childs JE, Schwartz BS, Ksiazek TG, et al. Risk factors associated with antibodies to leptospires in

inner-city residents of Baltimore: a protective role for cats. *Am J Public Health* 1992;82:597–599.

494. Greene CE, Sykes JE, Brown CA, et al. Leptospirosis. In: Greene CE, ed. *Infectious Diseases of the Dog and Cat*. Philadelphia: Saunders Elsevier, 2006, pp. 402–417.

495. Birnbaum N, Barr SC, Center SA, et al. Naturally acquired leptospirosis in 36 dogs: serological and clinicopathological features. *J Small Anim Pract* 1998;39:231–236.

496. Rentko VT, Clark N, Ross LA, et al. Canine leptospirosis. A retrospective study of 17 cases. *J Vet Intern Med* 1992;6:235–244.

497. Klaasen HL, Molkenboer MJ, Vrijenhoek MP, et al. Duration of immunity in dogs vaccinated against leptospirosis with a bivalent inactivated vaccine. *Vet Microbiol* 2003;95:121–132.

498. Harkin KR, Roshto YM, Sullivan JT, et al. Comparison of polymerase chain reaction assay, bacteriologic culture, and serologic testing in assessment of prevalence of urinary shedding of leptospires in dogs. *J Am Vet Med Assoc* 2003;222: 1230–1233.

499. Levett PN, Whittington CU. Evaluation of the indirect hemagglutination assay for diagnosis of acute leptospirosis. *J Clin Microbiol* 1998;36:11–14.

500. Brown K, Prescott J. Leptospirosis in the family dog: a public health perspective. *CMAJ* 2008;178: 399–401.

501. Vijayachari P, Sehgal SC. Recent advances in the laboratory diagnosis of leptospirosis and characterisation of leptospires. *Indian J Med Microbiol* 2006; 24:320–322.

502. Suputtamongkol Y, Niwattayakul K, Suttinont C, et al. An open, randomized, controlled trial of penicillin, doxycycline, and cefotaxime for patients with severe leptospirosis. *Clin Infect Dis* 2004;39: 1417–1424.

503. DuPont H, Dupont-Perdrizet D, Perie JL, et al. Leptospirosis: prognostic factors associated with mortality. *Clin Infect Dis* 1997;25:720–724.

504. Vinetz JM. A mountain out of a molehill: do we treat acute leptospirosis, and if so, with what? *Clin Infect Dis* 2003;36:1514–1515.

505. Minke JM, Bey R, Tronel JP, et al. Onset and duration of protective immunity against clinical disease and renal carriage in dogs provided by a bi-valent inactivated leptospirosis vaccine. *Vet Microbiol* 2009;137:137–145.

506. Schreiber P, Martin V, Najbar W, et al. Prevention of renal infection and urinary shedding in dogs by a *Leptospira* vaccination. *Vet Microbiol* 2005;108: 113–118.

507. Adesiyun AA, Hull-Jackson C, Mootoo N, et al. Sero-epidemiology of canine leptospirosis in Trinidad: serovars, implications for vaccination and public health. *J Vet Med B Infect Dis Vet Public Health* 2006;53:91–99.

508. Geisen V, Stengel C, Brem S, et al. Canine leptospirosis infections—clinical signs and outcome with different suspected *Leptospira* serogroups (42 cases). *J Small Anim Pract* 2007;48:324–328.

509. Lorber B. Listeria monocytogenes. In: Mandell GL, Bennett JE, Dolin R, eds. *Principles and Practice of Infectious Diseases*. Philadelphia: Elsevier, 2005.

510. Mylonakis E, Hohmann EL, Calderwood SB. Central nervous system infection with *Listeria monocytogenes*. 33 years' experience at a general hospital and review of 776 episodes from the literature. *Medicine (Baltimore)* 1998;77:313–336.

511. Siegman-Igra Y, Levin R, Weinberger M, et al. *Listeria monocytogenes* infection in Israel and review of cases worldwide. *Emerg Infect Dis* 2002;8: 305–310.

512. Beauregard M, Malkin KL. Isolation of *Listeria monocytogenes* from brain specimens of domestic animals in Ontario. *Can Vet J* 1971;12:221–223.

513. Decker RA, Rogers JJ, Lesar S. Listeriosis in a young cat. *J Am Vet Med Assoc* 1976;168:1025.

514. Schroeder H, van Rensburg IB. Generalised *Listeria monocytogenes* infection in a dog. *J S Afr Vet Med Assoc* 1993;64:133–136.

515. Loncarevic S, Artursson K, Johansson I. A case of canine cutaneous listeriosis. *Vet Dermatol* 1999; 10:69–71.

516. Sturgess CP. Listerial abortion in the bitch. *Vet Rec* 1989;124:177.

517. Iida T, Kanzaki M, Maruyama T, et al. Prevalence of *Listeria monocytogenes* in intestinal contents of healthy animals in Japan. *J Vet Med Sci* 1991;53: 873–875.

518. Svabić-Vlahović M, Pantić D, Pavićić M, et al. Transmission of *Listeria monocytogenes* from mother's milk to her baby and to puppies. *Lancet* 1988; 2:1201.

519. Turenne CY, Wallace R, Behr MA. *Mycobacterium avium* in the postgenomic era. *Clin Microbiol Rev* 2007;20:205–229.

520. Turenne CY, Semret M, Cousins DV, et al. Sequencing of hsp65 distinguishes among subsets of the *Mycobacterium avium* complex. *J Clin Microbiol* 2006;44:433–440.

521. Bruijnesteijn van Coppenraet LE, de Haas PE, Lindeboom JA, et al. Lymphadenitis in children is caused by *Mycobacterium avium hominissuis* and not related to 'bird tuberculosis'. *Eur J Clin Microbiol Infect Dis* 2008;27:293–299.

522. Haist V, Seehusen F, Moser I, et al. *Mycobacterium avium* subsp. *hominissuis* infection in 2 pet dogs, Germany. *Emerg Infect Dis* 2008;14:988–990.

523. Shitaye EJ, Grymova V, Grym M, et al. *Mycobacterium avium* subsp. *hominissuis* infection in a pet parrot. *Emerg Infect Dis* 2009;15:617–619.

524. Biet F, Boschiroli M, Thorel M, et al. Zoonotic aspects of *Mycobacterium bovis* and *Mycobacterium avium-intracellulare* complex (MAC). *Vet Res* 2005;36:411–436.

525. Weil ML, Cuttino JT, McCabe AM. Pure granulomatous nocardiosis; a new form of disseminated infectious granulomatosis with massive retroperitoneal lymphadenopathy due to *Nocardia intracellularis*, n. sp. *Pediatrics* 1949;3:345–352.

526. Hoop RK, Böttger EC, Pfyffer GE. Etiological agents of mycobacterioses in pet birds between 1986 and 1995. *J Clin Microbiol* 1996;34:991–992.

527. Manarolla G, Liandris E, Pisoni G, et al. Avian mycobacteriosis in companion birds: 20-year survey. *Vet Microbiol* 2009;133:323–327.

528. Ludwig E, Reischl U, Janik D, et al. Granulomatous pneumonia caused by *Mycobacterium genavense* in a dwarf rabbit (*Oryctolagus cuniculus*). *Vet Pathol* 2009;46:1000–1002.

529. Hughes MS, Ball NW, Love DN, et al. Disseminated *Mycobacterium genavense* infection in a FIV-positive cat. *J Feline Med Surg* 1999;1:23–29.

530. Kiehn TE, Hoefer H, Bottger EC, et al. *Mycobacterium genavense* infections in pet animals. *J Clin Microbiol* 1996;34:1840–1842.

531. Lucas J, Lucas A, Furber H, et al. *Mycobacterium genavense* infection in two aged ferrets with conjunctival lesions. *Aust Vet J* 2000;78:685–689.

532. Ristola MA, von Reyn CF, Arbeit RD, et al. High rates of disseminated infection due to nontuberculous mycobacteria among AIDS patients in Finland. *J Infect* 1999;39:61–67.

533. Greene CE, Gunn-Moore D. Infections caused by slow-growing mycobacteria. In: Greene CE, ed. *Infectious Diseases of the Dog and Cat*. Philadelphia: Saunders Elsevier, 2006, pp. 462–477.

534. Gordin FM, Horsburgh CRJ. *Mycobacterium avium* complex. In: Mandell GL, Bennett JE, Dolin R, eds. *Principles and Practice of Infectious Diseases*. Philadelphia: Elsevier, 2005, pp. 2897–2909.

535. Sugita Y, Ishii N, Katsuno M, et al. Familial cluster of cutaneous *Mycobacterium avium* infection resulting from use of a circulating, constantly heated bath water system. *Br J Dermatol* 2000;142: 789–793.

536. Chapman JS. Role of milk and livestock in the epidemiology of diseases due to atypical mycobacteria. *Rev Tuberc Pneumol (Paris)* 1970;34:17–24.

537. Eggers JS, Parker GA, Braaf HA, et al. Disseminated *Mycobacterium avium* infection in three miniature schnauzer litter mates. *J Vet Diagn Invest* 1997; 9:424–427.

538. Gow AG, Gow DJ. Disseminated *Mycobacterium avium* complex infection in a dog. *Vet Rec* 2008; 162:594–595.

539. Horn B, Forshaw D, Cousins D, et al. Disseminated *Mycobacterium avium* infection in a dog with chronic diarrhoea. *Aust Vet J* 2000;78:320–325.

540. Bauer N, Burkhardt S, Kirsch A, et al. Lymphadenopathy and diarrhea in a miniature schnauzer. *Vet Clin Pathol* 2002;31:61–64.

541. O'Toole D, Tharp S, Thomsen BV, et al. Fatal mycobacteriosis with hepatosplenomegaly in a young dog due to *Mycobacterium avium*. *J Vet Diagn Invest* 2005;17:200–204.

542. Malik R, Gabor L, Martin P, et al. Subcutaneous granuloma caused by *Mycobacterium avium* complex infection in a cat. *Aust Vet J* 1998;76:604–607.

543. Barry M, Taylor J, Woods JP. Disseminated *Mycobacterium avium* infection in a cat. *Can Vet J* 2002;43:369–371.

544. Griffin A, Newton AL, Aronson LR, et al. Disseminated *Mycobacterium avium* complex infection following renal transplantation in a cat. *J Am Vet Med Assoc* 2003;222:1097–1101, 1077–1098.

545. Knippel A, Hetzel U, Baumgärtner W. Disseminated *Mycobacterium avium-intracellulare* infection in a Persian cat. *J Vet Med B Infect Dis Vet Public Health* 2004;51:464–466.

546. Morita Y, Kimur H, Kozawa K, et al. Cutaneous infection in a cat caused by *Mycobacterium avium* complex serovar 6. *Vet Rec* 2003;152:120.

547. Millán J, Negre N, Castellanos E, et al. Avian mycobacteriosis in free-living raptors in Majorca Island, Spain. *Avian Pathol* 2010;39:1–6.

548. Foldenauer U, Curd S, Zulauf I, et al. Ante mortem diagnosis of mycobacterial infection by liver biopsy in a budgerigar (*Melopsittacus undulatus*). *Schweiz Arch Tierheilkd* 2007;149:273–276.

549. Schultheiss PC, Dolginow SZ. Granulomatous enteritis caused by *Mycobacterium avium* in a ferret. *J Am Vet Med Assoc* 1994;204:1217–1218.

550. Glanemann B, Schönenbrücher H, Bridger N, et al. Detection of *Mycobacterium avium* subspecies *paratuberculosis*-specific DNA by PCR in intestinal biopsies of dogs. *J Vet Intern Med* 2008;22: 1090–1094.

551. Naughton JF, Mealey KL, Wardrop KJ, et al. Systemic *Mycobacterium avium* infection in a dog diagnosed by polymerase chain reaction analysis of buffy coat. *J Am Anim Hosp Assoc* 2005;41:128–132.

552. O'Brien RJ, Geiter LJ, Snider DE. The epidemiology of nontuberculous mycobacterial diseases in the United States. Results from a national survey. *Am Rev Respir Dis* 1987;135:1007–1014.

553. Debrunner M, Salfinger M, Brändli O, et al. Epidemiology and clinical significance of

nontuberculous mycobacteria in patients negative for human immunodeficiency virus in Switzerland. *Clin Infect Dis* 1992;15:330–345.

554. Winthrop KL, McNelley E, Kendall B, et al. Pulmonary nontuberculous mycobacterial disease prevalence and clinical features; an emerging public health disease. *Am J Respir Crit Care Med* 2010; 182:977–982.

555. Iseman MD, Buschman DL, Ackerson LM. Pectus excavatum and scoliosis. Thoracic anomalies associated with pulmonary disease caused by *Mycobacterium avium* complex. *Am Rev Respir Dis* 1991;144:914–916.

556. Reichenbach J, Rosenzweig S, Döffinger R, et al. Mycobacterial diseases in primary immunodeficiencies. *Curr Opin Allergy Clin Immunol* 2001; 1:503–511.

557. Winter SM, Bernard EM, Gold JW, et al. Humoral response to disseminated infection by *Mycobacterium avium-Mycobacterium intracellulare* in acquired immunodeficiency syndrome and hairy cell leukemia. *J Infect Dis* 1985;151:523–527.

558. American Thoracic Society. Diagnosis and treatment of disease caused by nontuberculous mycobacteria. This official statement of the American Thoracic Society was approved by the Board of Directors, March 1997. Medical Section of the American Lung Association. *Am J Respir Crit Care Med* 1997;156:S1–25.

559. O'Reilly LM, Daborn CJ. The epidemiology of *Mycobacterium bovis* infections in animals and man: a review. *Tuber Lung Dis* 1995;76(Suppl. 1):1–46.

560. Ellis MD, Davies S, McCandlish IA, et al. *Mycobacterium bovis* infection in a dog. *Vet Rec* 2006;159:46–48.

561. de la Rua-Domenech R. Human *Mycobacterium bovis* infection in the United Kingdom: incidence, risks, control measures and review of the zoonotic aspects of bovine tuberculosis. *Tuberculosis (Edinb)* 2006; 86:77–109.

562. Ward AI, Smith GC, Etherington TR, et al. Estimating the risk of cattle exposure to tuberculosis posed by wild deer relative to badgers in England and Wales. *J Wildl Dis* 2009;45:1104–1120.

563. Coleman JD, Cooke MM. *Mycobacterium bovis* infection in wildlife in New Zealand. *Tuberculosis (Edinb)* 2001;81:191–202.

564. Moonan PK, Chatterjee SG, Lobue PA. The molecular epidemiology of human and zoonotic *Mycobacterium bovis*: the intersection between veterinary medicine and public health. *Prev Vet Med* 2009;88:226–227.

565. Ritacco V, de Kantor IN. Zoonotic tuberculosis in Latin America. *J Clin Microbiol* 1992;30:3299–3300.

566. Gay G, Burbidge HM, Bennett P, et al. Pulmonary *Mycobacterium bovis* infection in a dog. *N Z Vet J* 2000;48:78–81.

567. Monies B, Jahans K, de la Rua R. Bovine tuberculosis in cats. *Vet Rec* 2006;158:245–246.

568. Monies RJ, Cranwell MP, Palmer N, et al. Bovine tuberculosis in domestic cats. *Vet Rec* 2000;146: 407–408.

569. van der Burgt GM, Crawshaw T, Foster AP, et al. *Mycobacterium bovis* infection in dogs. *Vet Rec* 2009;165:634.

570. Isaac J, Whitehead J, Adams JW, et al. An outbreak of *Mycobacterium bovis* infection in cats in an animal house. *Aust Vet J* 1983;60:243–245.

571. Kaneene JB, Bruning-Fann CS, Dunn J, et al. Epidemiologic investigation of *Mycobacterium bovis* in a population of cats. *Am J Vet Res* 2002;63: 1507–1511.

572. Snider WR, Cohen D, Reif JS, et al. Tuberculosis in canine and feline populations. Study of high risk populations in Pennsylvania, 1966–1968. *Am Rev Respir Dis* 1971;104:866–876.

573. Shrikrishna D, de la Rua-Domenech R, Smith NH, et al. Human and canine pulmonary *Mycobacterium bovis* infection in the same household: re-emergence of an old zoonotic threat? *Thorax* 2009;64:89–91.

574. Twomey DF, Higgins RJ, Worth DR, et al. Cutaneous TB caused by *Mycobacterium bovis* in a veterinary surgeon following exposure to a tuberculous alpaca (*Vicugna pacos*). *Vet Rec* 2010;166:175–177.

575. Thoen C, Lobue P, de Kantor I. The importance of *Mycobacterium bovis* as a zoonosis. *Vet Microbiol* 2006;112:339–345.

576. de Lisle GW, Collins DM, Loveday AS, et al. A report of tuberculosis in cats in New Zealand, and the examination of strains of *Mycobacterium bovis* by DNA restriction endonuclease analysis. *N Z Vet J* 1990;38:10–13.

577. Wilkins MJ, Bartlett PC, Berry DE, et al. Absence of *Mycobacterium bovis* infection in dogs and cats residing on infected cattle farms: Michigan, 2002. *Epidemiol Infect* 2008;136:1617–1623.

578. Houde C, Dery P. *Mycobacterium bovis* sepsis in an infant with human immunodeficiency virus infection. *Pediatr Infect Dis J* 1988;7:810–812.

579. Malik R, Hughes MS, James G, et al. Feline leprosy: two different clinical syndromes. *J Feline Med Surg* 2002;4:43–59.

580. McIntosh DW. Feline leprosy: a review of forty-four cases from Western Canada. *Can Vet J* 1982;23: 291–295.

581. Rojas-Espinosa O, Løvik M. *Mycobacterium leprae* and *Mycobacterium lepraemurium* infections in domestic and wild animals. *Rev Off Int Epizoot* 2001; 20:219–251.

582. Passantino A, Macrì D, Coluccio P, et al. Importation of mycobacteriosis with ornamental fish: Medicolegal implications. *Travel Med Infect Dis* 2008;6: 240–244.

583. Adhikesavan LG, Harrington TM. Local and disseminated infections caused by *Mycobacterium marinum*: an unusual cause of subcutaneous nodules. *J Clin Rheumatol* 2008;14:156–160.

584. Pandian TK, Deziel PJ, Otley CC, et al. *Mycobacterium marinum* infections in transplant recipients: case report and review of the literature. *Transplant Infect Dis* 2008;10:358–363.

585. Faoagali JL, Muir AD, Sears PJ, et al. Tropical fish tank granuloma. *N Z Med J* 1977;85:332–335.

586. Zanoni RG, Florio D, Fioravanti ML, et al. Occurrence of *Mycobacterium* spp. in ornamental fish in Italy. *J Fish Dis* 2008;31:433–441.

587. Doedens RA, van der Sar AM, Bitter W, et al. Transmission of *Mycobacterium marinum* from fish to a very young child. *Pediatr Infect Dis J* 2008;27: 81–83.

588. Dompmartin A, Lorier E, de Raucourt S, et al. Sporotrichoid form of *M. marinum* infection in a patient treated with cyclosporin following kidney transplantation. *Ann Dermatol Venereol* 1991,118. 377–379.

589. Brown-Elliott BA, Wallace RJ. Infections caused by nontuberculous mycobacteria. In: Mandell GL, Bennett JE, Dolin R, eds. *Principles and Practice of Infectious Diseases*. Philadelphia: Elsevier, 2005, pp. 2909–2916.

590. Lewis FM, Marsh BJ, von Reyn CF. Fish tank exposure and cutaneous infections due to *Mycobacterium marinum*: tuberculin skin testing, treatment, and prevention. *Clin Infect Dis* 2003;37:390–397.

591. Parsons SD, Gous TA, Warren RM, et al. Pulmonary *Mycobacterium tuberculosis* (Beijing strain) infection in a stray dog. *J S Afr Vet Med Assoc* 2008;79: 95–98.

592. Erwin PC, Bemis DA, McCombs SB, et al. *Mycobacterium* tuberculosis transmission from human to canine. *Emerg Infect Dis* 2004;10:2258–2210.

593. Hackendahl NC, Mawby DI, Bemis DA, et al. Putative transmission of *Mycobacterium tuberculosis* infection from a human to a dog. *J Am Vet Med Assoc* 2004;225:1573–1577, 1548.

594. Une Y, Mori T. Tuberculosis as a zoonosis from a veterinary perspective. *Comp Immunol Microbiol Infect Dis* 2007;30:415–425.

595. Dye C, Scheele S, Dolin P, et al. Consensus statement. Global burden of tuberculosis: estimated incidence, prevalence, and mortality by country. WHO Global Surveillance and Monitoring Project. *JAMA* 1999;282:677–686.

596. Fitzgerald D, Haas DW. *Mycobacterium* tuberculosis. In: Mandell GL, Bennett JE, Dolin R, eds. *Principles and Practice of Infectious Diseases*. Philadelphia: Elsevier, 2005, pp. 2852–2886.

597. Valway SE, Sanchez MP, Shinnick TF, et al. An outbreak involving extensive transmission of a virulent strain of *Mycobacterium tuberculosis*. *N Engl J Med* 1998;338:633–639.

598. Hawthorne VM, Jarrett WF, Lauder I, et al. Tuberculosis in man, dog, and cat. *Br Med J* 1957; 2:675–678.

599. Liu S, Weitzman I, Johnson GG. Canine tuberculosis. *J Am Vet Med Assoc* 1980;177:164–167.

600. Turinelli V, Ledieu D, Guilbaud L, et al. *Mycobacterium tuberculosis* infection in a dog from Africa. *Vet Clin Pathol* 2004;33:177–181.

601. Snider WR, Cohen D, Reif JS, et al. Tuberculin sensitivity in a high-risk canine population. *Am J Epidemiol* 1975;102:185–190.

602. Schmidt V, Schneider S, Schlomer J, et al. Transmission of tuberculosis between men and pet birds: a case report. *Avian Pathol* 2008;37: 589–592.

603. Steinmetz HW, Rutz C, Hoop RK, et al. Possible human-avian transmission of *Mycobacterium tuberculosis* in a green-winged macaw (*Ara chloroptera*). *Avian Dis* 2006;50:641–645.

604. Daley CL. Update in tuberculosis 2009. *Am J Respir Crit Care Med* 2010;181:550–555.

605. Jafari C, Thijsen S, Sotgiu G, et al. Bronchoalveolar lavage enzyme-linked immunospot for a rapid diagnosis of tuberculosis: a Tuberculosis Network European Trials group study. *Am J Respir Crit Care Med* 2009;180:666–673.

606. Mazurek GH, Jereb J, Lobue P, et al. Guidelines for using the QuantiFERON-TB Gold test for detecting *Mycobacterium tuberculosis* infection, United States. *MMWR Recomm Rep* 2005;54:49–55.

607. Canadian Tuberculosis Committee (CTC). Updated recommendations on interferon gamma release assays for latent tuberculosis infection. An Advisory Committee Statement (ACS). *Can Commun Dis Rep* 2008;34:1–13.

608. Ashley BD, Noone M, Dwarakanath AD, et al. Fatal *Pasteurella dagmatis* peritonitis and septicaemia in a patient with cirrhosis: a case report and review of the literature. *J Clin Pathol* 2004;57:210–212.

609. Fajfar-Whetstone CJ, Coleman L, Biggs DR, et al. *Pasteurella multocida* septicemia and subsequent *Pasteurella dagmatis* septicemia in a diabetic patient. *J Clin Microbiol* 1995;33:202–204.

610. Ganiere JP, Escande F, Andre G, et al. Characterization of *Pasteurella* from gingival scrapings of dogs and cats. *Comp Immunol Microbiol Infect Dis* 1993;16: 77–85.

611. Freshwater A. Why your housecat's trite little bite could cause you quite a fright: a study of domestic felines on the occurrence and antibiotic susceptibility of *Pasteurella multocida*. *Zoonoses Public Health* 2008;55:507–513.

612. Zurlo JJ. *Pasteurella* species. In: Mandell GL, Bennett JE, Dolin R, eds. *Principles and Practice of Infectious Diseases*. Philadelphia: Elsevier, 2005, pp. 2687–2691.

613. Goldstein EJ, Baraff LJ, Meislin H, et al. Animal bites. *JACEP* 1978;7:417–418.

614. Antony SJ, Oglesby KA. Peritonitis associated with *Pasteurella multocida* in peritoneal dialysis patients—case report and review of the literature. *Clin Nephrol* 2007;68:52–56.

615. Boerlin P, Siegrist HH, Burnens AP, et al. Molecular identification and epidemiological tracing of *Pasteurella multocida* meningitis in a baby. *J Clin Microbiol* 2000;38:1235–1237.

616. Chun ML, Buekers TE, Sood AK, et al. Postoperative wound infection with *Pasteurella multocida* from a pet cat. *Am J Obstet Gynecol* 2003;188:1115–1116.

617. Cooke FJ, Kodjo A, Clutterbuck EJ, et al. A case of *Pasteurella multocida* peritoneal dialysis-associated peritonitis and review of the literature. *Int J Infect Dis* 2004;8:171–174.

618. Kumar A, Devlin HR, Vellend H. *Pasteurella multocida* meningitis in an adult: case report and review. *Rev Infect Dis* 1990;12:440–448.

619. Green BT, Ramsey KM, Nolan PE. *Pasteurella multocida* meningitis: case report and review of the last 11 y. *Scand J Infect Dis* 2002;34:213–217.

620. Kimura R, Hayashi Y, Takeuchi T, et al. *Pasteurella multocida* septicemia caused by close contact with a domestic cat: case report and literature review. *J Infect Chemother* 2004;10:250–252.

621. Kofteridis DP, Christofaki M, Mantadakis E, et al. Bacteremic community-acquired pneumonia due to *Pasteurella multocida*. *Int J Infect Dis* 2009;13:e81–e83.

622. Schmulewitz L, Chandesris MO, Mainardi JL, et al. Invasive *Pasteurella multocida* sinusitis in a renal transplant patient. *Transpl Infect Dis* 2008;10:206–208.

623. Chang K, Siu LK, Chen YH, et al. Fatal *Pasteurella multocida* septicemia and necrotizing fasciitis related with wound licked by a domestic dog. *Scand J Infect Dis* 2007;39:167–170.

624. Drenjancevic IH, Ivic D, Drenjancevic D, et al. Fatal fulminant sepsis due to a cat bite in an immunocompromised patient. *Wien Klin Wochenschr* 2008;120:504–506.

625. Liu W, Chemaly RF, Tuohy MJ, et al. *Pasteurella multocida* urinary tract infection with molecular evidence of zoonotic transmission. *Clin Infect Dis* 2003;36:E58–E60.

626. Clapp DW, Kleiman MB, Reynolds JK, et al. *Pasteurella multocida* meningitis in infancy. An avoidable infection. *Am J Dis Child* 1986;140:444–446.

627. Godey B, Morandi X, Bourdinière J, et al. Beware of dogs licking ears. *Lancet* 1999;354:1267–1268.

628. Cohen-Adam D, Marcus N, Scheuerman O, et al. *Pasteurella multocida* septicemia in a newborn without scratches, licks or bites. *Isr Med Assoc J* 2006;8:657–658.

629. London RD, Bottone EJ. *Pasteurella multocida*: zoonotic cause of peritonitis in a patient undergoing peritoneal dialysis. *Am J Med* 1991;91:202–204.

630. Youssef NM, El-Shamy HA, Abou-Donia HA, et al. A study of *Plesiomonas shigelloides* from human, pets and aquatic environments. *J Egypt Public Health Assoc* 1993;68:293–308.

631. Holmberg SD, Wachsmuth IK, Hickman-Brenner FW, et al. Plesiomonas enteric infections in the United States. *Ann Intern Med* 1986;105:690–694.

632. Lee AC, Yuen KY, Ha SY, et al. *Plesiomonas shigelloides* septicemia: case report and literature review. *Pediatr Hematol Oncol* 1996;13:265–269.

633. Schneider F, Lang N, Reibke R, et al. *Plesiomonas shigelloides* pneumonia. *Med Mal Infect* 2009;39:397–400.

634. Arai T, Ikejima N, Itoh T, et al. A survey of *Plesiomonas shigelloides* from aquatic environments, domestic animals, pets and humans. *J Hyg (Lond)* 1980;84:203–211.

635. Krovacek K, Eriksson LM, González-Rey C, et al. Isolation, biochemical and serological characterisation of *Plesiomonas shigelloides* from freshwater in Northern Europe. *Comp Immunol Microbiol Infect Dis* 2000;23:45–51.

636. Foster G, Patterson T, Pennycott T, et al. *Plesiomonas shigelloides*—an uncommon cause of diarrhoea in cats? *Vet Rec* 2000;146:411.

637. Jagger T, Keane S, Robertson S. *Plesiomonas shigelloides*—an uncommon cause of diarrhoea in cats? *Vet Rec* 2000;146:296.

638. González-Rey C, Svenson SB, Bravo L, et al. Serotypes and anti-microbial susceptibility of *Plesiomonas shigelloides* isolates from humans, animals and aquatic environments in different countries. *Comp Immunol Microbiol Infect Dis* 2004;27:129–139.

639. Davis WA, Chretien JH, Garagusi VF, et al. Snake-to-human transmission of *Aeromonas* (Pl) *shigelloides* resulting in gastroenteritis. *South Med J* 1978;71:474–476.

640. Gaastra W, Boot R, Ho HT, et al. Rat bite fever. *Vet Microbiol* 2009;133:211–228.

641. Washburn RG. *Streptobacillus moniliformis* (rat-bite fever. In: Mandell GL, Bennett JE, Dolin R, eds.

Principles and Practice of Infectious Diseases. Philadelphia: Elsevier, 2005, pp. 2708–2710.

642. Kimura M, Tanikawa T, Suzuki M, et al. Detection of *Streptobacillus* spp. in feral rats by specific polymerase chain reaction. *Microbiol Immunol* 2008; 52:9–15.

643. Arkless HA. Rat-bite fever at Albert Einstein Medical Center. *Pa Med* 1970;73:49.

644. Gilbert GL, Cassidy JF, Bennett NM. Rat-bite fever. *Med J Aust* 1971;2:1131–1134.

645. Taylor JD, Stephens CP, Duncan RG, et al. Polyarthritis in wild mice (*Mus musculus*) caused by *Streptobacillus moniliformis*. *Aust Vet J* 1994;71: 143–145.

646. Fordham JN, McKay-Ferguson E, Davies A, et al. Rat bite fever without the bite. *Ann Rheum Dis* 1992;51:411–412.

647. Rygg M, Bruun CF. Rat bite fever (*Streptobacillus moniliformis*) with septicemia in a child. *Scand J Infect Dis* 1992;24:535–540.

648. Prager L, Frenck RW. *Streptobacillus moniliformis* infection in a child with chickenpox. *Pediatr Infect Dis J* 1994;13:417–418.

649. Shvartsblat S, Kochie M, Harber P, et al. Fatal rat bite fever in a pet shop employee. *Am J Ind Med* 2004;45:357–360.

650. Wilkins EG, Millar JG, Cockcroft PM, et al. Rat-bite fever in a gerbil breeder. *J Infect* 1988;16: 177–180.

651. Wouters EG, Ho HT, Lipman LJ, et al. Dogs as vectors of *Streptobacillus moniliformis* infection? *Vet Microbiol* 2008;128:419–422.

652. Albedwawi S, LeBlanc C, Shaw A, et al. A teenager with fever, rash and arthritis. *CMAJ* 2006;175:354.

653. Elliott SP. Rat bite fever and *Streptobacillus moniliformis*. *Clin Microbiol Rev* 2007;20:13–22.

654. Signorini L, Colombini P, Cristini F, et al. Inappropriate footwear and rat-bite fever in an international traveler. *J Travel Med* 2002;9:275–276.

655. Raffin BJ, Freemark M. Streptobacillary rat-bite fever: a pediatric problem. *Pediatrics* 1979;64: 214–217.

656. Freels LK, Elliott SP. Rat bite fever: three case reports and a literature review. *Clin Pediatr* 2004;43:291–295.

657. Savage NL, Joiner GN, Florey DW. Clinical microbiological, and histological manifestations of *Streptobacillus moniliformis*-induced arthritis in mice. *Infect Immun* 1981;34:605–609.

658. Glastonbury JR, Morton JG, Matthews LM. *Streptobacillus moniliformis* infection in Swiss white mice. *J Vet Diagn Invest* 1996;8:202–209.

659. Centers for Disease Control and Prevention (CDC). Fatal rat-bite fever—Florida and Washington, 2003. *MMWR Morb Mortal Wkly Rep* 2005;53:1198–1202.

660. Nakagomi D, Deguchi N, Yagasaki A, et al. Rat-bite fever identified by polymerase chain reaction detection of *Streptobacillus moniliformis* DNA. *J Dermatol* 2008;35:667–670.

661. Taber LH, Feigin RD. Spirochetal infections. *Pediatr Clin North Am* 1979;26:377–413.

662. Pérez-Osorio CE, Zavala-Velázquez JE, Arias León JJ, et al. *Rickettsia felis* as emergent global threat for humans. *Emerg Infect Dis* 2008;14:1019–1023.

663. Zavala-Castro J, Zavala-Velázquez J, Walker D, et al. Severe human infection with *Rickettsia felis* associated with hepatitis in Yucatan, Mexico. *Int J Med Microbiol* 2009;299:529–533.

664. Karpathy SE, Hayes EK, Williams AM, et al. Detection of *Rickettsia felis* and *Rickettsia typhi* in an area of California endemic for murine typhus. *Clin Microbiol Infect* 2009;15(Suppl. 2):218–219.

665. Azad AF, Radulovic S, Higgins JA, et al. Flea-borne rickettsioses: ecologic considerations. *Emerg Infect Dis* 1997;3:319–327.

666. Higgins JA, Radulovic S, Schriefer ME, et al. *Rickettsia felis*: a new species of pathogenic rickettsia isolated from cat fleas. *J Clin Microbiol* 1996;34:671–674.

667. Nogueras MM, Pons I, Ortuño A, et al. Seroprevalence of *Rickettsia typhi* and *Rickettsia felis* in dogs from north-eastern Spain. *Clin Microbiol Infect* 2009; 15(Suppl. 2):237–238.

668. Wedincamp J, Foil LD. Infection and seroconversion of cats exposed to cat fleas (*Ctenocephalides felis* Bouché) infected with *Rickettsia felis*. *J Vector Ecol* 2000;25:123–126.

669. Adams JR, Schmidtmann ET, Azad AF. Infection of colonized cat fleas, *Ctenocephalides felis* (Bouché), with a rickettsia-like microorganism. *Am J Trop Med Hyg* 1990;43:400–409.

670. Parola P, Miller RS, McDaniel P, et al. Emerging rickettsioses of the Thai-Myanmar border. *Emerg Infect Dis* 2003;9:592–595.

671. Raoult D, La Scola B, Enea M, et al. A flea-associated Rickettsia pathogenic for humans. *Emerg Infect Dis* 2001;7:73–81.

672. Richter J, Fournier PE, Petridou J, et al. *Rickettsia felis* infection acquired in Europe and documented by polymerase chain reaction. *Emerg Infect Dis* 2002;8:207–208.

673. Renvoisé A, Joliot AY, Raoult D. *Rickettsia felis* infection in man, France. *Emerg Infect Dis* 2009;15: 1126–1127.

674. Zavala-Velázquez JE, Ruiz-Sosa JA, Sánchez-Elias RA, et al. *Rickettsia felis* rickettsiosis in Yucatán. *Lancet* 2000;356:1079–1080.

675. Raoult D. Introduction to rickettsioses and ehrlichioses. In: Mandell GL, Bennett JE, Dolin R, eds. *Principles and Practice of Infectious Diseases.* Philadelphia: Elsevier, 2005, pp. 2284–2287.

676. Walker DH, Raoult D. *Rickettsia rickettsii* and other spotted fever group *Rickettsiae*. In: Mandell GL, Bennett JE, Dolin P, eds. *Principles and Practice of Infectious Diseases*. Philadelphia: Elsevier, 2005, pp. 2287–2295.

677. Centers for Disease Control and Prevention (CDC). Fatal cases of Rocky Mountain spotted fever in family clusters—three states, 2003. *MMWR Morb Mortal Wkly Rep* 2004;53:407–410.

678. Chapman AS, Murphy SM, Demma LJ, et al. Rocky mountain spotted fever in the United States, 1997–2002. *Ann N Y Acad Sci* 2006;1078:154–155.

679. Greene CE, Levy JK. Immunocompromised people and shared human and animal infections: zoonoses, sapronoses and anthroponoses. In: Greene CE, ed. *Infectious Diseases of the Dog and Cat*. Philadelphia: Saunders Elsevier, 2006, pp. 1051–1068.

680. Elchos BN, Goddard J. Implications of presumptive fatal Rocky Mountain spotted fever in two dogs and their owner. *J Am Vet Med Assoc* 2003;223:1450–1452, 1433.

681. Gray JT, Hungerford LL, Fedorka-Cray PJ, et al. Extended-spectrum-cephalosporin resistance in *Salmonella enterica* isolates of animal origin. *Antimicrob Agents Chemother* 2004;48:3179–3181.

682. Low JC, Tennant B, Munro D. Multiple-resistant *Salmonella typhimurium* DT104 in cats. *Lancet* 1996;348:1391.

683. Van Immerseel F, Pasmans F, De Buck J, et al. Cats as a risk for transmission of antimicrobial drug-resistant *Salmonella*. *Emerg Infect Dis* 2004;10:2169–2174.

684. Wall PG, Threlfall EJ, Ward LR, et al. Multiresistant *Salmonella typhimurium* DT104 in cats: a public health risk. *Lancet* 1996;348:471.

685. Wright JG, Tengelsen LA, Smith KE, et al. Multidrug-resistant *Salmonella* Typhimurium in four animal facilities. *Emerg Infect Dis* 2005;11:1235–1241.

686. Pegues DA, Ohl ME, Miller SI. *Salmonella* species, including *Salmonella* Typhi. In: Mandell GL, Bennett JE, Dolin R, eds. *Principles and Practice of Infectious Diseases*. Philadelphia: Elsevier, 2005, pp. 2636–2654.

687. Mead PS, Slutsker L, Dietz V, et al. Food-related illness and death in the United States. *Emerg Infect Dis* 1999;5:607–625.

688. Bagcigil AF, Ikiz S, Dokuzeylu B, et al. Fecal shedding of *Salmonella* spp. in dogs. *J Vet Med Sci* 2007;69:775–777.

689. Cave NJ, Marks SL, Kass PH, et al. Evaluation of a routine diagnostic fecal panel for dogs with diarrhea. *J Am Vet Med Assoc* 2002;221:52–59.

690. Sokolow S, Rand C, Marks S, et al. Epidemiologic evaluation of diarrhea in dogs in an animal shelter. *Am J Vet Res* 2005;66:1018–1024.

691. Tsai HJ, Huang HC, Lin CM, et al. Salmonellae and campylobacters in household and stray dogs in northern Taiwan. *Vet Res Commun* 2007;31:931–939.

692. Joffe DJ, Schlesinger DP. Preliminary assessment of the risk of *Salmonella* infection in dogs fed raw chicken diets. *Can Vet J* 2002;43:441–442.

693. Morley P, Strohmeyer R, Tankson J, et al. Evaluation of the association between feeding raw meat and *Salmonella enterica* infections at a Greyhound breeding facility. *J Am Vet Med Assoc* 2006;228:1524–1532.

694. Lefebvre SL, Reid-Smith R, Boerlin P, et al. Evaluation of the risks of shedding Salmonellae and other potential pathogens by therapy dogs fed raw diets in Ontario and Alberta. *Zoonoses Public Health* 2008;55:470–480.

695. Centers for Disease Control and Prevention (CDC). Human salmonellosis associated with animal-derived pet treats—United States and Canada, 2005. *MMWR Morb Mortal Wkly Rep* 2006;55:702–705.

696. Strohmeyer R, Morley P, Hyatt D, et al. Evaluation of bacterial and protozoal contamination of commercially available raw meat diets for dogs. *J Am Vet Med Assoc* 2006;228:537–542.

697. Weese J, Rousseau J, Arroyo L. Bacteriological evaluation of commercial canine and feline raw diets. *Can Vet J* 2005;46:513–516.

698. Finley R, Ribble C, Aramini J, et al. The risk of salmonellae shedding by dogs fed *Salmonella*-contaminated commercial raw food diets. *Can Vet J* 2007;48:69–75.

699. Zhao S, McDermott PF, White DG, et al. Characterization of multidrug resistant *Salmonella* recovered from diseased animals. *Vet Microbiol* 2007;123:122–132.

700. Keymer IF. The unsuitability of non-domesticated animals as pets. *Vet Rec* 1972;91:373–381.

701. Hidalgo-Vila J, Díaz-Paniagua C, Pérez-Santigosa N, et al. *Salmonella* in free-living exotic and native turtles and in pet exotic turtles from SW Spain. *Res Vet Sci* 2008;85:449–452.

702. Cooke FJ, De Pinna E, Maguire C, et al. First report of human infection with *Salmonella enterica* serovar Apapa, associated with a pet lizard. *J Clin Microbiol* 2009;47:2672–2674.

703. Sareyyüpoğlu B, Ok AC, Cantekin Z, et al. Polymerase chain reaction detection of *Salmonella* spp. in fecal samples of pet birds. *Avian Dis* 2008;52:163–167.

704. Seepersadsingh N, Adesiyun AA. Prevalence and antimicrobial resistance of *Salmonella* spp. in pet mammals, reptiles, fish aquarium water, and birds in Trinidad. *J Vet Med B Infect Dis Vet Public Health* 2003;50:488–493.

705. Riley PY, Chomel BB. Hedgehog zoonoses. *Emerg Infect Dis* 2005;11:1–5.
706. Mermin J, Hutwagner L, Vugia D, et al. Reptiles, amphibians, and human *Salmonella* infection: a population-based, case-control study. *Clin Infect Dis* 2004;38(Suppl. 3):S253–S261.
707. Lamm SH, Taylor A, Gangarosa EJ, et al. Turtle-associated salmonellosis. I. An estimation of the magnitude of the problem in the United States, 1970–1971. *Am J Epidemiol* 1972;95:511–517.
708. Centers for Disease Control and Prevention (CDC). Multistate outbreak of human *Salmonella* infections associated with exposure to turtles—United States, 2007–2008. *MMWR Morb Mortal Wkly Rep* 2008; 57:69–72.
709. Centers for Disease Control and Prevention (CDC). Turtle-associated salmonellosis in humans—United States, 2006–2007. *MMWR Morb Mortal Wkly Rep* 2007;56:649–652.
710. Harris JR, Bergmire-Sweat D, Schlegel JH, et al. Multistate outbreak of *Salmonella* infections associated with small turtle exposure, 2007–2008. *Pediatrics* 2009;124:1388–1394.
711. Editorial team, Bertrand S, Rimhanen-Finne R, et al. *Salmonella* infections associated with reptiles: the current situation in Europe. *Euro Surveill* 2008; 13:pii18902.
712. Jones TF, Ingram LA, Fullerton KE, et al. A case-control study of the epidemiology of sporadic *Salmonella* infection in infants. *Pediatrics* 2006;118: 2380–2387.
713. Van Meervenne E, Botteldoorn N, Lokietek S, et al. Turtle-associated *Salmonella* septicaemia and meningitis in a 2-month-old baby. *J Med Microbiol* 2009;58:1379–1381.
714. Fuller C, Jawahir S, Leano F, et al. A multi-state *Salmonella* Typhimurium outbreak associated with frozen vacuum-packed rodents used to feed snakes. *Zoonoses Public Health* 2008;55:481–487.
715. Lee KM, McReynolds JL, Fuller CC, et al. Investigation and characterization of the frozen feeder rodent industry in Texas following a multistate *Salmonella* Typhimurium outbreak associated with frozen vacuum-packed rodents. *Zoonoses Public Health* 2008;55:488–496.
716. Centers for Disease Control and Prevention (CDC). Outbreak of multidrug-resistant *Salmonella typhimurium* associated with rodents purchased at retail pet stores—United States, December 2003-October 2004. *MMWR Morb Mortal Wkly Rep* 2005;54:429–433.
717. Swanson SJ, Snider C, Braden CR, et al. Multidrug-resistant *Salmonella enterica* serotype Typhimurium associated with pet rodents. *N Engl J Med* 2007; 356:21–28.
718. Clark C, Cunningham J, Ahmed R, et al. Characterization of *Salmonella* associated with pig ear dog treats in Canada. *J Clin Microbiol* 2001;39: 3962–3968.
719. Pitout JD, Reisbig MD, Mulvey M, et al. Association between handling of pet treats and infection with *Salmonella enterica* serotype newport expressing the AmpC beta-lactamase, CMY-2. *J Clin Microbiol* 2003;41:4578–4582.
720. Centers for Disease Control and Prevention (CDC). Multistate outbreak of human *Salmonella* infections caused by contaminated dry dog food—United States, 2006–2007. *MMWR Morb Mortal Wkly Rep* 2008;57:521–524.
721. Centers for Disease Control and Prevention (CDC). Update: recall of dry dog and cat food products associated with human *Salmonella* Schwarzengrund infections—United States, 2008. *MMWR Morb Mortal Wkly Rep* 2008;57:1200–1202.
722. Schotte U, Borchers D, Wulff C, et al. *Salmonella* Montevideo outbreak in military kennel dogs caused by contaminated commercial feed, which was only recognized through monitoring. *Vet Microbiol* 2007;119:316–323.
723. Centers for Disease Control and Prevention (CDC). African pygmy hedgehog-associated salmonellosis—Washington, 1994. *MMWR Morb Mortal Wkly Rep* 1995;44:462–463.
724. Craig C, Styliadis S, Woodward D, et al. African pygmy hedgehog—associated *Salmonella* tilene in Canada. *Can Commun Dis Rep* 1997;23:129–131, discussion 131–122.
725. Woodward DL, Khakhria R, Johnson WM. Human salmonellosis associated with exotic pets. *J Clin Microbiol* 1997;35:2786–2790.
726. Celum CL, Chaisson RE, Rutherford GW, et al. Incidence of salmonellosis in patients with AIDS. *J Infect Dis* 1987;156:998–1002.
727. Stam F, Römkens TE, Hekker TA, et al. Turtle-associated human salmonellosis. *Clin Infect Dis* 2003;37:e167–e169.
728. Chiu CH, Lin TY, Ou JT. Predictors for extraintestinal infection of non-typhoidal *Salmonella* in patients without AIDS. *Int J Clin Pract* 1999;53: 161–164.
729. Thamlikitkul V, Dhiraputra C, Paisarnsinsup T, et al. Non-typhoidal *Salmonella* bacteraemia: clinical features and risk factors. *Trop Med Int Health* 1996;1:443–448.
730. Lee WS, Puthucheary SD, Parasakthi N. Extraintestinal non-typhoidal *Salmonella* infections in children. *Ann Trop Paediatr* 2000;20:125–129.
731. Philbey AW, Brown FM, Mather HA, et al. Salmonellosis in cats in the United Kingdom: 1955 to 2007. *Vet Rec* 2009;164:120–122.

732. Sirinavin S, Garner P. Antibiotics for treating *Salmonella* gut infections. *Cochrane Database Syst Rev* 2000;CD001167.

733. Frazee B, Salz T, Lambert L, et al. Fatal community-associated methicillin-resistant *Staphylococcus aureus* pneumonia in an immunocompetent young adult. *Ann Emerg Med* 2005;46:401–404.

734. Kazakova S, Hageman J, Matava M, et al. A clone of methicillin-resistant *Staphylococcus aureus* among professional football players. *N Engl J Med* 2005;352:468–475.

735. Mertz P, Cardenas T, Snyder R, et al. *Staphylococcus aureus* virulence factors associated with infected skin lesions: influence on the local immune response. *Arch Derm* 2007;143:1259–1263.

736. Voyich J, Otto M, Mathema B, et al. Is Panton-Valentine leukocidin the major virulence determinant in community-associated methicillin-resistant *Staphylococcus aureus* disease? *J Infect Dis* 2006; 194:1761–1770.

737. Becker K, Friedrich AW, Lubritz G, et al. Prevalence of genes encoding pyrogenic toxin superantigens and exfoliative toxins among strains of *Staphylococcus aureus* isolated from blood and nasal specimens. *J Clin Microbiol* 2003;41:1434–1439.

738. Chambers HF, DeLeo FR. Waves of resistance: *Staphylococcus aureus* in the antibiotic era. *Nat Rev Microbiol* 2009;7:629–641.

739. Klevens RM, Morrison MA, Nadle J, et al. Invasive methicillin-resistant *Staphylococcus aureus* infections in the United States. *JAMA* 2007;298:1763–1771.

740. Campbell K, Vaughn A, Russell K, et al. Risk factors for community-associated methicillin-resistant *Staphylococcus aureus* infections in an outbreak of disease among military trainees in San Diego, California, in 2002. *J Clin Microbiol* 2004;42: 4050–4053.

741. Gilbert M, MacDonald J, Gregson D, et al. Outbreak in Alberta of community-acquired (USA300) methicillin-resistant *Staphylococcus aureus* in people with a history of drug use, homelessness or incarceration. *CMAJ* 2006;175:149–154.

742. Wulf M, Voss A. MRSA in livestock animals—an epidemic waiting to happen? *Clin Microbiol Infect* 2008;14:519–521.

743. Mainous A, Hueston W, Everett C, et al. Nasal carriage of *Staphylococcus aureus* and methicillin-resistant *S aureus* in the United States, 2001–2002. *Ann Fam Med* 2006;4:132–137.

744. Gorwitz RJ, Kruszon-Moran D, McAllister SK, et al. Changes in the prevalence of nasal colonization with *Staphylococcus aureus* in the United States, 2001–2004. *J Infect Dis* 2008;197:1226–1234.

745. Hanselman BA, Kruth SA, Rousseau J, et al. Methicillin-resistant *Staphylococcus aureus* coloniza-tion in schoolteachers in Ontario. *Can J Infect Dis Med Microbiol* 2008;19:405–408.

746. Datta R, Huang SS. Risk of infection and death due to methicillin-resistant *Staphylococcus aureus* in long-term carriers. *Clin Infect Dis* 2008;47:176–181.

747. Safdar N, Bradley EA. The risk of infection after nasal colonization with *Staphylococcus aureus*. *Am J Med* 2008;121:310–315.

748. Griffeth GC, Morris DO, Abraham JL, et al. Screening for skin carriage of methicillin-resistant coagulase-positive staphylococci and *Staphylococcus schleiferi* in dogs with healthy and inflamed skin. *Vet Dermatol* 2008;19:142–149.

749. Hanselman BA, Kruth SA, Rousseau J, et al. Coagulase positive staphylococcal colonization of people and their household pets. *Can Vet J* 2009;50:954–958.

750. Abraham J, Morris D, Griffeth G, et al. Surveillance of healthy cats and cats with inflammatory skin disease for colonization of the skin by methicillin-resistant coagulase-positive staphylococci and *Staphylococcus schleiferi* ssp. *schleiferi*. *Vet Dermatol* 2007;18:252–259.

751. Baptiste K, Williams K, Willams N, et al. Methicillin-resistant staphylococci in companion animals. *Emerg Infect Dis* 2005;11:1942–1944.

752. Boost M, O'Donoghue M, Siu K. Characterisation of methicillin-resistant *Staphylococcus aureus* isolates from dogs and their owners. *Clin Microbiol Infect* 2007;13:731–733.

753. Malik S, Coombs G, O'Brien F, et al. Molecular typing of methicillin-resistant staphylococci isolated from cats and dogs. *J Antimicrob Chemother* 2006;58:428–431.

754. Moodley A, Stegger M, Bagcigil A, et al. spa typing of methicillin-resistant *Staphylococcus aureus* isolated from domestic animals and veterinary staff in the UK and Ireland. *J Antimicrob Chemother* 2006; 58:1118–1123.

755. O'Mahony R, Abbott Y, Leonard F, et al. Methicillin-resistant *Staphylococcus aureus* (MRSA) isolated from animals and veterinary personnel in Ireland. *Vet Microbiol* 2005;109:285–296.

756. Weese J, Dick H, Willey B, et al. Suspected transmission of methicillin-resistant *Staphylococcus aureus* between domestic pets and humans in veterinary clinics and in the household. *Vet Microbiol* 2006; 115:148–155.

757. Epstein CR, Yam WC, Peiris JS, et al. Methicillin-resistant commensal staphylococci in healthy dogs as a potential zoonotic reservoir for community-acquired antibiotic resistance. *Infect Genet Evol* 2009;9:283–285.

758. Hanselman BA, Kruth S, Weese JS. Methicillin-resistant staphylococcal colonization in dogs enter-

ing a veterinary teaching hospital. *Vet Microbiol* 2007;126:277–281.

759. Kottler S, Middleton JR, Weese JS, et al. Prevalence of *Staphylococcus aureus* and MRSA carriage in three populations. 26th Annual Conference of the American College of Veterinary Internal Medicine. San Antonio, TX, 2008.

760. Loeffler A, Boag A, Sung J, et al. Prevalence of methicillin-resistant *Staphylococcus aureus* among staff and pets in a small animal referral hospital in the UK. *J Antimicrob Chemother* 2005;56:692–697.

761. Weese JS, Faires M, Rousseau J, et al. Cluster of methicillin-resistant *Staphylococcus aureus* colonization in a small animal intensive care unit. *J Am Vet Med Assoc* 2007;231:1361–1364.

762. Weese J, Rousseau J, Willey B, et al. Methicillin-resistant *Staphylococcus aureus* in horses at a veterinary teaching hospital: frequency, characterization, and association with clinical disease. *J Vet Intern Med* 2006;20:182–186.

763. Faires MC, Tater KC, Weese JS. An investigation of methicillin-resistant *Staphylococcus aureus* colonization in people and pets in the same household with an infected person or infected pet. *J Am Vet Med Assoc* 2009;235:540–543.

764. Loeffler A, Pfeiffer DU, Lloyd DH, et al. Methicillin-resistant *Staphylococcus aureus* carriage in UK veterinary staff and owners of infected pets: new risk groups. *J Hosp Infect* 2010;74:282–288.

765. van Loo I, Huijsdens X, Tiemersma E, et al. Emergence of methicillin-resistant *Staphylococcus aureus* of animal origin in humans. *Emerg Infect Dis* 2007;13:1834–1839.

766. van Rijen MM, Van Keulen PH, Kluytmans JA. Increase in a Dutch hospital of methicillin-resistant *Staphylococcus aureus* related to animal farming. *Clin Infect Dis* 2008;46:261–263.

767. Witte W, Strommenger B, Stanek C, et al. Methicillin-resistant *Staphylococcus aureus* ST398 in humans and animals, Central Europe. *Emerg Infect Dis* 2007; 13:255–258.

768. Nienhoff U, Kadlec K, Chaberny IF, et al. Transmission of methicillin-resistant *Staphylococcus aureus* strains between humans and dogs: two case reports. *J Antimicrob Chemother* 2009;64: 660–662.

769. Rich M, Roberts L. MRSA in companion animals. *Vet Rec* 2006;159:535–536.

770. Rankin S, Roberts S, O'Shea K, et al. Panton Valentine leukocidin (PVL) toxin positive MRSA strains isolated from companion animals. *Vet Microbiol* 2005;108:145–148.

771. Walther B, Wieler L, Friedrich A, et al. Methicillin-resistant *Staphylococcus aureus* (MRSA) isolated from small and exotic animals at a university hos-

pital during routine microbiological examinations. *Vet Microbiol* 2007;127:171–178.

772. Leonard F, Abbott Y, Rossney A, et al. Methicillin-resistant *Staphylococcus aureus* isolated from a veterinary surgeon and five dogs in one practice. *Vet Rec* 2006;158:155–159.

773. Manian FA. Asymptomatic nasal carriage of mupirocin-resistant, methicillin-resistant *Staphylococcus aureus* (MRSA) in a pet dog associated with MRSA infection in household contacts. *Clin Infect Dis* 2003;36:e26–e28.

774. van Duijkeren E, Wolfhagen MJ, Heck ME, et al. Transmission of a Panton-Valentine leucocidin-positive, methicillin-resistant *Staphylococcus aureus* strain between humans and a dog. *J Clin Microbiol* 2005;43:6209–6211.

775. Sing A, Tuschak C, Hörmansdorfer S. Methicillin-resistant *Staphylococcus aureus* in a family and its pet cat. *N Engl J Med* 2008;358:1200–1201.

776. Vitale C, Gross T, Weese J. Methicillin-resistant *Staphylococcus aureus* in cat and owner. *Emerg Infect Dis* 2006;12:1998–2000.

777. Hanselman B, Kruth S, Rousseau J, et al. Methicillin-resistant *Staphylococcus aureus* colonization in veterinary personnel. *Emerg Infect Dis* 2006;12: 1933–1938.

778. Wulf M, van Nes A, Eikelenboom-Boskamp A, et al. Methicillin-resistant *Staphylococcus aureus* in veterinary doctors and students, the Netherlands. *Emerg Infect Dis* 2006;12:1939–1941.

779. Moodley A, Nightingale EC, Stegger M, et al. High risk for nasal carriage of methicillin-resistant *Staphylococcus aureus* among Danish veterinary practitioners. *Scand J Work Environ Health* 2008; 34:151–157.

780. Burstiner L, Faires M, Weese JS. Methicillin-resistant *Staphylococcus aureus* colonization of veterinary personnel at a surgical conference. ASM-ESCMID Conference on Methicillin-Resistant Staphylococci in Animals, 2009.

781. Burstiner LC, Faires M, Weese JS. Methicillin-resistant *Staphylococcus aureus* colonization in personnel attending a veterinary surgery conference. *Vet Surg* 2010;39:150–157.

782. Zemlicková H, Fridrichová M, Tyllová K, et al. Carriage of methicillin-resistant *Staphylococcus aureus* in veterinary personnel. *Epidemiol Infect* 2009; 137:1233–1236.

783. Scott E, Duty S, Callahan M. A pilot study to isolate *Staphylococcus aureus* and methicillin-resistant *S aureus* from environmental surfaces in the home. *Am J Infect Control* 2008;36:458–460.

784. Murphy C, Reid-Smith RJ, Prescott JF, et al. Occurrence of antimicrobial resistant bacteria in healthy dogs and cats presented to private

veterinary hospitals in southern Ontario: a preliminary study. *Can Vet J* 2009;50:1047–1053.

785. Heller J, Armstrong SK, Girvan EK, et al. Prevalence and distribution of methicillin-resistant *Staphylococcus aureus* within the environment and staff of a university veterinary clinic. *J Small Anim Pract* 2009;50:168–173.

786. Morris D, Rook K, Shofer F, et al. Screening of *Staphylococcus aureus*, *Staphylococcus intermedius*, and *Staphylococcus schleiferi* isolates obtained from small companion animals for antimicrobial resistance: a retrospective review of 749 isolates (2003–04). *Vet Dermatol* 2006;17:332–337.

787. Owen MR, Moores AP, Coe RJ. Management of MRSA septic arthritis in a dog using a gentamicin-impregnated collagen sponge. *J Small Anim Pract* 2004;45:609–612.

788. Morris D, Mauldin E, O'Shea K, et al. Clinical, microbiological, and molecular characterization of methicillin-resistant *Staphylococcus aureus* infections of cats. *Am J Vet Res* 2006;67:1421–1425.

789. Faires M, Weese JS. Risk factors for methicillin-resistant *Staphylococcus aureus* infection in small animals. ASM Conference on Antimicrobial Resistance in Zoonotic and Foodborne Pathogens. Copenhagen, Denmark, 2008.

790. Faires M, Weese JS. Prevalence of inducible clindamycin resistant *Staphylococcus aureus* isolates from dogs and cats. ASM Conference on Antimicrobial Resistance in Zoonotic and Foodborne Pathogens, 2008;60.

791. Rich M, Deighton L, Roberts L. Clindamycin-resistance in methicillin-resistant *Staphylococcus aureus* isolated from animals. *Vet Microbiol* 2005; 111:237–240.

792. Frazee B, Lynn J, Charlebois E, et al. High prevalence of methicillin-resistant *Staphylococcus aureus* in emergency department skin and soft tissue infections. *Ann Emerg Med* 2005;45:311–320.

793. Moran G, Amii R, Abrahamian F, et al. Methicillin-resistant *Staphylococcus aureus* in community-acquired skin infections. *Emerg Infect Dis* 2005; 11:928–930.

794. Gabillot-Carré M, Roujeau J. Acute bacterial skin infections and cellulitis. *Curr Opin Infect Dis* 2007;20:118–123.

795. Labandeira-Rey M, Couzon F, Boisset S, et al. *Staphylococcus aureus* Panton-Valentine leukocidin causes necrotizing pneumonia. *Science* 2007;315: 1130–1133.

796. Miller L, Perdreau-Remington F, Rieg G, et al. Necrotizing fasciitis caused by community-associated methicillin-resistant *Staphylococcus aureus* in Los Angeles. *N Engl J Med* 2005;352: 1445–1453.

797. Centers for Disease Control and Prevention. Four pediatric deaths from community-acquired methicillin-resistant Staphylococcus aureus—Minnesota and North Dakota, 1997–1999. *JAMA* 1999;282:1123–1125.

798. Weese JS, Dick H, Willey B, et al. Suspected transmission of methicillin-resistant *Staphylococcus aureus* between domestic pets and humans in veterinary clinics and in the household. *Vet Microbiol* 2006;115: 148–155.

799. Loeffler A, Pfeiffer DU, Lindsay JA, et al. Lack of transmission of methicillin-resistant *Staphylococcus aureus* (MRSA) between apparently healthy dogs in a rescue kennel. *Vet Microbiol* 2010;141:178–181.

800. Barton M, Hawkes M, Moore D, et al. Guidelines for the prevention and management of community-associated methicillin-resistant *Staphylococcus aureus*: a perspective for Canadian health care practitioners. *Can J Infect Dis Med Microbiol* 2006;17(Suppl. C):4C–24C.

801. Devriese L, Vancanneyt M, Baele M, et al. *Staphylococcus pseudintermedius* sp. nov., a coagulase-positive species from animals. *Int J Syst Evol Microbiol* 2005;55:1569–1573.

802. Sasaki T, Kikuchi K, Tanaka Y, et al. Methicillin-resistant *Staphylococcus pseudintermedius* in a veterinary teaching hospital. *J Clin Microbiol* 2007;45: 1118–1125.

803. Fazakerley J, Nuttall T, Sales D, et al. Staphylococcal colonization of mucosal and lesional skin sites in atopic and healthy dogs. *Vet Dermatol* 2009;20: 179–184.

804. Hartmann FA, White DG, West SE, et al. Molecular characterization of *Staphylococcus intermedius* carriage by healthy dogs and comparison of antimicrobial susceptibility patterns to isolates from dogs with pyoderma. *Vet Microbiol* 2005;108:119–131.

805. Saijonmaa-Koulumies LE, Lloyd DH. Colonization of neonatal puppies by *Staphylococcus intermedius*. *Vet Dermatol* 2002;13:123–130.

806. Lilenbaum W, Esteves AL, Souza GN. Prevalence and antimicrobial susceptibility of staphylococci isolated from saliva of clinically normal cats. *Lett Appl Microbiol* 1999;28:448–452.

807. Lilenbaum W, Nunes EL, Azeredo MA. Prevalence and antimicrobial susceptibility of staphylococci isolated from the skin surface of clinically normal cats. *Lett Appl Microbiol* 1998;27:224–228.

808. Gronlund-Andersson U, Finn M, Kadlec K, et al. Methicillin-resistant *Staphylococcus pseudintermedius*; an emerging companion animal health problem. ASM-ESCMID Conference on Methicillin-Resistant Staphylococci in Animals, 2009;A-40.

809. Vengust M, Anderson M, Rousseau J, et al. Methicillin-resistant staphylococcal colonization in

clinically normal dogs and horses in the community. *Lett Appl Microbiol* 2006;43:602–606.

810. Weese JS, Frank LA, Reynolds LM, et al. Retrospective study of methicillin-resistant and methicillin-susceptible *Staphylococcus pseudintermedius* infections in dogs. ASM-ESCMID Conference on Methicillin-Resistant Staphylococci in Animals, 2009;A-67.

811. Lee J. *Staphylococcus intermedius* isolated from dog-bite wounds. *J Infect* 1994;29:105.

812. Vandenesch F, Célard M, Arpin D, et al. Catheter-related bacteremia associated with coagulase-positive *Staphylococcus intermedius*. *J Clin Microbiol* 1995;33:2508–2510.

813. Gerstadt K, Daly JS, Mitchell M, et al. Methicillin-resistant *Staphylococcus intermedius* pneumonia following coronary artery bypass grafting. *Clin Infect Dis* 1999;29:218–219.

814. Tanner M, Everett C, Youvan D. Molecular phylogenetic evidence for noninvasive zoonotic transmission of *Staphylococcus intermedius* from a canine pet to a human. *J Clin Microbiol* 2000;38:1628–1631.

815. Kikuchi K, Karasawa T, Piao C, et al. Molecular confirmation of transmission route of *Staphylococcus intermedius* in mastoid cavity infection from dog saliva. *J Infect Chemother* 2004;10:46–48.

816. Atalay B, Ergin F, Cekinmez M, et al. Brain abscess caused by *Staphylococcus intermedius*. *Acta Neurochir* 2005;147:347–348.

817. Talan DA, Staatz D, Staatz A, et al. Frequency of *Staphylococcus intermedius* as human nasopharyngeal flora. *J Clin Microbiol* 1989;27:2393.

818. Guardabassi L, Loeber M, Jacobson A. Transmission of multiple antimicrobial-resistant *Staphylococcus intermedius* between dogs affected by deep pyoderma and their owners. *Vet Microbiol* 2004;98:23–27.

819. Campanile F, Bongiorno D, Borbone S, et al. Characterization of a variant of the SCCmec element in a bloodstream isolate of *Staphylococcus intermedius*. *Microb Drug Resist* 2007;13:7–10.

820. van Duijkeren E, Houwers DJ, Schoormans A, et al. Transmission of methicillin-resistant *Staphylococcus intermedius* between humans and animals. *Vet Microbiol* 2008;128:213–215.

821. Cabassu J, Moissonnier P. Surgical treatment of a vertebral fracture associated with a haematogenous osteomyelitis in a dog. *Vet Comp Orthop Traumatol* 2007;20:227–230.

822. Cohn LA, Gary AT, Fales WH, et al. Trends in fluoroquinolone resistance of bacteria isolated from canine urinary tracts. *J Vet Diagn Invest* 2003;15:338–343.

823. Farrar ET, Washabau RJ, Saunders HM. Hepatic abscesses in dogs: 14 cases (1982–1994). *J Am Vet Med Assoc* 1996;208:243–247.

824. Gerding PA, McLaughlin SA, Troop MW. Pathogenic bacteria and fungi associated with external ocular diseases in dogs: 131 cases (1981–1986). *J Am Vet Med Assoc* 1988;193:242–244.

825. Holm BR, Rest JR, Seewald W. A prospective study of the clinical findings, treatment and histopathology of 44 cases of pyotraumatic dermatitis. *Vet Dermatol* 2004;15:369–376.

826. Zubeir I, Kanbar T, Alber J, et al. Phenotypic and genotypic characteristics of methicillin/oxacillin-resistant *Staphylococcus intermedius* isolated from clinical specimens during routine veterinary microbiological examinations. *Vet Microbiol* 2007;121: 170–176.

827. Girard C, Higgins R. *Staphylococcus intermedius* cellulitis and toxic shock in a dog. *Can Vet J* 1999; 40:501–502.

828. Weese JS, Poma R, James F, et al. *Staphylococcus pseudintermedius* necrotizing fasciitis in a dog. *Can Vet J* 2009;50:655–656.

829. Loeffler A, Linek M, Moodley A, et al. First report of multiresistant, mecA-positive *Staphylococcus intermedius* in Europe: 12 cases from a veterinary dermatology referral clinic in Germany. *Vet Dermatol* 2007;18:412–421.

830. Bemis DA, Jones RD, Frank LA, et al. Evaluation of susceptibility test breakpoints used to predict mecA-mediated resistance in *Staphylococcus pseudintermedius* isolated from dogs. *J Vet Diagn Invest* 2009;21:53–58.

831. Weese JS, Faires M, Brisson BA, et al. Infection with methicillin-resistant *Staphylococcus pseudintermedius* masquerading as cefoxitin susceptible in a dog. *J Am Vet Med Assoc* 2009;235:1064–1066.

832. Pottumarthy S, Schapiro J, Prentice J, et al. Clinical isolates of *Staphylococcus intermedius* masquerading as methicillin-resistant *Staphylococcus aureus*. *J Clin Microbiol* 2004;42:5881–5884.

833. Célard M, Vandenesch F, Darbas H, et al. Pacemaker infection caused by *Staphylococcus schleiferi*, a member of the human preaxillary flora: four case reports. *Clin Infect Dis* 1997;24:1014–1015.

834. Igimi S, Takahashi E, Mitsuoka T. *Staphylococcus schleiferi* subsp. *coagulans* subsp. nov., isolated from the external auditory meatus of dogs with external ear otitis. *Int J Syst Bacteriol* 1990;40:409–411.

835. Hernández JL, Calvo J, Sota R, et al. Clinical and microbiological characteristics of 28 patients with *Staphylococcus schleiferi* infection. *Eur J Clin Microbiol Infect Dis* 2001;20:153–158.

836. Frank L, Kania S, Hnilica K, et al. Isolation of *Staphylococcus schleiferi* from dogs with pyoderma. *J Am Vet Med Assoc* 2003;222:451–454.

837. Jones R, Kania S, Rohrbach B, et al. Prevalence of oxacillin- and multidrug-resistant staphylococci in

clinical samples from dogs: 1,772 samples (2001–2005). *J Am Vet Med Assoc* 2007;230:221–227.

838. Arciola CR, Campoccia D, An YH, et al. Prevalence and antibiotic resistance of 15 minor staphylococcal species colonizing orthopedic implants. *Int J Artif Organs* 2006;29:395–401.

839. Brebbia G, Boni L, Dionigi G, et al. Surgical site infections in day surgery settings. *Surg Infect (Larchmt)* 2006;7(Suppl. 2):S121–S123.

840. Koksal F, Yasar H, Samasti M. Antibiotic resistance patterns of coagulase-negative *Staphylococcus* strains isolated from blood cultures of septicemic patients in Turkey. *Microbiol Res* 2009;164:404–410.

841. Kluytmans J, Berg H, Steegh P, et al. Outbreak of *Staphylococcus schleiferi* wound infections: strain characterization by randomly amplified polymorphic DNA analysis, PCR ribotyping, conventional ribotyping, and pulsed-field gel electrophoresis. *J Clin Microbiol* 1998;36:2214–2219.

842. Kumar D, Cawley JJ, Irizarry-Alvarado JM, et al. Case of *Staphylococcus schleiferi* subspecies coagulans endocarditis and metastatic infection in an immune compromised host. *Transpl Infect Dis* 2007;9:336–338.

843. Galpérine T, Cazorla C, Blanchard E, et al. *Streptococcus canis* infections in humans: retrospective study of 54 patients. *J Infect* 2007;55:23–26.

844. Chaffer M, Friedman S, Saran A, et al. An outbreak of *Streptococcus canis* mastitis in a dairy herd in Israel. *N Z Vet J* 2005;53:261–264.

845. Iglauer F, Kunstýr I, Mörstedt R, et al. *Streptococcus canis* arthritis in a cat breeding colony. *J Exp Anim Sci* 1991;34:59–65.

846. Matsuu A, Kanda T, Sugiyama A, et al. Mitral stenosis with bacterial myocarditis in a cat. *J Vet Med Sci* 2007;69:1171–1174.

847. Pesavento PA, Bannasch MJ, Bachmann R, et al. Fatal *Streptococcus canis* infections in intensively housed shelter cats. *Vet Pathol* 2007;44:218–221.

848. Sura R, Hinckley LS, Risatti GR, et al. Fatal necrotising fasciitis and myositis in a cat associated with *Streptococcus canis*. *Vet Rec* 2008;162:450–453.

849. Lyskova P, Vydrzalova M, Mazurova J. Identification and antimicrobial susceptibility of bacteria and yeasts isolated from healthy dogs and dogs with otitis externa. *J Vet Med A Physiol Pathol Clin Med* 2007;54:559–563.

850. Takeda N, Kikuchi K, Asano R, et al. Recurrent septicemia caused by *Streptococcus canis* after a dog bite. *Scand J Infect Dis* 2001;33:927–928.

851. Bert F, Lambert-Zechovsky N. Septicemia caused by *Streptococcus canis* in a human. *J Clin Microbiol* 1997;35:777–779.

852. Miller C, Prescott J, Mathews K, et al. Streptococcal toxic shock syndrome in dogs. *J Am Vet Med Assoc* 1996;209:1421–1426.

853. Ingrey K, Ren J, Prescott J. A fluoroquinolone induces a novel mitogen-encoding bacteriophage in *Streptococcus canis*. *Infect Immun* 2003;71:3028–3033.

854. DeWinter L, Low D, Prescott J. Virulence of *Streptococcus canis* from canine streptococcal toxic shock syndrome and necrotizing fasciitis. *Vet Microbiol* 1999;70:95–110.

855. Pedersen K, Pedersen K, Jensen H, et al. Occurrence of antimicrobial resistance in bacteria from diagnostic samples from dogs. *J Antimicrob Chemother* 2007;60:775–781.

856. Stafford Johnson JM, Martin MW, Stidworthy MF. Septic fibrinous pericarditis in a cocker spaniel. *J Small Anim Pract* 2003;44:117–120.

857. Sykes JE, Kittleson MD, Pesavento PA, et al. Evaluation of the relationship between causative organisms and clinical characteristics of infective endocarditis in dogs: 71 cases (1992–2005). *J Am Vet Med Assoc* 2006;228:1723–1734.

858. Moyaert H, De Graef EM, Haesebrouck F, et al. Acquired antimicrobial resistance in the intestinal microbiota of diverse cat populations. *Res Vet Sci* 2006;81:1–7.

859. Lam MM, Clarridge JE, Young EJ, et al. The other group G *Streptococcus*: increased detection of *Streptococcus canis* ulcer infections in dog owners. *J Clin Microbiol* 2007;45:2327–2329.

860. Whatmore AM, Engler KH, Gudmundsdottir G, et al. Identification of isolates of *Streptococcus canis* infecting humans. *J Clin Microbiol* 2001;39:4196–4199.

861. Jacobs JA, de Krom MC, Kellens JT, et al. Meningitis and sepsis due to group G *Streptococcus*. *Eur J Clin Microbiol Infect Dis* 1993;12:224–225.

862. Carapetis JR, Steer AC, Mulholland EK, et al. The global burden of group A streptococcal diseases. *Lancet Infect Dis* 2005;5:685–694.

863. Centers for Disease Control and Prevention. Active bacterial core surveillance (ABCs) report, group A *Streptococcus*, 2002, 2003.

864. Copperman SM. Cherchez le chien: household pets as reservoirs of persistent or recurrent streptococcal sore throats in children. *N Y State J Med* 1982;82:1685–1687.

865. Huminer D. Streptococcal pharyngitis derived from dogs. *Postgrad Med* 1985;78:29–30.

866. Mayer G, Van Ore S. Recurrent pharyngitis in family of four. Household pet as reservoir of group A streptococci. *Postgrad Med* 1983;74:277–279.

867. Kurek C, Rutkowiak B. Dogs as carriers of *Streptococcus pyogenes* on the mucous membrane of the tonsil. *Przegl Epidemiol* 1971;25:263–267.

868. Crowder HR, Dorn CR, Smith RE. Group A *Streptococcus* in pets and group A streptococcal disease in man. *Int J Zoonoses* 1978;5:45–54.

869. Wilson KS, Maroney SA, Gander RM. The family pet as an unlikely source of group A beta-hemolytic streptococcal infection in humans. *Pediatr Infect Dis J* 1995;14:372–375.

870. Lefebvre SL, Waltner-Toews D, Peregrine AS, et al. Prevalence of zoonotic agents in dogs visiting hospitalized people in Ontario: implications for infection control. *J Hosp Infect* 2006;62:458–466.

871. Roos K, Holm SE, Ekedahl C. Treatment failure in acute streptococcal tonsillitis in children over the age of 10 and in adults. *Scand J Infect Dis* 1985; 17:357–365.

872. Falck G, Holm SE, Kjellander J, et al. The role of household contacts in the transmission of group A streptococci. *Scand J Infect Dis* 1997;29:239–244.

873. Bisno AL, Gerber MA, Gwaltney JM, et al. Practice guidelines for the diagnosis and management of group A streptococcal pharyngitis. Infectious Diseases Society of America. *Clin Infect Dis* 2002; 35:113–125.

874. Ladlow J, Scase T, Waller A. Canine strangles case reveals a new host susceptible to infection with *Streptococcus equi. J Clin Microbiol* 2006;44: 2664–2665.

875. Byun JW, Yoon SS, Woo GH, et al. An outbreak of fatal hemorrhagic pneumonia caused by *Streptococcus equi* subsp. *zooepidemicus* in shelter dogs. *J Vet Sci* 2009;10:269–271.

876. Kim MK, Jee H, Shin SW, et al. Outbreak and control of haemorrhagic pneumonia due to *Streptococcus equi* subspecies *zooepidemicus* in dogs. *Vet Rec* 2007;161:528–530.

877. Pesavento PA, Hurley KF, Bannasch MJ, et al. A clonal outbreak of acute fatal hemorrhagic pneumonia in intensively housed (shelter) dogs caused by *Streptococcus equi* subsp. *zooepidemicus. Vet Pathol* 2008;45:51–53.

878. Chalker VJ, Brooks HW, Brownlie J. The association of *Streptococcus equi* subsp. *zooepidemicus* with canine infectious respiratory disease. *Vet Microbiol* 2003;95:149–156.

879. Gibson D, Richardson G. Haemorrhagic streptococcal pneumonia in a dog. *Vet Rec* 2008;162:423–424.

880. Adams SJ. Peracute haemorrhagic pneumonia syndrome in dogs. *Vet Rec* 2008;162:599–600.

881. Barnham M, Kerby J, Chandler RS, et al. Group C streptococci in human infection: a study of 308 isolates with clinical correlations. *Epidemiol Infect* 1989;102:379–390.

882. Barnham M, Thornton TJ, Lange K. Nephritis caused by *Streptococcus zooepidemicus* (Lancefield group C). *Lancet* 1983;1:945–948.

883. Thorley AM, Campbell D, Moghal NE, et al. Post streptococcal acute glomerulonephritis secondary to sporadic *Streptococcus equi* infection. *Pediatr Nephrol* 2007;22:597–599.

884. Edwards AT, Roulson M, Ironside MJ. A milk-borne outbreak of serious infection due to *Streptococcus zooepidemicus* (Lancefield group C). *Epidemiol Infect* 1988;101:43–51.

885. Low DE, Young MR, Harding GK. Group C streptococcal meningitis in an adult. Probable acquisition from a horse. *Arch Intern Med* 1980;140: 977–978.

886. Abbott Y, Acke E, Khan S, et al. Zoonotic transmission of *Streptococcus equi* subsp. *zooepidemicus* from a dog to a handler. *J Med Microbiol* 2010;59: 120–123.

887. Bucher M, Meyer C, Grötzbach B, et al. Epidemiological data on pathogenic *Yersinia enterocolitica* in Southern Germany during 2000–2006. *Foodborne Pathog Dis* 2008;5:273–280.

888. Fukushima H, Nakamura R, Iitsuka S, et al. Presence of zoonotic pathogens (*Yersinia* spp., *Campylobacter jejuni, Salmonella* spp., and *Leptospira* spp.) simultaneously in dogs and cats. *Zentralbl Bakteriol Mikrobiol Hyg B* 1985;181:430–440.

889. Wooley RE, Shotts EB, McConnell JW. Isolation of *Yersinia enterocolitica* from selected animal species. *Am J Vet Res* 1980;41:1667–1668.

890. Hayashidani H, Kaneko K, Sakurai K, et al. Experimental infection with *Yersinia enterocolitica* serovar 0:8 in beagle dogs. *Vet Microbiol* 1995;47: 71–77.

891. Fredriksson-Ahomaa M, Korte T, Korkeala H. Transmission of *Yersinia enterocolitica* 4/O:3 to pets via contaminated pork. *Lett Appl Microbiol* 2001;32:375–378.

892. Greene CE. Yersiniosis. In: Greene CE, ed. *Infectious Diseases of the Dog and Cat*. Philadelphia: Saunders Elsevier, 2006, pp. 361–362.

893. Fredriksson-Ahomaa M, Stolle A, Korkeala H. Molecular epidemiology of *Yersinia enterocolitica* infections. *FEMS Immunol Med Microbiol* 2006;47: 315–329.

894. Szita J, Svidró A, Kubinyi M, et al. *Yersinia enterocolitica* infection of animals and human contacts. *Acta Microbiol Acad Sci Hung* 1980;27:103–109.

895. World Health Organization. *Plague Manual: Epidemiology, Distribution, Surveillance and Control*. Geneva, Switzerland: World Health Organization, 1999.

896. Eisen RJ, Borchert JN, Holmes JL, et al. Early-phase transmission of *Yersinia pestis* by cat fleas (*Ctenocephalides felis*) and their potential role as vectors in a plague-endemic region of Uganda. *Am J Trop Med Hyg* 2008;78:949–956.

897. Centers for Disease Control and Prevention (CDC). Human plague—four states, 2006. *MMWR Morb Mortal Wkly Rep* 2006;55:940–943.

898. Doll JM, Zeitz PS, Ettestad P, et al. Cat-transmitted fatal pneumonic plague in a person who traveled from Colorado to Arizona. *Am J Trop Med Hyg* 1994;51:109–114.

899. Feldmann H, Czub M, Jones S, et al. Emerging and re-emerging infectious diseases. *Med Microbiol Immunol* 2002;191:63–74.

900. Macy D. Plague. In: Greene CE, ed. *Infectious Diseases of the Dog and Cat*. Philadelphia: Saunders Elsevier, 2006, pp. 439–446.

901. Brinkerhoff RJ, Collinge SK, Bai Y, et al. Are carnivores universally good sentinels of plague? *Vector Borne Zoonotic Dis* 2008;9:491–497.

902. Eidson M, Thilsted JP, Rollag OJ. Clinical, clinicopathologic, and pathologic features of plague in cats: 119 cases (1977–1988). *J Am Vet Med Assoc* 1991;199:1191–1197.

903. Chomel BB, Jay MT, Smith CR, et al. Serological surveillance of plague in dogs and cats, California, 1979–1991. *Comp Immunol Microbiol Infect Dis* 1994;17:111–123.

904. Gage KL, Dennis DT, Orloski KA, et al. Cases of cat-associated human plague in the Western US, 1977–1998. *Clin Infect Dis* 2000;30:893–900.

905. Werner SB, Weidmer CE, Nelson BC, et al. Primary plague pneumonia contracted from a domestic cat at South Lake Tahoe, Calif. *JAMA* 1984;251:929–931.

906. Thornton DJ, Tustin RC, Pienaar BJ, et al. Cat bite transmission of *Yersinia pestis* infection to man. *J S Afr Vet Med Assoc* 1975;46:165–169.

907. Orloski K, Lathrop S. Plague: a veterinary perspective. *J Am Vet Med Assoc* 2003;222:444–448.

908. Gould LH, Pape J, Ettestad P, et al. Dog-associated risk factors for human plague. *Zoonoses Public Health* 2008;55:448–454.

909. Mann JM, Martone WJ, Boyce JM, et al. Endemic human plague in New Mexico: risk factors associated with infection. *J Infect Dis* 1979;140:397–401.

910. Hull HF, Montes JM, Mann JM. Septicemic plague in New Mexico. *J Infect Dis* 1987;155:113–118.

911. Meyer KF. Pneumonic plague. *Bacteriol Rev* 1961;25:249–261.

912. Orloski KA, Eidson M. *Yersinia pestis* infection in three dogs. *J Am Vet Med Assoc* 1995;207:316–318.

913. Rust JH, Cavanaugh DC, O'Shita R, et al. The role of domestic animals in the epidemiology of plague. I. Experimental infection of dogs and cats. *J Infect Dis* 1971;124:522–526.

914. Watson RP, Blanchard TW, Mense MG, et al. Histopathology of experimental plague in cats. *Vet Pathol* 2001;38:165–172.

915. Meyer KF, Quan SF, McCrumb FR, et al. Effective treatment of plague. *Ann N Y Acad Sci* 1952;55:1228–1274.

916. Smadel JE, Woodward TE, Amies CR, et al. Antibiotics in the treatment of bubonic and pneumonic plague in man. *Ann N Y Acad Sci* 1952;55:1275–1284.

917. Garner JS. Guideline for isolation precautions in hospitals. The Hospital Infection Control Practices Advisory Committee. *Infect Control Hosp Epidemiol* 1996;17:53–80.

918. Fukushima H, Gomyoda M. Restriction endonuclease analysis of plasmid DNA of *Yersinia pseudotuberculosis* infections in Shimane Prefecture, Japan. *Zentralbl Bakteriol* 1995;282:498–506.

919. Fukushima H, Gomyoda M. Intestinal carriage of *Yersinia pseudotuberculosis* by wild birds and mammals in Japan. *Appl Environ Microbiol* 1991;57:1152–1155.

920. Keymer IF, Gibson EA, Reynolds DJ. Zoonoses and other findings in hedgehogs (*Erinaceus europaeus*): a survey of mortality and review of the literature. *Vet Rec* 1991;128:245–249.

921. Mackintosh CG, Henderson T. Potential wildlife sources of *Yersinia pseudotuberculosis* for farmed deer (*Cervus elaphus*). *N Z Vet J* 1984;32:208–210.

922. Fukushima H, Nakamura R, Iitsuka S, et al. Prospective systematic study of *Yersinia* spp. in dogs. *J Clin Microbiol* 1984;19:616–622.

923. Obwolo MJ, Gruffydd-Jones TJ. *Yersinia pseudotuberculosis* in the cat. *Vet Rec* 1977;100:424–425.

924. Spearman JG, Hunt P, Nayar PS. *Yersinia pseudotuberculosis* infection in a cat. *Can Vet J* 1979;20:361–364.

925. Weber J, Finlayson NB, Mark JB. Mesenteric lymphadenitis and terminal ileitis due to *Yersinia pseudotuberculosis*. *N Engl J Med* 1970;283:172–174.

926. Butler T, Dennis DT. *Yersinia* species, including plague. In: Mandell GL, Bennett JE, Dolin R, eds. *Principles and Practice of Infectious Diseases*. Philadelphia: Elsevier, 2005, pp. 2691–2701.

927. Bourdin M. Pseudotuberculosis in man: possible epidemiological role of the cats. *Comp Immunol Microbiol Infect Dis* 1979;1:243–251.

928. Fukushima H, Gomyoda M, Ishikura S, et al. Cat-contaminated environmental substances lead to *Yersinia pseudotuberculosis* infection in children. *J Clin Microbiol* 1989;27:2706–2709.

929. Tertti R, Granfors K, Lehtonen OP, et al. An outbreak of *Yersinia pseudotuberculosis* infection. *J Infect Dis* 1984;149:245–250.

3

Viral Diseases

J. Scott Weese and Martha B. Fulford

Introduction

Viral zoonoses from companion animals are very rare in developed countries but can result in a significant burden of disease in some areas. This is best exemplified by rabies, which is exceedingly rare in most developed countries but which kills tens of thousands of people yearly in other areas. Despite the rarity of viral zoonoses, tremendous efforts are put into the prevention and control of some diseases, and sporadic infections and outbreaks of various pathogens continue to cause significant morbidity and mortality.

Cowpox

Introduction

Cowpox is often considered mainly of historical interest, relating to Jenner's observation about cowpox infection providing protection from smallpox. In reality, cowpox is endemic in rodents in some regions, and human disease can occur from contact with wild rodents, pet rodents, and cats. It may be an emerging zoonosis in some areas, particularly in certain areas of Europe.

Companion Animal Zoonoses. Edited by J. Scott Weese and Martha B. Fulford. © 2011 Blackwell Publishing Ltd.

Etiology

Cowpox virus is a DNA virus of the *Orthopoxvirus* genus that is similar to monkeypox and smallpox. While originally associated with cattle, rodents are the natural reservoir, and various animal species can be affected.[1,2] Cattle, along with cats, zoo animals, and humans, are accidental hosts.[3] Most infections are now diagnosed in cats and zoo animals, and cowpox has not been isolated from cattle in the past three decades.[4]

Geographic distribution/epidemiology

Human cowpox infections are uncommon and have predominantly been reported in Europe, western parts of the former Soviet Union, and parts of Northern and Central Asia.[2,3,5] Most cases are identified in the late summer and fall.[6] Similarly, most feline infections occur in late summer,[7] likely coinciding with times when rodent populations are highest and suggesting that cats may be a sentinel for cowpox activity in wild rodents.[4]

Cowpox is transmitted by direct contact with an infected animal. Cowpox virus is believed to have relatively low infectivity for humans, and direct contact of skin lesions or mucous membranes with virus is required for infection.[6,8] The degree of contact required for infection is not known. In one report of rat-associated cowpox, all four infected humans had been scratched.[5]

Increasing attention is being paid to the role of cats and pet rodents in zoonotic transmission of cowpox. Cats are among the most commonly infected nonreservoir species and may be the most important source of human infection because of the close contact they often have with people.[6,9,10] Up to 5% of domestic cats have antibodies to cowpox in some regions,[11] indicating the high frequency of exposure and presumably low incidence of clinical disease in cats. Pet rats may also be important sources of human infection.[12,13] Clusters of infections have been associated with rats purchased from pet stores.[3,5] While pet rat-associated cowpox infections have typically been single sporadic cases, larger numbers, including outbreaks, can occur if rat breeding or distribution facilities are infected, resulting in the sale of large numbers of infected rats. Duration of shedding of cowpox virus is relatively short (2–3 weeks), and persistent infections do not occur. It is thought that the risk of human cowpox infections has increased because of cessation of smallpox vaccination, which would have provided cross-protection.[2]

Animals

Clinical presentation

Feline cowpox starts as a pruritic, bite-like lesion over the front limbs or head.[6] Concurrent systemic disease with fever and lethargy may be present. Secondary lesions subsequently develop. Lesions are typical for poxvirus infections with progression to ulcerated papules and vesicles up to 1 cm in diameter.[6] Self-trauma may produce more extensive lesions. Severe infections, including pneumonia and fatal generalized disease, have been reported but are rare.[14,15]

Classical pox-like skin lesions can be observed in rats, with fatal infection occurring in some cases; however, transmission can occur from rats without obvious skin lesions.[3,5] Signs of respiratory disease have also been reported.[5]

Diagnosis

Electron microscopy and virus isolation can be used for diagnosis.

Management

Cowpox infection in animals is typically self-limited. No specific treatments are available. Severe infections such as viral pneumonia can occur but are rare.[6] Supportive therapy may be required in moderate to severe cases.

Humans

Clinical presentation

The incubation period is usually 3–7 days but can be as long as 14 days.[11] In people, cowpox infection usually produces lesions on the hands and face.[6] Lesions rarely occur at other body sites. Lesions are typical "pox" lesions. An initial macular lesion progresses through papular, vesicular, and pustular stages before forming a hard black crust. Lesions are painful, and edema and erythema are common around the location of the lesion.[6] Only a single lesion is present in most cases but multiple lesions can be caused by multiple inoculations or auto-inoculation.[6] Vascular or lymphatic spread is possible but rare. Influenza-like symptoms such as fever and fatigue, as well as lymphadenopathy, are common. Conjunctivitis may also be present. Severe, even fatal, disease can occur in immuno-compromised individuals and people with severe eczema.[6] Virus-associated pneumonia may occur but is rare. Incubation period may be longer and disease milder in people that have been previously vaccinated against smallpox.[3]

Diagnosis

Diagnosis of cowpox can involve electron microscopy, virus isolation, or molecular testing.[11] Minimal effort should be paid to relating infection to contact with cattle, since cattle are an uncommon source of infection. More attention should be paid to querying contact with cats and pet rats,[6] particularly close contact with animals with skin lesions or newly acquired pet rats.

Management

Cowpox is typically a relatively mild self-limited disease. Serious disease, including disseminated infection, is most common in children, immunocompromised individuals, and people with eczema.[6,11] Treatment is usually supportive. There are no antiviral drugs licensed for treatment of cowpox infections. Corticosteroids are contraindicated. Cowpox lesions typically resolve within 6–8 weeks, often with scarring, which may be permanent. Lesions should be covered until the scab falls off to reduce the risk of transmission to other individuals and autoinoculation.[6] Considering the cross-protection that typically occurs between orthopoxviruses, smallpox vaccination after exposure to cowpox could be considered but is probably unwarranted because of the typically mild and self-limited nature of disease, as opposed to monkeypox, another orthopoxvirus but one that can cause serious disease.

Prevention

With the decrease in population protection against smallpox and the increase in popularity of pet rats and cats, cowpox has the potential to be an emerging problem in areas where the virus is endemic in wild rodents and/or in rodent-breeding facilities. Pet owners and veterinarians in endemic regions should be aware of the potential for cowpox in cats and pet rats, and ensure that animals with skin lesions are investigated.

Overall, the risk of transmission to humans is relatively low,[16] particularly if general infection control protocols are used. It has been reported that no human case has ever occurred in someone caring for an infected cat after the infection was diagnosed.[6] Proper hygiene practices, particularly hand hygiene, and bite avoidance should reduce the risk of cowpox transmission from animals. Contact with infected animals should be avoided. Cats are an important source of human infection, and cowpox should be considered in any cat with skin lesions in an endemic area. The same should apply to rats with skin lesions. Gloves should be worn when handling cats and rats with skin lesions, and hands should be washed immediately after glove removal. If skin lesions are identified on a rat, particularly over the feet, ears, or tail, prompt veterinary examination is indicated. Rats with skin lesions should not be purchased. Cats and pet rats should not have contact with wild rodents. Wild rats should not be caught and kept

as pets. Rat owners should understand good handling practices to reduce the risk of bites and to ensure that any bites are promptly and thoroughly cleaned.

Identification of cowpox in pet rats should result in a public health investigation of the source because of the potential for pet stores or rat breeding facilities to widely disseminate cowpox.

There is no evidence of transmission of cowpox between humans; however, basic hygiene practices are warranted, particularly avoiding contact with skin lesions.

European bat lyssavirus (EBLV)

Introduction

EBLV is a Rhabdovirus that is related to rabies virus. Like rabies virus, EBLV can cause fatal neurological disease in humans and animals, but unlike rabies, human infections are rare, with only three fatal infections ever reported.[17–19]

Exposure is most commonly associated with bats; however, the potential for transmission from companion animals cannot be overlooked.

Etiology

This *Lyssavirus* from the Rhabdoviridae family is naturally found in insectivorous bat species. EBLV is divided into two groups: EBLV-1 and EBLV-2. Bat-to-human transmission has been reported for both types, while reported natural infections of other mammals have involved EBLV-1.[19] Experimental infection of foxes and ferrets with EBVL-2 did not result in disease.[20–22] In contrast, disease was produced in sheep following experimental infection with either EBLV-1 or EBLV-2.[23]

Geographic distribution/epidemiology

While much less is known about EBLV compared with rabies virus, EBLV is endemic in the bat population in some regions, with most reports coming from western Europe.[24–27] The prevalence of infection of bats can be high (20–29%) in some regions.[26,28] Among domestic animals, cats may be at highest risk of exposure, presumably through catching infected bats. EBLV has also been identified in other "spillover" species, including stone martens[29] and sheep.[23]

Humans are at greatest risk of EBLV infection from direct contact with infected bats. Risk of transmission of EBLV from other wild or domestic animal species is believed to be low but not non-existent. The risk is probably greatest from cats based on the potential for this species to be exposed to infected bats and subsequently have close contact with humans. As with rabies, transmission of EBLV requires contact of nonintact skin or mucous membranes with EBLV-contaminated secretions, which could occur with bites. Guidelines for determining what constitutes rabies exposure apply equally to EBLV exposure; however, the true risks may be lower as it is believed that infected bats (and perhaps other species such as cats) only excrete small amounts of virus in saliva.[28]

Animals

Clinical presentation

There is limited clinical information about EBLV infection in companion animals, all of which pertains to cats. Clinical presentation is likely similar to rabies. The limited case reports of EBLV in cats have reported rapid death;[24] however, it cannot be stated with certainty that rapid progression to death occurs in all cases, as is the case with rabies. Therefore, gradual deterioration should not result in exclusion of the possibility of EBLV infection.

Diagnosis

Diagnosis can be challenging. EBLV should be suspected in all mammals with an acute onset of neurological disease in regions where the virus has been identified. Definitive diagnosis can be difficult, and persistence may be required. Rabies direct immunofluorescence antibody test and antigen capture enzyme-linked immunosorbent assay (ELISA) can be performed, but results may be inconsistent, even between tests on the same animal.[24] Virus isolation is diagnostic for EBLV infection but failure to isolate EBLV does not rule out infection. Polymerase chain reaction (PCR) to detect EBLV RNA is also diagnostic but not foolproof. The use of multiple tests is therefore recommended on EBLV suspects if results of initial testing are negative.

Management

There are no known treatment options. EBLV infection is presumably invariably fatal.

Humans

Clinical presentation

Clinical signs are similar to those described below for rabies.[17,18]

Diagnosis

Tests used to diagnose rabies virus infection can be used for EBLV. PCR detection of EBLV-specific RNA sequences can be used to differentiate EBLV from rabies.

Management

Available, but limited, data suggest that pre- and postexposure treatment protocols for rabies are effective for the prevention of EBLV infection.[24] More details are provided in the Rabies section below. Clinical EBLV infection is fatal.[30]

Prevention

There are no specific measures for the prevention of EBLV. Considering the rarity of disease in humans and the very low likelihood of transmission of EBLV from secondary hosts (i.e., cats), specific strategies are probably not indicated. Rabies vaccination of people at higher risk of exposure to potentially infected wildlife and domestic animals is reasonable, as per standard rabies practices. Routine wound care following bites from wild or domestic animals is likely an important measure. While the risks of transmission are low, a bite or similar high-risk exposure from an infected (or potentially infected) animal should result in an investigation as per rabies guidelines to determine if postexposure prophylaxis (PEP) is indicated. If so, standard rabies protocols would apply.

Measures to reduce human and animal contact with bats should be undertaken.

Hantavirus

Hantaviruses are a group of RNA viruses from the Bunyaviridae family. Unlike other Bunyaviridae, they do not require an insect vector. Rather, hantaviruses are adapted to survive in different rodent reservoirs, which are able to transmit the virus through direct and indirect routes. Numerous different hantaviruses are known, and these have different geographic ranges, reservoir hosts, and clinical effects. Sin Nombre virus is the most important hantavirus in North America and causes hantavirus pulmonary syndrome. In South America, Andes, Laguna Negra, and Juquitiba viruses predominate. Hantaan virus is an important Old World hantavirus that causes hemorrhagic fever with renal syndrome, predominantly in Asia.

All hantaviruses are associated with wild rodent reservoirs. Various rodent species can be involved; however, each hantavirus tends to have a single major reservoir species. For example, the deer mouse is the main reservoir of Sin Nombre virus.[31]

Hantavirus pulmonary syndrome is a severe and rapidly progressive condition that starts with fever and progresses to severe increases in pulmonary vascular permeability and shock. Death occurs in approximately 40–46% of cases with most deaths occurring very early in the disease.[32,33] Hemorrhagic fever with renal syndrome is characterized by fever, thrombocytopenia, and acute renal failure.[34] Mortality rates are lower than for hantavirus pulmonary syndrome, with death in approximately 5% of cases. Lower mortality rates (<1%) have been reported for Puumala virus.[34]

Transmission is mainly through inhalation of hantavirus from urine, feces, saliva, or nesting materials of infected animals. Human infections are often linked to inhalation of hantavirus after disturbing rodent nests in enclosed spaces or cleaning areas heavily contaminated with rodent urine and feces. Bite-associated transmission is rare but has been reported.[35,36]

Serum antibodies against hantavirus can be found in up to 9.6% of cats and 3.5% of dogs in some regions;[37,38] however, clinical disease has not been reported in companion animals. Exposure of cats to this virus is not surprising in endemic areas because of the potential exposure to infected rodent reservoir species while hunting. Even though serological evidence of exposure can be found in pets, hantavirus transmission has never been reported from domestic pets, and rodent species typically kept as pets are not known to be hantavirus carriers.

Human infection from infected nonrodent pets is extremely unlikely. Concern was raised at one point due to a Chinese study that indicated cat ownership was associated with Hantaan virus infection.[39] However, no subsequent studies have implicated cats or other pet species. The risk from cats that have been exposed is presumably very low, and there is no evidence that exposed cats shed hantavirus. Infections from pets would ultimately have to have come from infected wild animal reservoirs, and identification of hantavirus exposure in a pet is probably more useful as an indication of the potential for human exposure from the same source rather than a concern about pet–human infection.

While hantavirus infection of pet rodent species has not been reported, it cannot be completely dismissed. Captive pet rodents would need to be exposed through contact with infected wild rodents. Household rodent control to prevent contact of pets, especially pet rodents, with wild animal reservoirs is important for hantavirus as well as other zoonotic pathogens such as lymphocytic choriomeningitis virus (LCMV), and should be a standard precaution taken by all pet rodent owners. Contact with wild rodents should be avoided and wild rodents should never be kept as pets.

Herpes simplex virus (HSV)

Human herpesviruses 1 and 2, also known as HSV, are common human viruses that, like many other herpesviruses, are neurotropic and able to establish latent infection in neuronal cells. Clinically, infections in humans are characterized by labial, genital, oral, and, less commonly, ocular lesions. More severe consequences such as encephalitis, radiculitis, and transverse myelitis can occur but are rare.

Humans are the primary host of this virus and up to 80% seroprevalence has been reported for HSV-1 and up to 20% for HSV-2, although a much lower percentage of the population will be actively shedding virus at any given time. Despite being predominantly a human virus, it can infect other animals, particularly nonhuman primates. Infection of companion animals is rare but has been reported in rabbits, rats, mice, and chinchillas, typically with fatal outcomes.[40-42] Documented cases of rabbit infections have been associated with human-to-rabbit transmission from women with active labial and facial infections. Humans have presumably been the source of infections in rodent species, although a link to infected people has not always been reported.

Concern has been expressed that infected pets could be a source of infection for humans.[41] Overall, the risk of herpes simplex transmission between people and pets is presumably low, particularly since the few reports of herpes simplex infection in pets have involved rather short courses of disease without external lesions. Conjunctivitis can be a component of disease[41] however, so there is the potential for infection at an exposed external site.

While the risk of transmission is very low, it is prudent to emphasize routine hygiene measures in people with herpes simplex infections. In particular, people with active lesions should avoid direct or indirect contact of lesion sites with pets and ensure that they perform proper hand hygiene after contact with lesions. The risks are probably greatest for the pets of infected people because of the known potential for human-to-pet transmission and often-fatal nature of infection in pets.

Human immunodeficiency virus (HIV)

HIV is a retrovirus and the cause of acquired immunodeficiency syndrome (AIDS) in humans. This virus is not able to cause infection in domestic animals, regardless of the route of exposure. Exposure of dogs and cats to blood from an infected human, through bites, scratches, or licking open sores, cannot result in the transmission of HIV from human to pet. Concern is periodically raised about the ability of animals (especially dogs) to transmit HIV through bites. While there is a theoretical possibility that an animal could transfer

HIV by biting an infected person (drawing blood) and immediately biting another individual, the likelihood of HIV transmission is exceptionally low. HIV is poorly stable outside the human body and would be rapidly inactivated in the mouth of a biting cat or dog. There have been no reported cases of documented or suspected pet involvement in HIV transmission, despite close tracking of new HIV cases.

Influenza: avian

Introduction

Avian influenza has received much attention because of concerns about the potential for an influenza pandemic. Most of the attention has been focused on highly pathogenic avian influenza (HPAI) A H5N1 because of unprecedented high mortality poultry outbreaks in Asia, Europe, the Middle East, and Africa, along with sporadic but severe human infections.[43] While a human H5N1 pandemic has not developed, the severity of human disease associated with this strain, its recurring presence in humans and animals in various regions, and the ever-present potential for recombination and increased transmissibility in humans support ongoing concerns. The emergence of new avian influenza strains in humans and animals is a serious threat and one that will not decrease in the foreseeable future. Ultimately, there are potential issues regarding companion animals and avian influenza, but pets should at worst play a minor role in the propagation of infection and little to no role as a source of recombinant viruses.

Etiology

Influenza viruses are single-stranded RNA viruses of the Orthomyxoviridae family. Influenza viruses are divided into three types: A, B, and C. Influenza B and C are human influenza types and therefore not of zoonotic disease concern. Influenza A can infect birds, humans, and other animal species. Influenza strains are further classified on the basis of antigenicity of two surface glycoproteins: hemagglutinin (H) and neuraminidase (N). Currently,

16 different H and 9 different N types are recognized.[43]

Influenza viruses have high mutation rates, which results in "antigenic drift"; minor antigenic changes that occur over time from point mutations in H and N genes. More profound changes can occur through reassortment between human and animal influenza A viruses or direct animal-to-human transmission of novel strains.[43] This is termed "antigenic shift." It only occurs in influenza A viruses, and accordingly, pandemics are only caused by novel influenza A strains.

Influenza A viruses are also divided into "low pathogenic avian influenza (LPAI)" and "HPAI" based on their pathogenicity in birds, as well as specific molecular criteria.[43] LPAI does not usually cause disease in wild birds but may cause mild disease in domestic poultry. Human infections are rare and mild.[43,44] HPAI can cause devastating outbreaks in poultry as well as mild to severe infections in humans and other animal species.[43,45-48]

Geographic distribution/epidemiology

Aquatic waterbirds are the natural hosts for all known influenza A strains, harboring virus strains with all combinations of H and N.[43,49] Non-avian species can be infected by some avian influenza viruses, but this is restricted to a limited number of subtypes and strains with broad host ranges are rare.[49]

H5N1 avian influenza has caused most of the concern in recent years. This virus has been reported to infect at least 172 different vertebrate species[49] and is a significant zoonotic disease concern in some regions. The first reported human H5N1 influenza infections were in Hong Kong in 1997.[47,50] Four hundred thirty-three infections were subsequently identified in 15 countries from 2003 to 2009,[51] mainly in southeast Asia and associated with the ongoing panzootic in poultry. Spread of H5N1 to Europe and Africa has been attributed to migratory birds, a mode of transmission that is very difficult to control.

Most human H5N1 infections have been linked to contact with sick domestic poultry.[52,53] In most developed countries, few individuals have close contact with domestic poultry. Accordingly, other sources of transmission are of greater concern should avian influenza become established. Human-to-human transmission is one possible means of transmission. Currently, H5N1 influenza is very poorly transmitted between people, with the few documented human-to-human transmissions occurring in people with close and prolonged contact with infected individuals. Mutation of H5N1 influenza, recombination with a human influenza virus, and emergence of a new and more readily transmissible strain are the main concerns. Pet-to-human transmission of avian influenza has not been documented but should not be dismissed because of the susceptibility of some pet species to avian influenza viruses and documented transmission of avian influenza between or within domestic animal species. It has been suggested that exposure of people in the United States to H5N1 influenza is more likely to occur via contact with infected companion animals than wild birds or poultry.[54]

The risk may be greatest with cats because of their susceptibility to influenza viruses, their tendency to roam and encounter wild birds, and their close contact with humans. Natural infection of domestic, feral, and zoo cats with H5N1 has been widely reported, predominantly in Asia but also in Europe.[52,55-59] Mortality rates are high among affected animals, with rapid progression and neurological disease being common. In contrast, 20% seroprevalence was identified in stray cats near poultry markets in Java and Sumatra,[60] suggesting common mild, or at least survivable, disease in that population. The likelihood of exposure and infection of stray cats in areas with active H5N1 is still unclear, with studies of stray cats in areas of Europe failing to identify any seropositive animals.[53,61] Cats can be experimentally infected with H5N1 influenza virus and can subsequently transmit the virus to other cats with direct contact, raising concern about cats as a source of human infection.[62] Transmission of H5N1 from experimentally infected cats to dogs was not identified in another study.[63] Household pet cats are unlikely to be a major reservoir of H5N1; however, the virus could plausibly circulate in the feral cat population, with pet cats acting as a bridge to the human population.

Ferrets are highly susceptible to influenza A viruses and have been used as a model of avian influenza. Experimental coinfection of ferrets with H5N1 and human H3N2 resulted in production of reassortant viruses,[64] indicating that ferrets could be both a source of human infection and potentially serve as a "mixing vessel" for influenza.

Pet birds are an obvious concern with respect to avian influenza, but there have been few reports of avian influenza in pet bird species (both captive and in the wild). Natural infection was identified in a parrot from Suriname in a quarantine facility in the United Kingdom, although no clinical signs were present.[65] Severe disease can be induced experimentally in budgerigars.[66] Pet pot-bellied pigs are also of concern because of the high susceptibility of swine to influenza viruses of various origins, but H5N1 infections have not been reported.

Dogs appear to be relatively resistant to infection with avian influenza but infections with H5N1 and H3N2 avian influenza have been reported. Fatal H5N1 infection developed in a dog that ate a contaminated chicken carcass.[67] High seroprevalence was identified in dogs in a village in Thailand, but no information about clinical status is available. Experimental studies confirm some degree of susceptibility to H5N1 influenza. Mild disease was reproduced experimentally using H5N1, but disease was less severe than in cats inoculated with the same dose, indicating a decreased susceptibility.[63] While concern has been expressed regarding dogs as a source of human infection, a small study of experimentally infected dogs did not identify any transmission of H5N1 influenza to in-contact dogs and cats.[63] Another study only identified short-term virus shedding with low titers following experimental infection,[68] providing further support to thoughts that the risk of dogs as sources of infection is low. Outbreaks of severe respiratory disease in dogs caused by H3N2 influenza of avian origin are periodically reported.[69] Nasal H3N2 shedding has been identified, raising concern about the potential for dogs to transmit H3N2 to other dogs or humans, but this has not been demonstrated.

The route of infection of H5N1 in, and between, companion animal species has not been adequately investigated. Experimental studies have identified direct-contact transmission in cats and ferrets, although the types, duration, and intensity of contact required for transmission are not known. Close contact with an infected swan resulted in transmission of infection (but not disease) in a small percentage of exposed cats.[52] Oral exposure can also occur, as shown through natural infections of animals fed carcasses from poultry that had died of H5N1 influenza[55,56,67] and induction of infection in cats fed experimentally inoculated chicks.[70] The ability of cats to become infected from ingesting sick birds highlights the potential role of indoor–outdoor cats in bringing H5N1 influenza into the household, since cats can catch large numbers of birds and sick birds would be easier to catch. Infected cats can shed influenza virus through both the respiratory and gastrointestinal tracts.

Animals

Clinical presentation

The type of disease produced is highly dependent on the animal species. There are several main clinical syndromes that can be produced. In some species (e.g., birds of the Galliformes order), sudden death is the main sign. Cats and some bird species display primarily neurological abnormalities and a high mortality rate. More prolonged systemic disease often with multiorgan failure and death is more common in ferrets and with experimental infection of some other laboratory species. Others, including pigs, are highly resistant, displaying few to no signs of infection.[49] In dogs, conjunctivitis and fever have been reported following experimental infection.[63]

Diagnosis

The availability of specific tests for H5N1 is variable. PCR can be used to identify avian influenza viruses from oropharyngeal, nasal, or rectal swabs, but specific methods to differentiate different strains are required. Virus isolation can also be performed, but because of the human health implications and required high level of biosecurity (BSL-3), many veterinary diagnostic laboratories are unable to try to isolate avian influenza. Demonstration of seroconversion is diagnostic but retrospective, and requires the use of tests targeted against the specific strain. Immunohistochemical testing of tissues can also be performed.[56]

Management

Supportive care is the only treatment measure available at this time. The efficacy of antiviral agents in the treatment of natural avian influenza infection in companion animals is unclear. Empirical therapy with antiviral drugs such as oseltamivir has been discussed, but there are ethical concerns about the use of these drugs in animals because of the potential emergence of resistance and thus decreased effectiveness in humans.

Humans

Clinical presentation

The severity of clinical disease will vary greatly with the avian influenza strain that is involved. Most attention has been paid to H5N1 influenza because of its continued presence in some regions and severity of disease. The incubation period of H5N1 is usually 2–5 days, but can be 7 days or more.[51] Fever is the main initial sign and can be accompanied by cough, malaise, myalgia, headache, sore throat, conjunctivitis, abdominal pain, vomiting, and diarrhea.[51] The clinical course is usually rapid and severe, with progression of respiratory disease leading to shortness of breath, dyspnea, tachypnea, and chest pain.[45,46,51,71] Respiratory failure commonly develops, with acute respiratory distress syndrome developing in some patients. Secondary bacterial pneumonia may complicate disease and worsen the already poor prognosis. Potential extrapulmonary complications include heart failure, encephalitis, renal failure, and disseminated intravascular coagulation.[51]

Diagnosis

The gold standard is isolation and characterization of influenza virus from respiratory specimens.[43] Because of the time and specialized facilities required for culture, PCR for viral RNA in throat or nasal swabs is the main clinical diagnostic test.[51] Specific testing is required to differentiate avian influenza from other influenza A viruses, and protocols for detection of H5N1 are well established. Virus isolation is available through specialized laboratories. Isolation is important with early or atypical cases to permit characterization of the virus, and is less important in outbreak situations, when the presence of the strain in the population is known and where rapid diagnosis of disease in the individual patient is more important. Rapid diagnostic tests for influenza A are available but have been reported to have poor sensitivity and specificity for H5N1, and are not recommended.[72] Seroconversion is diagnostic but retrospective. Immunohistochemical staining can be performed on autopsy tissue specimens.

Management

Supportive care and antiviral therapy are the main components of treatment. Aggressive supportive measures may be required based on the severity of disease. Early treatment with oseltamivir or zanamivir is recommended.[73] Optimal dosing regimens are not known and resistance can emerge during treatment,[51] but preliminary data indicate that early treatment may reduce the incidence of severe disease and improve survival.[46,48,73,74]

The prognosis is guarded because of the severity of disease and rapidity of progression, with death in approximately 60% of infected individuals.[51] Very high mortality rates occur in patients with extrapulmonary manifestations.

Prevention

The likelihood of pets being an important source of avian influenza is low, but measures should be taken to reduce any risks that could be present due to the serious nature of infection. Consideration must be given to management of pets during times that avian influenza is endemic in a region. Measures to reduce the chance of exposure of pets, particularly pet birds, cats, and ferrets, to wild birds should be implemented. Of greatest importance is keeping pets inside, a simple act that would greatly reduce any risk of infection. Animals should never be fed raw poultry that may have been infected with avian influenza.

If a person in the household has (or is suspected or having) avian influenza, their pets should be observed closely for signs of infection. Contact between potentially infected people and their pets should be restricted. Pets should be kept inside and not allowed to have contact with other individuals.

Pets that are suspected of being infected should be strictly quarantined. Ideally, infected pets should be kept away from other household members, both human and animal, by restricting them to one room or area of the house. Physical contact with the pet should be minimized, and close contact with respiratory secretions or feces must be avoided. The potential for fecal shedding, at least in cats, should be emphasized because people may focus on avoiding respiratory tract exposure. The environment is likely a minimal source of exposure, but attention to hygiene when handling high-risk items like food bowls, water bowls, and litter boxes is required.

Precautions should be taken when handling avian influenza suspects in veterinary clinics. Companion animals that may be infected should be handled as little as possible, and in such a manner as to reduce the risk of close contact and aerosolization of respiratory secretions and feces. Chemical restraint should be considered in fractious or unpredictable animals or when close work around the mouth is required. Feces, saliva, and respiratory secretions should be considered high risk and unprotected contact with corresponding body sites or areas contaminated by those fluids must be avoided. Use of a face shield or mask and eye protection is indicated. Animals should be housed in isolation. Routine cleaning and disinfection practices should be adequate if performed properly.

Widespread culling is often used to address avian influenza in poultry. While the potential seriousness of avian influenza in humans needs to be considered, the short-term nature of influenza infection, the lack of a postinfection carrier state, the small number of people that most pets have contact with, emotional attachment to pets, and the relative ease of applying strict quarantine to a small number of pets in a household indicate that infection control practices should be considered instead of euthanasia.

The likelihood of pet birds introducing avian influenza into a region is miniscule but not zero. Legal or illegal importation of pet birds could plausibly result in transmission of avian influenza. Importation of birds should never be performed from areas where avian influenza is active.

Thorough diagnostic testing should be performed on any newly imported bird that becomes ill with signs consistent with influenza or that dies suddenly.

Influenza: pandemic H1N1 influenza

There is no specific type of pandemic influenza virus and the role of companion animals in previous human influenza pandemics is minimal to nonexistent. The 2009 novel H1N1 influenza pandemic involved a new influenza A H1N1 virus that possessed genes from humans, swine, and birds. Infections in a small number of pets were identified and caused significant concern among some individuals. Serious, including fatal, disease was identified in pet ferrets. Experimentally, pandemic H1N1 was more pathogenic than seasonal H1N1 in ferrets, and infected ferrets shed pandemic H1N1 more abundantly than seasonal H1N1.[75] Disease ranging from mild flu-like disease to fatal disease was also diagnosed in a small number of pet cats. However, there were few anecdotal reports and, at the time of writing, only one published report describing H1N1 influenza in a cat.[76] Furthermore, a study of 99 French cats with respiratory disease failed to identify H1N1 by real-time PCR.[77] There were also anecdotal reports of illness in dogs. Identification of disease in pets, particularly ferrets and cats, was not particularly surprising given the known susceptibility of ferrets to influenza viruses and reports of feline infections during H5N1 influenza outbreaks. Concerns were also expressed about pet birds and pot-bellied pigs because of the background of this virus and its ability to infect swine and poultry, but at the time of writing, infections of those species had not been identified.

The small number of diagnosed infections in some pets was not particularly surprising when one considered the scope of the problem in humans, with huge numbers of infected individuals and the fact that the majority of households in many affected countries have household pets. Accordingly, tens of thousands of pets, if not many more, potentially exposed to this virus yet only a small number developed illness. It is not known whether any of these infected animals were able to shed the virus, but the risk of pets as sources of influenza was probably limited as the most likely source of exposure of household pets would be infected humans. By the time a pet was exposed and infected, other household members would have likely already been exposed to the same source that infected the pet. It is currently impossible to state that there is no risk of pets as sources of infection, and concerns would be greatest among animals that are allowed to go outdoors and have opportunities to be exposed to other animals and humans.

The role of pets should be considered during influenza pandemics, and many of the measures taken to reduce the risk of transmission by humans in the household would also be reasonably applied to pets. People with influenza should avoid close contact with pets, just as they would for humans. Close and prolonged face-to-face contact should be prevented. Pets should not be allowed to sleep on beds. Hand hygiene should be emphasized. During an epidemic or pandemic where the role of pets has not been definitively established, pets from infected households should be prevented from having contact with other animals. Cats should be kept indoors, regardless of the status of the household, so that cats from infected households do not transmit the infection to other cats, and so cats from uninfected households do not acquire influenza and bring it back to a naive household. The risk of either of these events occurring is probably very low, but in the absence of objective evidence indicating no risk, these basic measures should be considered.

If influenza that could possibly infect pets is circulating, veterinarians should be aware of the potential but very low risk of infection of companion animals. Information about contact with people with influenza or unsupervised outdoor access should be queried for cases presenting with an acute onset of respiratory disease or flu-like illness and potentially infected animals should be handled with contact and respiratory precautions. Potentially infectious animals should be admitted directly to an examination room or isolation to prevent exposure of people or animals in the admitting area. Veterinary clinics should have a policy in place to discourage employees from coming to work if they have influenza-like illness, more for prevention of human–human transmission than transmission to animals.

Lymphocytic choriomeningitis virus (LCMV)

Introduction

LCMV is a rodent-associated virus that can cause disease ranging from mild flu-like illness to aseptic meningitis or severe meningoencephalitis. Transmission from pet rodents can occur, with most reported cases from hamsters. The consequences of infection of pregnant women can be severe, with a possibility of fetal death or developmental defects. Infections can also be severe in people with compromised immune systems.

Etiology/epidemiology

LCMV is an arenavirus, a single-stranded, enveloped RNA virus. It is likely distributed worldwide, although definitive evidence of human infection is only available for Europe and the Americas.[78] Like other arenaviruses, LCMV is a rodent-associated virus. Wild house mice are the primary reservoir and the source of most human infections.[79] Pet hamsters or guinea pigs are not considered natural reservoirs for LCMV but can be infected.[79] Hamsters account for the vast majority of pet-associated cases. Whether that is because of increased susceptibility to infection or higher viral shedding, or whether it is simply because hamsters are common pets and have closer contact with people has not been clarified. The potential risk associated with other pet rodents (i.e., mice, rats, chinchillas, gerbils) is unclear, but it is plausible that they could also be a source of infection.

Infected animals can shed LCMV in feces, urine, and saliva, and transmission can occur from direct contact or inhalation of virus from these sources.[80] Infected pet rodents can shed virus in urine for up to 8 months.[81] The mode of infection and specific risk factors have not been well investigated. It is believed that inhalation of infectious aerosols is the most common method of infection, followed by direct contact and bites;[78] however, it is unclear whether the relative importance of these different routes of infection are different for pet rodents compared with wild rodents. It is certainly possible that direct contact and bites are more important for pet-associated disease because close human–rodent contact is more common with pets that wild rodents.

Large outbreaks of LCMV have been identified associated with pet rodents from single distributors. In 1974, 181 human LCMV infections in 12 U.S. states were linked to a single distributor.[82] Other outbreaks have also been reported, typically linked to single hamster breeders or distributors.[83,84] Active LCMV infection was identified in 3.4% of hamsters from one U.S. distributor in yet another investigation.[79] Mixing of healthy and infected animals in the same cage or room, poor hand hygiene practices, placing new animals in cages that have not been cleaned and disinfected, and reusing items such as water bottles and food bowls without disinfecting can lead to transmission in animal distribution centers, pet stores, and other facilities.[79]

Infections have also been reported in pet store workers. Aseptic meningitis was diagnosed in a pet store employee who had handled various rodent species, and serological evidence of previous infection was identified in one other employee.[85] Thirteen percent of healthy employees of an Austrian zoological garden were seropositive,[86] suggesting that subclinical infection of individuals working with captive rodents may be relatively common.

Multiple instances of organ transplantation-associated infection, typically with fatal outcomes, have been reported.[87–89] Most cases were linked to pet hamsters.[88,89] Maternal–fetal transmission can also occur.[87]

Animals

Clinical presentation

Clinical signs are not typically present.

Diagnosis

Virus isolation or PCR are the main tests. Testing is rarely performed and almost always used in the context of investigation of human infections.

Management

There is no treatment to eradicate LCMV infection in rodents.

Humans

Clinical presentation

Asymptomatic infections or mild disease occur in approximately 30% of infected individuals.[90] However, given seroprevalence data from some rodent-contact groups, it is possible that asymptomatic or mild infections are much more common than is realized.

Most people with clinically apparent disease have aseptic meningitis or meningoencephalitis.[90] The incubation period is typically 6–13 days but may be as long as 3 weeks.[91] Biphasic disease is encountered, with an initial flu-like illness phase of fever, myalgia, malaise, headache, photophobia, nausea, vomiting, sore throat, and cough. This may progress to development of neurological disease with aseptic meningitis to severe encephalitis or meningoencephalitis.[91] Fever is not typically present by the time neurological disease develops.[90]

Infection during the first or second trimester of pregnancy can result in developmental defects including chorioretinitis, hydrocephalus, psychomotor retardation, and fetal death.[79,80,92] In transplant patients, fatal hemorrhagic fever-like disease has been reported.[87]

Diagnosis

Identification of rodent contact should be part of a standard history for people with central nervous system (CNS) disease.[93] Congenital infection should be considered in infants and children with unexplained hydrocephalus, micro- or macroencephalopathy, intracranial calcifications, chorioretinitis, and nonimmune hydrops.[90] Diagnosis of congenital LCMV infection is based on serological testing of the mother and infant using immunofluorescent antibody testing or ELISA.[80]

In patients with neurological disease, a mononuclear pleocytosis may be present in cerebrospinal fluid (CSF). Other laboratory findings are nonspecific. Virus can be isolated from blood, CSF, or urine. Isolation is usually more successful in blood early in disease and CSF later in disease.[78] Rarely, LCMV can be isolated from nasopharyngeal samples.[91] PCR can also be performed on CSF. Positive results for any of these tests are diagnostic. Demonstration of seroconversion through immunofluorescent testing or ELISA is also diagnostic but time-consuming. Detection of anti-LCMV IgM in serum or CSF is a faster method and is supplanting other tests.[78]

Management

Supportive, symptomatic therapy is the main component of management.

Overall, the case fatality rate is less than 1%; however, mortality is greater in certain groups, particularly people with transplant-associated infection. One person that survived transplant-associated LCMV infection was treated with ribavirin and reduction of immunosuppressive therapy;[87] however, it cannot be stated with confidence that the treatment was responsible for survival.

Prevention

Overall, the risk of exposure to LCMV from pet rodents is low. The greatest risk would be shortly after purchase[79] since infection is more likely to be acquired during distribution than in the household.

Wild mice are presumably the ultimate source of LCMV infection in pet rodents. Contact of pet and wild rodents could result in transmission of LCMV from wild rodents to pets, and should therefore be prevented in rodent-breeding facilities, distribution facilities, pet stores, and households. Good general wild rodent control practices are required. Pet rodents should not be allowed to roam freely in a house where wild rodents may be present.

Ideally, pet rodent distributors would periodically test for LCMV, but this is probably unlikely to occur. Serological testing of rodents is not reliable as some animals that are actively shedding LCMV can be seronegative.[79] Since routine testing is impractical, efforts should be directed toward reducing the risk of entry of LCMV into a pet rodent population.

Protocols for reducing the risk of LCMV exposure and transmission must be developed and followed in distribution centers and pet stores. This involves prevention of mixing of different groups of rodents and rodents from different sources,

good general hygiene practices, good management practices, and proper cleaning and disinfection of cages and other items. Depopulation has been used in response to identification of LCMV in pet rodent distribution centers and pet stores.[79,82,85]

Ideally, people should not purchase rodents that have come from large distributors. While this does not remove any risk, it probably decreases the likelihood of LCMV exposure.

While the role of bites in LCMV transmission is uncertain, measures to avoid bites should be undertaken. Bites from hamsters and other small rodents are not uncommon and are often the result of improper handling. All pet rodent owners should be competent in safe handling practices. Children should be taught how to safely handle pet rodents, and any interactions between young children and pet rodents should be supervised. Pet rodents should not be allowed to roam freely in bedrooms overnight or to sleep in beds with people.

Pregnant women should avoid all contact with rodents and areas potentially contaminated with feces, urine, or other secretions.[79,80,94] They should also avoid obtaining a new pet rodent during pregnancy. Immunocompromised individuals should take similar precautions.

Screening of pet rodents in households is not indicated because the likelihood of infection is low and because of the limitations with testing that are described above. Screening of rodents prior to purchase is similarly not recommended. If the concern about LCMV infection in a household member is so great that screening is considered, then rodents are likely inappropriate pets regardless of screening results.

Monkeypox virus

Introduction

Since the eradication of smallpox, monkeypox has been called the most important poxvirus infection of humans,[95] and it is a perfect example of the unpredictable nature of zoonotic diseases, as well as the risks posed by importation of exotic animal species and mixing of exotic and domestic animals. Monkeypox is a wildlife-associated zoonotic disease in Western and Central Africa, primarily in humid lowland evergreen tropical forest regions,[95] but emerged as a pet-associated zoonotic disease in the United States in 2003. While perhaps a remarkable event that is unlikely to recur in the pet population, awareness of monkeypox and broader issues of emerging diseases associated with animal transportation is important.

Etiology

Monkeypox virus is a double-stranded DNA virus from the Poxviridae family and *Orthopoxvirus* genus, along with cowpox and variola virus (smallpox). There are two main monkeypox virus clades: Western Africa and Central Africa, with the Central Africa clade being more virulent.[95] As with cowpox, its name is misleading. Despite being first isolated from a monkey, rodents (particularly squirrels) are believed to be the main natural reservoirs.

Geographic distribution/epidemiology

Monkeypox virus was first identified in 1957 in monkeys in a Copenhagen zoo and was later identified in outbreaks of disease in monkeys in zoos in Europe and the United States.[95] Human infections were not reported until the 1970s in Western and Central Africa,[96,97] during smallpox eradication campaigns with their intensive investigation of anyone with skin lesions.

There is much that is unknown about the ecology and epidemiology of monkeypox virus. The range of host species in not known. Transmission of monkeypox from animals to humans has been proven for orangutans, cynomolgus monkeys, rope squirrels, and prairie dogs, while monkeypox virus has been isolated from a wider range of rodents.[95] Transmission is predominantly from direct contact with an infected animal. Close contact through capturing, handling, and eating wild animals has been associated with infection in African outbreaks.[98,99] Bites and exposure to respiratory excretions, secretions, and droplets can also transmit monkeypox.[100] Human-to-human transmission can occur, although the secondary attack rate among humans is only 3%, much lower than with smallpox (80%).[95] The low secondary attack rate indicates that sustained spread will not occur in

susceptible human populations.[98] People are most infectious during the first week of the rash and are infectious until the last scab is shed. Duration of infectivity is not well known for other species but clinically infected animals presumably have a similar pattern. Long-term shedding by healthy individuals of some reservoir species has not been excluded.

Until 2003, monkeypox virus was only known to be present in humans in Central and Western Africa. In those regions, monkeypox occurs as sporadic infections with occasional outbreaks and is primarily associated with direct animal-to-human transmission. Concerns regarding pets and monkeypox arose in the United States in 2003 with a large outbreak of monkeypox in people that had not travelled nor had contact with monkeys. Ultimately, 72 cases were identified, with laboratory confirmation in 37.[101-103] Eighteen individuals were hospitalized but disease was only classified as severe in two children. One child developed encephalitis and the other severely painful cervical and tonsillar lymphadenopathy with extensive lesions in the oropharynx.[104] This outbreak was linked to importation of African rodents, transmission to prairie dogs in an animal distribution facility, and subsequent infection of humans through contact with infected prairie dogs. A Gambian giant pouched rat, three dormice, and two rope squirrels were identified as infected, but not all animals imported from Africa during that period were tested. This outbreak was remarkable for more than the fact that it was the first identification of monkeypox outside of its endemic area. It involved many people across the United States and transmission of monkeypox virus to humans from a species (prairie dogs) that was not previously known to be susceptible. Human infections were associated with contact with infected animals and no human-to-human transmission was noted. While the incidence of disease in people exposed to infected prairie dogs was reasonably high, close contact appeared to have been required for transmission. Daily exposure to a sick prairie dog, cleaning cages and bedding of a sick prairie dog, and touching a sick prairie dog were risk factors in one study.[100] In another investigation of 70 persons in veterinary facilities and a childcare center that had contact with two infected prairie dogs, 13% developed disease: 4/4 people with extensive direct contact, 5/26 (19%) with moderate contact, and 0/40 schoolchildren that had limited contact.[105] People with "complex" exposure (e.g., bite or scratch plus direct contact) were more likely to have more pronounced signs of systemic disease and require hospitalization than those with other types of contact.[106] Transmission from casual contact with animals was not identified in any study. Other species, including gerbils, hamsters, chinchillas, hedgehogs, opossums, and ground-hogs were also infected, although they were not identified as sources of human infection.

Occupational infection occurred in 12 veterinary personnel, pet store employees, and animal distributor employees.[107] Working directly with animals, caring for a prairie dog, caring for an animal within 6 ft. of a prairie dog, and feeding a sick prairie dog were associated with monkeypox virus infection, while having never handled a sick prairie dog was protective. Sporadic use of personal protective equipment was reported, which undoubtedly played a major role in occupational infection.

Animals

Clinical presentation

In monkeys, generalized skin eruptions are present, with papules mainly on the trunk, face, palms, and soles.[95] Papules progress through the vesicle stage, scab, then fall off approximately 10 days after the first signs of skin disease. The severity of disease varies between primate species.

In prairie dogs, severe disease, including extensive skin lesions, oral lesions, anorexia, wasting, coughing, swollen eyelids, ocular discharge, and respiratory distress, is common.[108,109] Mortality rates are high; 67% of naturally infected prairie dogs died in one report,[108] while all died in an experimental study following intraperitoneal challenge.[110]

Diagnosis

Monkeypox can be diagnosed by detection of the virus in skin lesions by PCR, virus isolation, immunological testing, or electron microscopy. Seroconversion is also diagnostic.

Management

There are no specific treatment measures. Supportive therapy may be required.

Humans

Clinical presentation

After an incubation period of approximately 12 days (range 7–17), a prodromal phase with headache, fever, sweating, malaise, back pain, and lymphadenopathy may develop.[104] Within a few days, a maculopapular rash develops, mainly on the trunk, with possible extension to the palms and soles of the feet (Figure 3.1). Oral, lingual, and genital lesions occur in a small percentage of cases. As with typical poxvirus diseases, the lesions progress through macular, papular, vesicular, and pustular stages before scabs form and desquamate over 14–21 days.[104]

Complications can develop but do so in a minority of cases. These include secondary skin or soft tissue infection (19% of cases), pneumonitis (12%), ocular lesions (4–5%), and encephalitis (<1%).[111] Disease is usually less severe in people that have previously been vaccinated against smallpox since cross-protection is typically present among different orthopoxviruses.[95]

Diagnosis

In the face of known exposure, clinical signs are highly suggestive. Definitive diagnosis requires

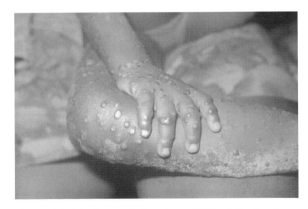

Figure 3.1 Monkeypox lesions in a child (public domain, Centers for Disease Control and Prevention).

laboratory confirmation, and despite the relative rarity of this illness in developed countries, efforts have been put into optimal diagnostic testing because of the potential use of this virus as a bioterrorism agent and because of the clinical similarity of smallpox, a bioterrorism agent of critical concern.

Identification of monkeypox virus in skin lesions by PCR or virus isolation can be used for diagnosis. Detection of seroconversion or the presence of IgM are also diagnostic provided assays are able to adequately discriminate monkeypox virus from other orthopoxviruses.[104] Immunological testing of tissues is suggestive but cross-reaction with other orthopoxviruses is a concern. Electron microscopy can be used to rule out parapoxviruses such as orf and vesicular stomatitis, because of the distinct differences in appearance.[104]

Management

Supportive therapy is the mainstay of treatment. Pre- and postexposure smallpox vaccination was used in the 2003 U.S. outbreak, and vaccination is recommended within 4 days of close contact with a confirmed monkeypox case.[112] Cidofovir has been suggested as a treatment option but the efficacy is unclear, and it should only be considered in severe infections because of the significant toxicity of the drug.[112] The potential effect of vaccinia immunoglobulin is not known, but it could be considered as a treatment or for prophylactic use in an exposed person with severe deficiency in T-cell function, in whom smallpox vaccination would be contraindicated.[104]

Fatality rates in African outbreaks tend to range from 4% to 33%,[95,98] with more deaths in children.[98] Disease in the American outbreak appeared to be milder than typically reported in endemic areas. There were no deaths, but two children required intensive care. Whether this reflects differences in viral strains or other factors such as the type of health care provided is unclear. Involvement of the less virulent Western Africa clade[113] in the American outbreak is probably the cause.

Prevention

Importation of rodents from Africa should be avoided because of the potential for subclinical monkeypox virus carriage. Regulations against importation of African rodents were implemented in some countries following the 2003 outbreak, which should substantially decrease the risk of further pet-associated disease. However, since the full host range of this virus is not known, it is possible that other host species could be legally imported. Further, there is a thriving international black market involving illegal importation of pets, and no country can be absolutely certain that African rodents are not being imported.

Transmission of monkeypox to veterinary personnel highlights the occupational risks that veterinary personnel are exposed to with emerging infectious diseases. Since monkeypox should now be rare to nonexistent in pets in most regions, infection control efforts should focus on general practices to reduce the risk of exposure to various pathogens, including rare, exotic, or emerging pathogens. It is likely that many of the veterinary personnel infections that occurred during the U.S. outbreak could have been prevented with good adherence to routine infection control practices such as the use of proper protective outerwear (barrier precautions, including gloves) and proper hand hygiene. Similar routine practices, particularly hand hygiene, should also be used by others in animal contact environments such as animal distribution centers and pet stores.

Smallpox vaccination is an effective preventive measure and the CDC recommends preexposure vaccination of people who investigate human or animal monkeypox cases, as well as laboratory workers who may be exposed.[112] Vaccination of people in contact with companion animals should not be necessary if proper importation restrictions and quarantine are in place.

Nipah virus

Nipah virus is a paramyxovirus that was first identified in Malaysia in 1998 in a large outbreak of febrile encephalitis in humans with a high (32%) mortality rate.[114,115] It has also been identified in Singapore, Bangladesh, and India.[116] Fruit bats are the reservoir;[117] however, human infection is from contact with other infected animal species. In initial outbreaks, most infected individuals had contact with pigs within 2 weeks of the onset of disease and pigs have been identified as the main source of human infection.[115] Other species can also be infected, and natural infection of cats and dogs has been identified.[117] Experimentally infected cats can shed Nipah virus via the nasopharynx and urine, suggesting the potential for transmission.[118] Additionally, one study reported an association between contact with sick or dying dogs and Nipah virus infection in humans.[119] This could represent a risk to humans from dogs infected with Nipah virus, but could also indicate common-source exposure. Serological study of dogs in endemic regions indicated that dog-to-dog transmission was unlikely and that dogs are not an amplifying reservoir for Nipah virus.[120] No seropositive animals were identified in a study of feral cats in Malaysia, leading the authors to conclude that the risk posed by feral cats is low.[121] Concern still exists about the potential for dogs and cats to transmit Nipah virus in endemic areas, but this mainly involves contact with sick animals, particularly dogs, that have been infected from contact with infected pigs. Dogs are not believed to be able to sustain Nipah virus in the absence of infected pigs[120] and, at best, play a peripheral role in transmission.

In areas where Nipah virus is present, contact of dogs and cats with pigs should be prevented. Pets should also not be fed raw pork or bones from pigs that may have been infected.[120] Culling of pigs is one method used to control outbreaks, but there is no indication to cull other species such as dogs or cats.

Rabies

Introduction

Rabies is often at the forefront when people consider zoonotic diseases. This viral disease can infect all mammals and is endemic throughout much of the world. Human rabies is largely a preventable disease through vaccination and proper postexposure treatment; however, access to treatment is variable and rabies still kills tens of thousands of people, mostly in developing countries. Even in regions with a low incidence of human infection, rabies can also have significant social and economic impacts.

Etiology

Rabies virus is an enveloped RNA virus in the Rhabdoviridae family and *Lyssavirus* genus. Rabies virus can be divided into different genotypes, which are subsequently divided into variants that correspond to specific regions or animal hosts.

Geographic distribution/epidemiology

Rabies is present throughout much of the world. In any given region, there is typically a predominant rabies virus variant that is adapted to a specific host reservoir. In North America, rabies is predominantly maintained in foxes, coyotes, raccoons, skunks, or bats, with different variants in different regions. In Europe, bat and fox rabies are most common, except in Turkey where canine rabies predominates.[122] Canine rabies variant predominates in areas of South America, Africa, and Asia.

Rabies-free areas are defined by the World Health Organization (WHO) as regions with no cases of indigenously acquired infection by a lyssavirus in humans or animals (including bats) in the previous 2 years and the presence of an adequate surveillance system to detect cases.[123] Some areas consider themselves rabies free more specifically through the absence of infections caused by rabies virus despite the presence of EBLV.

All mammals are susceptible to infection; however, there is some degree of species specificity with some species more prone to infection than others with certain variants. For example, cats are more resistant to infection with canine rabies virus than dogs, but they are more prone to infection with some strains from wildlife.[122]

Pathophysiology

Rabies virus infection occurs when the virus is inoculated into wounds or onto mucosal surfaces. Transmission cannot occur through intact skin. After gaining entry into the body, rabies virus replicates in muscle cells, infecting the muscle spindle. It then infects the nerve innervating the spindle and subsequently spreads centripetally to the CNS. After CNS infection, the virus spreads to the rest of the body by peripheral nerves. Highest viral concentrations are in the saliva, from shedding from sensory nerve endings in the oral mucosa and replication of rabies virus in the salivary glands.

The incubation period can be prolonged. The site of inoculation and amount of inoculated virus are presumably key determinants of incubation period. Clinical signs typically develop 2–3 months after exposure, but the range in humans may be from 2 weeks to 6 years.[123]

Transmission

Bites from rabid animals are the main source of infection (Table 3.1), accounting for the vast majority of human and animal rabies cases. High levels of rabies virus are shed in the saliva of infected individuals, which leads to a high risk of exposure from bites. Several factors may affect the likelihood of infection, with the main determining factor being the amount of saliva inoculated into the body. Multiple bites are probably higher risk than single bites. Bites through heavy clothing may be lower risk than bites directly through unprotected skin as clothing could remove some of the saliva from the teeth.[124] Bites around the face are more likely to cause disease and to have a shorter incubation period than bites of more peripheral areas.

Nonbite exposure is possible but is very rare. Exposure is possible, although unlikely, from contamination of open wounds or mucous membranes with saliva or infected neural tissue.[125] Scratches that penetrate the skin can be a source of exposure. Rabies virus is not shed through the claws; however, scratches create the opportunity for inadvertent or undetected inoculation of saliva into the body. Other routes of transmission not relevant to companion animals include transplantation of cornea, solid organs, and vascularized tissues from infected donors,[126–128] and inhalation of large amounts of aerosolized virus in laboratories. The environment is not considered a source of exposure, as rabies virus is quite labile. Transplacental infection has been reported in skunks, a human, and a cow,[129–131] and it is reasonable to assume that it could occur in any mammalian species.

Internationally, dogs are the main source of human rabies, accounting for over 99% of cases.[123] In developed countries, human exposure to rabies virus is most commonly from wildlife,[132] but pets are still a concern. Pets belonging to the exposed individual and pets owned by other individuals can be involved, as well as stray animals. The relative risk of these groups is probably dictated largely by the availability and use of routine rabies vaccination in pets. A Chinese study of human rabies associated with postexposure prophylaxis (PEP)

Table 3.1　World Health Organization guidelines for type of contact, exposure, and recommended postexposure prophylaxis.[123]

Category	Type of contact with confirmed rabid animal or animal unavailable for testing	Type of exposure	Recommended postexposure prophylaxis
I	Touching, feeding of animal Licking intact skin	None	None, if history is reliable
II	Nibbling uncovered skin Minor scratches or abrasions without bleeding	Minor	Administer vaccine immediately: if exposure was from an apparently healthy pet or in low-risk area, observation and delaying treatment may be warranted
III	Transdermal bites, scratches, licks on broken skin Contamination of mucous membrane with saliva (i.e., licks) Exposure to bats	Severe	Administered RIG and vaccine immediately Stop treatment if animal remains healthy through a 10-day observation period or if rabies test from a reliable lab using appropriate techniques is negative

failure reported that 48% of people were infected by their dogs and 18% were infected by other individuals' dogs, while only 18% were infected by stray dogs and 15% were infected by other species.[133]

Rabies in pets

Rabies is extremely rare in household pets in many regions, presumably due to a combination of widespread and efficacious vaccination and limited contact with wildlife reservoirs. Not surprisingly, most rabies cases in pets occur in areas where rabies is endemic in wildlife and are associated with the region's dominant wildlife variant. Risk factors for rabies in pets have not been clearly investigated, but presumably, factors associated with contact with wildlife such as being allowed to roam freely or living in an area that is hospitable to wildlife are important.

In areas that do not have canine rabies virus variant, cats tend to be more commonly affected; there were 294 reported feline cases compared with 75 canine cases in the United States in 2008.[134] This probably relates to increased roaming behavior by cats and lower vaccination rates compared with dogs, since rabies vaccination is required for licensing of dogs, but not cats, in most regions.

Importation of pets from endemic areas can result in importation of rabies if adequate protocols are not in place. An example of this was diagnosis of rabies in a dog imported from Iraq as part of a program reuniting U.S. military personnel with dogs they had "adopted."[135]

Rabies is extremely rare in other household pet species but can occur. Often, people dismiss concerns about rabies in small mammals like rabbits, rats, hamsters, and guinea pigs because of the impression that exposure to a rabid animal would result in death of these small mammals. However, rabies infection has been identified in various small pet mammals, including rabbits, hamsters, rats, and guinea pigs,[133,136,137] resulting in human exposure.

Rabies in humans

The number of human cases is staggering for a disease that can be controlled with proper vaccina-

tion and PEP. Rabies deaths in Africa and Asia have been estimated at 55,000 per year, with most deaths occurring in rural regions.[123] Beyond the obvious impact of mortality, rabies can have a significant burden from side effects of PEP, costs of medical care, time required to access medical care in some regions, and psychological impacts.[123] Overall, rabies is estimated to cost in excess of US$500 million in Africa and Asia.[123]

In contrast, human rabies rates are extremely low in most other regions and human infections are rarely associated with companion animals. Only three human cases were reported in the United States in 2002 and two in 2008, all associated with bat variants.[138,139] Despite the low incidence of human infection, economic impacts remain high with an estimated US$300 million cost of rabies prevention annually in the United States and US$261 million in Europe.[123]

Young individuals are at highest risk of exposure. People under 20 years of age were reported as being overrepresented among rabies infections in China,[133] and the WHO reports that children under 15 years of age account for approximately 50% of exposures in canine rabies endemic areas.[123]

Animals

Clinical presentation

Rabies is typically divided into two types: furious and paralytic. These are reasonable generalizations; however, it is important to remember that rabies can cause a wide range of clinical signs and that rabies must be considered in any animal with an acute onset of behavioral changes or lower motor neuron paralysis.

Often, there is a prodromal phase that lasts 2–3 days. Nervousness, anxiety, and fever may be noted during this time, as well as early behavioral changes.[122] It has been reported that most animals will lick the site of inoculation,[122] likely because of some degree of neuralgia. Pupillary dilation may be evident. In the classical situation, there is then progression to the furious phase, with 1–7 days of markedly abnormal behavior. Varying degrees of restlessness, aggression, excitability, photophobia, hyperesthesia, and psychotic behavior are displayed. In contrast, some may prefer to hide in a dark or quiet location. During this stage, animals may become very unpredictable and aggressive, particularly when disturbed in a cage or hiding place. As this phase progresses, incoordination, disorientation, and seizures develop. Death may occur before the paralytic stage, which is typically short. It is characterized by progressive lower motor neuron paralysis with ultimate involvement of the entire CNS. With brainstem involvement, an inability to swallow produces salivation, a classical sign of rabies that is most common in dogs. Unfortunately, if salivation is the first observed sign, owners or veterinarians may place their hands in the mouth looking for an obstruction, foreign body, or other lesion, thereby exposing themselves to rabies. Coma and respiratory paralysis soon follow, resulting in death.

Diagnosis

Definitive antemortem diagnosis is currently impossible. Clinical signs can be suggestive although other neurological diseases can produce similar signs. A history of exposure, identification of a bite wound, or lack of rabies vaccination provide an increased index of suspicion. Examination of the pet for a bite wound is useful; however, given the potential time frame between exposure and disease and the potential for exposure from very minor bites (especially from bats), failure to identify a wound by no means excludes the possibility of rabies. Rapid *in vivo* testing of the live animal would be preferred because of the invariably fatal nature of rabies in animals and the desire to obtain a definitive diagnosis to guide decisions about euthanasia, but until that is available, the clinician's index of suspicion along with other factors, such as owner wishes and human exposure, must guide decisions. Once a high index of suspicion of rabies is present, euthanasia is warranted. This is particularly true when there has been human exposure, and diagnosis will determine the need for PEP.

Fluorescent antibody testing of brain tissue is the gold standard for diagnosis;[123] however, it is not infallible and the accuracy is dependent on the expertise of the person performing the test, the quality of antirabies conjugate, the quality of the sample, and available equipment.[123] Testing of the brain stem, thalamus, cerebellum, and the hippocampus should be performed for optimal sensitivity.[123] Virus isolation can be used as a confirmatory test and to characterize the virus, but is not a useful tool clinically because of the time required. Molecular techniques such as PCR are becoming increasingly popular for rapid diagnosis of infectious diseases; however, PCR for diagnosis of rabies is not currently recommended.[123]

Management

Rabies in animals is not treatable. The use of aggressive protocols such as the "Wisconsin protocol" that has been used in humans is not indicated because of the extremely low likelihood of success, long-term nature of treatment and rehabilitation, and the ongoing risk of exposure of caretakers. Once rabies is strongly suspected, euthanasia is warranted. Definitive diagnosis should always be sought after euthanasia through submission of the brain for rabies testing.

Humans

Clinical presentation

Initial signs of rabies are vague and include fever, headache, and malaise.[124] Abnormal sensation at the site of infection may be noted.[140] A wide range of neurological abnormalities then develop. These can include behavioral changes, personality changes, blurred or double vision, and fatigue. Myoedema, temporary mounding of muscle struck with a reflex hammer, is common.[141] Rabies is often not considered in individuals at this stage of disease unless a history of exposure was reported. This prodromal stage tends to last 4–10 days and is followed by more specific and severe signs. It is at this point that rabies is classically divided into furious and paralytic ("dumb") forms. The furious form is characterized by agitation, severe behavioral abnormalities, delirium, and hydrophobia.[124] Hydrophobia does not truly represent a fear of water. Rather, it is severe laryngospasm triggered by stimuli such as trying to drink water or swallow saliva. Seizures, periodic hyperactivity, ataxia, pupillary dilation, hypersalivation, hyperhidrosis, cardiac arrhythmias, and other signs may also be observed.[124] Coma and respiratory failure eventually develop.

The paralytic form may develop subsequent to the furious form or be the first sign of rabies. The paralytic form resembles ascending paralysis or symmetric quadriparesis.[124] Patients do not have hydrophobia, hyperactivity, or seizures. Headache and neck stiffness may be present with normal sensorium. As this form progresses, confusion develops, and there is rapid progression to coma.

Diagnosis

Clinical signs are not adequate for a diagnosis of rabies, even with a history of an animal bite or other exposure. The "classical" presentation of a patient with hydrophobia and associated signs following a bite from a known rabid animal is rare, and the history of exposure is not often present at the time of initial presentation. Early clinical signs are vague, and as the disease progresses, differentiation from other causes of encephalitis is not necessarily easy. Hematology is typically unremarkable. Cerebrospinal fluid findings are nonspecific, with a mild lymphocytic pleocytosis and modest hyperproteinemia sometimes identified.[124] CT is usually normal, particularly early in disease.[123] MRI can be used to rule out various other potential causes. Additionally, in the presence of typical clinical signs, ill-defined, mild hypersignal T2 images involving the brain stem, hippocampus, hypothalamus, deep and subcortical white matter, and deep and cortical gray matter are strongly supportive of rabies.[123] Definitive diagnosis requires specific laboratory testing.

Fluorescent antibody testing is the gold standard[123] and is the preferred test for both biopsy and autopsy specimens. Samples are usually taken from the nuchal area of the neck and should include hair follicles.[123] Multiple (at least 20) sections must be examined.

PCR-based testing has been used to detect rabies virus in saliva, CSF, and urine, with positive results most common in the saliva.[142] Testing of brain biopsies is possible, but brain biopsy taken solely for rabies testing is not recommended.[142] PCR testing of hair samples from excised skin with hair follicles from the nape of the neck has also yielded positive results.[142] An added advantage of PCR is the ability to determine the rabies virus variant.[143] Positive results of PCR testing can be useful as long

as there is adequate quality control; however, the implications of a positive result, potentially including withdrawal of aggressive care, indicate that such testing must have an extremely high positive predictive value. PCR should never be used as the sole diagnostic test and results should be considered in the context of clinical signs and other diagnostic testing results.[123] Negative results of PCR testing do not rule out rabies.[142]

Detection of serum antibodies in nonvaccinated patients can provide a strong suspicion of rabies; however, antibodies do not appear until an average of 8 days after the onset of clinical signs,[123] which limits the clinical value of this type of test. Detection of any antibody level in CSF is highly suggestive of rabies.

Virus isolation can be attempted from saliva, CSF, or tears, with variable results. Positive results are diagnostic, but negative results do not exclude the possibility of rabies.

Management

Rabies has the highest case-fatality rate of any recognized infectious disease[123] and was previously considered "invariably fatal." Now, it is considered "almost invariably fatal" following survival of a small number of individuals. At least five patients who received preexposure prophylaxis or PEP and subsequently developed clinical signs of rabies have survived, though most had neurological sequelae.[123,140] A teenager from Wisconsin who did not receive any treatment prior to the onset of clinical signs survived following treatment with drug-induced coma, ventilator support, and intravenous ribavirin.[140] This "Wisconsin protocol" has been subsequently used on other affected individuals, with the only successful report being in a teenager who received four doses of vaccine before the onset of clinical signs. Successful treatment of people who did not receive any PEP prior to the onset of disease has not yet been reproduced.

With both furious and paralytic rabies, the course of disease from initial signs to coma is usually 2–14 days, with death typically occurring approximately 18 days after the onset of disease.[124] Intensive supportive care can prolong survival but the prognosis is grave, particularly in individuals who received no PEP.

Prevention

Determination of exposure

Any bite from a mammal that penetrates the skin should be considered a possible exposure and should be investigated further. Identification of the animal is critical because in the absence of evidence that the animal does not have rabies, it must be assumed that the person was exposed.

Nonbite exposure rarely causes rabies, but occasional reports of infection indicate that PEP should be considered in certain situations.[125] The most relevant nonbite exposures with pets are contamination of open wounds or mucous membranes with saliva. There is conflicting information regarding the approach to scratches. Scratches that may have inoculated saliva into the wound are clearly an exposure. WHO guidelines[123] are more aggressive in the treatment of scratches than the U.S. Advisory Committee on Immunization Practices, which states that PEP is not indicated following a scratch unless it met the definition of saliva or other potentially infectious materials being introduced into fresh open cuts on skin or mucous membranes.[125] This is a rather subjective statement and what constitutes an indication that saliva or potentially infectious material has been inoculated is not clearly explained.

Medical care should be sought for any potential exposure to determine if PEP is required. Determination of the need for PEP can be difficult in some situations. Factors that must be considered include the nature of exposure, the likelihood of rabies in the animal (e.g., prevalence in the animal species in the area, animal behavior, or other clinical signs), availability of the animal for observation or testing, and the vaccination history of the animal. In situations where rabies is considered unlikely and where the animal is available for observation or testing, waiting until the end of the quarantine period or for test results is reasonable. Situations that would lead to more prompt initiation of PEP would include a high index of suspicion of rabies, unavailability of the animal for observation or testing, high likelihood of exposure (e.g., significant bite), and bites to the head or neck. There are no objective guidelines, and considering the severity of disease and relative safety of PEP, prudence dictates that one should err on the side of caution and begin PEP promptly if there is any doubt. A history of rabies vaccination of an animal does not guarantee that the animal is not rabid, and vaccination history, while important to consider, should never be used to indicate no risk of exposure. The behavior of the animal should also be considered but not relied on as a sole determinant of risk because of the highly variable nature of rabies.

Quarantine and observation of a pet that has bitten a person

Rabies virus is present in high levels in the saliva of infected animals. While rabies may have a long incubation period, rabies virus only begins to be secreted in the saliva a few days prior to the onset of illness. Any dog, cat, or ferret that has bitten someone should be kept under observation for 10 days. The reason for this is that an animal that is shedding rabies virus in the saliva will invariably develop clinical signs of rabies within 10 days. Any animal that is still alive and clinically normal 10 days after biting someone was therefore not infectious at the time of the bite. The methods used for observation, ranging from formal quarantine to observation by owners in the household, vary between jurisdictions. Preferably, animals are kept under the care of a veterinarian so that they can be closely observed and to reduce the risk of the animal disappearing. If an animal that is being observed cannot be accounted for after 10 days, then it must be assumed to have had rabies. Care must be taken when allowing owners to observe animals in the household, because the implications of the animal running away can be major. If the animal dies or must be euthanized during the 10-day period, rabies testing of brain tissue must be performed, regardless of the reason for death or euthanasia.

While there is confidence in the 10-day observation period in dogs, cats, and ferrets, the natural progression of rabies is not adequately understood for other pet mammals. It cannot be stated with confidence that all individuals of those species will develop signs of disease or die within the 10-day period.[123] This complicates measures as there are no clear recommendations for species other than cats, dogs, and ferrets. WHO guidelines state that people exposed to mammals other than dogs and cats should receive PEP unless the animal is eutha-nized and tested.[123] However, that can be seen as an extreme measure in household pet species, par-ticularly in situations where the index of suspicion is low. Prompt euthanasia and testing is reasonable if the animal is displaying signs of disease poten-tially attributable to rabies. In other situations, observation of the animal is a reasonable measure, as long as all parties are aware that objective data are not available and that there would be some degree of risk involved. Despite the lack of infor-mation, it is quite likely that most or all pet mammals that were infectious at the time of a bite would develop clinical signs of rabies and/or die during a 10-day quarantine.

Management of bites

Treatment should begin as soon as possible after exposure.[123] Bite wounds should be cleaned thor-oughly with water, soap, and a virucidal antiseptic such as povidone iodine or ethanol.[123] This should be done as soon as possible after exposure and for at least 15 minutes.

Postexposure prophylaxis (PEP)

Prompt and proper treatment of exposed individu-als is highly effective at preventing rabies. Strict adherence to WHO guidelines is believed to virtu-ally guarantee protection from disease,[123] a level of confidence rarely expressed for prophylaxis for any disease, let alone a highly fatal disease such as rabies.

Once it is determined that PEP is indicated, treat-ment should be initiated as soon as possible after exposure because of the potential for a short incu-bation period. However, PEP administration is considered a medical urgency, not emergency,[125] and time should be taken to properly assess the situation and the need for PEP. If PEP is started before rabies testing results are available, and results are negative, PEP can be discontinued. While prompt treatment is recommended, PEP should not be denied to anyone who presents even months after a potential exposure because of the potential for a very long incubation time.[123] Pregnancy, infancy, old age, and concurrent disease are not contraindications to PEP.[123]

PEP involves intramuscular administration of a single dose of rabies immunoglobulin (RIG) and rabies vaccination on days 0, 3, 7, 14, and 28. Recently, the U.S. Advisory Committee on Immunization Practices recommended that four doses of vaccine be given instead of five, on days 0, 3, 7, and 14.[144] Cell culture or purified embryo-nated egg vaccines should be used instead of nerve-tissue vaccines, for reasons discussed below under Rabies Vaccination.

While RIG is usually given on day 0, if that is not possible, it can be administered up to day 7 of PEP.[125] After that point, it is not indicated because an antibody response to vaccination is assumed to have occurred. Guidelines are different for indi-viduals that have been previously vaccinated against rabies. Those individuals do not receive RIG and are revaccinated on days 0 and 3.[125]

Failure to access PEP is a pressing concern. In a study of rabies cases in China, 67% of patients did not seek any form of treatment after being bitten while a further 20% treated the wound them-selves.[133] Almost 50% of people that sought medical care did not receive RIG and rabies vaccine. Five cases of rabies in individuals that received proper PEP within 24 hours of exposure were identified. The cause of PEP failure was not determined though improper vaccine storage by patients was suspected.[133] Similarly, a study of rabies deaths in Pakistan reported that all people failing PEP did not receive RIG.[145] Any failure of PEP should be promptly and thoroughly investigated to identify the potential cause(s), which could include inap-propriate administration, incomplete treatment, immunodeficiency, low vaccine potency, or poten-tial emergence of a new rabies virus variant.[123]

There are numerous possible barriers to PEP. One is a lack of reporting of bites, especially minor bites, and identification of need. Serious bites that require medical care are not required for rabies transmission. Rabies virus can be transmitted by seemingly minor bites, and in such cases, people who do not understand concerns about rabies may simply not seek medical care and be offered treat-ment. In some regions, access to PEP is sporadic because of vaccine or RIG shortages or unavail-ability, or lack of understanding of the issues by frontline healthcare workers. Cost of PEP is also a significant concern and is a potential barrier to treatment. This is of particular concern in developing countries, as there may be a high economic burden in a country with endemic rabies. Economic concerns also exist in developed countries, particularly when individuals are required to pay the high costs of PEP. The approach to funding PEP likely has an impact on compliance.

The type of PEP that is available also varies among countries, and the relative risks of adverse effects may affect both compliance and the overall economic impact of rabies exposure. Nerve-tissue vaccines are still in widespread use in some countries because of the low production cost, but they can be associated with severe and long-term adverse effects at a much higher incidence than other vaccine types.[123]

Human vaccination (preexposure prophylaxis)

Rabies vaccination of humans is recommended for people at frequent or high risk of exposure. Typically, vaccination is recommended for veterinary personnel, wildlife control personnel, humane society personnel, animal rehabilitators, and people working in research or diagnostic labs that handle tissues from rabies suspects or rabies virus.[123,125] Vaccination may also be warranted for people travelling to areas with high rabies rates, especially if they may have contact with feral animals or wildlife. In veterinary clinics, all personnel that might have contact with rabies suspects should be vaccinated. If lay staff such as receptionists may occasionally have contact with animals, such as assisting carrying sick animals into the clinic or restraining animals, they should be vaccinated. Problems may arise with short-term staff such as co-op students, volunteers, or similar and often transient personnel. The approach to these individuals is difficult. Ideally, they would all be vaccinated; however, that is probably unlikely based on cost and aversion to vaccines for short-term placements in veterinary clinics. If unvaccinated persons are permitted to work in a clinic, clear guidelines must be in place to prevent any contact with potential rabies suspects. A difficulty with this is the highly variable presentation of rabies and the potential for exposure before rabies is considered a possibility. As exposure can never be completely prevented, these personnel (and their parents, in the case of minors) must be adequately informed of the risk of rabies exposure.

A variety of vaccines are available, and the quality and safety of rabies vaccines have greatly improved but this is still variable, and vaccines of questionable safety and efficacy are still used in some regions. A relatively easy and cost-effective approach to rabies vaccine production has involved production of vaccine in nervous tissues. Vaccines produced using this approach have high rates of adverse effects and variable immunogenicity, and the WHO Expert Consultation Group has strongly recommended that the use of nerve-tissue vaccines be discontinued.[123] They are still used in some developing countries, although many such countries have discontinued the production of these vaccines and import cell culture or purified embryonated egg vaccines.

Vaccine is administered on days 0, 7, and either 21 or 28 in the deltoid region (or anterolateral thigh in young children).[123] Intramuscular vaccination is considered the gold standard, but intradermal vaccination is an appealing option because of the low volume of vaccine that is used. This decreases the cost of vaccination and allows for more efficient use of available vaccine when there are vaccine shortages. A study of intramuscular versus intradermal vaccination reported lower antibody levels in individuals vaccinated by the intradermal route, but the authors felt that this did not affect the level of protection.[146] Duration of immunity is a potential concern. In one study, 79% of people vaccinated intramuscularly had protective immunity 2–2.5 years after vaccination versus 51% of intradermally vaccinated individuals.[147] Another study reported protective antibody titers in 93–98% of intramuscularly vaccinated individuals versus 83–95% of people vaccinated intradermally.[148] Proper training of personnel administering intradermal vaccination is critical. Not all products that are used intramuscularly are considered safe and efficacious when used intradermally.[123] Intradermal vaccination should not be used in individuals receiving malaria prophylaxis.[123] The use of chloroquine should also be delayed for at least 1 month after intradermal vaccination.[149] Immunocompromised individuals and people taking corticosteroids may also have an unpredictable response to intradermal vaccination and should be vaccinated intramuscularly. Pregnancy is not a contra-indication to vaccination.[125]

Testing of rabies titers

All individuals that are at increased risk of rabies exposure, as discussed above, should have the rabies antibody titers checked periodically. Standard recommendations are to check titers in vaccinated individuals that are at frequent risk of exposure every 2 years.[125] That includes veterinary personnel working in regions where rabies is endemic. People at continuous risk of exposure, such as people working in laboratories handling large quantities of virus, should have titers checked every 6 months.[123] Testing of titers of vaccinated individuals such as veterinarians in low endemic areas is not required.[125] A single booster should be administered to anyone whose rabies titer drops below 0.5 IU/mL.[123]

There is no indication for titer testing of vaccinated individuals that have been exposed, since the same two-dose PEP regimen would be prescribed regardless of the titer. Titers should be tested following preexposure prophylaxis of immunocompromised individuals to determine if they adequately responded to vaccination.[125] Routine testing of other vaccinated individuals is not indicated.

Reducing rabies exposure

A common misconception is that "indoor pets" are not at risk of rabies exposure, sometimes leading to reluctance to vaccinate. This is incorrect, and rabies exposure or infection of indoor pets certainly can (and does) occur. Indoor pets can escape and become exposed. Wildlife can also enter houses, something that is of particular concern with bats. Even small rodents in cages have acquired rabies, and no mammal in an area where rabies is endemic can be assumed to be at no risk of exposure.

Efforts to reduce rabies in wildlife, such as the use of aerial rabies vaccine baits, can have a major impact on wildlife rabies[150] and, correspondingly, the risk of human and pet exposure. Other measures to reduce contact with wildlife are also important. Outdoor yard environments should not

be hospitable to wildlife and feeding wildlife, either purposefully or indirectly through leaving pet food outside, should be avoided. Ideally, pets should not be left unsupervised outdoors and should not be housed outdoors overnight. Pets that are housed outdoors in rabies endemic areas should be in an environment that is inaccessible to wildlife or, at a minimum, an environment that deters wildlife. Rabbits housed outdoors should be double caged whenever possible.[136]

Control of feral animals, particularly dogs, is critical. This is of particular importance in countries with hyperendemic rabies mainly associated with feral dogs, but is also useful in any region where rabies may be present. Feral animals represent an important reservoir and a source of human and pet exposure. Measures such as vaccination of feral animals have been used. Public education to decrease feeding of feral animals may help control the population and reduce contact between animals and humans.

Vaccination of pets

Because rabies exposure is a low but ever-present risk in areas where the virus is present in wildlife, vaccination is a critical component of both pet and human rabies control. Vaccination is highly effective but not infallible. Rabies has been diagnosed in properly vaccinated dogs and cats,[151] although this is very rare. All dogs, cats, and ferrets should be vaccinated against rabies.[125,152] Vaccination of other mammalian pets would be desirable but is complicated by a lack of licensed vaccines and clear guidelines.

Parenteral modified live vaccines were used in dogs and cats originally, but were sometimes associated with development of rabies, especially in cats. While later versions of these vaccines were more effective with fewer side effects and a very low likelihood of vaccine-induced disease, they have largely been replaced by other vaccine types and modified live vaccines are no longer available in most regions. Parenteral killed vaccines are able to produce an effective immune response through the use of adjuvants and high viral content. An injectable canarypox virus-vector rabies vaccine is available for cats in some countries and is preferred because of concerns regarding adverse reactions to killed vaccines.

Because of the potential for interference by maternal antibodies, animals must be at least 3 months of age prior to vaccination. Two months has been suggested as the minimum age for cats vaccinated with recombinant vaccine.[123] A booster is then administered 1 year later. The timing of subsequent vaccine boosters has been a controversial area in veterinary medicine. Traditionally, annual revaccination of dogs and cats has been recommended; however, concerns about vaccine-associated sarcomas in cats, other vaccine reactions, anecdotal fears of various immune-mediated diseases, and cost led to reassessment of vaccine recommendations. After the initial series of two vaccines (initial plus booster 1 year later), revaccination should be performed every 1–3 years. Every 3-year vaccination is considered acceptable and is recommended unless local regulations mandate yearly vaccination. A rabies vaccine with a 3-year label claim must be used. Animals are considered protected by 28 days after vaccination.[152] Accordingly, animals exposed to rabies within the first 28 days of initial vaccination should be considered unvaccinated. Animals are considered protected immediately after booster vaccination, even animals that are overdue for vaccination.[152]

Delivery of rabies vaccination in developed countries is somewhat controversial. Some areas have used low-cost or free rabies clinics to attempt to maximize vaccine coverage among pets, particularly pets that do not receive routine veterinary care. The potential benefit of these programs in terms of increasing rabies vaccination coverage in the pet population is sometimes countered with concerns about the lack of proper examination or preventive medicine associated with vaccine clinics and the potential associated impacts on animal health. There is no consensus regarding these programs. From the rabies standpoint, these programs certainly have a positive impact on vaccination rates and that must be considered carefully against the potential negative effects. Free vaccination may be critical in developing countries where the cost of veterinary care is prohibitive to large percentages of the population. Even partially subsidized vaccination may not achieve optimal vaccine coverage.[153]

Testing rabies titers in pets

Apart from demonstrating that a pet has been vaccinated and mounted an immune response for importation into a rabies-free country, there is no indication for testing rabies titers since results do not necessarily correlate with protection from disease.[122,152] Titers should not be used to determine whether to revaccinate.

Management of pets that may have been exposed to rabies

There are variable approaches to animals that have been exposed to rabies, depending on the type of exposure, vaccination status of the animal, and jurisdiction. As with exposure of humans, identification of the offending animal and determination of its disease status is important. If the animal cannot be identified and determined to be rabies free, one must assume that the pet has been exposed.

For unvaccinated dogs and cats, euthanasia or strict 6-month quarantine is recommended, with a single dose of vaccine given at the start of the quarantine or 1-month prior to the end of quarantine.[152] The harsh nature of this has led to consideration of PEP protocols for pets. A study of experimentally infected dogs reported that all dogs vaccinated on days 0, 3, 7, 14, and 35 after exposure developed rabies, while monoclonal antibody administration on day 0 alone protected 4/5 dogs and a combination of monoclonal antibody and vaccination protected 5/5 dogs.[154] Another study using experimentally challenged dogs indicated that vaccination of dogs on days 0, 3, 7, and 28, or on days 0, 5, and 28 prevented rabies.[155] Based on the size of these studies and the conflicting results, plus the significant public health concerns regarding rabies, there is no clear answer about PEP in pets. From a medical standpoint, vaccination of exposed pets as part of the quarantine process is logical. Postexposure vaccination should never be used in place of proper quarantine. Reliance on PEP without quarantine is difficult to justify at this time given the small size of studies and lack of any field studies evaluating these approaches. The WHO discourages the use of RIG in animals,[123] although the reasons for this are not explained.

The approach to previously vaccinated animals is more variable between regions and can involve different lengths of strict quarantine or owner observation; however, prompt revaccination and 45 days of owner observation is recommended.[152] Animals that are overdue for revaccination should be handled on a case-by-case basis.

If any animal under quarantine or owner observation develops signs consistent with rabies, it should be euthanized and tested.

Eradication of canine rabies

Eradication of canine rabies is feasible and has been achieved in the United States and Canada, some areas of South America, western Europe, and Japan.[123] Considering over 99% of human rabies cases are from dogs and that 50% of the world's population lives in canine rabies endemic areas, eradication of canine rabies is a desirable goal. Vaccination is the key component of rabies eradication, and the WHO recommends that, to eliminate canine rabies, 70% vaccine coverage should be obtained.[123] There are many challenges to achieving this goal. Regions with endemic canine rabies are often resource limited; cost of vaccination may be prohibitive and veterinary care is of limited availability. Large numbers of dogs may be difficult to access in endemic regions because of large feral populations. Oral rabies vaccine baiting may be a supplementary strategy in such regions.[123] Feral animal population control is a component of rabies control, but population control and culling are not synonymous, and culling of feral dogs alone is not an effective rabies control measure.[123]

It is important to note that elimination of canine rabies does not mean that dogs cannot acquire or transmit rabies. Elimination of canine rabies involves removal of the canine rabies variant. Dogs will still be susceptible to rabies from other sources and can still infect humans. However, elimination of canine rabies can greatly reduce the prevalence of rabies in the dog population, particularly in countries where canine rabies is endemic in large feral populations, and where rabies from other sources is rare.

Handling of animal rabies suspects

Extreme care must be taken when handling rabies suspects because of their often aggressive and unpredictable behavior. Rabies suspects should be isolated and handled as little as possible. Only people that have been vaccinated against rabies and who have ample experience handling aggressive or unpredictable animals should be involved. Time and planning are required for any contact, and careful consideration should be given to the type of physical or chemical restraint that is to be used. The use of catchpoles and heavy gloves is recommended whenever needed. Liberal use of chemical restraint should be considered. Barrier precautions should be used for any procedure, consisting of a gown (or other form of dedicated protective outerwear) and gloves. Face protection or mask and eye protection should be used if there is a reasonable potential for splattering of saliva, such as when trying to catch or restrain a fractious rabid animal. If a procedure cannot be performed safely, it should not be performed. The use of a pole syringe or other remote means of sedating may be required and should be used in lieu of any risky physical restraint measures.

After euthanasia, rabies testing is required. Procedures for this will vary with jurisdiction. If the head or brain must be removed for submission, this should be done with care. Contact with blood is not a concern, but severing the head will result in exposure to potentially infectious nervous tissue. Power tools should never be used, and care should be taken when handling sharps. If the brain must be removed, extreme care must be taken. This should be done in an isolated area where there is no personnel traffic. As mentioned, power tools should never be used, nor should any tool requiring excessive force that could result in splattering or aerosolization of infectious materials. The entire brain should be submitted. Samples should be kept at refrigeration temperatures but not frozen.[152]

Rabies virus can remain viable inside an animal carcass for several days at 20°C and longer if refrigerated,[122] so proper handling practices must be continued after death or euthanasia.

Rabies-free areas

Most regions that are free of rabies have strict quarantine measures in place to prevent the introduction of rabies into the country. Aggressive measures such as strict 6-month quarantine have increasingly been replaced by specific requirements for proof of vaccination, serological testing, and a certificate of good health, which is logical, given the very low likelihood of rabies in pets that travel.

Severe acute respiratory syndrome (SARS)

SARS is a severe respiratory disease that emerged in dramatic fashion in China in late 2002.[156] It quickly spread outside of Asia and caused outbreaks in various countries, eventually causing disease in 30 countries in five continents.[157] This disease, subsequently shown to be caused by the SARS coronavirus (SCV), causes fever and severe lower respiratory tract disease with severe pneumonia or acute respiratory distress syndrome. Mechanical ventilation is often required and[158] mortality rates range from 3.8% to 30%.[157–159]

Bats were ultimately identified as the natural reservoirs of SCV,[160] but initial human cases were believed to have been acquired from wild game, particularly palm civets.[161] High seroprevalence rates were identified in civets in animal markets,[162] implicating those markets as key sources of infection. Subsequent human-to-human transmission involved direct contact, infectious aerosols, or fomites,[157,158] although there was considerable debate about the potential for true airborne transmission. Human hospitals were the source of a large percentage of cases, with infection of both patients and healthcare workers. Transmission from aerosols from sewage was implicated in a large outbreak in an apartment complex in Hong Kong.[163] Transmission during air flight was also documented.[164]

Infected cats, both clinically ill and healthy, were identified in an apartment complex in Hong Kong that had more than 100 infected humans.[165] Experimental infection has been achieved in cats and ferrets.[166,167] Infected cats and ferrets, both healthy and clinically ill, can shed SCV from the respiratory tract.[166] Furthermore, infected cats and ferrets were able to transmit SCV to other cats and ferrets that they were housed with.[166] In hindsight, this should raise concerns as it indicates a potential for cats and ferrets to become at least short-term reservoirs of SCV and theoretical sources of transmission to humans.

Given the rarity of the disease and the lack of clear information pertaining to risks from compan-ion animals, there is currently minimal concern about the role of pets in SARS transmission. SARS may be more important as a reminder that pets need to be considered in the emergence of new infectious diseases, since the potential role of companion animals received little consideration during initial SARS outbreaks. Considering it is now known that cats and ferrets are susceptible to the virus and can shed appreciable quantities of virus, it is perhaps fortunate that these (and possibly other) pet species were not apparently involved in disease transmission. Concerns about the lack of consideration of pets in voluntary quarantine, as was employed in SARS control in some regions, have been expressed,[168] and the potential role of pets in emerging zoonoses such as SARS must be considered proactively.

Should SARS reemerge in humans, infected individuals should restrict contact with pets, just as they would with other humans. If close contacts are being quarantined because of potential SCV exposure, the same guidelines should apply to pets.

References

1. Chantrey J, Meyer H, Baxby D, et al. Cowpox: reservoir hosts and geographic range. *Epidemiol Infect* 1999;122:455–460.
2. Vorou RM, Papavassiliou VG, Pierroutsakos IN. Cowpox virus infection: an emerging health threat. *Curr Opin Infect Dis* 2008;21:153–156.
3. Campe H, Zimmermann P, Glos K, et al. Cowpox virus transmission from pet rats to humans, Germany. *Emerg Infect Dis* 2009;15:777–780.
4. Kaysser P, von Bomhard W, Dobrzykowski L, et al. Genetic diversity of feline cowpox virus, Germany 2000–2008. *Vet Microbiol* 2010;141:282–288.
5. Ninove L, Domart Y, Vervel C, et al. Cowpox virus transmission from pet rats to humans, France. *Emerg Infect Dis* 2009;15:781–784.
6. Baxby D, Bennett M, Getty B. Human cowpox 1969–93: a review based on 54 cases. *Br J Dermatol* 1994;131:598–607.
7. Pfeffer M, Pfleghaar S, von Bomhard D, et al. Retrospective investigation of feline cowpox in Germany. *Vet Rec* 2002;150:50–51.
8. Baxby D, Bennett M. Cowpox: a re-evaluation of the risks of human cowpox based on new epidemiological information. *Arch Virol Suppl* 1997;13:1–12.

9. Casemore DP, Emslie ES, Whyler DK, et al. Cowpox in a child, acquired from a cat. *Clin Exp Dermatol* 1987;12:286–287.

10. Pether JV, Trevains PH, Harrison SR, et al. Cowpox from cat to man. *Lancet* 1986;1:38–39.

11. Damon I. Orthopoxviruses: vaccinia (smallpox vaccine), variola (smallpox), monkeypox and cowpox). In: Mandell GL, Bennett JE, Dolin R, eds. *Principles and Practice of Infectious Diseases*, 6th ed. Philadelphia: Elsevier, 2005, pp. 1742–1751.

12. Hönlinger B, Huemer HP, Romani N, et al. Generalized cowpox infection probably transmitted from a rat. *Br J Dermatol* 2005;153:451–453.

13. Wolfs TF, Wagenaar JA, Niesters HG, et al. Rat-to-human transmission of cowpox infection. *Emerg Infect Dis* 2002;8:1495–1496.

14. Schöniger S, Chan DL, Hollinshead M, et al. Cowpox virus pneumonia in a domestic cat in Great Britain. *Vet Rec* 2007;160:522–523.

15. Schulze C, Alex M, Schirrmeier H, et al. Generalized fatal cowpox virus infection in a cat with transmission to a human contact case. *Zoonoses Public Health* 2007;54:31–37.

16. Baxby D, Bennett M. Low risk from feline cowpox. *Lancet* 1990;336:1070–1071.

17. Fooks AR, McElhinney LM, Pounder DJ, et al. Case report: isolation of a European bat lyssavirus type 2a from a fatal human case of rabies encephalitis. *J Med Virol* 2003;71:281–289.

18. Nathwani D, McIntyre PG, White K, et al. Fatal human rabies caused by European bat lyssavirus type 2a infection in Scotland. *Clin Infect Dis* 2003; 37:598–601.

19. European Centre for Disease Prevention and Control. Expert consultation on rabies post-exposure prophylaxis. Stockholm, Sweden, 2009.

20. Cliquet F, Picard-Meyer E, Barrat J, et al. Experimental infection of foxes with European bat lyssaviruses type-1 and 2. *BMC Vet Res* 2009; 5:19.

21. Vos A, Müller T, Cox J, et al. Susceptibility of ferrets (*Mustela putorius furo*) to experimentally induced rabies with European bat lyssaviruses (EBLV). *J Vet Med B Infect Dis Vet Public Health* 2004;51:55–60.

22. Vos A, Müller T, Neubert L, et al. Rabies in red foxes (*Vulpes vulpes*) experimentally infected with European bat lyssavirus type 1. *J Vet Med B Infect Dis Vet Public Health* 2004;51:327–332.

23. Brookes SM, Klopfleisch R, Müller T, et al. Susceptibility of sheep to European bat lyssavirus type-1 and -2 infection: a clinical pathogenesis study. *Vet Microbiol* 2007;125:210–223.

24. Dacheux L. European bat lyssavirus transmission among cats, Europe. *Emerg Infect Dis* 2009;15: 280–284.

25. Freuling C, Grossmann E, Conraths FJ, et al. First isolation of EBLV-2 in Germany. *Vet Microbiol* 2008;131:26–34.

26. Van der Poel WH, Van der Heide R, Verstraten ER, et al. European bat lyssaviruses, The Netherlands. *Emerg Infect Dis* 2005;11:1854–1859.

27. Vázquez-Morón S, Juste J, Ibáñez C, et al. Endemic circulation of European bat lyssavirus type 1 in serotine bats, Spain. *Emerg Infect Dis* 2008;14: 1263–1266.

28. Takumi K, Lina PH, van der Poel WH, et al. Public health risk analysis of European bat lyssavirus infection in The Netherlands. *Epidemiol Infect* 2009;137:803–809.

29. Müller T, Cox J, Peter W, et al. Spill-over of European bat lyssavirus type 1 into a stone marten (*Martes foina*) in Germany. *J Vet Med B Infect Dis Vet Public Health* 2004;51:49–54.

30. Stantic-Pavlinic M. Public health concerns in bat rabies across Europe. *Euro Surveill* 2005;10: 217–220.

31. Centers for Disease Control and Prevention. All about hantaviruses. 2006. www.cdc.gov/ncidod/diseases/hanta/hps/noframes/FAQ.htm. Accessed December 29, 2009.

32. Jonsson CB, Hooper J, Mertz G. Treatment of hantavirus pulmonary syndrome. *Antiviral Res* 2008; 78:162–169.

33. Rivers MN, Alexander JL, Rohde RE, et al. Hantavirus pulmonary syndrome in Texas: 1993–2006. *South Med J* 2009;102:36–41.

34. Peters CJ. Bioterrorism: viral hemorrhagic fevers. In: Mandell GL, Bennett JE, Dolin R, eds. *Principles and Practice of Infectious Diseases*, 6th ed. Philadelphia: Elsevier, 2005, pp. 3626–3629.

35. Douron E, Moriniere B, Matheron S, et al. HFRS after a wild rodent bite in the Haute-Savoie—and risk of exposure to Hantaan-like virus in a Paris laboratory. *Lancet* 1984;1:676–677.

36. St Jeor SC. Three-week incubation period for hantavirus infection. *Pediatr Infect Dis J* 2004;23:974–975.

37. Bennett M, Lloyd G, Jones N, et al. Prevalence of antibody to hantavirus in some cat populations in Britain. *Vet Rec* 1990;127:548–549.

38. Malecki TM, Jillson GP, Thilsted JP, et al. Serologic survey for hantavirus infection in domestic animals and coyotes from New Mexico and northeastern Arizona. *J Am Vet Med Assoc* 1998;212:970–973.

39. Xu ZY, Tang YW, Kan LY, et al. Cats—source of protection or infection? A case-control study of hemorrhagic fever with renal syndrome. *Am J Epidemiol* 1987;126:942–948.

40. Gruber A, Pakozdy A, Weissenböck H, et al. A retrospective study of neurological disease in 118 rabbits. *J Comp Pathol* 2009;140:31–37.

41. Wohlsein P, Thiele A, Fehr M, et al. Spontaneous human herpes virus type 1 infection in a chinchilla (*Chinchilla lanigera* f. dom.). *Acta Neuropathol* 2002;104:674–678.

42. Müller K, Fuchs W, Heblinski N, et al. Encephalitis in a rabbit caused by human herpesvirus-1. *J Am Vet Med Assoc* 2009;235:66–69.

43. Ortiz JR, Uyeki TM. Avian influenza A (H5N1) virus. In: Scheld WM, ed. *Emerging Infections 7.* Washington, DC: ASM Press, 2007, pp. 1–22.

44. Butt KM, Smith GJ, Chen H, et al. Human infection with an avian H9N2 influenza A virus in Hong Kong in 2003. *J Clin Microbiol* 2005;43:5760–5767.

45. Buchy P, Mardy S, Vong S, et al. Influenza A/H5N1 virus infection in humans in Cambodia. *J Clin Virol* 2007;39:164–168.

46. Kandun IN, Tresnaningsih E, Purba WH, et al. Factors associated with case fatality of human H5N1 virus infections in Indonesia: a case series. *Lancet* 2008;372:744–749.

47. Ku AS, Chan LT. The first case of H5N1 avian influenza infection in a human with complications of adult respiratory distress syndrome and Reye's syndrome. *J Paediatr Child Health* 1999;35:207–209.

48. Liem NT, Tung CV, Hien ND, et al. Clinical features of human influenza A (H5N1) infection in Vietnam: 2004–2006. *Clin Infect Dis* 2009;48:1639–1646.

49. Cardona CJ, Xing Z, Sandrock CE, et al. Avian influenza in birds and mammals. *Comp Immunol Microbiol Infect Dis* 2009;32:255–273.

50. Subbarao K, Klimov A, Katz J, et al. Characterization of an avian influenza A (H5N1) virus isolated from a child with a fatal respiratory illness. *Science* 1998;279:393–396.

51. Uyeki TM. Human infection with highly pathogenic avian influenza A (H5N1) virus: review of clinical issues. *Clin Infect Dis* 2009;49:279–290.

52. Leschnik M, Weikel J, Möstl K, et al. Subclinical infection with avian influenza A (H5N1) virus in cats. *Emerg Infect Dis* 2007;13:243–247.

53. Marschall J, Hartmann K. Avian influenza A H5N1 infections in cats. *J Feline Med Surg* 2008;10:359–365.

54. Ayyalasomayajula S, DeLaurentis DA, Moore GE, et al. A network model of H5N1 avian influenza transmission dynamics in domestic cats. *Zoonoses Public Health* 2008;55:497–506.

55. Keawcharoen J, Oraveerakul K, Kuiken T, et al. Avian influenza H5N1 in tigers and leopards. *Emerg Infect Dis* 2004;10:2189–2191.

56. Songserm T, Amonsin A, Jam-on R, et al. Avian influenza H5N1 in naturally infected domestic cat. *Emerg Infect Dis* 2006;12:681–683.

57. Thanawongnuwech R, Amonsin A, Tantilertcharoen R, et al. Probable tiger-to-tiger transmission of avian influenza H5N1. *Emerg Infect Dis* 2005;11:699–701.

58. Yingst SL, Saad MD, Felt SA. Qinghai-like H5N1 from domestic cats, northern Iraq. *Emerg Infect Dis* 2006;12:1295–1297.

59. Klopfleisch R, Wolf PU, Uhl W, et al. Distribution of lesions and antigen of highly pathogenic avian influenza virus A/Swan/Germany/R65/06 (H5N1) in domestic cats after presumptive infection by wild birds. *Vet Pathol* 2007;44:261–268.

60. ProMED-mail. Avian influenza: Indonesia (feline), Japan, Hungary. International Society for Infectious Diseases.2007. www.promedmail.org/pls/otn/f?p=2400:1202:2932787583139744:NO:F2400_P1202_CHECK_DISPLAY,F2400_P1202_PUB_MAIL_ID:X,36080. Accessed December 29, 2009.

61. Paltrinieri S, Spagnolo V, Giordano A, et al. Influenza virus type A serosurvey in cats. *Emerg Infect Dis* 2007;13:662–664.

62. Rimmelzwaan G, van Riel D, Baars M, et al. Influenza A virus (H5N1) infection in cats causes systemic disease with potential novel routes of virus spread within and between hosts. *Am J Pathol* 2006;168:176–183.

63. Giese M, Harder TC, Teifke JP, et al. Experimental infection and natural contact exposure of dogs with avian influenza virus (H5N1). *Emerg Infect Dis* 2008;14:308–310.

64. Jackson S, Van Hoeven N, Chen LM, et al. Reassortment between avian H5N1 and human H3N2 influenza viruses in ferrets: a public health risk assessment. *J Virol* 2009;83:8131–8140.

65. ProMED-mail. Avian influenza—Eurasia: Russia, UK, Sweden. 2005. www.promedmail.org/pls/otn/f?p=2400:1202:2932787583139744:NO:F2400_P1202_CHECK_DISPLAY,F2400_P1202_PUB_MAIL_ID:X,30789. Accessed December 29, 2009.

66. Perkins LE, Swayne DE. Comparative susceptibility of selected avian and mammalian species to a Hong Kong-origin H5N1 high-pathogenicity avian influenza virus. *Avian Dis* 2003;47:956–967.

67. Songserm T, Amonsin A, Jam-on R, et al. Fatal avian influenza A H5N1 in a dog. *Emerg Infect Dis* 2006;12:1744–1747.

68. Maas R, Tacken M, Ruuls L, et al. Avian influenza (H5N1) susceptibility and receptors in dogs. *Emerg Infect Dis* 2007;13:1219–1221.

69. Song D, Kang B, Lee C, et al. Transmission of avian influenza virus (H3N2) to dogs. *Emerg Infect Dis* 2008;14:741–746.

70. Kuiken T, Rimmelzwaan G, van Riel D, et al. Avian H5N1 influenza in cats. *Science* 2004;306:241.

71. Oner AF, Bay A, Arslan S, et al. Avian influenza A (H5N1) infection in eastern Turkey in 2006. *N Engl J Med* 2006;355:2179–2185.

72. Global Influenza Programme. Expert consultation on diagnosis of H5N1 avian influenza infections in humans. *Influenza Other Respir Viruses* 2007;1:131–138.

73. Writing Committee of the Second World Health Organization Consultation on Clinical Aspects of Human Infection with Avian Influenza A (H5N1) Virus, Abdel-Ghafar AN, Chotpitayasunondh T, et al. Update on avian influenza A (H5N1) virus infection in humans. *N Engl J Med* 2008;358:261–273.

74. Yu H, Gao Z, Feng Z, et al. Clinical characteristics of 26 human cases of highly pathogenic avian influenza A (H5N1) virus infection in China. *PLoS One* 2008;3:e2985.

75. Munster VJ, de Wit E, van den Brand JM, et al. Pathogenesis and transmission of swine-origin 2009 A(H1N1) influenza virus in ferrets. *Science* 2009;325:481–483.

76. Sponseller BA, Strait E, Jergens A, et al. Influenza A pandemic (H1N1) 2009 virus infection in domestic cat. *Emerg Infect Dis* 2010;16:534–537.

77. Pingret JL, Rivière D, Lafon S, et al. Epidemiological survey of H1N1 influenza virus in cats in France. *Vet Rec* 2010;166:307.

78. Peters CJ. Lymphocytic choriomeningitis virus, Lassa virus, and the South American hemorrhagic fevers. In: Mandell GL, Bennett JE, Dolin R, eds. *Principles and Practice of Infectious Diseases*, 6th ed. Philadelphia: Elsevier, 2005, pp. 2090–2096.

79. Centers for Disease. Control and Prevention (CDC). Update: interim guidance for minimizing risk for human lymphocytic choriomeningitis virus infection associated with pet rodents. *MMWR Morb Mortal Wkly Rep* 2005;54:799–801.

80. Barton LL, Mets MB, Beauchamp CL. Lymphocytic choriomeningitis virus: emerging fetal teratogen. *Am J Obstet Gynecol* 2002;187:1715–1716.

81. Skinner HH, Knight EH, Buckley LS. The hamster as a secondary reservoir host of lymphocytic choriomeningitis virus. *J Hyg* 1976;76:299–306.

82. Gregg MB. Recent outbreaks of lymphocytic choriomeningitis in the United States of America. *Bull World Health Organ* 1975;52:549–553.

83. Biggar RJ, Woodall JP, Walter PD, et al. Lymphocytic choriomeningitis outbreak associated with pet hamsters. Fifty-seven cases from New York State. *JAMA* 1975;232:494–500.

84. Maetz HM, Sellers CA, Bailey WC, et al. Lymphocytic choriomeningitis from pet hamster exposure: a local public health experience. *Am J Public Health* 1976;66:1082–1085.

85. Ceianu C, Tatulescu D, Muntean M, et al. Lymphocytic choriomeningitis in a pet store worker in Romania. *Clin Vaccine Immunol* 2008;15:1749.

86. Juncker-Voss M, Prosl H, Lussy H, et al. Screening for antibodies against zoonotic agents among employees of the Zoological Garden of Vienna, Schönbrunn, Austria. *Berl Munch Tierarztl Wochenschr* 2004;117:404–409.

87. Centers for Disease Control and Prevention (CDC). Brief report: lymphocytic choriomeningitis virus transmitted through solid organ transplantation—Massachusetts, 2008. *MMWR Morb Mortal Wkly Rep* 2008;57:799–801.

88. Amman B. Pet rodents and fatal lymphocytic choriomeningitis in transplant patients. *Emerg Infect Dis* 2007;13:719–725.

89. Fischer SA, Graham MB, Kuehnert MJ, et al. Transmission of lymphocytic choriomeningitis virus by organ transplantation. *N Engl J Med* 2006;354:2235–2249.

90. Barton LL, Mets MB. Congenital lymphocytic choriomeningitis virus infection: decade of rediscovery. *Clin Infect Dis* 2001;33:370–374.

91. American Academy of Pediatrics. *Red Book: 2009 Report of the Committee on Infectious Diseases*, 28th ed. Elk Grove Village, IL: American Academy of Pediatrics, 2009.

92. Jamieson DJ, Kourtis AP, Bell M, et al. Lymphocytic choriomeningitis virus: an emerging obstetric pathogen? *Am J Obstet Gynecol* 2006;194:1532–1536.

93. Deibel R, Woodall JP, Decher WJ, et al. Lymphocytic choriomeningitis virus in man. Serologic evidence of association with pet hamsters. *JAMA* 1975;232:501–504.

94. Ackermann R. Risk to humans through contact with golden hamsters carrying lymphocytic choriomeningitis virus. *Dtsch Med Wochenschr* 1977;102:1367–1370.

95. Essbauer S, Pfeffer M, Meyer H. Zoonotic poxviruses. *Vet Microbiol* 2009;140:229–236.

96. Jezek Z, Marennikova SS, Mutumbo M, et al. Human monkeypox: a study of 2,510 contacts of 214 patients. *J Infect Dis* 1986;154:551–555.

97. Foster SO, Brink EW, Hutchins DL, et al. Human monkeypox. *Bull World Health Organ* 1972;46:569–576.

98. Hutin YJ, Williams RJ, Malfait P, et al. Outbreak of human monkeypox, Democratic Republic of Congo, 1996 to 1997. *Emerg Infect Dis* 2001;7:434–438.

99. Meyer H, Perrichot M, Stemmler M, et al. Outbreaks of disease suspected of being due to human monkeypox virus infection in the Democratic Republic of Congo in 2001. *J Clin Microbiol* 2002;40:2919–2921.

100. Reynolds MG, Davidson WB, Curns AT, et al. Spectrum of infection and risk factors for human monkeypox, United States, 2003. *Emerg Infect Dis* 2007;13:1332–1339.

101. Centers for Disease Control and Prevention (CDC). Multistate outbreak of monkeypox—Illinois, Indiana, and Wisconsin, 2003. *MMWR Morb Mortal Wkly Rep* 2003;52:537–540.

102. Reed K, Melski J, Graham M, et al. The detection of monkeypox in humans in the Western Hemisphere. *N Engl J Med* 2004;350:342–350.

103. Sejvar JJ, Chowdary Y, Schomogyi M, et al. Human monkeypox infection: a family cluster in the midwestern United States. *J Infect Dis* 2004;190: 1833–1840.

104. Nalca A, Rimoin AW, Bavari S, et al. Reemergence of monkeypox: prevalence, diagnostics, and countermeasures. *Clin Infect Dis* 2005;41: 1765–1771.

105. Kile JC, Fleischauer AT, Beard B, et al. Transmission of monkeypox among persons exposed to infected prairie dogs in Indiana in 2003. *Arch Pediatr Adolesc Med* 2005;159:1022–1025.

106. Reynolds MG, Yorita KL, Kuehnert MJ, et al. Clinical manifestations of human monkeypox influenced by route of infection. *J Infect Dis* 2006;194: 773–780.

107. Croft DR, Sotir MJ, Williams CJ, et al. Occupational risks during a monkeypox outbreak, Wisconsin, 2003. *Emerg Infect Dis* 2007;13:1150–1157.

108. Guarner J, Johnson BJ, Paddock CD, et al. Monkeypox transmission and pathogenesis in prairie dogs. *Emerg Infect Dis* 2004;10:426–431.

109. Langohr IM, Stevenson GW, Thacker HL, et al. Extensive lesions of monkeypox in a prairie dog (*Cynomys* sp). *Vet Pathol* 2004;41:702–707.

110. Xiao SY, Sbrana E, Watts DM, et al. Experimental infection of prairie dogs with monkeypox virus. *Emerg Infect Dis* 2005;11:539–545.

111. Di Giulio DB, Eckburg PB. Human monkeypox: an emerging zoonosis. *Lancet Infect Dis* 2004;4: 15–25.

112. Centers for Disease Control and Prevention. Updated interim CDC guidance for use of smallpox vaccine, cidofovir, and vaccinia immune globulin (VIG) for prevention and treatment in the setting of an outbreak of monkeypox infections. 2008. www.cdc.gov/ncidod/monkeypox/treatmentguidelines.htm. Accessed December 29, 2009.

113. Sbrana E, Xiao SY, Newman PC, et al. Comparative pathology of North American and central African strains of monkeypox virus in a ground squirrel model of the disease. *Am J Trop Med Hyg* 2007;76:155–164.

114. Chua KB, Goh KJ, Wong KT, et al. Fatal encephalitis due to Nipah virus among pig-farmers in Malaysia. *Lancet* 1999;354:1257–1259.

115. Goh KJ, Tan CT, Chew NK, et al. Clinical features of Nipah virus encephalitis among pig farmers in Malaysia. *N Engl J Med* 2000;342:1229–1235.

116. Lo MK, Rota PA. The emergence of Nipah virus, a highly pathogenic paramyxovirus. *J Clin Virol* 2008;43:396–400.

117. Field HE, Young P, Yob JM, et al. The natural history of Hendra and Nipah viruses. *Microbes Infect* 2001;3:307–314.

118. Middleton DJ, Westbury HA, Morrissy CJ, et al. Experimental Nipah virus infection in pigs and cats. *J Comp Pathol* 2002;126:124–136.

119. Parashar UD, Sunn LM, Ong F, et al. Case-control study of risk factors for human infection with a new zoonotic paramyxovirus, Nipah virus, during a 1998–1999 outbreak of severe encephalitis in Malaysia. *J Infect Dis* 2000;181:1755–1759.

120. Mills JN, Alim AN, Bunning ML, et al. Nipah virus infection in dogs, Malaysia, 1999. *Emerg Infect Dis* 2009;15:950–952.

121. Epstein JH, Abdul Rahman S, Zambriski JA, et al. Feral cats and risk for Nipah virus transmission. *Emerg Infect Dis* 2006;12:1178–1179.

122. Greene CE, Rupprecht CE. Rabies and other lyssavirus infections. In: Greene CE, ed. *Infectious Diseases of the Dog and Cat*, 3rd ed. Philadelphia: Saunders Elsevier, 2006, pp. 167–183.

123. World Health Organization. WHO Expert Consultation on Rabies. Geneva, Switzerland, 2005.

124. Bleck TP, Rupprecht CE. Rhabdoviruses. In: Mandell GL, Bennett JE, Dolin R, eds. *Principles and Practice of Infectious Diseases*, 6th ed. Philadelphia: Elsevier, 2005, pp. 2047–2054.

125. Centers for Disease Control and Prevention. Human rabies prevention, United States, 2008. Recommendations of the Advisory Committee on Immunization Practices. *MMWR* 2008;57:1–28.

126. Burton EC, Burns DK, Opatowsky MJ, et al. Rabies encephalomyelitis: clinical, neuroradiological, and pathological findings in 4 transplant recipients. *Arch Neurol* 2005;62:873–882.

127. Hellenbrand W, Meyer C, Rasch G, et al. Cases of rabies in Germany following organ transplantation. *Euro Surveill* 2005;10:213–217.

128. Srinivasan A, Burton EC, Kuehnert MJ, et al. Transmission of rabies virus from an organ donor to four transplant recipients. *N Engl J Med* 2005;352:1103–1111.

129. Howard DR. Transplacental transmission of rabies virus from a naturally infected skunk. *Am J Vet Res* 1981;42:691–692.

130. Martell MA, Montes FC, Alcocer R. Transplacental transmission of bovine rabies after natural infection. *J Infect Dis* 1973;127:291–293.

131. Sipahioğlu U, Alpaut S. Transplacental rabies in humans. *Mikrobiyol Bul* 1985;19:95–99.

132. Balsamo GA, Ratard R, Claudet A. The epidemiology of animal bite, scratch, and other potential rabies exposures, Louisiana. *J La State Med Soc* 2009;161:260–265.

133. Si H, Guo ZM, Hao YT, et al. Rabies trend in China (1990–2007) and post-exposure prophylaxis in the Guangdong province. *BMC Infect Dis* 2008;8:113.

134. Blanton JD, Palmer D, Christian KA, et al. Rabies surveillance in the United States during 2007. *J Am Vet Med Assoc* 2008;233:884–897.

135. Centers for Disease. Control and Prevention (CDC). Rabies in a dog imported from Iraq—New Jersey, June 2008. *MMWR Morb Mortal Wkly Rep* 2008;57:1076–1078.

136. Eidson M, Matthews SD, Willsey AL, et al. Rabies virus infection in a pet guinea pig and seven pet rabbits. *J Am Vet Med Assoc* 2005;227:932–935. 918.

137. ProMED-mail. Rabies, Hamster-Russia (Voronej). International Society for Infectious Diseases.2004. www.promedmail.org/pls/otn/f?p=2400:1202: 3590251627295062:NO:F2400_P1202_CHECK_ DISPLAY,F2400_P1202_PUB_MAIL_ID:X,27290. Accessed December 29, 2009.

138. Blanton JD, Robertson K, Palmer D, et al. Rabies surveillance in the United States during 2008. *J Am Vet Med Assoc* 2009;235:676–689.

139. Krebs JW, Wheeling JT, Childs JE. Rabies surveillance in the United States during 2002. *J Am Vet Med Assoc* 2003;223:1736–1748.

140. Centers for Disease Control and Prevention (CDC). Recovery of a patient from clinical rabies—Wisconsin, 2004. *MMWR Morb Mortal Wkly Rep* 2004;53:1171–1173.

141. Lopez A, Miranda P, Tejada E, et al. Outbreak of human rabies in the Peruvian jungle. *Lancet* 1992;339:408–411.

142. Hemachudha T, Wacharapluesadee S. Antemortem diagnosis of human rabies. *Clin Infect Dis* 2004;39:1085–1086.

143. Nadin-Davis SA. Polymerase chain reaction protocols for rabies virus discrimination. *J Virol Methods* 1998;75:1–8.

144. Rupprecht CE, Briggs D, Brown CM, et al. Evidence for a 4-dose vaccine schedule for human rabies post-exposure prophylaxis in previously non-vaccinated individuals. *Vaccine* 2009;27:7141–7148.

145. Parviz S, Chotani R, McCormick J, et al. Rabies deaths in Pakistan: results of ineffective post-exposure treatment. *Int J Infect Dis* 2004;8:346–352.

146. Dreesen DW, Fishbein DB, Kemp DT, et al. Two-year comparative trial on the immunogenicity and adverse effects of purified chick embryo cell rabies vaccine for pre-exposure immunization. *Vaccine* 1989;7:397–400.

147. Jaijaroensup W, Limusanno S, Khawplod P, et al. Immunogenicity of rabies postexposure booster injections in subjects who had previously received intradermal preexposure vaccination. *J Travel Med* 1999;6:234–237.

148. Fishbein DB, Dreesen DW, Holmes DF, et al. Human diploid cell rabies vaccine purified by zonal centrifugation: a controlled study of antibody response and side effects following primary and booster pre-exposure immunizations. *Vaccine* 1989;7:437–442.

149. Committee to Advise on Tropical Medicine and Travel. Statement on travellers and rabies vaccine. *CCDR* 2002;28:1–12.

150. Sterner RT, Meltzer MI, Shwiff SA, et al. Tactics and economics of wildlife oral rabies vaccination, Canada and the United States. *Emerg Infect Dis* 2009;15:1176–1184.

151. Murray KO, Holmes KC, Hanlon CA. Rabies in vaccinated dogs and cats in the United States, 1997–2001. *J Am Vet Med Assoc* 2009;235:691–695.

152. NASPHV, Prevention CfDCa, Epidemiologists CoSaT, et al. Compendium of measures to prevent disease associated with animals in public settings, 2009: National Association of State Public Health Veterinarians, Inc. (NASPHV). *MMWR Recomm Rep* 2009;58:1–21.

153. Durr S, Mindekem R, Kaninga Y, et al. Effectiveness of dog rabies vaccination programmes: comparison of owner-charged and free vaccination campaigns. *Epidemiol Infect* 2009;137:1558–1567.

154. Hanlon CA, Niezgoda M, Rupprecht CE. Postexposure prophylaxis for prevention of rabies in dogs. *Am J Vet Res* 2002;63:1096–1100.

155. Manickama R, Basheer MD, Jayakumar R. Postexposure prophylaxis (PEP) of rabies-infected Indian street dogs. *Vaccine* 2008;26:6564–6568.

156. Zhong NS, Zheng BJ, Li YM, et al. Epidemiology and cause of severe acute respiratory syndrome (SARS) in Guangdong, People's Republic of China, in February, 2003. *Lancet* 2003;362:1353–1358.

157. Cheng VC, Lau SK, Woo PC, et al. Severe acute respiratory syndrome coronavirus as an agent of emerging and reemerging infection. *Clin Microbiol Rev* 2007;20:660–694.

158. Poutanen SM, Low DE, Henry B, et al. Identification of severe acute respiratory syndrome in Canada. *N Engl J Med* 2003;348:1995–2005.

159. Zhong N. Management and prevention of SARS in China. *Philos Trans R Soc Lond B Biol Sci* 2004; 359:1115–1116.

160. Li W, Shi Z, Yu M, et al. Bats are natural reservoirs of SARS-like coronaviruses. *Science* 2005;310: 676–679.

161. Song HD, Tu CC, Zhang GW, et al. Cross-host evolution of severe acute respiratory syndrome coronavirus in palm civet and human. *Proc Natl Acad Sci U S A* 2005;102:2430–2435.

162. Tu C, Crameri G, Kong X, et al. Antibodies to SARS coronavirus in civets. *Emerg Infect Dis* 2004; 10:2244–2248.

163. Chu CM, Cheng VC, Hung IF, et al. Viral load distribution in SARS outbreak. *Emerg Infect Dis* 2005;11:1882–1886.

164. Olsen SJ, Chang HL, Cheung TY, et al. Transmission of the severe acute respiratory syndrome on aircraft. *N Engl J Med* 2003;349:2416–2422.

165. Abbott A. Pet theory comes to the fore in fight against SARS. *Nature* 2003;423:576.

166. Martina B, Haagmans B, Kuiken T, et al. Virology: SARS virus infection of cats and ferrets. *Nature* 2003;425:915.

167. van den Brand JM, Haagmans BL, Leijten L, et al. Pathology of experimental SARS coronavirus infection in cats and ferrets. *Vet Pathol* 2008;45:551–562.

168. Weese J, Kruth S. Pets in voluntary household quarantine. *Emerg Infect Dis* 2006;12:1029–1030.

4 Fungal Diseases

J. Scott Weese and Martha B. Fulford

Introduction

Fungal diseases may actually be among the most common pet-associated zoonoses, although the vast majority of this is caused by dermatophytes. While dermatophytosis (ringworm) is the most common fungal zoonosis and is typically mild and self-limited, some fungal pathogens can cause serious, including fatal, disease, particularly in immunocompromised individuals. Fortunately, these are rare, and the overall risk of serious fungal disease is low. An additional group of pathogens that deserves consideration is fungi that can infect both animals and humans from the same environmental source, but with little to no risk of interspecies transmission. In those situations, pets may be useful as sentinels for human exposure but pose minimal risk to humans.

Aspergillus spp.

Aspergillus spp. are hyaline molds that are ubiquitous in the environment. *Aspergillus fumigatus* is most commonly associated with infection. These fungal species grow on organic matter, and conidia

(spores) are released into the air. People and animals are exposed by inhalation and probably inhale hundreds of conidia on a daily basis.[1] Despite widespread exposure, infections are rare and, in humans, most commonly occur in immunocompromised individuals.

Aspergillosis can be highly variable, from subclinical infection to acute, fatal invasive disease. Invasive disease is very rare in immunocompetent individuals, but aspergillosis is a major cause of morbidity and mortality in immunocompromised patients. It is most common in hematopoietic stem cell transplant recipients and persons with hematologic malignancies, but can occur in a wide spectrum of immunocompromised or critically ill individuals.

In animals, nasal aspergillosis is the most common clinical presentation, occurring predominantly in immunocompetent individuals. Disseminated disease is rare but has been reported. In dogs, there is not a clear association between immunocompromised hosts and disseminated infection. In contrast, most cats with disseminated infection are immunocompromised from conditions such as feline leukemia virus infection, feline infectious peritonitis, panleukopenia, or glucocorticoid therapy.[2]

Transmission of *Aspergillus* from companion animals to humans has not been reported. Humans and animals may be infected from the same environmental sources. There are minimal concerns regarding zoonotic transmission of *Aspergillus*, even to immunocompromised individuals. Regardless, prudence dictates that immunocompromised individuals should take added precautions when handing animals with *Aspergillus* infections. These would consist largely of restricting close contact with infected animals, careful attention to hand hygiene, not allowing infected pets to sleep on beds, avoiding contact with the infected site, keeping the infected site covered with a barrier dressing whenever possible, and avoiding contact with potentially contaminated items such as bandage materials. Identification of aspergillosis in a household pet of an immunocompromised individual should probably trigger investigation of possible high-risk sources of infection in the household, to determine whether any interventions are required to reduce the risk of human infection from the same source that infected the animal.

Blastomycosis

Blastomycosis is a fungal disease caused by the dimorphic yeast *Blastomyces dermatitidis*. Dogs are highly susceptible, but disease can also occur in other domestic species. It is most common in the United States in Mississippi, Missouri, the Ohio River valley, and mid-Atlantic states, and in Canada in focal areas of Ontario, Quebec, and Manitoba. It has also been reported in other areas of North America and in parts of Europe, Asia, Latin America, and Africa. *B. dermatitidis* can exist in two forms: a yeast form and a mold form. It is the yeast form that causes infections, but this form cannot be transmitted by direct contact or aerosols. The mold form is the highly infectious form that is present at ambient temperatures in the environment. While routine contact with infected animals poses no risk, animal-to-human transmission of blastomycosis has been reported following a dog bite.[3] It has also occurred following inoculation of *Blastomyces* into the finger of a veterinarian from a needlestick injury during fine-needle aspiration of an infected site in a dog.[4] Bite avoidance, proper bite wound management, and safe handling of sharps are the main preventive measures. The main role of dogs in human disease may be as

sentinels of infection because of their high susceptibility.

Coccidioidomycosis

The dimorphic soil-borne fungi *Coccidioides immitis* and *Coccidioides posadasii* are the cause of coccidioidomycosis. This disease is mainly reported in humans, dogs, and cats, predominantly in the southwestern United States, northern Mexico, and scattered regions of Central America, Colombia, Venezuela, Paraguay, and Argentina. *C. immitis* is only found in California, while *C. posadasii* accounts for infections in all other regions.

In humans, infection is usually self-limited or asymptomatic in immunocompetent individuals.[5,6] When disease is present, pulmonary disease with an influenza-like illness predominates. Malaise, fever, cough, myalgia, headache, and chest pain are the most common clinical signs.[5] A maculopapular rash, erythema multiforme, erythema nodosum, or arthralgia may also develop in a reasonable percentage of individuals. Disseminated infection is a rare but potentially devastating form of disease that occurs in approximately 0.5% of infections in the general population but at a much higher rate in immunocompromised individuals, such as those with HIV/AIDS, people on chronic corticosteroid therapy, people undergoing chemotherapy, and allogenic transplant recipients.[7] Dissemination to bone, skin, joints, the central nervous system (CNS), lungs, and/or skin may occur.[5]

Clinical aspects are similar in dogs, with most infections being subclinical, and clinical infections typically characterized by lower respiratory tract infection. Disseminated disease can result in a range of clinical signs, depending on the organ system that is involved. Skin lesions are commonly found in cats, along with fever, weight loss, and inappetence.[8]

Infection occurs through contact with arthroconidia, the infective form, either directly or indirectly from soil. Coccidioidomycosis is generally considered to be nontransmissible between animals and humans because infective arthroconidia do not typically develop in infected tissues. There is a report of coccidioidomycosis in a veterinarian that was associated with necropsy of a horse with disseminated disease.[9] Inhalation of tissue-phase endospores, potentially associated with inadvertently cutting through an infected area with a band saw, was postulated as the reason for infection. In general, direct animal–human transmission does not occur. There is a recent report describing coccidioidomycosis in a veterinary technician who was bitten by a cat with disseminated disease.[10] The technician was bitten on the arm and approximately 2 weeks later, developed severe erythema, inflammation, and lymphangitis of the entire arm. No other cases of suspected zoonotic transmission have been reported.

People caring for animals with wounds infected by *Coccidioides* should probably be cautious when handling bandage material based on the theoretical possibility that arthroconidia could develop in that environment. While the risk is probably low, the use of eye or face protection, a mask, and gloves, along with close attention to standard hygiene practices, would be prudent. Careful attention to necropsy procedures is required in animals that have died of this disease. The use of face or eye and respiratory protection during necropsy may be prudent. While presumably very rare, bites from animals with disseminated coccidioidomycosis should be considered a possible source of infection, and medical advice should be obtained. There is little evidence regarding a role for postexposure prophylaxis in such an event, and the most likely recommended course would be careful monitoring.

Cryptococcosis

Cryptococcosis is an uncommon but important disease of humans and animals. It is primarily caused by *Cryptococcus neoformans*, an encapsulated yeast that can be found virtually worldwide. *Cryptococcus gattii* (*C. neoformans* var. *gattii*) is also pathogenic to humans and animals, and is found mainly in rural areas of Australia, Vancouver Island and the associated British Columbia mainland in Canada, and Washington and Oregon states in the United States. Other species such as *Cryptococcus albidus*, *Cryptococcus laurentii*, and *Cryptococcus curvatus* are less frequent causes of infection.

Immunocompetent individuals may develop *C. neoformans* infection but disease is most frequent and severe in immunocompromised individuals. People with renal failure, diabetes, or alcoholism,[11] or those treated with tumor necrosis factor alpha antagonists[12] may also be at increased risk. HIV/AIDS patients are at particular risk, and variations in cryptococcosis rates are usually closely associated with HIV/AIDS rates in the population. Almost all human cases are associated with environmental exposure, though there are reports of pet bird-associated cryptococcosis, likely through inhalation of yeast passed in feces.[12-14] In contrast, *C. gattii* infections occur mainly in immunocompetent individuals, both human and animal. There is currently no evidence indicating a potential role of animals in human *C. gattii* infection.

Cryptococcal infection occurs mainly via inhalation of yeast cells, with subsequent hematogenous dissemination. Gastrointestinal infection and inoculation into broken skin have also been reported but are likely rare.

Both *C. neoformans* and *C. gattii* can infect domestic mammals, particularly cats. Direct transmission of *Cryptococcus* spp. from mammals to humans is of minimal concern as aerosolization of infective yeast cells does not occur from infected sites. Inoculation of tissue infected with *C. neoformans* into laboratory animals has resulted in transmission of infection, indicating that there is the possibility of zoonotic transmission from needlestick or surgical injuries. Accordingly, proper sharps handling practices are important. The greatest role of mammals in human cryptococcosis may be as sentinels, as has been best shown with *C. gattii*.[15]

The main concern regarding zoonotic transmission of *Cryptococcus* involves *C. neoformans* and pet birds. The risk posed from pet birds is probably minimal in average households. A case of cryptococcal meningitis associated with a pet bird has been reported in an immunocompetent person.[13] Of some concern is that this individual did not report close contact with the bird or its cage, yet both bird and human harbored indistinguishable isolates of *C. neoformans*. It has been shown that *C. neoformans* can be isolated from the air near bird cages, indicating that close contact is not necessarily required for the transmission of infection.[16] The risk to immunocompromised individuals has not been adequately investigated, although *C. neoformans* infections in such patients have been linked to pet birds.[12,14] Because of reports of infection associated with pet birds, the potential for life-threatening disease, and some reports of a high prevalence of *C. neoformans* shedding by captive birds,[17] it has been recommended that high-risk individuals avoid having pet birds in living spaces and participating in activities related to pet bird care.[11,18] It is unclear whether this broad prohibition on bird ownership is required. The risks to high-risk individuals, particularly those with HIV/AIDS, must be carefully considered alongside potential benefits of bird ownership.

One additional area of potential concern is the keeping of birds in healthcare facilities, particularly long-term care facilities. The presence of high-risk individuals in these facilities would presumably create some degree of risk, and it is unclear whether this risk is justifiable in such a population. Since it has been recommended that high-risk people avoid pet birds, the presence of pet birds in long-term care facilities and similar facilities should be reevaluated.

If birds are to be kept indoors, the risk of zoonotic infection can likely be minimized by keeping birds in cages, ensuring that high-risk individuals do not have contact with bedding materials and cleaning of cages either away from rooms where high-risk individuals are or when they are not present in the room. Lightly spraying bedding with water may help reduce the risk of aerosolization of infectious yeast cells during handling of bedding. Routine testing of birds for *Cryptococcus* shedding is impractical because of the lack of information about shedding patterns, cost, and the lengthy time that can be required to isolate cryptococci.

Dermatophytosis (ringworm)

Introduction

Ringworm is a fungal disease caused by dermatophytes. It is considered by some to be the most common zoonotic disease in the world. Dermatophytes are classified into three groups. Zoophilic species are normally found in animals,

many of which can be transmitted to humans. Anthropophilic species are normally found in humans. Geophilic species are soil-inhabiting saprophytes. With the exception of *Microsporum gypseum*, dermatophytes that cause zoonotic ringworm are zoophilic, particularly *Microsporum canis*, *Trichophyton verrucosum*, *Trichophyton equinum*, and *Trichophyton mentagrophytes*. *M. canis* is probably the most prevalent zoophilic species worldwide.[19]

Etiology

Dermatophytes have different preferred hosts, although most are able to infect multiple species. Dogs and cats are most commonly infected with *M. canis*, *T. mentagrophytes*, or *M. gypseum*, while *T. verrucosum* mainly affects cattle and *T. equinum* predominates in horses. All can be transmitted to humans. It has been estimated that zoonotic species account for 20–50% of human infections.

Geographic distribution/epidemiology

Dermatophytes are present worldwide; however, there are geographic differences in species distribution. Colonization or subclinical infection with dermatophytes is common, particularly in cats. *M. canis* can be found in 3–36% of healthy dogs and 0–54% of healthy cats.[20–27] Higher rates, up to 100%, can be found in certain groups such as stray cats.[24] In addition to stray cats, cats less than 1 year of age and cats from multi-cat facilities have higher carriage rates.[24,25] Long-haired animals may be predisposed as hair mats can interfere with normal grooming and provide a hospitable environment for fungal growth, although data on hair length as a risk factor are conflicting.[25,27] Dogs are less commonly affected than cats, and affected dogs are usually puppies. Other household pet species that have been reported to carry or transmit dermatophytes include guinea pigs,[28] hamsters,[21] hedgehogs,[29,30] and psittacine birds.[21]

Dermatophytes are highly transmissible. A study of households with cats infected with *M. canis* reported that 50% of household contacts, 44% of adults, and 80% of children subsequently became infected.[31] Zoophilic dermatophytes do not usually spread between people, though multiple household members may be infected from the same animal source.

Cats are the main companion animal source of dermatophytes, probably because of the higher prevalence of infection compared with other companion animal species and the closeness of interaction between cats and people. Transmission from other companion animal species can also occur, particularly from clinically infected animals. Transmission of anthropophilic species from humans to pets is rare but can occur.

Pathophysiology

Dermatophytes are present in large numbers on hair and skin cells shed by infected individuals, and clinical signs of dermatophytosis do not need to be present for an animal to be infectious. Transmission is primarily by direct contact with arthrospores from an infected individual or contaminated environment, but arthrospores are small enough to be spread over short distances in the air. Fleas can also carry arthrospores between individuals. Common-contact items such as furniture or bedding can also spread dermatophytes.

Development of infection requires contact of arthrospores with nonintact skin, as arthrospores cannot penetrate intact skin, but minor skin trauma or damage from moisture can be adequate to allow infection to develop.[32] Disease is more common in hot, humid environments because these conditions favor dermatophyte survival and moisture-associated skin maceration. Once established, dermatophytes proliferate in keratinous tissue and invade hair, skin, and nails. The incubation period is approximately 1–3 weeks.

Animals

Clinical presentation

Clinical signs can be highly variable. The most common signs are hair loss, scaling, and crusting.[32] Disease may range from nonpruritic to highly pruritic with significant skin trauma from scratching. The classical ring-shaped lesion with a clearing center and active leading edges may be present but does not develop in all cases. In cats, lesions can be focal or multifocal to generalized. Scaling and hair loss may be extensive. Scaling and erythema of the pinnae are common. Severe cases may mimic pemphigus foliaceus. In dogs, focal or multifocal hair loss is the most common sign. Dogs will more often develop classical focal lesions than cats, with widespread lesions being less common than in cats.

Diagnosis

Due to the variability in clinical presentation and similarity to other dermatologic diseases, clinical signs alone are not diagnostic. Wood's light examination is often used as a screening tool. This test has reasonable specificity but limited sensitivity as only approximately one-half of M. canis will fluoresce and other dermatophyte species will not. A true positive result is a bright "apple green" color along the hair shafts. While the positive predictive value of the characteristic fluorescence is probably reasonable, all animals should also be tested by culture. Wood's lamp testing is probably most useful during an outbreak with a known fluorescing strain of M. canis.

Identification of dermatophytes can be done by microscopic examination of hairs plucked from the animal and suspended in mineral oil or, preferably, wet mounted in 10–20% potassium hydroxide overnight and heated gently for 10 minutes.[32] The use of this technique is probably limited, particularly in inexperienced personnel and is best used as a follow-up of positive Wood's lamp screening.

Culture is used for definitive diagnosis and should be routinely attempted. False-positive and false-negative results can occur, and there can be a long turnaround time. The ideal method for sample collection is the brush method, using a new toothbrush, which is vigorously brushed over the area of suspected lesions for 2–3 minutes. The brush is then submitted for fungal culture.

Management

In otherwise healthy animals, infection is usually self-limited; however, it may take up to 2–3 months for natural resolution. Because of the potential for transmission of infection during this period, treatment is recommended. Treatment of subclinically infected animals is also recommended to reduce the risk of transmission. Topical therapy is preferred, and body clipping may be required to facilitate proper application of antifungals. Care must be taken to avoid widespread environmental contamination and personnel exposure during clipping because of the potential for widespread dissemination of infected hairs. Sedation should be considered, particularly in cats. Clipping the animal while the clipped area is enclosed in a garbage or biohazard bag will help reduce the spread of infected hairs. Vacuuming during clipping could be useful if the vacuum is equipped with a functioning HEPA filter. Enilconazole, lime sulfur, and miconazole are the most commonly used topical therapies. Treatments should be directed at the entire hair coat, not just visible lesions. Combined topical and systemic therapy can shorten the course of disease but is usually reserved for recurrent infections, immunocompromised animals, or in outbreaks.[32] Numerous systemic agents are available, including griseofulvin, ketoconazole, itraconazole, fluconazole, and terbinafine, depending on the animal species. Terbinafine is an excellent option but may be cost prohibitive in multiple animal situations. Ideally, treatment should continue until two weekly or biweekly cultures, started 2–4 weeks after initiation of treatment, are negative.[32]

Humans

Clinical presentation

In humans, the term *tinea* is used to refer to dermatophytosis, followed by a description of the site of infection. Tinea corporis, often referred to as ringworm, is characterized by one or more circular lesions with scaling and crusting, a prominent leading edge that may contain pustules or follicular papules and a clear or resolving center (Figure 4.1).[19] The trunk and legs are most commonly affected. There may be varying degrees of pruritis. Infection with zoophilic species typically causes more inflammation and pustules. Dermatophytes are more common in tropical regions. In temperate regions, these most often occur in children and with zoophilic species. Elderly and immunocompromised individuals are at increased risk.

Tinea capitis is characterized by scaling of the scalp with variable erythema, inflammation, and alopecia. It is most common in 4- to 11-year-old

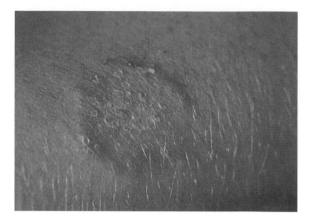

Figure 4.1   Classical ringworm lesion caused by *Trichophyton mentagrophtes* (public domain, Centers for Disease Control and Prevention, photo credit Dr. Lucille Georg).

children. Endemic infections are usually associated with anthropophilic species, but zoophilic infections can occur.

Disseminated or deep dermatophytosis is uncommon and mainly occurs in immunocompromised people, particularly those with HIV/AIDS.[33,34] Reports of disseminated disease caused by zoophilic species are very limited. It is caused by invasion of dermatophytes into subcutaneous tissues and lymphatics, potentially followed by further systemic spread. This condition can be fatal, particularly if there is CNS involvement.

Tinea pedis (athlete's foot) and tinea cruris (jock itch) are dermatophytoses but are not zoonotic; they are caused by anthropophilic species.

Diagnosis

Principles of diagnosis are similar to that presented for animals above. Samples for culture are collected from scrapings or clippings of lesions. Sampling the edge of skin lesion and infected nails is important. In addition to making a definitive diagnosis, identification of the dermatophyte involved can be useful to infer the source—human versus animal. This is particularly important in situations where a household-wide intervention is planned, and it is important to determine whether animals need to be concurrently tested and treated.

Management

Topical antifungal therapy is commonly used, but systemic treatment may be needed for nail and hair infections. Topical keratolytics such as Whitfield's ointment (salicyclic and benzoic acids) are often used on hairless areas. Terbinafine and various members of the imidazole group (clotrimazole, econazole, miconazole) are also commonly used topical agents for tinea corporis. With larger lesions, oral terbinafine, itraconazole, or fluconazole may be used. Oral griseofulvin is less commonly used for tinea corporis but is the main treatment of tinea capitis; however, this drug is no longer available in some jurisdictions. Six to eight weeks of griseofulvin treatment is usually required. Shorter treatment times have been recommended for imidazoles and tinea corporis.

Prevention

The main method for the prevention of zoonotic transmission of ringworm is avoiding contact with infected animals. This is complicated by the potential for some animals to carry dermatophytes without any clinical signs.

In households where a pet has been diagnosed with ringworm, treatment of all pets in the household should be considered given the likelihood that other pets have been, or will be, infected. This would decrease the risk of human exposure by transmission of dermatophytes between pets during the treatment period.

In situations where ringworm has been diagnosed in a person, veterinary examination of the pet is indicated. Automatic treatment of the pet is not recommended as human infection could have been from another source and transmission of anthropophilic species from human to pet is unlikely. If clinical signs consistent with dermatophytosis are present or dermatophytes are identified through diagnostic testing, treatment of all pets is indicated.

During treatment, infected household pets should be confined to a single room without carpeting to facilitate containment of dermatophyte transmission and facilitate environmental cleaning.

Treatment of all individuals in a house, both human and pet, is a reasonable (but not necessarily

required) approach to single cases of ringworm in a person caused by zoophilic dermatophytes and is certainly indicated with multiperson or recurrent disease. In the absence of identification of the dermatophyte involved in human disease (zoophilic vs. anthropophilic), treating animals without prior testing is somewhat debatable, although it is probably not contraindicated.

Dermatophytes can survive in the environment for prolonged periods of time, up to 18 months in one study.[32] Environmental cleaning and disinfection are important but difficult. Various disinfectants have been shown to be effective against dermatophytes; however, this is based on in vitro testing on the mycelial form or microconidia, not infective arthrospores, and does not consider the effects on organic debris (skin, hair) with which dermatophytes are usually associated. There may, therefore, be poor correlation between in vitro and in vivo efficacy. Bleach (1:10–1:100 dilution of household bleach)[32] is commonly used as it is readily available and cost-effective. However, bleach is noxious and not appropriate for many surfaces such as carpets. Other disinfectants, such as accelerated stabilized hydrogen peroxide and peroxygens, are recommended by some, though efficacy data are sparse. Regardless of the disinfectant used, a minimum contact time of 10 minutes is required, with some disinfectants requiring more. An additional approach is the use of 0.2% enilconazole spray, which is commercially available in some regions and approved for use in catteries. Given the difficulty of effective disinfection, comprehensive environmental disinfection is not usually performed, or truly needed[32] with limited infections occurring in a contained environment. Proper management of animals and people, and thorough cleaning are probably adequate. With larger numbers of infected individuals and longer time frames, the need for comprehensive environmental disinfection increases. Thorough environmental management is critical in shelters, catteries, and other multi-animal facilities. Removal of debris is essential, yet there is limited information about how to do so effectively and safely. Vacuuming areas where infected animals have been can remove infective particles, yet the use of vacuums without HEPA filters could simply disseminate dermatophytes throughout the environment. It is reasonable to recommend that only HEPA-filtered vacuums be used. Steam cleaning is a potentially viable alternative as moistening of infective particles would presumably reduce the risk of dissemination. High-pressure power washing should be avoided because of the potential for aerosolization of dermatophytes. Consideration must be given to other surfaces and objects with which infected animals may have had contact. Animals' bedding, toys, cages, and other items should be cleaned and disinfected. Cleaning followed by chemical disinfection and washing in hot water followed by hot-air drying are potential strategies. Items that cannot be adequately decontaminated should be discarded, if possible. Replacement of furnace filters and use of HEPA filters during the treatment and decontamination period may help reduce airborne dissemination.

In catteries or multi-cat households, where the risk of ringworm is greatest, routine screening (culture) of new animals, prior to allowing them to have contact with other animals is prudent. Prophylactic bathing in antifungals may be considered when animals have originated from a high-risk facility.

In veterinary clinics, animals with ringworm should be isolated and handled with contact precautions, consisting of a disposable gown or other form of dedicated outerwear and gloves. Hands should be washed after gloves are removed. Environmental cleaning and disinfection are critical, and should be performed considering the issues presented above. All items that have been in contact with an infected animal or its environment should be disinfected or discarded.

An *M. canis* vaccine is available in some regions but is generally not recommended because of poor evidence of efficacy.

Encephalitozoon cuniculi

Introduction

E. cuniculi is a microsporidial organism that was rarely identified as a cause of disease in the pre-HIV era, but which is now recognized as an opportunistic infection in immunocompromised individuals. It is an important cause of neurological disease in rabbits.

Etiology

E. cuniculi is a microsporidian organism that can be found in rabbits worldwide, as well as in a range of other mammalian species.[35] Microsporidia are unicellular, obligate intracellular eukaryotes that have emerged as important opportunistic pathogens in immunocompromised individuals, particularly people with HIV/AIDS.[35] Three different strains of *E. cuniculi* are recognized: I, II, and III, which are also designated "rabbit," "mouse," and "dog" strains.[35]

Life cycle

Microsporidia have a proliferative merogenic stage, followed by a sporogenic stage. The sporogenic stage is characterized by small (1–4μm) infective spores that are highly resistant to environmental effects and disinfectants.[35] Spores contain a unique apparatus, a "polar tube," which extrudes from the spore, and penetrates a potential new host cell, into which it transfers its sporoplasm and nucleus. It can also use this mechanism to infect the host cell from endocytosed spores within phagosomes.[35] Merogeny, the proliferative stage, occurs next as the sporoplasm develops into meronts, which multiply into multinucleate plasmodial forms. Sporogeny follows, during when the meront cell membranes thicken to form sporonts, which give rise to sporoblasts, then mature spores.[36] The cell then ruptures, releasing spores.

Geographic distribution/epidemiology

E. cuniculi can be found worldwide. Infections have been reported as far back as 1959,[37] though the reliance on morphological diagnosis means that it cannot be definitively stated that *E. cuniculi* was actually the cause in those older reports or whether other microsporidia may have been involved instead. Historically, infections have been very rare, with an apparent increasing incidence based largely on increasing numbers of people that are immunocompromised from HIV/AIDS, organ transplantation, or idiopathic CD4+ T-lymphocyte deficiency.[35,38–40] The incidence of microsporidial infections in HIV/AIDS patients has likely declined in recent years in developed countries because of access to highly active antiretroviral therapy (HAART). Infections can also occur in immunocompetent individuals, but these are rare.

First identified in rabbits, E. cuniculi has since been reported in over 20 mammalian species, including humans. Exposure and seroconversion is common in some species, particularly rabbits, where seroprevalences of 23–75% have been reported.[41–44] The current prevalence of E. cuniculi in research rabbits is relatively low because of efforts to create disease-free colonies, with screening and high hygienic standards, but infection remains endemic in pet rabbits.[35] The seroprevalence is lower in wild rabbit populations, likely due to decreased animal density and likelihood of exposure.[45] Zero to thirty-eight percent seroprevalence has been reported in healthy dogs, with most studies reporting 0% prevalence, even among very large study populations.[46–50] Less information is available about cats; 24% seroprevalence was reported in one study.[49] Experimental infection with the rabbit strain of E. cuniculi was achieved in newborn kittens and postweaning kittens first infected with feline leukemia virus, with development of E. cuniculi renal and brain lesions.[51] It is, however, difficult to extrapolate these experimental results to natural exposure. While it appears that at least some cats may be susceptible to E. cuniculi, the lack of reports of clinical disease suggests that cats are relatively resistant to the organism.

E. cuniculi DNA has also been detected in feces of 13% of healthy pet birds,[52] but the relevance of this to both birds and humans is unknown. While E. cuniculi clearly infects rodents, epidemiological data involving pet rodents are scarce, and little is known about seroprevalence, shedding, or the potential for zoonotic transmission from those animals.

In general, infection with E. cuniculi does not result in clinical disease. In particular, it frequently exists as a latent, subclinical infection in rabbits.[48] However, clinical infections can occur in domestic animals, particularly rabbits, dogs, and pet rodents. The course of infection is usually slow. In rabbits, it typically takes weeks to months to develop a significant spore burden in tissues, and even with high levels, clinical disease may not be apparent.[45] Infection seems to occur in the kidneys first, with subsequent spread to the brain.[45] Serum antibodies are usually detectable within 3 weeks of initial infection, which is prior to the ability to detect intracellular organisms or excretion of the organism in urine.[45,53] Brain lesions are usually only detectable 8 weeks or more after seroconversion.

Spores can be shed in various body fluids, particularly feces, urine, and respiratory secretions,[36] with urine likely the main mode of dissemination.[45] Spores can be detected in urine 38–63 days after experimental infection, with intermittent low-level shedding thereafter.[45,53] Ingestion of spores is the main route of infection. Infection may also occur via inhalation of spores.[53] Transplacental and intrauterine infection can also occur, at least in some species, such as rabbits.[35] Because of the environmental tolerance of the organism, waterborne infection is theoretically possible but unproven.[35,36]

Human infections have typically been considered rare, but it is possible that mild infections are more common but overlooked.[36] A small percentage of the healthy human population has antibodies against E. cuniculi, indicating previous exposure. Seroprevalence data are variable and reports range from 3.9% to 42%, with higher rates in immunocompromised individuals and people with a history of other tropical disease or visiting tropical countries.[35,48,49] Seropositivity tends to be more common in younger (≤19 years of age) individuals, with rates declining thereafter over time.[48] Strains I (rabbit strain) and III (dog strain) are of greatest concern in terms of human infection from companion animals.[54,55]

Given the data on the prevalence of E. cuniculi in humans versus animals, as well as molecular epidemiological data, it is unlikely that this organism is a natural pathogen of humans. While direct animal–human transmission has not been documented, human E. cuniculi infections are presumed to be zoonotic in origin.[35] Published information regarding zoonotic transmission, however, is rather circumstantial. Patients infected with dog and rabbit strains have reported exposure to dogs and rabbits, respectively.[40,55–57] Studies confirming indistinguishable organisms from humans and their associated animal contacts have not yet been reported. In one report, dogs were implicated as the source of infection of an HIV-infected individual by virtue of the person's occupation as a dog groomer,[58] a supposition that is certainly weak. In other reports, it has been noted that infected individuals had previous contact with rabbits or dogs,[40,55–57] something that clearly cannot provide much evidence of transmission. Identification of seroconversion in a child exposed to an infected puppy provides more support.[59]

Animals

Clinical presentation

In rabbits, *E. cuniculi* causes infections ranging from inapparent to severe neurological disease. Onset of disease may be more likely following a stressful event.[45] The most common clinical manifestation is neurological disease, with predominantly vestibular signs.[41,44,60] Onset is usually sudden. Head tilt, ataxia, paresis or paralysis, and head tremors are common.[41,42,44] Behavioral changes, aggression, or cranial nerve deficits are less commonly identified.[45] Ocular and renal disease may also develop, along with, or independent of, neurological disease.[42,44] Ocular signs are usually unilateral and consist of uveitis and cataracts.[42,45] Most renal infections are mild or subclinical, but renal failure can develop.

In dogs, encephalitis–nephritis syndrome is most common and is characterized by blindness, stunted growth, and nephritis.[47,61,62] Depression, inappetence, and weight loss may be seen initially, followed by progressive neurological disease with ataxia, hypermetria, central blindness, and circling.[61] Most affected animals are less than 1 year of age; in one report, 17/19 affected dogs were 4–10 weeks of age.[61,62]

Diagnosis

Definitive antemortem diagnosis is difficult because clinical signs are not pathognomonic, and there are limitations in available diagnostic tests. Presumptive diagnosis (particularly in rabbits) is usually made based on clinical signs, exclusion of other possible causes, and serological testing. The high seroprevalence rate in healthy rabbits complicates assessment of serological testing, thereby pre-

cluding definitive diagnosis. Negative serological results have a good negative predictive value because it is rare to have clinical infection without a detectable antibody response.[45] Serological testing may be of more value in dogs than rabbits because of the lower prevalence in healthy dogs in most regions, but the apparent predominance of disease in young (and immunologically immature) puppies may affect its reliability.[61] Evaluation of acute and convalescent titers for seroconversion is not useful because of the late and gradual onset of disease with respect to time of exposure.

Detection of intracellular spores in urine, feces, or tissues is preferred but can be problematic. Samples of kidney and brain would provide the highest yield, but obviously these are not readily accessible in live animals. Spores can sometimes be detected in the feces or urine of infected animals.[61] Modified trichrome staining or chitin-staining fluorophores can be used for microscopic detection of spores,[61] though access to either of these methods and personnel with experience in detecting microsporidia is limited. Detection of spores in urine or feces is supportive of the diagnosis if appropriate clinical signs are present, although it is not absolutely diagnostic because some animals can shed spores in the absence of disease.

Though not commonly available, polymerase chain reaction (PCR) can be performed on urine or other body fluids to detect spores. Even when available, the usefulness of PCR is unclear, since the presence of *E. cuniculi* DNA in body fluids does not correlate well with disease.[63,64] Additionally, negative urine results do not exclude encephalitozoonosis because spores may be shed intermittently.[45]

Histopathology is a good diagnostic tool for biopsy or postmortem specimens.[60] However, *E. cuniculi* spores do not stain well with the routinely used H&E stain and can be missed, particularly if pathologists are not aware of the potential for microsporidial disease or have little experience in identifying these unique organisms.

Management

There is limited objective information regarding treatment. In rabbits with neurological disease, three components must be considered: elimination of the organism, reduction of inflammation, and control of seizures. Variable response has been reported to albendazole, fenbendazole, and corticosteroids,[42] with fenbendazole recommended as the drug of choice in rabbits.[45] Recent evidence suggests that meloxicam may be very useful. Recovery without treatment has also been documented.[42]

There is no information regarding optimal treatments for renal failure, and general supportive care and fenbendazole are likely the most reasonable options. Response of uveitis to conservative therapy is unlikely, although successful treatment with systemic and topical administration of dexamethasone and oxytetracycline has been reported.[44] Prompt removal of the lens in combination with medical therapy is the most effective treatment.[65] Enucleation may be required in chronic cases.[45]

The prognosis is reasonable for rabbits with neurological disease. In one study, 54% of rabbits with neurological disease recovered, usually within a few days.[44] The prognosis is poor if renal failure is present.[44]

No objective information is available regarding treatment in dogs. A similar approach to that taken in rabbits is reasonable, although disease in dogs is often more insidious and advanced by the time E. cuniculi is considered, and the prognosis should be considered poor in affected dogs.

Humans

Clinical presentation

E. cuniculi infection can result in a wide range of syndromes in immunocompromised individuals, including peritonitis, hepatitis, urethritis, prostatitis, nephritis, sinusitis, keratoconjunctivitis, cystitis, diarrhea, and disseminated infection, but granulomatous encephalitis is the classic presentation.[36] It has been described as mimicking Toxoplasma encephalitis, an important differential diagnosis in immunocompromised patients.[40] Infections of immunocompetent individuals are extremely rare.[66]

Diagnosis

Definitive antemortem diagnosis can be difficult. Spores can be identified in various body fluids using specific strains such has modified trichrome staining, Warthin–Starry silver staining, or chitin-staining fluorophores.[36] Depending on the location of infection, urine or cerebrospinal fluid, as well as specimens of intestinal and biliary epithelium, corneal or conjunctival epithelium, renal tubular epithelium, upper or lower respiratory tract epithelium, or uroepithelium may be appropriate for testing.[36] Biopsy or autopsy specimens can also be tested using various stains. PCR is of increasing availability and is a sensitive and specific method.[35,67] Serology has been considered to be of minimal use because of low specificity, though the use of tests directed against polar tube antigens may be more helpful for the retrospective diagnosis of E. cuniculi.[68]

Management

Albendazole is the treatment of choice.[36] Improvement in immune function is critical but not always possible. Infections in people without a known immunocompromising disorder should prompt further investigation, particularly HIV testing.

Prevention

Routine screening of pet rabbits has been "strongly advised";[41] however, this may be difficult to justify. When one considers the apparently low incidence of disease in humans, the likely very low risk in immunocompetent individuals, and the high prevalence in healthy animals, screening is questionable. Further, eradication therapy has not been described for healthy rabbits shedding E. cuniculi, so the actual response to test results is unclear. Removal of positive animals from the household is not a reasonable recommendation, and given limitations in diagnostic testing, one cannot state with certainty that a negative animal is truly negative (or will stay negative). Therefore, efforts are probably better directed at practical household infection control measures to reduce the risk of exposure should the animal be shedding E. cuniculi. In particular, immunocompromised individuals should avoid contact with rabbit urine or feces, should not clean rabbit cages, and should pay attention to good personal hygiene (especially hand hygiene). If cage cleaning must be performed by a high-risk individual, gloves should be worn, care should be taken to avoid aerosolizing debris, the cage should be disinfected after cleaning, and hands should be washed thoroughly after removal of gloves. Rabbits that are not reliably litter-box trained should not be allowed to roam freely in households.

Animals that are clinically affected should be assumed to be shedding *E. cuniculi* spores in urine, though it is uncertain that they are infectious at the time of clinical infection. The risk to immunocompetent humans is low, but reasonable measures should be implemented to reduce the risk of exposure of humans and other animals. This primarily involves avoiding exposure to rabbit urine through the use of proper protective clothing and personal hygiene. Cages and areas potentially contaminated with urine should be properly cleaned and disinfected. Isolation of infected animals is desirable to reduce indirect transmission via personnel or fomites, but proper use of barrier precautions should allow for adequate containment of infected animals in general household or veterinary clinic housing areas. Posttreatment testing is of little value because of the potential for intermittent shedding and questionable sensitivity of tests to detect shedding.

The spores of *E. cuniculi* are highly tolerant of environmental effects and can survive in the environment for prolonged periods of time.[35,48] They are susceptible to heat (boiling for 5 minutes, autoclaving, 85°C for 2–6 minutes), as well as many disinfectants, including 70% ethanol, 1% hydrogen peroxide, and 0.01% sodium hypochlorite (bleach).[45,48]

Encephalitozoon hellem

E. hellem is a rare cause of microsporidial infection in humans and animals, with only a limited number of infections reported in people, almost all with HIV/AIDS.[35] It is unknown whether this *Encephalitozoon* species is less prevalent, less virulent, or more difficult to diagnose, but it is probably truly a rare cause of infection. It has only been reported in a few immunocompetent individuals,[69] and in all cases, it was found as a coinfection with another pathogen, so its clinical relevance was unclear.

In HIV/AIDS patients, disseminated and ocular infections are most commonly reported, though

respiratory infections can also occur.[70,71] Punctate keratoconjunctivitis is likely the most common clinical manifestation of infection.[36] The organism can also be found in a small percentage (1.6%) of asymptomatic immunocompromised individuals.[72,73]

The epidemiology of *E. hellem* is poorly understood. *E. hellem* has been detected in various bird species, particularly psittacines, both healthy and ill.[74–80] A study of captive Psittaciformes, Passeriformes, and Columbiformes from pet stores, breeders, and households identified *E. hellem* in 8.3% of 287 birds, involving a variety of different species.[52] Coinfection with other microsporidia may occur.[52,81] Chronic subclinical infection is possible and fecal shedding by birds (at least budgerigars) may be sporadic, so single samples may underestimate the prevalence of shedding.[81] The clinical relevance of *E. hellem* in birds is often unclear, although it has been implicated in fatal enteritis in some bird species.[75,76] *E. hellem* has also been found in other animal species, such as Egyptian fruit bats and European brown hares.[82,83]

The mode of transmission is not known, but fecal–oral transmission is likely considering that the organism can be shed in feces. Additionally, reports of respiratory disease suggest that inhalation of spores, perhaps from infectious fecal aerosols, is another potential route of transmission.

Evidence of zoonotic risk is minimal at this point. Naturally and experimentally infected birds can shed *E. hellem* in feces, though the clinical relevance of this is unclear, particularly to immunocompetent individuals. Zoonotic transmission has been suggested in some cases by virtue of an infected person having contact with pet birds,[56,84,85] but objective evidence is currently lacking. Despite the apparent rarity of disease and relatively weak evidence of zoonotic infection from pets, fecal shedding of *E. hellem* by pet psittacines with subsequent human infection is certainly possible, and is one of many reasons for immunocompromised individuals, particularly those with HIV/AIDS or impaired T-lymphocyte function, to restrict contact with pet birds and avoid contact with bird feces. There is no evidence indicating that screening of pet birds for *E. hellem* is indicated, useful, or practical. Concerns about this organism are best countered by careful attention to hygiene practices, particularly avoiding contact with feces and restricting contact between immunocompromised individuals and pet birds.

Enterocytozoon bieneusi

Introduction

This organism is the most common cause of microsporidial infections in humans,[35] predominantly causing diarrhea in people that are immunocompromised as a result of HIV/AIDS. It can also be found in various animal species, including healthy dogs and cats. The role of pets in human infections is unclear and probably minimal, but the potential for zoonotic transmission in households cannot be dismissed.

Etiology

Microsporidia are an incredibly diverse group of unicellular, obligate intracellular eukaryotes that can infect a diverse range of mammals and insects and which have emerged as important opportunistic pathogens in people with HIV/AIDS.[35] Originally, microsporidia were classified within the Archezoa, along with *Giardia*, trichomonads, and *Entamoeba*; however, more recent evidence indicates that they are actually highly derived fungi.[35] The life cycle is as described for *E. cuniculi* above.

Geographic distribution/epidemiology

E. bieneusi is present worldwide.[35] Clinical infections are largely confined to people that are immunocompromised due to HIV/AIDS; however, occasional cases have also been reported in individuals that are immunocompromised for other reasons, particularly organ transplantation.[86,87] Though rare, infections have been diagnosed in apparently immunocompetent, HIV-negative people,[88,89] and it has been suggested that this may be an underreported problem in such individuals because of the typical mild nature of disease, difficulty in diagnosing infection, and lack of routine testing in individuals with mild community-associated diarrhea.[88] In immunocompetent people,

the elderly may be at greatest risk because of the potential for age-related decreases in immune function, although this has not been proven.[35] *E. bieneusi* can also be recovered from a small percentage of nondiarrheic individuals, as was found in a study reporting the organism in feces of 3% of people with HIV/AIDS.[90]

Though first identified in humans, *E. bieneusi* has subsequently been detected in various animal species, particularly pigs.[35,52,91–96] High rates of colonization have been identified in some groups of healthy pigs, particularly in weaner pigs.[97] It was subsequently found in other species such as calves, a goat, a llama, hedgehogs, birds, various fur-bearing animals, horses, and nonhuman primates.[35,52,92–96]

E. bieneusi can be detected in the feces of healthy dogs and cats.[98–100] Prevalence data are limited, but the organism or its DNA has been detected in the feces of 15% of stray dogs in Colombia,[101] 1.7% of stray dogs and 5% pet shop dogs in Japan,[102] and 8.3% of farm dogs in Switzerland.[100] Similarly, *E. bieneusi* DNA was identified in 17% of stray cats in Colombia[103] and 8.3% of cats in Switzerland.[100] Study of pets in households is lacking. Fecal shedding was also identified in 12.5% of captive birds, from a wide range of Psittaciformes, Passeriformes, and Columbiformes.[52] Colonization was reported in 5% of guinea pigs, with an unusual strain that probably originates in guinea pigs but which can also infect humans.[88]

Genotypes found in dogs and cats can be the same as those found in people,[98–103] giving rise to concerns about the potential for zoonotic transmission. Dogs were suggested as the source of infection of an HIV-positive individual infected with both *E. bieneusi* and *E. cuniculi*;[58] however, that was based solely on the person's occupation as a dog groomer, and there is little objective information supporting that hypothesis. The most convincing evidence of zoonotic transmission was a case report that detected the same strain of *E. bieneusi* in an immunocompetent child with intestinal microsporidiosis and in 7/8 pet guinea pigs in the household.[88]

The role of pets in human infections is probably limited, although significant knowledge gaps exist regarding the epidemiology of this pathogen, and the potential for pet-associated infections cannot be excluded.

Risk factors for *E. bieneusi* colonization and infection have not been well characterized, but poor sanitary conditions are presumed to be an important risk factor.[90] Fecal–oral, oral–oral, inhalation of infectious aerosols, and ingestion of contaminated food have all been suggested as possible sources of transmission.[35] The incubation period is unknown.

Animals

Little is known about the potential role of *E. bieneusi* in disease of companion animals. At this time, there is no information indicating whether this organism is a pathogen in pet species. Diagnosis would be as discussed for humans below. No information is available about treatment.

Humans

Clinical presentation

Diarrhea is the most common problem in HIV/AIDS patients, with up to 50% prevalence reported in some groups of diarrheic patients.[35] Diarrhea may range from self-limited to persistent, likely depending in large part on the individual's immune status. Chronic diarrhea may be more common, or, more specifically, *E. bieneusi* may be more commonly involved in chronic versus acute diarrhea.[104,105] Malabsorption and weight loss may also be components of intestinal *E. bieneusi* infection.[5,88] Respiratory disease, particularly rhinitis and bronchitis, has been described, but is uncommon.

Diagnosis

Diagnosis can be difficult because of the small size of the organism and the difficulty of identifying it using visualization techniques. An experienced microscopist can detect microsporidial spores from feces and duodenal aspirates using chromotrope-based stains.[5] Spores can also be detected histologically in intestinal biopsy specimens, but this is obviously not amenable for routine diagnosis in diarrheic individuals. Spores can be identified in tissue sections using various stains, including Giemsa, Gram, periodic acid-Schiff (PAS), and acid-fast. Careful examination is required as spores are easy to miss because of their small size, low stain uptake, and minimal associated inflammatory response in infected tissues.[5] None of these visualization techniques are able to differentiate different microsporidia. PCR has the potential to be a much more sensitive and specific diagnostic tool and will likely become more widely used.

Management

Improvement in immune function is a critical factor and could be the most important aspect of treatment in some individuals. Administration of highly active antiretroviral therapy to HIV/AIDS patients with *E. bieneusi* diarrhea can itself result in remission.[106] If infection is reported in someone without a known immunodeficiency, testing for HIV infection should be done. There is limited objective information regarding optimal treatments. Fumagillin appears to be the drug of choice.[5] Albendazole, the main treatment for *Enterocytozoon intestinalis* infection, is not effective against *E. bieneusi*. In immunocompetent individuals, infection is probably most often mild and self-limited.[88]

Prevention

It is difficult to make objective recommendations for dealing with people that have acquired *E. bieneusi* infection. Testing of pets could be performed, but it is unclear whether the results would be useful. Identification of the organism in pets would not differentiate whether pets were the source of infection, whether humans infected them, whether there may have been a common source of infection, or whether the two are completely unrelated. Genotyping the organism and demonstrating the same strain in a person and a pet provides more information but still cannot differentiate route of transmission or exclude common-source infection. Furthermore, there is currently no information pertaining to the treatment of colonized animals, and treatment of carriers would probably not be indicated. Therefore, testing would not result in any specific information or action, so it is difficult to justify. In human hospitals, contact precautions are recommended only for diapered and incontinent children with *E. bieneusi* diarrhea.[5]

Isolation of affected individuals in households is not warranted but general hygiene practices should be emphasized to reduce the risk of human–human and human–animal transmission.

Screening of healthy pets in households with high-risk individuals is not recommended. Optimal screening methods are not known, nor is adequate information available about the epidemiology of the organism to interpret results. A single negative result could provide a false sense of security, particularly if there is intermittent shedding, frequent reinfection, or suboptimal test sensitivity. There is no indication that positive pets should be removed from households or treated. Furthermore, measures that would be recommended for handling positive pets (avoiding contact with feces, hand hygiene) should be implemented regardless of the pets' *E. bieneusi* status.

The role of the environment in transmission is unclear. Considering the potential fecal–oral route of transmission and association of infection with poor sanitary conditions, the household or hospital environment could be a source of infection, but the true risk is unknown. Microsporidial spores are highly tolerant of environmental effects and disinfectants, and could potentially survive for prolonged periods of time in the environment. They can be inhibited by several disinfectants, including 1 : 30 bleach, 70% ethanol, quaternary ammoniums, and hydrogen peroxide.[107,108]

Histoplasmosis

Histoplasma capsulatum is a dimorphic fungus that is disseminated widely throughout temperate and subtropical regions. Human disease is mainly caused by *H. capsulatum* var. *capsulatum* and *H. capsulatum* var. *duboisii*. *Histoplasma* spp. are similar to other dimorphic yeast in that they live in the environment in the highly infective mold (micelial) phase and are present in the body during infections in the yeast phase. Human exposure is often related to airborne infection from areas contaminated with bird and bat guano. Various clinical presentations can result, including pulmonary and disseminated forms. It has become an important opportunistic infection in immunocompromised individuals, particularly individuals with HIV/AIDS.[109,110]

Of the domestic animals, cats appear to be most prone to infection. Disseminated disease is common and signs may be rather nonspecific. In dogs, disseminated disease with significant gastrointestinal involvement is most common. Histoplasmosis does not appear to have a strong link to immunocompromised dogs and cats. In humans, infection is more common in immunocompromised individuals, though histoplasmosis also occurs in immunocompetent hosts.

Because the yeast phase that is present in infected tissues is minimally infective, direct transmission between animals and humans is very unlikely. Animal-to-human transmission has not been reported. It is plausible that infection could be transmitted by inoculation of yeast phase into a person, as was reported with blastomycosis caused by needlestick injuries. Bite transmission of *Histoplasma* cannot be dismissed but is certainly rare, if it occurs. Proper sharps handling and bite avoidance are prudent in case zoonotic transmission is possible in these limited circumstances. The greatest implication of diagnosis of histoplasmosis in a pet is an indication that humans might also have been exposed from the same source.

Malassezia pachydermatis

Malassezia spp. are lipophilic yeasts that reside predominantly on the skin of mammals. They are common commensals in many species but can cause infections, particularly of the skin. Of the 11 known *Malassezia* spp., only *M. pachydermatis* is associated with rare zoonotic transmission. Most human *Malassezia* infections are caused by species that are human commensals, such as *Malassezia furfur*.

Dogs are considered the natural host of *M. pachydermatis*.[111] Colonization rates of 8–42% have been reported for healthy dogs, with variation in rates between body sites.[111–115] Colonization is most common in the external ear canal, lip, interdigital skin, and anus, and can be occasionally found in the nose and vagina.[116] Low numbers of *Malassezia* are typically present on healthy skin,[117] but numbers can increase greatly in animals with underlying skin disease, particularly allergic disease.[111] This yeast is an opportunistic pathogen that typically causes disease following alterations in the skin's protective mechanisms and an important cause of dermatitis (particularly on the face and in cutaneous folds) and otitis externa.[118] Clinical signs are variable, from erythema and mild pruritis to severe pruritis, alopecia, greasy exudation, and scaling. Secondary excoriation, lichenification, and hyperpigmentation can occur. West Highland white terriers, Basset hounds, poodles, Australian silky terriers, and American cocker spaniels appear to be overrepresented.[118]

While most of the attention regarding *M. pachydermatis* involves dogs, colonization of the external ear of 25–40% of healthy cats has been reported.[114,119]

Because of high colonization rates and frequent contact of humans with the skin of animals, the potential for transmission of *M. pachydermatis* is high. A study of dog owners reported identification of *M. pachydermatis* from the hands of 6% of owners of healthy dogs and 39% of owners of dogs with *M. pachydermatis* dermatitis or otitis.[111] Despite the high likelihood of human exposure to *M. pachydermatis*, the incidence of zoonotic disease is low.

In humans, the greatest risk appears to involve compromised neonates, particularly bloodstream infections in low-birth-weight children receiving intravenous lipid solutions.[120] Outbreaks of invasive *M. pachydermatis* infection have been reported in neonatal intensive care units (NICUs).[120,121] One of these was associated with *M. pachydermatis* colonization of healthcare workers' dogs, and it was hypothesized that *M. pachydermatis* was introduced to the NICU by the hands of dog-owning healthcare workers.[120] Bloodstream infection was also reported in a person with acute myeloid leukemia who had undergone allogenic bone marrow transplantation.[122] Community-onset *M. pachydermatis* infections are very rare.

Because *M. pachydermatis* is a commensal organism that can be found in clinically healthy dogs, complete avoidance of exposure is impossible, especially in the community. While the risk of disease is low in the general population, concerns about zoonotic transmission are reasonable in high-risk populations like hospitalized individuals that have contact with therapy, service, or visitation animals. The lipophilic nature of this organism may be the reason it has been associated with bloodstream infections in people receiving intravenous lipid solutions. Therefore, it is prudent to ensure that there is no direct or indirect contact of dogs with patients receiving intravenous lipids, or at least ensure that contact with the catheter site is strictly prevented and there is close attention to hand hygiene. This would be especially important in patients receiving home total parenteral nutrition (TPN) who have a dog in the house or who have regular contact with dogs. There are no clear guidelines for management of infected or colonized dogs in the community. Given the very low incidence of disease, particularly in immunocompetent individuals, aggressive control measures are not indicated. An emphasis on hygiene, particularly hand hygiene, is probably the most important infection control tool.

Proper diagnosis and treatment of infected animals is required to reduce the period during which infected animals are likely to be carrying a large burden of *M. pachydermatis*. A systematic review concluded that the optimal topical treatment of *M. pachydermatis* dermatitis in dogs is 2% micondazole nitrate and 2% chlorhexidine, twice weekly for 3 weeks.[118] Less evidence was available for systemic therapies, but it was concluded that there is fair evidence of efficacy of two systemic treatments, ketoconazole (10 mg/kg/day) and itraconazole (5 mg/kg/day) for 3 weeks. Objective infection control recommendations are lacking. Good attention to hygiene practices, particularly hand hygiene, is probably the most critical factor. No information is available regarding the risk to immunocompromised individuals in the community. Given the low incidence of disease, aggressive measures are not likely required. Proper hand hygiene after having contact with dogs, avoiding contact with ears, and avoiding contact with sites of skin and/or ear infection are prudent. Screening of healthy pets is not indicated. No recommendations have been made for treatment of colonized (healthy) animals, and it is difficult to envision a situation where that would be indicated.

Pneumocystis

Pneumocystis is a genus of saprophytic fungi that were originally thought to be protozoa. Since its classification as a fungus, it has become clear that this genus contains a group of related species that are rather host specific. *Pneumocystis jiroveci* (formerly *Pneumocystis carinii* f. sp. *hominis*) resides in humans and is the main human health concern. Almost all other mammalian species may harbor at least one *Pneumocystis* species that is not found in other mammals.[123]

Pneumocystis spp. have a tropism for the lung, and in most individuals, colonize alveolar spaces without invading. Human infections with *P. jiroveci* almost exclusively occur in immunocompromised individuals, in whom pneumonia and disseminated infection may develop. While essentially nonpathogenic to immunocompetent individuals, it can cause life-threatening pulmonary infection in immunocompromised patients, including patients receiving high doses of corticosteroids. It is particularly important in people with HIV/AIDS, and *Pneumocystis* pneumonia is considered an AIDS-defining infection in HIV-positive individuals.[124]

Infections of domestic animals are uncommonly reported and typically occur in immunocompromised individuals.[125,126] Colonization with *Pneumocystis* spp. has been identified in various animal species, including cats, mice, guinea pigs, rabbits, and sheep.[127]

Despite the widespread dissemination of *Pneumocystis* spp. in animals and earlier concerns about the potential for zoonotic transmission, improved ability to characterize *Pneumocystis* spp. from animals and humans has led to the conclusion that pneumocystosis is not a zoonotic disease.[128,129]

Sporotrichosis

Introduction

Sporotrichosis is an uncommon fungal disease that affects humans and various animal species, particularly cats. It has often been considered to be of minimal zoonotic potential, but recent evidence indicates that transmission of infection from cats to humans may be a concern. Populations at greatest risk for zoonotic sporotrichosis include veterinarians, veterinary technicians, and owners of infected animals, particularly cats.

Etiology

Sporotrichosis is caused by the dimorphic yeast *Sporothrix schenckii*. As with other dimorphic yeast,

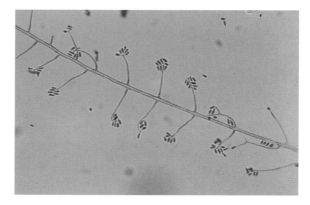

Figure 4.2   *Sporothrix schenkii* mold form from the environment (public domain, Centers for Disease Control and Prevention).

S. schenckii grows in the mycelian (mold) form at ambient temperatures (Figure 4.2) and as a yeast at mammalian body temperatures.

Geographic distribution/epidemiology

S. schenckii can be found worldwide, but most cases of disease are reported in North America. It prefers environments rich in decaying organic debris. Transmission is primarily through traumatic inoculation of tissues with soil or vegetation contaminated with the mold phase. After deposition of *S. schenckii* into tissues, the organism converts into the yeast form. It then reproduces and invades locally, and can also spread via lymphatics.

Disease in animals is most often associated with hunting dogs and dogs and cats that are allowed to roam outdoors. Direct zoonotic transmission can occur through bites or scratches, or contact with draining lesions. Transmission from cats has been reported in the absence of a penetrating wound, and there is increasing evidence that cats may be important sources of sporotrichosis, at least in some regions.[130-133] Caring for sick cats was the main risk factor in evaluation of an outbreak of sporotrichosis in Brazil.[132] Contamination of multiple body sites is typical in infected cats, which may account for the association with zoonotic transmission. One study reported isolation of *S. schenckii* from 66% of nasal cavities, 42% of oral cavities, and 40% of nail beds of cats with sporotrichosis.[134] This clearly demonstrates the potential for transmission associated with bites and scratches. *S. schenckii* has also been isolated from the oral cavity of a small percentage (~4%) of healthy cats that live with infected cats.[135] Isolation of *S. schenckii* from the nasal cavities or nail beds of healthy cats (2%) independent of contact with infected cats was reported in Peru.[136] It is probable that colonization of healthy cats is rare in areas with lower endemic rates. Zoonotic transmission of *S. schenckii* to a veterinarian caring for an infected cat has also been reported.[137]

Animals

Clinical presentation

There are three clinical forms, cutaneous, cutaneolymphatic, and disseminated, with more than one form possibly presenting at the same time. In dogs, cutaneous or cutaneolymphatic disease is most common. Cutaneous sporotrichosis is characterized by multiple dermal and subcutaneous nodules, usually on the trunk or head. Nasal masses may also be present. Ulceration is common and often accompanied by purulent exudates and crusting. In the cutaneolymphatic form, nodules usually start in the distal aspect of one limb, then ascend via lymphatics. Firm nodules are palpable and may ulcerate and drain purulent debris. Regional lymphadenopathy is often present.

The clinical presentation in cats is usually different from that in dogs. Lesions are typically first noted on distal aspects of the limbs, head, and tail base—sites that may be traumatized by thorny vegetation or during cat fights. The initial presentation is often similar to that caused by cat-bite abscesses, draining tracts with localized inflammation. Lymphatic involvement is rarely evident clinically but can be detected at necropsy. The affected areas may then expand and become ulcerated, with associated drainage and crusting. Normal grooming behavior may spread infection to other body sites. Disseminated infection is much more common in cats compared with dogs, and primarily involves the lungs and liver. Coinfection with feline immunodeficiency virus (FIV) may be a risk factor for disseminated disease, but this has not been proven.

Diagnosis

Sporotrichosis is often first suspected based on the appearance of the lesions and lack of response to antibacterial therapy. Cytological examination of exudates may be strongly suggestive, through visualization of pleomorphic yeast-like organisms within macrophages or extracellularly using Wright's stain. The use of PAS or Gomori's methenamine silver (GMS) staining can confirm the presence of a fungus.[134] Visualization of yeast is common in cats but rare in dogs, and negative cytology does not rule out sporotrichosis.[134] Fungal culture can be confirmatory. Samples of exudates from a deep draining tract or pieces of deep, infected tissue are preferred. Histopathology can be a useful adjunctive test, and nodular to diffuse pyogranulomatous inflammation is characteristic. As with cytology, organisms are more commonly found in specimens from cats than dogs. Fluorescent antibody testing of affected tissues can be diagnostic and is particularly useful in dogs. Serological tests are available, but antibodies may simply indicate previous exposure, not active infection.

Management

Supersaturated sodium iodide is commonly used for treatment in dogs. Ketoconazole or itraconazole can be used in dogs that are intolerant of sodium iodide therapy. Treatment of cats can be more difficult because cats are less likely to tolerate sodium iodide therapy. Ketoconazole can be similarly problematic so itraconazole is often used. Months of therapy are required. Concurrent antimicrobial therapy is often required because of secondary bacterial infection.

Humans

Clinical presentation

There are four main forms: lymphocutaneous, fixed cutaneous, disseminated, and extracutaneous. The lymphocutaneous form is most common and is characterized by multiple necrotic, nodular cutaneous lesions, typically over the distal extremities, which follow the lymphatics. Local spread to bones and joints can occur. The fixed cutaneous form has similar appearing skin lesions, but the lesions remain confined to the site of inoculation. Disseminated infection is most common in immunocompromised individuals, alcoholics, and people with comorbidities such as diabetes mellitus, hematologic malignancy, and chronic obstructive pulmonary disease. Visceral, meningeal, and pulmonary sporototrichosis may result. Extracutaneous sporotrichosis is rare and is a deep infection caused by inhalation of *S. schenckii*. Arthritis and tenosynovitis are the most common manifestations.

Diagnosis

Culture is the main diagnostic tool. Histopathology may also be used, but the typically low organism numbers decrease its sensitivity. Antibody testing can be performed but is rarely used clinically because of low diagnostic value.

Management

Detailed information on treatment is available in guidelines published by the Infectious Disease Society of America.[138] Cutaneous sporotrichosis is treated with systemic antifungals, typically itraconazole. Terbinafine or potassium iodide may be used in poorly responsive cases. Fluconazole is usually reserved for patients intolerant of other options. While potentially more toxic, amphotericin B is recommended for extensive or life-threatening infections. Months of therapy are required.

Prevention

Most infections are environmentally acquired, and prevention of zoonotic infections largely involves prevention and proper care of bites and scratches. Prompt cleaning of bite and scratch wounds presumably decreases the risk of disease by removing *S. schenckii* that has been deposited in tissues.

Particular care should be taken around animals with sporotrichosis (and likely also animals in contact with infected animals) because of the high likelihood that they are carrying *S. schenckii* in their mouths and nail beds. In addition to bite and scratch avoidance, measures should be taken to reduce the risk of direct transmission of *S. schenckii*

from the infected site. Transmission can occur without a penetrating wound, so care should be taken around the animal and its environment. Contact with the infected site and bandage material should be avoided as much as possible. If contact is required, such as for bandage changes, the site should be handled carefully while wearing gloves. Hands should be washed thoroughly after glove removal. The same precautions should be taken when handling contaminated bandage material or other items that may have been contaminated, including bedding and cages. Infected sites should be covered with a barrier dressing if at all possible. *S. schenckii* can also be found in feces of infected cats, so careful handling of feces and the use of good hand hygiene is important. The risk of transmission from dogs appears to be much lower, perhaps because *S. schenckii* numbers seem to be lower in affected dogs.

In regions with high levels of endemic sporotrichosis and large feral cat populations, restriction of contact between people and domestic cats with feral cats is important, along with measures to control the feral cat population.

There has been minimal investigation of the susceptibility of *S. schenckii* to disinfectants, but based on extrapolation from other fungi, it is likely susceptible to oxidizing agents (bleach, accelerated stabilized hydrogen peroxide, peroxygens) and some quaternary ammoniums.

References

1. Richarson MD, Hope W. Aspergillus. In: Anaissie EJ, McGinnis MR, Pflaller MA, eds. *Clinical Mycology*, 2nd ed. London: Churchill Livingston Elseview, 2009, pp. 271–296.
2. Day MJ. Canine disseminated aspergillosis. In: Greene CE, ed. *Infectious Diseases of the Dog and Cat*, 3rd ed. Philadelphia: Saunders Elsevier, 2006, pp. 620–626.
3. Gnann JW, Bressler GS, Bodet CA, et al. Human blastomycosis after a dog bite. *Ann Intern Med* 1983;98:48–49.
4. Ramsey D. Blastomycosis in a veterinarian. *J Am Vet Med Assoc* 1994;205:968.
5. American Academy of Pediatrics. *Red Book: 2009 Report of the Committee on Infectious Diseases*, 28th ed. Elk Grove Village, IL: American Academy of Pediatrics, 2009.

6. Smith CE, Saito MT, Beard RR, et al. Histoplasmin sensitivity and coccidioidal infection: 1. Occurrence of cross-reactions. *Am J Public Health Nations Health* 1949;39:722–736.

7. Galgiana J. *Coccidioides* species. In: Mandell GL, Bennett JE, Dolin R, eds. *Principles and Practice of Infectious Diseases*. Philadelphia: Saunders, 2005, pp. 3040–3051.

8. Greene RT. Coccidioidomycosis and paracoccidioidomycosis. In: Greene CE, ed. *Infectious Diseases of the Dog and Cat*. Philadelphia: Saunders Elsevier, 2006, pp. 598–608.

9. Kohn GJ, Linné SR, Smith CM, et al. Acquisition of coccidioidomycosis at necropsy by inhalation of coccidioidal endospores. *Diagn Microbiol Infect Dis* 1992;15:527–530.

10. Gaidici A, Saubolle MA. Transmission of coccidioidomycosis to a human via a cat bite. *J Clin Microbiol* 2009;47:505–506.

11. Viviani MA, Tortorano AM. Cryptococcus. In: Anaissie EJ, McGinnis MR, Pfaller MA, eds. *Clinical Mycology*. London: Churchill Livingstone Elsevier, 2009, pp. 231–250.

12. Shrestha RK, Stoller JK, Honari G, et al. Pneumonia due to *Cryptococcus neoformans* in a patient receiving infliximab: possible zoonotic transmission from a pet cockatiel. *Respir Care* 2004;49:606–608.

13. Lagrou K, Van Eldere J, Keuleers S, et al. Zoonotic transmission of *Cryptococcus neoformans* from a magpie to an immunocompetent patient. *J Intern Med* 2005;257:385–388.

14. Nosanchuk JD, Shoham S, Fries BC, et al. Evidence of zoonotic transmission of *Cryptococcus neoformans* from a pet cockatoo to an immunocompromised patient. *Ann Intern Med* 2000;132:205–208.

15. MacDougall L, Kidd SE, Galanis E, et al. Spread of *Cryptococcus gattii* in British Columbia, Canada, and detection in the Pacific Northwest, USA. *Emerg Infect Dis* 2007;13:42–50.

16. Staib F. Sampling and isolation of *Cryptococcus neoformans* from indoor air with the aid of the Reuter Centrifugal Sampler (RCS) and guizotia abyssinica creatinine agar. A contribution to the mycological-epidemiological control of *Cr. neoformans* in the fecal matter of caged birds. *Zentralbl Bakteriol Mikrobiol Hyg B* 1985;180:567–575.

17. Lugarini C, Goebel CS, Condas LA, et al. *Cryptococcus neoformans* isolated from passerine and psittacine bird excreta in the state of Paraná, Brazil. *Mycopathologia* 2008;166:61–69.

18. Centers for Disease Control and Prevention. *Cryptococcus* (cryptococcosis). 2008. http://www.cdc.gov/nczved/dfbmd/disease_listing/cryptococcus_gi.html.

19. Hay RJ. Dermatophytosis and other superficial mycoses. In: Mandell GL, Bennett JE, Dolin R, eds. *Principles and Practice of Infectious Diseases*. Philadelphia: Elsevier, 2005, pp. 3051–3062.

20. Brilhante RS, Cavalcante CS, Soares-Junior FA, et al. High rate of *Microsporum canis* feline and canine dermatophytoses in Northeast Brazil: epidemiological and diagnostic features. *Mycopathologia* 2003;156:303–308.

21. Cabañes FJ, Abarca ML, Bragulat MR. Dermatophytes isolated from domestic animals in Barcelona, Spain. *Mycopathologia* 1997;137:107–113.

22. Cafarchia C, Romito D, Capelli G, et al. Isolation of *Microsporum canis* from the hair coat of pet dogs and cats belonging to owners diagnosed with *M. canis* tinea corporis. *Vet Dermatol* 2006;17:327–331.

23. Guzman-Chavez RE, Segundo-Zaragoza C, Cervantes-Olivares RA, et al. Presence of keratinophilic fungi with special reference to dermatophytes on the haircoat of dogs and cats in México and Nezahualcoyotl cities. *Rev Latinoam Microbiol* 2000; 42:41–44.

24. Iorio R, Cafarchia C, Capelli G, et al. Dermatophytoses in cats and humans in central Italy: epidemiological aspects. *Mycoses* 2007;50:491–495.

25. Mancianti F, Nardoni S, Cecchi S, et al. Dermatophytes isolated from symptomatic dogs and cats in Tuscany, Italy during a 15-year-period. *Mycopathologia* 2002;156:13–18.

26. Moriello KA, DeBoer DJ. Fungal flora of the coat of pet cats. *Am J Vet Res* 1991;52:602–606.

27. Moriello KA, DeBoer DJ. Fungal flora of the haircoat of cats with and without dermatophytosis. *J Med Vet Mycol* 1991;29:285–292.

28. Drouot S, Mignon B, Fratti M, et al. Pets as the main source of two zoonotic species of the *Trichophyton mentagrophytes* complex in Switzerland, *Arthroderma vanbreuseghemii* and *Arthroderma benhamiae*. *Vet Dermatol* 2009;20:13–18.

29. Rosen T. Hazardous hedgehogs. *South Med J* 2000; 93:936–938.

30. Riley PY, Chomel BB. Hedgehog zoonoses. *Emerg Infect Dis* 2005;11:1–5.

31. Pepin GA, Oxenham M. Zoonotic dermatophytosis (ringworm). *Vet Rec* 1986;118:110–111.

32. de Boer DJ, Moriello KA. Cutaneous fungal infections. In: Greene CE, ed. *Infectious Diseases of the Dog and Cat*, 3rd ed. St. Louis, MO: Saunders Elsevier, 2006, pp. 550–569.

33. Lowinger-Seoane M, Torres-Rodríguez JM, Madrenys-Brunet N, et al. Extensive dermatophytoses caused by *Trichophyton mentagrophytes* and *Microsporum canis* in a patient with AIDS. *Mycopathologia* 1992;120:143–146.

34. Porro AM, Yoshioka MC, Kaminski SK, et al. Disseminated dermatophytosis caused by *Microsporum gypseum* in two patients with the acquired immunodeficiency syndrome. *Mycopathologia* 1997; 137:9–12.

35. Mathis A, Weber R, Deplazes P. Zoonotic potential of the microsporidia. *Clin Microbiol Rev* 2005;18: 423–445.

36. Weiss LM. Microsporidia. In: Mandell GL, Bennett JE, Dolin R, eds. *Principles and Practice of Infectious Diseases*, 6th ed. Philadelphia: Elsevier, 2005, pp. 3237–3253.

37. Matsubayashi H, Koike T, Mikata I, et al. A case of *Encephalitozoon*-like body infection in man. *AMA Arch Pathol* 1959;67:181–187.

38. Orenstein JM, Russo P, Didier ES, et al. Fatal pulmonary microsporidiosis due to *Encephalitozoon cuniculi* following allogeneic bone marrow transplantation for acute myelogenous leukemia. *Ultrastruct Pathol* 2005;29:269–276.

39. Tosoni A, Nebuloni M, Ferri A, et al. Disseminated microsporidiosis caused by *Encephalitozoon cuniculi* III (dog type) in an Italian AIDS patient: a retrospective study. *Mod Pathol* 2002;15:577–583.

40. Weber R, Deplazes P, Flepp M, et al. Cerebral microsporidiosis due to *Encephalitozoon cuniculi* in a patient with human immunodeficiency virus infection. *N Engl J Med* 1997;336:474–478.

41. Dipineto L, Rinaldi L, Santaniello A, et al. Serological survey for antibodies to *Encephalitozoon cuniculi* in pet rabbits in Italy. *Zoonoses Public Health* 2008;55: 173–175.

42. Harcourt-Brown FM, Holloway HK. *Encephalitozoon cuniculi* in pet rabbits. *Vet Rec* 2003;152: 427–431.

43. Igarashi M, Oohashi E, Dautu G, et al. High seroprevalence of *Encephalitozoon cuniculi* in pet rabbits in Japan. *J Vet Med Sci* 2008;70:1301–1304.

44. Künzel F, Gruber A, Tichy A, et al. Clinical symptoms and diagnosis of encephalitozoonosis in pet rabbits. *Vet Parasitol* 2008;151:115–124.

45. Künzel F, Joachim A. Encephalitozoonosis in rabbits. *Parasitol Res* 2009;106:299–309.

46. Akerstedt J. Serological investigation of canine encephalitozoonosis in Norway. *Parasitol Res* 2003; 89:49–52.

47. Lindsay DS, Goodwin DG, Zajac AM, et al. Serological survey for antibodies to *Encephalitozoon cuniculi* in ownerless dogs from urban areas of Brazil and Colombia. *J Parasitol* 2009;95:760–763.

48. Furuya K. Spore-forming microsporidian encephalitozoon: current understanding of infection and prevention in Japan. *Jpn J Infect Dis* 2009;62: 413–422.

49. Halánová M, Cisláková L, Valencáková A, et al. Serological screening of occurrence of antibodies to *Encephalitozoon cuniculi* in humans and animals in Eastern Slovakia. *Ann Agric Environ Med* 2003;10: 117–120.

50. Hollister WS, Canning EU, Viney M. Prevalence of antibodies to *Encephalitozoon cuniculi* in stray dogs as determined by an ELISA. *Vet Rec* 1989;124: 332–336.

51. Pang VF, Shadduck JA. Susceptibility of cats, sheep, and swine to a rabbit isolate of *Encephalitozoon cuniculi*. *Am J Vet Res* 1985;46:1071–1077.

52. Kasicková D, Sak B, Kvác M, et al. Sources of potentially infectious human microsporidia: molecular characterisation of microsporidia isolates from exotic birds in the Czech Republic, prevalence study and importance of birds in epidemiology of the human microsporidial infections. *Vet Parasitol* 2009;165:125–130.

53. Cox JC, Hamilton RC, Attwood HD. An investigation of the route and progression of *Encephalitozoon cuniculi* infection in adult rabbits. *J Protozool* 1979;26:260–265.

54. Rossi P, La Rosa G, Ludovisi A, et al. Identification of a human isolate of *Encephalitozoon cuniculi* type I from Italy. *Int J Parasitol* 1998;28:1361–1366.

55. Didier ES, Visvesvara GS, Baker MD, et al. A microsporidian isolated from an AIDS patient corresponds to *Encephalitozoon cuniculi* III, originally isolated from domestic dogs. *J Clin Microbiol* 1996;34:2835–2837.

56. Mathis A, Michel M, Kuster H, et al. Two *Encephalitozoon cuniculi* strains of human origin are infectious to rabbits. *Parasitology* 1997;114(Pt. 1): 29–35.

57. Teachey DT, Russo P, Orenstein JM, et al. Pulmonary infection with microsporidia after allogeneic bone marrow transplantation. *Bone Marrow Transplant* 2004;33:299–302.

58. Weitzel T, Wolff M, Dabanch J, et al. Dual microsporidial infection with *Encephalitozoon cuniculi* and *Enterocytozoon bieneusi* in an HIV-positive patient. *Infection* 2001;29:237–239.

59. Didier ES, Didier PJ, Snowden KF, et al. Microsporidiosis in mammals. *Microbes Infect* 2000; 2:709–720.

60. Csokai J, Gruber A, Künzel F, et al. Encephalitozoonosis in pet rabbits (*Oryctolagus cuniculus*): pathohistological findings in animals with latent infection versus clinical manifestation. *Parasitol Res* 2009;104:629–635.

61. Snowden KF, Lewis BC, Hoffman J, et al. *Encephalitozoon cuniculi* infections in dogs: a case series. *J Am Anim Hosp Assoc* 2009;45:225–231.

62. Botha WS, van Dellen AF, Stewart CG. Canine encephalitozoonosis in South Africa. *J S Afr Vet Assoc* 1979;50:135–144.

63. Csokai J, Joachim A, Gruber A, et al. Diagnostic markers for encephalitozoonosis in pet rabbits. *Vet Parasitol* 2009;163:18–26.

64. Jass A, Matiasek K, Henke J, et al. Analysis of cerebrospinal fluid in healthy rabbits and rabbits with clinically suspected encephalitozoonosis. *Vet Rec* 2008;162:618–622.

65. Fechle LM, Sigler RL. Phacoemulsification for the management of *Encephalitozoon cuniculi*-induced phacoclastic uveitis in a rabbit. *Vet Ophthalmol* 2002;5:211–215.

66. Bergquist NR, Stintzing G, Smedman L, et al. Diagnosis of encephalitozoonosis in man by serological tests. *Br Med J (Clin Res Ed)* 1984;288:902.

67. Notermans DW, Peek R, de Jong MD, et al. Detection and identification of *Enterocytozoon bieneusi* and *Encephalitozoon* species in stool and urine specimens by PCR and differential hybridization. *J Clin Microbiol* 2005;43:610–614.

68. van Gool T, Biderre C, Delbac F, et al. Serodiagnostic studies in an immunocompetent individual infected with *Encephalitozoon cuniculi*. *J Infect Dis* 2004; 189:2243–2249.

69. Schwartz DA, Visvesvara GS, Diesenhouse MC, et al. Pathologic features and immunofluorescent antibody demonstration of ocular microsporidiosis (*Encephalitozoon hellem*) in seven patients with acquired immunodeficiency syndrome. *Am J Ophthalmol* 1993;115:285–292.

70. Scaglia M, Sacchi L, Croppo GP, et al. Pulmonary microsporidiosis due to *Encephalitozoon hellem* in a patient with AIDS. *J Infect* 1997;34:119–126.

71. Schwartz DA, Visvesvara GS, Leitch GJ, et al. Pathology of symptomatic microsporidial (*Encephalitozoon hellem*) bronchiolitis in the acquired immunodeficiency syndrome: a new respiratory pathogen diagnosed from lung biopsy, bronchoalveolar lavage, sputum, and tissue culture. *Hum Pathol* 1993;24:937–943.

72. Chabchoub N, Abdelmalek R, Mellouli F, et al. Genetic identification of intestinal microsporidia species in immunocompromised patients in Tunisia. *Am J Trop Med Hyg* 2009;80:24–27.

73. Scaglia M, Gatti S, Sacchi L, et al. Asymptomatic respiratory tract microsporidiosis due to *Encephalitozoon hellem* in three patients with AIDS. *Clin Infect Dis* 1998;26:174–176.

74. Snowden K, Logan K. Molecular identification of *Encephalitozoon hellem* in an ostrich. *Avian Dis* 1999;43:779–782.

75. Black SS, Steinohrt LA, Bertucci DC, et al. *Encephalitozoon hellem* in budgerigars (*Melopsittacus undulatus*). *Vet Pathol* 1997;34:189–198.

76. Snowden K, Daft B, Nordhausen RW. Morphological and molecular characterization of *Encephalitozoon hellem* in hummingbirds. *Avian Pathol* 2001;30: 251–255.

77. Suter C, Mathis A, Hoop R, et al. *Encephalitozoon hellem* infection in a yellow-streaked lory (*Chalcopsitta scintillata*) imported from Indonesia. *Vet Rec* 1998;143:694–695.

78. Pulparampil N, Graham D, Phalen D, et al. *Encephalitozoon hellem* in two eclectus parrots (*Eclectus roratus*): identification from archival tissues. *J Eukaryot Microbiol* 1998;45:651–655.

79. Slodkowicz-Kowalska A, Graczyk TK, Tamang L, et al. Microsporidian species known to infect humans are present in aquatic birds: implications for transmission via water? *Appl Environ Microbiol* 2006;72:4540–4544.

80. Tocidlowski ME, Cornish TE, Loomis MR, et al. Mortality in captive wild-caught horned puffin chicks (*Fratercula corniculata*). *J Zoo Wildl Med* 1997;28:298–306.

81. Sak B, Kašičková D, Kváč M, et al. Microsporidia in exotic birds: intermittent spore excretion of *Encephalitozoon* spp. in naturally infected budgerigars (*Melopsittacus undulatus*). *Vet Parasitol* 2009.

82. Childs-Sanford SE, Garner MM, Raymond JT, et al. Disseminated microsporidiosis due to *Encephalitozoon hellem* in an Egyptian fruit bat (*Rousettus aegyptiacus*). *J Comp Pathol* 2006;134:370–373.

83. De Bosschere H, Wang Z, Orlandi PA. First diagnosis of *Encephalitozoon intestinalis* and *E. hellem* in a European brown hare (*Lepus europaeus*) with kidney lesions. *Zoonoses Public Health* 2007;54:131–134.

84. Yee RW, Tio FO, Martinez JA, et al. Resolution of microsporidial epithelial keratopathy in a patient with AIDS. *Ophthalmology* 1991;98:196–201.

85. Friedberg DN, Didier ES, Yee RW. Microsporidal keratoconjunctivitis. *Am J Ophthalmol* 1993;116: 380–381.

86. Goetz M, Eichenlaub S, Pape GR, et al. Chronic diarrhea as a result of intestinal microsposidiosis in a liver transplant recipient. *Transplantation* 2001;71:334–337.

87. Weber R, Bryan RT. Microsporidial infections in immunodeficient and immunocompetent patients. *Clin Infect Dis* 1994;19:517–521.

88. Cama VA, Pearson J, Cabrera L, et al. Transmission of *Enterocytozoon bieneusi* between a child and guinea pigs. *J Clin Microbiol* 2007;45:2708–2710.

89. Wanke CA, DeGirolami P, Federman M. *Enterocytozoon bieneusi* infection and diarrheal disease in patients who were not infected with human immunodeficiency virus: case report and review. *Clin Infect Dis* 1996;23:816–818.

90. Bern C, Kawai V, Vargas D, et al. The epidemiology of intestinal microsporidiosis in patients with

HIV/AIDS in Lima, Peru. *J Infect Dis* 2005;191: 1658–1664.

91. Deplazes P, Mathis A, Müller C, et al. Molecular epidemiology of *Encephalitozoon cuniculi* and first detection of *Enterocytozoon bieneusi* in faecal samples of pigs. *J Eukaryot Microbiol* 1996;43:93S.

92. Haro M, Izquierdo F, Henriques-Gil N, et al. First detection and genotyping of human-associated microsporidia in pigeons from urban parks. *Appl Environ Microbiol* 2005;71:3153–3157.

93. Reetz J, Rinder H, Thomschke A, et al. First detection of the microsporidium *Enterocytozoon bieneusi* in non-mammalian hosts (chickens). *Int J Parasitol* 2002;32:785–787.

94. Rinder H, Thomschke A, Dengjel B, et al. Close genotypic relationship between *Enterocytozoon bieneusi* from humans and pigs and first detection in cattle. *J Parasitol* 2000;86:185–188.

95. Santin-Duran M, Fayer R, Cortes Vecino JA. A zoonotic genotype of *Enterocytozoon bieneusi* in horses. *J Parasitol* 2009. Epub ahead of print.

96. Sulaiman IM, Fayer R, Lal AA, et al. Molecular characterization of microsporidia indicates that wild mammals harbor host-adapted *Enterocytozoon* spp. as well as human-pathogenic *Enterocytozoon bieneusi*. *Appl Environ Microbiol* 2003;69:4495–4501.

97. Breitenmoser AC, Mathis A, Bürgi E, et al. High prevalence of *Enterocytozoon bieneusi* in swine with four genotypes that differ from those identified in humans. *Parasitology* 1999;118(Pt. 5):447–453.

98. Dengjel B, Zahler M, Hermanns W, et al. Zoonotic potential of *Enterocytozoon bieneusi*. *J Clin Microbiol* 2001;39:4495–4499.

99. Lobo ML, Xiao L, Cama V, et al. Genotypes of *Enterocytozoon bieneusi* in mammals in Portugal. *J Eukaryot Microbiol* 2006;53(Suppl. 1):S61–S64.

100. Mathis A, Breitenmoser AC, Deplazes P. Detection of new *Enterocytozoon* genotypes in faecal samples of farm dogs and a cat. *Parasite* 1999;6: 189–193.

101. Santín M, Cortés Vecino JA, Fayer R. *Enterocytozoon bieneusi* genotypes in dogs in Bogota, Colombia. *Am J Trop Med Hyg* 2008;79:215–217.

102. Abe N, Kimata I, Iseki M. Molecular evidence of *Enterocytozoon bieneusi* in Japan. *J Vet Med Sci* 2009;71:217–219.

103. Santín M, Trout JM, Vecino JA, et al. *Cryptosporidium*, *Giardia* and *Enterocytozoon bieneusi* in cats from Bogota (Colombia) and genotyping of isolates. *Vet Parasitol* 2006;141:334–339.

104. Sobottka I, Schwartz DA, Schottelius J, et al. Prevalence and clinical significance of intestinal microsporidiosis in human immunodeficiency virus-infected patients with and without diarrhea in Germany: a prospective coprodiagnostic study. *Clin Infect Dis* 1998;26:475–480.

105. Grohmann GS, Glass RI, Pereira HG, et al. Enteric viruses and diarrhea in HIV-infected patients. Enteric Opportunistic Infections Working Group. *N Engl J Med* 1993;329:14–20.

106. Carr A, Marriott D, Field A, et al. Treatment of HIV-1-associated microsporidiosis and cryptosporidiosis with combination antiretroviral therapy. *Lancet* 1998;351:256–261.

107. Ortega YR, Torres MP, Van Exel S, et al. Efficacy of a sanitizer and disinfectants to inactivate *Encephalitozoon intestinalis* spores. *J Food Prot* 2007;70:681–684.

108. Jordan CN, Dicristina JA, Lindsay DS. Activity of bleach, ethanol and two commercial disinfectants against spores of *Encephalitozoon cuniculi*. *Vet Parasitol* 2006;136:343–346.

109. Baddley JW, Sankara IR, Rodriquez JM, et al. Histoplasmosis in HIV-infected patients in a southern regional medical center: poor prognosis in the era of highly active antiretroviral therapy. *Diagn Microbiol Infect Dis* 2008;62:151–156.

110. Mata-Essayag S, Colella MT, Roselló A, et al. Histoplasmosis: a study of 158 cases in Venezuela, 2000–2005. *Medicine (Baltimore)* 2008;87:193–202.

111. Morris DO. *Malassezia pachydermatis* carriage in dog owners. *Emerg Infect Dis* 2005;11:83–88.

112. Lefebvre S, Waltner-Toews D, Peregrine A, et al. Prevalence of zoonotic agents in dogs visiting hospitalized people in Ontario: implications for infection control. *J Hosp Infect* 2006;62:458–466.

113. Prado MR, Brilhante RS, Cordeiro RA, et al. Frequency of yeasts and dermatophytes from healthy and diseased dogs. *J Vet Diagn Invest* 2008;20:197–202.

114. Cafarchia C, Gallo S, Capelli G, et al. Occurrence and population size of *Malassezia* spp. in the external ear canal of dogs and cats both healthy and with otitis. *Mycopathologia* 2005;160:143–149.

115. Cafarchia C, Gallo S, Romito D, et al. Frequency, body distribution, and population size of *Malassezia* species in healthy dogs and in dogs with localized cutaneous lesions. *J Vet Diagn Invest* 2005;17: 316–322.

116. Bond R, Saijonmaa-Koulumies LE, Lloyd DH. Population sizes and frequency of *Malassezia pachydermatis* at skin and mucosal sites on healthy dogs. *J Small Anim Pract* 1995;36:147–150.

117. Kennis RA, Rosser EJ, Olivier NB, et al. Quantity and distribution of *Malassezia* organisms on the skin of clinically normal dogs. *J Am Vet Med Assoc* 1996;208:1048–1051.

118. Negre A, Bensignor E, Guillot J. Evidence-based veterinary dermatology: a systematic review of interventions for *Malassezia* dermatitis in dogs. *Vet Dermatol* 2009;20:1–12.

119. Dizotti CE, Coutinho SD. Isolation of *Malassezia pachydermatis* and *M. sympodialis* from the external

ear canal of cats with and without otitis externa. *Acta Vet Hung* 2007;55:471–477.

120. Chang HJ, Miller HL, Watkins N, et al. An epidemic of *Malassezia pachydermatis* in an intensive care nursery associated with colonization of health care workers' pet dogs. *N Engl J Med* 1998;338:706–711.

121. Chryssanthou E, Broberger U, Petrini B. *Malassezia pachydermatis* fungaemia in a neonatal intensive care unit. *Acta Paediatr* 2001;90:323–327.

122. Lautenbach E, Nachamkin I, Schuster MG. *Malassezia pachydermatis* infections. *N Engl J Med* 1998;339:270; author reply 271.

123. Pfaller MA, Anaissie EJ. Pneumocystis. In: Anaissie EJ, McGinnis MR, Pfaller MA, eds. *Clinical Mycology*, 2nd ed. London: Churchill Liningstone Elsevier, 2009, pp. 385–402.

124. Antiretroviral Therapy Cohort Collaboration (ART-CC), Mocroft A, Sterne JA, et al. Variable impact on mortality of AIDS-defining events diagnosed during combination antiretroviral therapy: not all AIDS-defining conditions are created equal. *Clin Infect Dis* 2009;48:1138–1151.

125. Hagiwara Y, Fujiwara S, Takai H, et al. *Pneumocystis carinii* pneumonia in a Cavalier King Charles Spaniel. *J Vet Med Sci* 2001;63:349–351.

126. Watson PJ, Wotton P, Eastwood J, et al. Immunoglobulin deficiency in Cavalier King Charles Spaniels with *Pneumocystis pneumonia*. *J Vet Intern Med* 2006;20:523–527.

127. Settnes OP, Hasselager E. Occurrence of *Pneumocystis carinii* Delanoë & Delanoë, 1912 in dogs and cats in Denmark. *Nord Vet Med* 1984;36:179–181.

128. Miller R, Huang L. *Pneumocystis jirovecii* infection. *Thorax* 2004;59:731–733.

129. Sinclair K, Wakefield AE, Banerji S, et al. *Pneumocystis carinii* organisms derived from rat and human hosts are genetically distinct. *Mol Biochem Parasitol* 1991;45:183–184.

130. Barros MB, Costa DL, Schubach TM, et al. Endemic of zoonotic sporotrichosis: profile of cases in children. *Pediatr Infect Dis J* 2008;27:246–250.

131. Barros MB, Schubach Ade O, do Valle AC, et al. Cat-transmitted sporotrichosis epidemic in Rio de Janeiro, Brazil: description of a series of cases. *Clin Infect Dis* 2004;38:529–535.

132. Barros MB, Schubach AO, Schubach TM, et al. An epidemic of sporotrichosis in Rio de Janeiro, Brazil: epidemiological aspects of a series of cases. *Epidemiol Infect* 2008;136:1192–1196.

133. Oliveira-Neto MP, Mattos M, Lazera M, et al. Zoonotic sporothricosis transmitted by cats in Rio de Janeiro, Brazil. A case report. *Dermatol Online J* 2002;8:5.

134. Rosser EJ, Dunstan RW. Sporotrichosis. In: Greene CE, ed. *Infectious Diseases of the Dog and Cat*, 3rd ed. Philadelphia: Elsevier, 2009, pp. 608–612.

135. Schubach TM, de Oliveira Schubach A, dos Reis RS, et al. *Sporothrix schenckii* isolated from domestic cats with and without sporotrichosis in Rio de Janeiro, Brazil. *Mycopathologia* 2002;153:83–86.

136. Kovarik CL, Neyra E, Bustamante B. Evaluation of cats as the source of endemic sporotrichosis in Peru. *Med Mycol* 2008;46:53–56.

137. Reed KD, Moore FM, Geiger GE, et al. Zoonotic transmission of sporotrichosis: case report and review. *Clin Infect Dis* 1993;16:384–387.

138. Kauffman CA, Hajjeh R, Chapman SW. Practice guidelines for the management of patients with sporotrichosis. For the Mycoses Study Group. Infectious Diseases Society of America. *Clin Infect Dis* 2000;30:684–687.

5 Pets and Immunocompromised Individuals

Jason Stull

Introduction

Pet ownership is common. Although the proportion varies by continent and country, most studies have reported that the majority of households own pets (Table 5.1).[1–11] Cats and dogs are the most frequently owned pets, but other species are often reported. The disease risks associated with pet ownership are poorly defined, but for many, zoonotic pathogens risks are highest among specific groups, particularly young children, the elderly, pregnant women, and immunocompromised individuals. Despite this increased risk, pet ownership remains common in these groups. In fact, households with children are more likely to have one or more pets than those without children.[4,12–14] Likewise, animal ownership by immunocompromised individuals appears to be similar to that of the general public.[15,16]

With medical progress and technology, an increasing number of people live with some degree of reduced immune function, and the resulting increased susceptibility to infection. People may be immunocompromised for various reasons, including disease (e.g., human immunodeficiency virus [HIV]/acquired immunodeficiency syndrome [AIDS]), treatment (e.g., cytotoxic chemotherapy, surgery, immunosuppressive therapy following organ transplantation), or other factors (e.g., comorbidities, advanced age). Estimates suggest that the proportion of individuals with some degree of immunodeficiency is high (up to 20% in the United States),[17] with this proportion continuing to increase. As such, animals are frequently a part of households with one or more individuals who are immunosuppressed. While immunocompromised individuals have an increased risk of particular pet-associated zoonotic diseases, they can also greatly benefit from animal companionship. Understanding both the infectious disease risks of pet contact, as well as the health benefits of animal companionship are critical in fully evaluating the impact of pets on the health of immunocompromised individuals and making sound recommendations to effectively reduce disease risks.

The human–animal bond

Distress and social isolation have accompanying psychological changes that can reduce a person's health. Depression and anxiety, for example, can lead to increased activity of the sympatho-adrenal-medulla system and hypothalamic–pituitary–adrenal axis, resulting in increased catecholamine

Companion Animal Zoonoses. Edited by J. Scott Weese and Martha B. Fulford. © 2011 Blackwell Publishing Ltd.

Table 5.1 Proportion of households reporting pet animal ownership by country.

Region/country	Any pet*	Dog*	Cat*	Other*
Africa				
Zimbabwe[1]	NR	62.0	NR	
Australia[2,3]	63	37.8	25.0–25.8	Cat and/or dog (53)
Europe				
Ireland[4]	NR	35.6	10.4[†]	
Italy[5]	46	32.7	15.1	
United Kingdom[6,7]	NR	23–30.6	19–25.5	Indoor fish (10), rabbit (2.6), indoor bird (2.5), guinea pig (1.6), hamster (1.1), horse (0.5), turtle (0.9), gerbil (0.3), snake (0.4), lizard (0.5), rat (0.3)
North America				
Canada[8,9]	56 (cat or dog)	30–32.3	28–35.5	Fish (12), bird (5), rabbit (2), hamster (2), lizard (1), horse (1), guinea pig (1), snake (1), frog (1), turtle (1), ferret (1), gerbil (1)
United States[10]	NR	37.2	32.4	Bird (3.9), horse (1.8)
South America				
Brazil (São Paulo)[11]	NR	52.5	NR	

* Proportion reporting owning one or more.
† Does not include outdoor only.
NR Not measured in the study.

release, corticosteroid release, and decreased myocardial perfusion. This can result in numerous systemic effects, such as immune dysfunction and cardiovascular instability.[18] Activities and relationships that improve psychosocial status and reduce distress and stress responses may thus result in improved human health.

The term "human–animal bond" is used to describe the relationship between people and their pets, and this relationship can influence their respective psychological and physiological states. The mental and physical benefits of the human–animal bond (i.e., pet ownership and companionship) are well established through studies in a variety of age groups and among groups with varying immune functions. The emotional bond between owners and pets can be as important to the owner as human relationships and provide similar psychological benefits.[19] Furthermore, numerous positive health outcomes including reduction in distress, anxiety, loneliness, and depression are associated with animal interaction.[18] Ownership of some animal species (e.g., dogs), increases exercise and thus directly improves owner's health.[18]

Children brought up with companion animals have better social skills, self-esteem, and empathy than children without pets.[20–22] A survey among children with pets found that children were as likely to talk to their pets about their emotions and secret experiences as with their siblings.[13] In adults and the elderly, studies have documented an association between pets and improved health, including a reduced risk of cardiovascular disease,[23] higher survival rates from myocardial infarction,[24] and improved psychological and physical well-being among the elderly.[25]

It is not surprising that the importance of the human–animal bond and its benefits are also well documented in individuals who are immunocompromised. Such individuals may spend considerable time alone, and thus are especially vulnerable to mental and physical illness.[16,18,26,27] Among individuals infected with HIV, domestic animals are often perceived as family members, serve as sources of support and affection, and protect against loneliness.[15,26,27] Siegel et al. reported that among HIV-infected persons, those with AIDS who owned pets reported less depression than persons with AIDS who did not own pets.[16]

Pet-associated zoonotic disease

Despite the established benefits of pet ownership and interaction, companion animals are a potential source of human diseases, as has been highlighted throughout this book. Numerous pet-related risk factors for the acquisition and transmission of zoonotic agents have been identified, including animal species, diet, age, immunity (both natural and vaccine induced), prior antibiotic use, opportunity for exposure (e.g., travel, level of confinement, hospitalization), and immunosuppression.[28] Human-related risk factors for the acquisition of zoonotic agents and clinical course of infection include diet, age, immunity, prior antibiotic use, opportunity for exposure (e.g., hospitalization, occupation, recreational activities), personal hygiene, and immunosuppression.[28] Additional information on pathogen, pet, and human factors is available elsewhere in this text. Here, we focus on the role of human immunosuppression on pet-associated zoonotic disease. The immune system plays a critical role in infectious disease prevention, with defects in one or more components resulting in increased susceptibility to a number of infections. As such, immunocompromised individuals are often at an increased risk of zoonotic diseases, may suffer more severe sequelae, experience symptoms for a longer duration, or experience more severe or unexpected complications than immunocompetent individuals.[17,28–35]

Role of the host immune system in zoonotic disease prevention

A properly functioning immune system is essential for effective defense against infectious organisms. Innate immunity (e.g., phagocytes, complement, natural killer cells, cytokines) and adaptive immunity (e.g., B lymphocytes with resulting antibodies, helper T lymphocytes, cytotoxic T lymphocytes) are both important for responding to invading organisms. In general, cell-mediated (T cell) immunity is primarily responsible for responding to viral, atypical mycobacterial, fungal, and intracellular bacterial infections. Antibody-mediated (B-cell, humoral) immunity is critical for responding to extracellular bacteria, enteric bacteria and viruses, and some parasites.[36] Defects in one or more of these components of the immune system

can lead to serious disorders, termed immunodeficiencies, resulting in an increased risk of pathogen-induced morbidity or mortality. Because the nature of immunodeficiency varies, all immunocompromised individuals are not at the same degree of risk, either in general or for specific pathogens. It is important to remember that, while immunocompromised individuals are often discussed as a single group, they are truly a heterogeneous population with variable risks. The level of infection risk and particular pathogens of greatest risk are a function of the degree of immunosuppression and specific immune components affected.

Immunodeficiencies are broadly classified as either congenital or acquired. Congenital (primary) immunodeficiencies are genetic X-linked or primary autosomal defects that include defects in innate immunity (e.g., phagocytes or complement), defects in B-cell development and activation, defects in T-cell activation and function, and severe combined immunodeficiencies (SCIDs; deficiencies of both B and T cells). Estimates suggest that in the United States, approximately 1 in 500 individuals is born with a defect in one or more components of the immune system; however, only a small proportion are affected severely enough to result in life-threatening complications.[28,36]

Acquired immunodeficiencies are much more common causes of immune dysfunction.[36] Acquired (secondary) immunodeficiencies develop as a consequence of nongenetic causes. Numerous biological disorders, normal physiological states (e.g., pregnancy), and drugs cause various degrees of immunosuppression. Acquired immunodeficiencies include (1) drug- and radiation-associated immunosuppression (via reduced lymphocyte precursors and activation), (2) infectious diseases (e.g., HIV), (3) metabolic diseases (e.g., diabetes mellitus; metabolic derangements inhibiting lymphocyte maturation and function), (4) splenectomy (via decreased phagocytosis of microbes), (5) hematopoietic and solid organ cancers, and (6) physiological factors (e.g., malnutrition, extremes of age, and pregnancy).[28,36,37]

Based on the numbers of organ transplant recipients and individuals infected with HIV, it is estimated that 3.6% of the U.S. human population has an acquired immunodeficiency.[38,39] When additional groups are added, such as the elderly and pregnant women, up to 20% of the U.S. population has some degree of immunosuppression.[17] Similar statistics likely apply to most developed countries, and it is likely this proportion will increase in future years due to advances in life-prolonging treatments, such as chemotherapeutic agents and immunosuppressive drugs.

Factors associated with occurrence and severity of human immunosuppression

Most immunodeficiencies are acquired, with many occurring as a result of infection with HIV or due to hematopoietic and solid organ cancers or their treatments. For hematopoietic and solid organ cancers, several variables have been determined to be important predictors for immunosuppression and risk factors for subsequent opportunistic infection, including age at diagnosis, CD4+ count or percentage, disease duration and stage, dose, duration, sequence and type of therapy used, number of previous regimens of therapy, time since organ/stem cell transplantation, breech in mucocutaneous integrity (e.g., vascular and urinary catheters), use of prophylaxis (e.g., antimicrobials and immunoglobulin), and use of immunomodulators (e.g., growth factors).[40–42] For organ transplant recipients, the greatest risk of infection occurs during the first 6 months after transplantation (the time prior to tapering of immunosuppressive therapy) or when immunosuppression is augmented following episodes of transplant rejection.[43] During this period, there are defined windows when particular pathogens from specific sources tend to occur (e.g., within the first month of transplant: preexisting organisms [colonization], antimicrobial-resistant species, hospital-associated pathogens;[44,45] 1–6 months posttransplant: viral pathogens and reactivated infections; greater than 6 months posttransplant: community-acquired pneumonia and urinary tract infections).[42] Similarly, recipients of hematopoietic stem cell transplants follow a predictable course of immunosuppression: (1) damaged mucocutaneous barriers and neutropenia during the first 30 days posttransplant, (2) impaired cellular immunity between 31 and 100 days posttransplant, and (3) impaired cellular and humoral immunity after 100 days posttransplant. For at least 1 year after transplantation, indi-

viduals remain predisposed to opportunistic infections.[46] Individuals are presumed immunocompetent at 24 months posttransplant, assuming they are not on immunosuppressive therapy and do not have graft-versus-host disease.[31] Research to date suggests CD4+ counts provide the best marker for the restoration of immune competence following transplant,[46] although in children, CD4+ percentage is preferable as the actual cell count is heavily influenced by age.[47]

Since its identification in the early 1980s, HIV infection has been responsible for a large proportion of individuals with acquired immunodeficiencies. HIV infection results in a depletion of CD4+ helper T cells and functional impairment of macrophages, thereby increasing susceptibility to a number of opportunistic infections, including cryptosporidiosis, recurrent *Salmonella* septicemia, and reactivation of latent toxoplasmosis. The recent adoption of highly active antiretroviral therapy (HAART) has had a dramatic effect on reducing immunosuppression in HIV-infected individuals.[48] The decrease in immunosuppression and use of antimicrobial prophylaxis has resulted in a significant reduction in the incidence of opportunistic infections (e.g., bacteremia decreased from 11.8 cases per 100 person-years to 6.3 cases per 100 person-years [$p = 0.0001$][49] and recurrent nontyphoid *Salmonella* bacteremia decreased from 70 cases per 100 person-years to 3 cases per 100 person-years [$p < 0.001$]).[50] A combination of CD4+ percentage or counts and HIV-1 viral load appears to be the best predictor of future disease progression and mortality in both HIV-infected adults and children.[51]

Pet-associated zoonotic pathogens affecting immunosuppressed individuals

Although many pathogens are capable of being transmitted from animals to humans, the pathogens cited as a particular concern for pet-associated infections are less numerous. Key pet-associated pathogens relevant to immunocompromised individuals are presented in Table 5.2. These pathogens vary in their environmental stability, mode of transmission, and animal prevalence, as well as characteristics that may differ for immunocompetent and compromised individuals, including

Table 5.2   Examples of pet-associated infections particularly relevant to immunocompromised individuals.

Infectious agent	Frequency or risk in immunocompromised individuals	Common clinical manifestations in general population (and immunocompromised)	Other comments
Toxoplasma gondii	Moderate; incidence of *Toxoplasma* encephalitis of 2.2% in HIV-infected individuals[76]	Subclinical or self-limited febrile illness (greater risk for in utero infection, encephalitis)	Most cases among transplant recipients caused by reactivation (3–26 weeks posttransplant); food and environment are main sources of human infection
Cryptosporidium spp.	Moderate; 3–6% of HIV-infected individuals; risk increases with degree of immunosuppression and is largely limited to those with impaired T-cell function (e.g., acute leukemia and lymphoma)[77]	Subclinical or self-limiting diarrhea (chronic intractable diarrhea, shortened survival; symptoms dependent on immune status and genotype/ species of infection)[78]	All species identified in companion animals should be considered potentially zoonotic in immunocompromised individuals[37,78]
Salmonella spp.	Low; incidence of bacteremia 20- to 100-fold higher among HIV-infected than among HIV uninfected individuals[50]	Self-limiting diarrhea, vomiting (higher rates of bacteremia, severe systemic and localized infections)[79]	Chemotherapy-triggered reactivation of asymptomatic colonization occurs[80]
Campylobacter jejuni	Low; greater rate in patients with hematologic malignancy versus without malignancy (incidence rate ratio=2.17)[56]	Self-limiting diarrhea, vomiting, fever (relapses of septicemia and diarrhea)	
Bartonella henselae	Low, but perhaps underdiagnosed	Lymphadenopathy and fever (bacteremia; proliferative lesions on the skin, liver, or spleen)	Hospitalization rate for general pediatric population under 5 years is 0.86 per 100,000 children[32]
Giardia intestinalis	Low	Subclinical or mild diarrhea (chronic diarrhea, weight loss)	
Bordetella bronchiseptica	Rare	Generally none (respiratory disease in children with lung transplants, those treated with immunosuppressive drugs, and HIV infected)[37]	
Capnocytophaga canimorsus	Rare	Generally none (sepsis, disseminated intravascular coagulation, death especially among asplenic persons, those of advanced age, or alcoholics)	Most relevant for splenectomized or functionally asplenic individuals

human prevalence, infectious dose necessary to colonize or infect individuals, severity of sequelae, and duration of sequelae.[17,28–35] Some pet-associated pathogens occur predominantly in immunocompromised individuals (e.g., *Capnocytophaga canimorsus*), while others occur in both immunocompetent and compromised individuals with the severity of illness or risk of infection increased in those with immune suppression (e.g., *Salmonella* spp.).

As most of these pathogens are potentially transmitted through several routes and from various sources, it is difficult to determine the burden of disease in people attributable to pets. In the studies that have attempted to define the epidemiology of these diseases, the pet-associated disease burden in immunocompromised individuals is often difficult to quantify as they (1) lack a control group (e.g., case series),[52–55] (2) do not assess pet exposure for those with and without disease,[56–59] or (3) do not target immunocompromised individuals.[60,61] The author is aware of two studies that do attempt to evaluate pet-associated disease burden in immunocompromised individuals through observational study designs.[62,63] These two studies attempted to evaluate the role of pet/animal exposure among HIV-infected individuals in *Cryptosporidium* infection[63] and infection with enteric parasites (coccidia, protozoa, and helminths).[62] Exposure to animals during the previous 3 months was a significant risk factor for the detection of enteric parasites (odds ratio [OR]=8.8 [95% confidence interval {CI}: 3.8–21.7; $p<0.001$]),[62] and dog ownership was nearly significant (OR=2.19, $p=0.05$) in *Cryptosporidium* infection.[63] Unfortunately, several methodological issues, including small sample size,[63] potential misclassification bias by combining zoonotic and nonzoonotic species into a single outcome variable[62,63] and by combining different animal species (e.g., dogs, cows, pigs), and types of contact into a single exposure variable,[62] make it difficult to appropriately interpret these studies and generalize findings to other populations. The true scope of pet-associated zoonoses in immunocompromised individuals is poorly understood.

Zoonotic disease knowledge, attitudes, and practices of immunocompromised individuals

A key component to successful disease prevention programs is ensuring those at risk receive accurate, timely advice on methods to remove or reduce risk. Several studies have evaluated zoonotic disease knowledge, pet ownership attitudes, and disease prevention practices for the general population or medical professionals (e.g., physicians and veterinarians).[64–72] These studies have revealed that many individuals in the general population

lack even basic knowledge about zoonotic diseases (e.g., only 63% of household heads believed diseases of pets could be transmitted to humans;[72] only 56% of dog owners in a Texas U.S. survey knew intestinal helminths could be transmitted from dogs to humans)[69] and the majority of veterinarians and physicians did not regularly discuss zoonotic disease risks with clients/patients.[64–66,68] Few studies have specifically targeted the knowledge base and practices of immunocompromised individuals, but available data suggest that animal-ownership practices of immunocompromised individuals are similar to those of the general public.[15,16] A previous study[15] revealed that 46% (187/408) of HIV-infected adults were living or had lived with a companion animal in the past 5 years (dog 38%, cat 15%, fish 8%, bird 8%, reptile 3%, rodent 2%; categories not mutually exclusive). Of those with pets, 25% had more than one pet. In addition, only 10% of respondents reported being informed about zoonotic diseases by healthcare workers. The lack of physician-derived education for immunocompromised individuals may, in part, be due to physicians not being aware of patients' pet ownership or contact habits.[65] Physicians are usually aware of their patient's immune status and, if knowledgeable on the subject and inquire about pet ownership and contact, are able to educate and inform the patient about preventing zoonotic diseases. This does not appear to be the case for the veterinary profession. In a study conducted by Grant and Olsen, 66% (205/310) of veterinarians were not aware of their clients' immune status.[64] Without knowledge of a client's immune status, targeted education about zoonotic disease prevention is difficult. The above studies highlight the need for targeted education for immunocompromised individuals and the importance of critically evaluating and improving physician- and veterinarian-based education efforts to this group.

Existing recommendations for reducing zoonotic pathogen transmission from pets to immunocompromised individuals

Several resources provide recommendations for reducing zoonotic pathogen transmission from pets to immunocompromised individuals. These guidelines, based on clinical experience and knowledge of the mode(s) and general risk factors for transmission, are presented in both national guidelines for the treatment and prevention of particular diseases[31,32] and review articles.[17,34,73–75] Given the established health benefits of animal ownership and reluctance of most individuals to give up their pets, resources now highlight the importance of following a number of simple animal-contact precautions, and reserve discouraging animal ownership and contact only for particular high-risk circumstances (e.g., animals considered to be frequently colonized or infected with enteric zoonotic pathogens such as young animals, animals with diarrhea, and particular animal species, such as reptiles and amphibians). Pet contact guidelines can be categorized into (1) pet health and husbandry practices, (2) personal hygiene, and (3) types and ages of animals (Table 5.3). Despite the availability of existing guidelines, it is unclear how

Table 5.3 General recommendations for reducing zoonotic pathogen transmission from pets to immunocompromised individuals.[17,31,32,34,73–75,81,82]

Personal hygiene
- Wash hands after handling animals or their environment; supervise hand washing for children under 5 years
- Avoid contact with pets' feces
- Avoid contact with animal-derived pet treats
- Promptly wash bites and scratches from animals
- Do not allow pets to lick open wounds or cuts
- Wear shoes, socks, long pants, and long-sleeved shirts when farming or working in gardens
- Wear gloves to clean aquariums; do not dispose of aquarium water in bathroom or kitchen sinks
- Ensure playground sandboxes are kept covered when not in use

Types and ages of animals
- Avoid contact with dogs and cats less than 6 months of age or strays (avoid acquiring a cat less than 1 year of age)
- Avoid contact with animals with diarrhea
- Avoid contact with young farm animals (e.g., petting zoos)
- Avoid contact with reptiles, amphibians, rodents, ferrets, baby poultry (chicks and ducklings), and anything that has been in contact with these animals; preferably, these animals should be kept out of the households of immunocompromised individuals
- Reptiles, amphibians, rodents, and baby poultry should not be permitted to roam freely through a home or living area and should be kept out of kitchens and food preparation areas
- Exercise caution when playing with cats to limit scratches; keep cats' nails short (declawing in not a recommended procedure)
- When acquiring a new pet, seek larger, mature animals from established vendors as these pose a lower risk than other types of animals
- Avoid contact with exotic pets and nonhuman primates
- When visiting other households with pets, take the same precautions with those pets
- Consider waiting to acquire a new pet until after the patient is on stable immune suppression (solid organ transplant recipients: at least 1 year after transplant; stem cell transplant recipients: at least 6 months after transplant); those who work with animals (veterinarians, laboratory workers, pet store employees, farmers, or slaughterhouse workers) should minimize working during periods of maximal immunosuppression
- Consider limiting contact with animals in medical settings (e.g., therapy and visitation animals)

Pet health and husbandry
- Spay/neuter to reduce the likelihood of infectious pathogen transmission through reproductive tract secretions
- Keep cats indoors; change litter boxes daily (preferably done by an immunocompetent person) and keep cats away from kitchens or other areas where food preparation and eating occur
- Keep dogs confined when possible; walk on leash to prevent hunting, coprophagia, and garbage eating
- Feed only canned or dried commercial food or well-cooked home-prepared food; any dairy products should be pasteurized
- Prohibit access to nonpotable water, such as surface water or toilet bowls
- Routine preventative care, including steps to control and prevent ecto- and endoparasites as indicated by the area
- Clean bird cage linings daily; wear disposable gloves (+/– surgical mask) when handling
- Clean small rodent cages frequently
- Regularly (e.g., weekly) launder pet bedding
- Seek veterinary care at first sign of illness in an animal

often these recommendations are provided to patients. A recent survey distributed to all pediatric oncology centers in the United Kingdom ($n = 22$) found that only four of the centers stated they used published or locally developed materials when providing guidelines for pet ownership.[67]

Conclusions

Pets play an important role in health and disease of immunocompromised individuals. Although a number of pathogens can be transmitted to immunocompromised people from their pets, the cost versus benefit of pet ownership must be thoughtfully considered. Following existing guidelines can reduce the risk of zoonoses. With an increasing number of immunocompromised individuals in the population, many with pets, it is more important than ever for both physicians and veterinarians to obtain information on household pet- and human-related risk factors for zoonotic transmission and to educate patients/clients. Early and frequent zoonotic disease discussions with pet owners can help them make informed decisions and implement appropriate precautions. Veterinarians and physicians should work together as part of the overall healthcare team to optimize the health and welfare of people and their pets.

References

1. Butler JR, Bingham J. Demography and dog-human relationships of the dog population in Zimbabwean communal lands. *Vet Rec* 2000;147(16):442–446.
2. Baldock FC, Alexander L, More SJ. Estimated and predicted changes in the cat population of Australian households from 1979 to 2005. *Aust Vet J* 2003;81(5): 289–292.
3. Hill M. *Contribution of the Pet Care Industry to Australian Economy*. North Sydney, NSW, Australia: Australian Companion Animal Council, 2006, 6th ed. Accessed April 3, 2010.
4. Downes M, Canty MJ, More SJ. Demography of the pet dog and cat population on the island of Ireland and human factors influencing pet ownership. *Prev Vet Med* 2009;92(1–2):140–149.
5. Slater MR, Di Nardo A, Pediconi O, et al. Cat and dog ownership and management patterns in central Italy. *Prev Vet Med* 2008;85(3–4):267–294.
6. Murray JK, Browne WJ, Roberts MA, et al. Number and ownership profiles of cats and dogs in the UK. *Vet Rec* 2010;166(6):163–168.
7. Pet Food Manufacturer's Association. Pet population figures 10. 2010. www.pfma.org.uk/overall/pet-population-figures-.htm. Accessed April 3, 2010.
8. Perrin T. The business of urban animals survey: the facts and statistics on companion animals in Canada. *Can Vet J* 2009;50(1):48–52.
9. Leger Marketing. *Canadians and Their Pets*. Montreal, Quebec, Canada: Leger Marketing, 2002. Accessed April 3, 2010.
10. American Veterinary Medical Association. *U.S. Pet Ownership & Demographics Sourcebook*. Schaumburg, IL: American Veterinary Medical Association, 2007.
11. Alves MC, Matos MR, Reichmann Mde L, et al. Estimation of the dog and cat population in the state of Sao Paulo. *Rev Saude Publica* 2005;39(6):891–897.
12. Brandt JC, Grabill CM. Communicating with special populations: children and older adults. *Vet Clin North Am Small Anim Pract* 2007;37(1):181–198.
13. Melson GF. Child development and the human–companion animal bond. *Am Behav Sci* 2003; 47(1):31–39.
14. Leslie BE, Meek AH, Kawash GF, et al. An epidemiological investigation of pet ownership in Ontario. *Can Vet J* 1994;35(4):218–222.
15. Conti L, Lieb S, Liberti T, et al. Pet ownership among persons with AIDS in three Florida counties. *Am J Public Health* 1995;85(11):1559–1561.
16. Siegel JM, Angulo FJ, Detels R, et al. AIDS diagnosis and depression in the multicenter AIDS cohort study: the ameliorating impact of pet ownership. *AIDS Care* 1999;11(2):157–170.
17. Trevejo RT, Barr MC, Robinson RA. Important emerging bacterial zoonotic infections affecting the immunocompromised. *Vet Res* 2005;36(3): 493–506.
18. Friedmann E, Son H. The human–companion animal bond: how humans benefit. *Vet Clin North Am Small Anim Pract* 2009;39(2):293–326.
19. McNicholas J, Gilbey A, Rennie A, et al. Pet ownership and human health: a brief review of evidence and issues. *BMJ* 2005;331(7527):1252–1254.
20. Reaser JK, Clark EE, Jr., Meyers NM. All creatures great and minute: a public policy primer for companion animal zoonoses. *Zoonoses Public Health* 2008; 55(8–10):385–401.
21. Poresky RH, Hendrix C. Differential effects of pet presence and pet-bonding on young children. *Psychol Rep* 1990;67(1):51–54.
22. Melson GF, Schwarz RL, Beck AM. Importance of companion animals in children's lives—implications for veterinary practice. *J Am Vet Med Assoc* 1997; 211(12):1512–1518.

23. Patronek GJ, Glickman LT. Pet ownership protects against the risks and consequences of coronary heart disease. *Med Hypotheses* 1993;40(4):245–249.

24. Friedmann E, Thomas SA. Pet ownership, social support, and one-year survival after acute myocardial infarction in the cardiac arrhythmia suppression trial (CAST). *Am J Cardiol* 1995;76(17):1213–1217.

25. Raina P, Waltner-Toews D, Bonnett B, et al. Influence of companion animals on the physical and psychological health of older people: an analysis of a one-year longitudinal study. *J Am Geriatr Soc* 1999;47(3):323–329.

26. Castelli P, Hart LA, Zasloff RL. Companion cats and the social support systems of men with AIDS. *Psychol Rep* 2001;89(1):177–187.

27. Carmack BJ. The role of companion animals for persons with AIDS/HIV. *Holist Nurs Pract* 1991;5(2):24–31.

28. Robinson RA. Zoonoses and immunosuppressed populations. In: Macpherson CNL, Meslin FX, Wandeler AI, eds. *Dogs, Zoonoses, and Public Health.* New York: CABI, 2001, pp. 273–297.

29. Celum CL, Chaisson RE, Rutherford GW, et al. Incidence of salmonellosis in patients with AIDS. *J Infect Dis* 1987;156(6):998–1002.

30. Sorvillo FJ, Lieb LE, Waterman SH. Incidence of campylobacteriosis among patients with AIDS in Los Angeles County. *J Acquir Immune Defic Syndr* 1991;4(6):598–602.

31. Centers for Disease Control and Prevention, Infectious Disease Society of America, American Society of Blood and Marrow Transplantation. Guidelines for preventing opportunistic infections among hematopoietic stem cell transplant recipients. *MMWR Recomm Rep* 2000;49(RR-10):1–125, CE1–7.

32. Mofenson LM, Brady MT, Danner SP, et al. Guidelines for the prevention and treatment of opportunistic infections among HIV-exposed and HIV-infected children: recommendations from CDC, the National Institutes of Health, the HIV Medicine Association of the Infectious Diseases Society of America, the Pediatric Infectious Diseases Society, and the American Academy of Pediatrics. *MMWR Recomm Rep* 2009;58(RR-11):1–166.

33. Ciepielewska D, Zelenay E. Salmonelloses in children with proliferative haematological diseases. *Mater Med Pol* 1991;23(3):223–225.

34. Glaser CA, Angulo FJ, Rooney JA. Animal-associated opportunistic infections among persons infected with the human immunodeficiency virus. *Clin Infect Dis* 1994;18(1):14–24.

35. Hohmann EL. Nontyphoidal salmonellosis. *Clin Infect Dis* 2001;32(2):263–269.

36. Abbas AK, Lichtman AH, Pillai S. Congenital and acquired immunodeficiencies. In: Abbas AK, Lichtman AH, Pillai S, eds. *Cellular and Molecular Immunology*, 6th ed. Philadelphia: Saunders, 2007, pp. 463–488.

37. Mani I, Maguire JH. Small animal zoonoses and immunocompromised pet owners. *Top Companion Anim Med* 2009;24(4):164–174.

38. Taylor LH, Latham SM, Woolhouse ME. Risk factors for human disease emergence. *Philos Trans R Soc Lond B Biol Sci* 2001;356(1411):983–989.

39. Kemper AR, Davis MM, Freed GL. Expected adverse events in a mass smallpox vaccination campaign. *Eff Clin Pract* 2002;5(2):84–90.

40. Morrison VA. Management of infectious complications in patients with chronic lymphocytic leukemia. *Hematology Am Soc Hematol Educ Program* 2007;40(1):332–338.

41. Engelhard D, Akova M, Boeckh MJ, et al. Bacterial infection prevention after hematopoietic cell transplantation. *Bone Marrow Transplant* 2009;44(8):467–470.

42. Fishman JA, Infectious AST. Diseases Community of Practice. Introduction: infection in solid organ transplant recipients. *Am J Transplant* 2009;9(Suppl. 4):S3–S6.

43. Fishman JA. Infection in solid-organ transplant recipients. *N Engl J Med* 2007;357(25):2601–2614.

44. Garzoni C. AST Infectious Diseases Community of Practice. Multiply resistant gram-positive bacteria methicillin-resistant, vancomycin-intermediate and vancomycin-resistant *Staphylococcus aureus* (MRSA, VISA, VRSA) in solid organ transplant recipients. *Am J Transplant* 2009;9(Suppl. 4):S41–S49.

45. Dubberke ER, Riddle DJ. AST Infectious Diseases Community of Practice. *Clostridium difficile* in solid organ transplant recipients. *Am J Transplant* 2009;9(Suppl. 4):S35–S40.

46. Mackall C, Fry T, Gress R, et al. Background to hematopoietic cell transplantation, including post transplant immune recovery. *Bone Marrow Transplant* 2009;44(8):457–462.

47. Gona P, Van Dyke RB, Williams PL, et al. Incidence of opportunistic and other infections in HIV-infected children in the HAART era. *JAMA* 2006;296(3):292–300.

48. Hung CC, Chang SC. Impact of highly active antiretroviral therapy on incidence and management of human immunodeficiency virus-related opportunistic infections. *J Antimicrob Chemother* 2004;54(5):849–853.

49. Tumbarello M, Tacconelli E, Donati KG, et al. HIV-associated bacteremia: how it has changed in the highly active antiretroviral therapy (HAART) era. *J Acquir Immune Defic Syndr* 2000;23(2):145–151.

50. Hung C, Hung M, Hsueh P, et al. Risk of recurrent nontyphoid *Salmonella* bacteremia in HIV-infected

patients in the era of highly active antiretroviral therapy and an increasing trend of fluoroquinolone resistance. *Clin Infect Dis* 2007;45(5):e60–e67.

51. Ylitalo N, Brogly S, Hughes MD, et al. Risk factors for opportunistic illnesses in children with human immunodeficiency virus in the era of highly active antiretroviral therapy. *Arch Pediatr Adolesc Med* 2006; 160(8):778–787.

52. Colford JM, Jr., Tager IB, Hirozawa AM, et al. Cryptosporidiosis among patients infected with human immunodeficiency virus. Factors related to symptomatic infection and survival. *Am J Epidemiol* 1996;144(9):807–816.

53. Gruenewald R, Blum S, Chan J. Relationship between human immunodeficiency virus infection and salmonellosis in 20- to 59-year-old residents of New York City. *Clin Infect Dis* 1994;18(3):358–363.

54. Novak R, Feldman S. Salmonellosis in children with cancer: review of 42 cases. *Am J Dis Child* 1979;133(3): 298–300.

55. Dworkin MS, Sullivan PS, Buskin SE, et al. *Bordetella bronchiseptica* infection in human immunodeficiency virus-infected patients. *Clin Infect Dis* 1999;28(5): 1095–1099.

56. Gradel KO, Norgaard M, Dethlefsen C, et al. Increased risk of zoonotic *Salmonella* and *Campylobacter* gastroenteritis in patients with haematological malignancies: a population-based study. *Ann Hematol* 2009;88(8):761–767.

57. Sorvillo F, Beall G, Turner PA, et al. Seasonality and factors associated with cryptosporidiosis among individuals with HIV infection. *Epidemiol Infect* 1998; 121(1):197–204.

58. Rongkavilit C, Rodriguez ZM, Gomez-Marin O, et al. Gram-negative bacillary bacteremia in human immunodeficiency virus type 1-infected children. *Pediatr Infect Dis J* 2000;19(2):122–128.

59. Rao Ajjampur SS, Asirvatham JR, Muthusamy D, et al. Clinical features & risk factors associated with cryptosporidiosis in HIV infected adults in India. *Indian J Med Res* 2007;126(6):553–557.

60. Studahl A, Andersson Y. Risk factors for indigenous *Campylobacter* infection: a Swedish case-control study. *Epidemiol Infect* 2000;125(2):269–275.

61. Tenkate TD, Stafford RJ. Risk factors for *Campylobacter* infection in infants and young children: a matched case-control study. *Epidemiol Infect* 2001;127(3): 399–404.

62. Dwivedi KK, Prasad G, Saini S, et al. Enteric opportunistic parasites among HIV infected individuals: associated risk factors and immune status. *Jpn J Infect Dis* 2007;60(2–3):76–81.

63. Glaser CA, Safrin S, Reingold A, et al. Association between *Cryptosporidium* infection and animal exposure in HIV-infected individuals. *J Acquir Immune Defic Syndr Hum Retrovirol* 1998;17(1):79–82.

64. Grant S, Olsen CW. Preventing zoonotic diseases in immunocompromised persons: the role of physicians and veterinarians. *Emerg Infect Dis* 1999;5(1):159–163.

65. von Matthiessen PW, Sansone RA, Meier BP, et al. Zoonotic diseases and at-risk patients: a survey of veterinarians and physicians. *AIDS* 2003;17(9): 1404–1406.

66. Lipton BA, Hopkins SG, Koehler JE, et al. A survey of veterinarian involvement in zoonotic disease prevention practices. *J Am Vet Med Assoc* 2008;233(8): 1242–1249.

67. Hemsworth S, Pizer B. Pet ownership in immunocompromised children—a review of the literature and survey of existing guidelines. *Eur J Oncol Nurs* 2006;10(2):117–127.

68. Stull JW, Carr AP, Chomel BB, et al. Small animal deworming protocols, client education, and veterinarian perception of zoonotic parasites in western Canada. *Can Vet J* 2007;48(3):269–276.

69. Bingham GM, Budke CM, Slater MR. Knowledge and perceptions of dog-associated zoonoses: Brazos County, Texas, USA. *Prev Vet Med* 2010;93(2–3): 211–221.

70. Pfukenyi DM, Chipunga SL, Dinginya L, et al. A survey of pet ownership, awareness and public knowledge of pet zoonoses with particular reference to roundworms and hookworms in Harare, Zimbabwe. *Trop Anim Health Prod* 2010;42(2):247–252.

71. Villar RG, Connick M, Barton LL, et al. Parent and pediatrician knowledge, attitudes, and practices regarding pet-associated hazards. *Arch Pediatr Adolesc Med* 1998;152(10):1035–1037.

72. Fontaine RE, Schantz PM. Pet ownership and knowledge of zoonotic diseases in De Kalb County, Georgia. *Anthrozoos* 1988;3(1):45–49.

73. Avery RK, Michaels MG. Strategies for safe living following solid organ transplantation. *Am J Transplant* 2009;9(Suppl. 4):S252–S257.

74. Angulo FJ, Glaser CA, Juranek DD, et al. Caring for pets of immunocompromised persons. *Can Vet J* 1995;36(4):217–222.

75. Pickering LK, Marano N, Bocchini JA, et al. Exposure to nontraditional pets at home and to animals in public settings: risks to children. *Pediatrics* 2008; 122(4):876–886.

76. Maschke M, Kastrup O, Esser S, et al. Incidence and prevalence of neurological disorders associated with HIV since the introduction of highly active antiretroviral therapy (HAART). *J Neurol Neurosurg Psychiatry* 2000;69(3):376–380.

77. Hunter PR, Nichols G. Epidemiology and clinical features of *Cryptosporidium* infection in immunocom-

promised patients. *Clin Microbiol Rev* 2002;15(1): 145–154.

78. Cama VA, Ross JM, Crawford S, et al. Differences in clinical manifestations among *Cryptosporidium* species and subtypes in HIV-infected persons. *J Infect Dis* 2007;196(5):684–691.

79. Kotton CN. Zoonoses in solid-organ and hematopoietic stem cell transplant recipients. *Clin Infect Dis* 2007;44(6):857–866.

80. Delaloye J, Merlani G, Petignat C, et al. Nosocomial nontyphoidal salmonellosis after antineoplastic chemotherapy: reactivation of asymptomatic coloniza-

tion? *Eur J Clin Microbiol Infect Dis* 2004;23(10): 751–758.

81. NASPHV, Centers for Disease Control and Prevention, Council of State and Territorial Epidemiologists, American Veterinary Medical Association. Compendium of measures to prevent disease associated with animals in public settings, 2009: National Association of State Public Health Veterinarians, Inc. (NASPHV). *MMWR Recomm Rep* 2009;58(RR-5):1–21.

82. Yokoe D, Casper C, Dubberke E, et al. Safe living after hematopoietic cell transplantation. *Bone Marrow Transplant* 2009;44(8):509–519.

6 Pet Bites

Martha B. Fulford

Introduction

It has been estimated that there are over 72 million dogs, 81 million cats, and 11 million birds living in households in the United States.[1] In addition, there are many less traditional pets described that encompass a variety of smaller mammals, such as rabbits and various rodents, fish, and reptiles. Unfortunately, along with the many benefits of pet ownership, there are potential risks, including that of sustaining a bite.

In 2001, over 360,000 people were treated in a U.S. emergency room for a dog bite-related injury with just over 42% occurring in children under the age of 15.[4] It has been estimated that dog and cat bites are responsible for around 1% of ER visits annually. A study reviewing 1994 data estimated that almost 4.5 million animal bites occurred annually; with just over 750,000 of the bite recipients seeking medical attention, either in an ER or other medical facility.[5] Sixty percent of bites are from dogs and an estimated 10–20% are from cats.[2]

Animal bites can result in trauma that can range from superficial lacerations, to deeper tears, fractured bones, and crush injuries. Some bites can penetrate into joint spaces or body cavities. In addition to the damage to tissue, there is also a risk of infection.

Dog bites

While any dog might potentially bite a human, the breeds that are the most commonly reported are pit bull terriers, rottweilers, and German shepherds.[5,6] The relative risk from individual breeds is an area of considerable debate, as is whether any breed-associated risk arises from genetics (nature) or training (nurture). While some studies identify high-risk breeds, either for absolute number of bites, the relative percentage of bites, or the likelihood to cause severe injury, it is important to recognize that dogs of any breed can bite, and bites of dogs of any size can cause serious injury or infection. Bites from larger dogs are more likely to result in severe crush injury and penetrate body cavities or joint spaces. Young children are more likely to be bitten in the head or upper body area, while adults are most likely to be bitten on the hand.[2] The majority of dog bites are from dogs known to the victim, with 80% of the dog bites incurred by children and adolescents caused by a family or neighborhood dog.[3]

Cat bites

In contrast to dog bites, victims of cat bites are more often adults and more likely to be women. Bites are most often in the arms or face and usually

Companion Animal Zoonoses. Edited by J. Scott Weese and Martha B. Fulford. © 2011 Blackwell Publishing Ltd.

provoked (although the person may not recognize they are provoking the cat). Though there are less data regarding breeds of cats with a propensity to bite, one study from Spain found that Siamese cats inflicted 43% of reported cat bites. In most areas, domestic short-haired cats are the predominant "breed," and little information about breed-specific risk is available.

As with dogs, the majority of bites, 68%, were from cats known to the victim.[7] The long, very narrow teeth of a cat can cause deep penetrating wounds that are more prone to infection. If the bite is near a bone or joint, there is a higher risk of a septic arthritis or tenosynovitis as a result of puncture into the periosteum or joint space. Cat scratches are a particular risk for the transmission of *Bartonella henselae*.

Rodent bites

The incidence of bites caused by pet rodents is unknown, but anecdotally, it appears to be relatively high. Rodents, by virtue of their generally small size, are unlikely to cause significant trauma when they bite. However, these bites need to be considered as there are certain specific infections associated with rodents. Rat bites may result in rat-bite fever, caused by either *Streptobacillus moniliformis* or *Spirillum minus*. Lymphocytic choriomeningitis virus, a virus found in several rodent species, has been associated with hamster bites. Secondary infections from various opportunistic bacteria from the rodent's oral cavity or the person's skin can also develop.

Microbiology

Bite infections are usually polymicrobial caused by a mix of aerobic and anaerobic organisms[8] that originate from the mouth of the biting animal and from the skin of the victim. Some of the more common aerobes found include streptococci, staphylococci (including methicillin-resistant *Staphylococcus aureus* [MRSA]), *Moraxella*, and *Neisseria*. Common anaerobes include *Bacteroides*, *Fusobacterium*, and *Prevotella*. *Pasteurella* was the most common pathogen from both dog and cat bites, with a predominance of *Pasteurella canis* from dogs and *Pasteurella multocida* subspecies *multocida* and *septica* from cats.[8] Less common, but of clinical

Table 6.1 Oral microflora that can be associated with bite infections.[8–10]

Animal	Oral flora
Dog	*Pasteurella* spp. including *P. canis*, *Staphylococcus aureus* (including MRSA), *Staphylococcus pseudintermedius*, *Streptococcus* spp., *Moraxella* spp., *Neisseria* spp., *Capnocytophaga canimorsus*, *Fusobacterium* spp., *Bacteroides* spp., *Porphyromonas* spp., *Prevotella* spp., *Clostridium* spp.
Cat	*Pasteurella multocida*, other *Pasteurella* spp., *Streptococcus* spp., *Staphylococcus* spp., *Moraxella* spp., *Fusobacterium* spp., *Bacteroides* spp., *Porphyromonas* spp.
Rat	Mixed aerobes and anaerobes, including *Streptobacillus moniliformis* and *Spirillum minus*
Primates/human	*Streptococcus* spp. (including *Streptococcus pyogenes*), Enterobacteriaceae, *Eikenella corrodens*, *Neisseria* spp., *Enterococcus*, *Staphylococcus* spp., anaerobic gram-negative bacilli including *Fusobacterium* spp., B virus (Cercopithecine herpesvirus 1) (monkeys only)
Fish/marine animals	Organisms found in marine environment, including *Vibrio* and *Aeromonas* spp.
Reptiles	Mixed aerobes and anaerobes, including *Salmonella* spp.

significance, is *Capnocytophaga canimorsus* that can cause fulminant infection in immunocompromised hosts following a dog bite or lick. Table 6.1 summarizes some of the more common pathogens found in different animal bite infections.

Assessment and management

Initial management of a bite injury involves a careful history, examination of the bite and associated structures and assessment for the risk of infection. The history should include the type of animal, whether it was a provoked or an unprovoked bite, any unusual behavior on the part of the animal (to help determine rabies risk), and vaccination history of the animal (if available). The animal should be identified and the owner should be contacted if possible, so that information regarding the animal's health status and rabies vaccination can be obtained. The pertinent history taken from the victim should include medical history with a focus on any risk factors for immune suppression (e.g., splenectomy, diabetes), medications and allergies, and tetanus immunization status.

The initial assessment of the bite involves careful assessment of the wound and the type of damage (e.g., crush injury, laceration, puncture) and involvement of any underlying structures. The time of the bite with respect to the time of presentation should be noted. Careful examination for any damage to nerves or vessels must be done. Both the wound and surrounding tissue need to be inspected for any signs of local infection and note should be made of any signs of systemic infection such as fever or lymphadenopathy.

Depending on the location and depth of the injury, there may be a need for specific diagnostic tests. If there is suspected bone or joint involvement, radiographs should be taken to assess for joint disruption or bone fractures. A radiograph might also be helpful to rule out any foreign bodies. Bites that are infected should be imaged to assess for the degree of tissue injury, for any evidence of subcutaneous gas as well as looking for bony injury. Certain bites to the head, especially a dog bite to the head of an infant or small child, may result in a skull fracture or cause a penetrating injury with subsequent brain abscess formation. Such injuries should be evaluated with a CT scan or MRI of the head. There is little value in culturing an uninfected bite. However, if there are signs of infection, tissue should be sent for both aerobic and anaerobic culture.[9–13]

As bites may be deceptively deep, especially bites from felines, or have significant tissue injury, local anesthesia of the area should be considered to permit more thorough exploration and cleansing. The wound should be scrupulously cleaned and irrigated with water or normal saline.[14] For larger bites, the use of a syringe or IV catheter can be used for deeper irrigation. Any devitalized tissue should be debrided, and any dirt or foreign material should be removed (e.g., teeth, fabric from clothing).[9–13]

Following irrigation and debridement, wound closure can be considered. Bites to the face are usually closed for cosmetic reasons. These wounds have a lower risk of infection, possibly due to an excellent vascular supply and lack of dependent edema.[2,10,13] Plastic surgery assessment should be obtained for any significant facial injury. If less than 12 hours old, a superficial laceration from a dog bite that is not on a hand or foot can also be considered for primary closure.[13] Other bite injuries are best left open and allowed to close by secondary intention. They should be examined daily for any signs of infection.[9–13]

All patients presenting with bites should be assessed for the need for tetanus toxoid immunization and for rabies postexposure prophylaxis.

Bites should be reported to the appropriate public health authorities. This is important to ensure that proper actions are taken with respect to potential rabies exposure, as well as documenting the bite to identify animals or owners that are recurrent offenders.

Antimicrobials

Antimicrobials used to treat an infected bite wound need to be broad spectrum with good aerobic and anaerobic activity. For dog and cat bites, the antimicrobial or antimicrobial combination needs to have excellent activity against *Pasteurella* spp. See Table 6.2 for recommended treatment regimens.

Table 6.2 Antimicrobial options for the treatment of animal bites.[9–13]

Antibiotic	Alternative regimen
Oral	
Amoxicillin/clavulanic acid	Fluoroquinolone or doxycycline or trimethoprim/ sulfamethoxazole *plus* metronidazole or clindamycin
Intravenous	
Ampicillin–sulbactam Piperacillin– tazobactam Ticarcillin–clavulanate	Carbapenem (imipenem– cilastatin, meropenem, ertapenem)
Third-generation cephalosporin *plus* metronidazole	Fluoroquinolone *plus* metronidazole

Table 6.3   General recommendations for reducing the risk of bites.

Select pet/breed suitable for your lifestyle and home environment (may require consultation with veterinarian, animal behaviorist, etc.).

Exclude animals with a history of aggression—either in that specific animal or in the breed.

If possible, spend time with the animal before buying or adopting it.

Spay/neuter dogs.

For dogs, socialize and train them appropriately. Teach them submissive behaviors (e.g., exposing abdomen, giving up food without growling).

Do not play aggressive games with animals.

Delay acquiring dog or other pet if a child is fearful or apprehensive.

Be careful bringing an animal, especially a young animal, into a household with an infant or very young child.

Never leave an infant or young child unattended with an animal.

Teach children basic rules for interactions with dogs/other animals:
    Do not approach an unknown animal.
    Never run from the animal or scream at the animal.
    Remain very still if approached by unknown dog/animal.
    Avoid direct eye contact with an animal like a dog.
    Do not disturb an eating or sleeping animal.
    Do not disturb an animal that is looking after its young.
    Do not pet a dog or other animal without letting it see you first.
    If bitten or scratched, immediately tell an adult.

Adapted from Centers for Disease Control and Prevention.[3]

There is no consensus on the use of antimicrobial prophylaxis following a bite to prevent infection. Current recommendations are for the use of prophylactic antibiotics for certain high-risk injuries: wounds that are primarily closed (e.g., on the face), deep punctures (especially those from cat bites), injuries requiring surgical repair (e.g., certain crush injuries, avulsion injuries), wounds on the hands, and wounds in the immunocompromised.[12,13] The choice of antibiotic would be similar to those used for treatment. Any antibiotic regimen selected must have good aerobic and anaerobic activity and, in the case of cat and dog bites, excellent activity against *Pasteurella* spp.

Bite prevention

Ideally, no companion animal would ever bite. Unfortunately, bites do occur, but there are measures that can be used to minimize the risk. Examples of these are listed in Table 6.3. Most of the recommendations are specifically aimed at pre-venting dog bites, but the strategies can be applied to any animal.

References

1. American Veterinary Medical Association. *U.S. Pet Ownership and Demographics Sourcebook.* 2007. www. avma.org/reference/marketstats/ownership.asp. Accessed May 14, 2010.
2. Oehler RL, Velez AP, Mizrachi M, et al. Bite-related and septic syndromes caused by cats and dogs. *Lancet Infect Dis* 2009;9:439–447.
3. Centers for Disease Control and Prevention. Nonfatal dog bite-related injuries treated in hospital emergency departments—United States, 2001. *MMWR Morb Mortal Wkly Rep* 2003;52(26):605–610.
4. Sacks JJ, Kresnow M, Houston B. Dog bites: how big a problem? *Inj Prev* 1996;2:52–54.
5. Shuler CM, DeBess EE, Lapidus JA, et al. Canine and human factors related to dog bite injuries. *J Am Vet Med Assoc* 2008;232:542–546.
6. Sacks JJ, Sinclair L, Gilchrist J, et al. Breeds of dogs involved in fatal human attacks in the United States

between 1979 and 1998. *J Am Vet Med Assoc* 2000;217: 836–840.

7. Palacio J, Leon-Artozqui M, Pastor-Villalba E, et al. Incidence of and risk factors for cat bites: a first step in prevention and treatment of feline aggression. *J Feline Med Surg* 2007;9:188–195.

8. Talan DA, Citron DM, Abrahamian FM, et al. Bacteriologic analysis of infected dog and cat bites. *N Engl J Med* 1999;340(2):85–92.

9. Brook I. Microbiology and management of human and animal bite wound infections. *Prim Care* 2003;30: 25–39.

10. Dendle C, Looke D. Management of mammalian bites. *Aust Fam Physician* 2009;38(11):868–874.

11. Brinker D, Hancox JD, Bernardon SO. Assessment and initial treatment of lacerations, mammalian bites, and insect stings. *AACN Clin Issues* 2003;14(4): 401–410.

12. Fleisher GR. The management of bite wounds. *N Engl J Med* 1999;340(2):138–140.

13. Endom EE. *Initial management of animal and human bites*. 2010. www.uptodate.com. Accessed May 13, 2010.

14. Moscati RM, Mayrose J, Reardon RF, et al. A multi-center comparison of tap water versus sterile water for wound irrigation. *Acad Emerg Med* 2007;14(5): 404–409.

Index

Note: Page numbers in italics refer to Figures; those in bold to Tables.

Companion Animal Zoonoses. Edited by J. Scott Weese and
Martha B. Fulford. © 2011 Blackwell Publishing Ltd.